Cognitive Neurorehabilitation

This is the first truly comprehensive survey of cognitive rehabilitation, spanning the spectrum from basic science to functional outcome. It offers a critical review of theoretical and methodological issues relating to specific rehabilitation procedures and also to programme organization and management. The international team of expert authors consider the multiple determinants contributing to the success of cognitive rehabilitation and present the most scientifically sound methods of practice.

The book is based on the twin premises that basic science is the foundation of rehabilitation and that successful outcome is dependent on the specificity of the rehabilitation. In demonstrating this, the book goes beyond cognitive rehabilitation treatments to cover biological issues such as the course of recovery, psychological status such as mood and motivation, social context such as the family environment, and historical factors such as education and age.

With its emphasis on scientific principles, multidisciplinary practice, and functional outcome, this book will serve as an essential resource for all scientists and clinicians concerned with cognitive deficits secondary to altered brain functioning, and particularly to psychologists, neurologists, psychiatrists, occupational therapists and physical therapists. It will also serve as a stimulus to the further development of cognitive rehabilitation as a discipline based on the complex influences of brain plasticity and behavioural change.

Donald T. Stuss is Director of the Rotman Research Institute at the Baycrest Centre for Geriatric Care, Toronto.

Gordon Winocur is Senior Scientist at the Rotman Research Institute.

Ian H. Robertson is Senior Scientist at the MRC Cognition and Brain Sciences Unit, Cambridge, UK.

Cognitive Neurorehabilitation

Edited by

Donald T. Stuss

Rotman Research Institute,
Baycrest Centre for Geriatric Care, Toronto, Canada
University of Toronto

Gordon Winocur

Rotman Research Institute,
Baycrest Centre for Geriatric Care, Toronto, Canada
Trent University and University of Toronto

and

Ian H. Robertson

Department of Psychology, Trinity College,
Dublin, Ireland

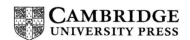

CAMBRIDGE
UNIVERSITY PRESS

PUBLISHED BY THE PRESS SYNDICATE OF THE UNIVERSITY OF CAMBRIDGE
The Pitt Building, Trumpington Street, Cambridge, United Kingdom

CAMBRIDGE UNIVERSITY PRESS
The Edinburgh Building, Cambridge CB2 2RU, UK   www.cup.cam.ac.uk
40 West 20th Street, New York, NY 10011–4211, USA   www.cup.org
10 Stamford Road, Oakleigh, Melbourne 3166, Australia
Ruiz de Alarcón 13, 28014 Madrid, Spain

First published 1999

Printed in the United Kingdom at the University Press, Cambridge

Typeset in Utopia 8/12pt in QuarkXPress™   [SE]

A catalogue record for this book is available from the British Library

Library of Congress Cataloguing in Publication data

Cognitive neurohabilitation / edited by Donald T. Stuss, Gordon
Winocur, and Ian H. Robertson.
p.   cm.
Includes index.
ISBN 0 521 58102 8 hb
1. Cognition disorders–Patients–Rehabilitation.   2. Brain
damage–Patients–Rehabilitation.   I. Stuss, Donald T.
II. Winocus, Gordon.   III. Robertson, Ian. 1951–   .
RC553.C64C654   1999
617.4′810443–dc21   98–43624 CIP

ISBN 0 521 58102 8 hardback

Every effort has been made in preparing this book to provide accurate and up-to-date information which is in accord with accepted standards and practice at the time of publication. Nevertheless, the authors, editors and publisher can make no warranties that the information contained herein is totally free from error, not least because clinical standards are constantly changing through research and regulation. The authors, editors and publisher therefore disclaim all liability for direct or consequential damages resulting from the use of material contained in this book. Readers are strongly advised to pay careful attention to information provided by the manufacturer of any drugs or equipment that they plan to use.

Contents

List of contributors   *page* vii

Preface   xi

Acknowledgements   xiii

Introduction and overview   1

Part I Mechanisms and principles of recovery

Introduction   5
Gordon Winocur

1 Neuroplasticity and recovery of function after
   brain injury   9
   Bryan Kolb and Robbin Gibb

2 Intracerebral transplantation and regeneration:
   practical implications   26
   **Heather Dickinson-Anson, Isabelle Aubert and
   Fred H. Gage**

3 The use of neuroimaging in neurorehabilitative
   research   47
   Cheryl L. Grady and Shitij Kapur

4 Principles of compensation in cognitive
   neurorehabilitation   59
   Roger A. Dixon and Lars Bäckman

5 Brain damage, sex hormones and recovery   73
   Donald G. Stein, Robin L. Roof and Zoltan L. Fulop

6 The psychosocial environment and cognitive
   rehabilitation in the elderly   94
   Deirdre Dawson, Gordon Winocur and Morris Moscovitch

Part II Pharmacological approaches

Introduction   111
Donald T. Stuss

7 Pharmacological strategies for neuroprotection
   and rehabilitation   113
   Amy F.T. Arnsten and Douglas H. Smith

8 Neuropharmacological contributions to the
   rehabilitation of patients with traumatic brain
   injury   136
   John W. Cassidy

9 Pharmacological interventions in Alzheimer's
   disease   153
   Fredda L. Leiter and Jeffrey L. Cummings

Part III Clinical and management issues

Introduction   173
Donald T. Stuss

10 Cognitive rehabilitation: leadership and
    management of the clinical programme   175
    Virginia M. Mills and Michael P. Alexander

11 Neuropsychological rehabilitation in the
    interdisciplinary team: the postacute stage   188
    Anne-Lise Christensen and Carla Caetano

12 Outcome measurement in cognitive
    neurorehabilitation   201
    Nadina Lincoln

13 Constraint-induced movement therapy: new
    approaches to outcome measurement in
    rehabilitation   215
    Gitendra Uswatte and Edward Taub

14 Mood and motivation in rehabilitation   230
    Anthony Feinstein

15 Motivation and awareness in cognitive
    neurorehabilitation   240
    George P. Prigatano

16 Family education and family partnership in
    cognitive rehabilitation   252
    Guy-B. Proulx

Part IV Neurorehabilitation techniques

Introduction   263
Ian H. Robertson

17 The role of theory in aphasia therapy: art or
    science?   265
    Robert T. Wertz

18 Traumatic brain injury: natural history and
    efficacy of cognitive rehabilitation   279
    Douglas I. Katz and Virginia M. Mills

19 The rehabilitation of attention   302
    Ian H. Robertson

20 The rehabilitation of executive disorders   314
    Catherine A. Mateer

21 Memory rehabilitation in brain-injured people 333
    Barbara A. Wilson

22 Memory rehabilitation in the elderly   347
    Elizabeth L. Glisky and Martha L. Glisky

Epilogue. The future of cognitive rehabilitation 362
Ian H. Robertson, Donald T. Stuss and Gordon Winocur

Index   367

Contributors

Michael P. Alexander
Behavioral Neurology, Kirstein 2
Beth Israel Deaconess Medical Center
330 Brookline Avenue
Boston, MA 02215
USA

Amy F.T. Arnsten
Section of Neurobiology
Yale Medical School
C303 SHM
P.O. Box 208001
New Haven, CT 06520–8001
USA

Isabelle Aubert
The Salk Institute for Biological Studies
Laboratory of Genetics
P.O. Box 85800
10010 North Torrey Pines Road
San Diego, CA 92186–5800
USA

Lars Bäckman
Stockholm Gerontology Research Center
P.O. Box 6400
S-113 82
Stockholm
Sweden

Carla Caetano
Center for Hjerneskade
Copenhagen University, Amager
Njalsgade 88
DK-2300, Copenhagen S
Denmark

John W. Cassidy
Neurobehavioral Programs
Neurobehavioral Associate
7400 Fannin Street, #1280
Houston, TX 77054
USA

Anne-Lise Christensen
Center for Hjerneskade
Copenhagen University, Amager
Njalsgade 88
DK-2300, Copenhagen S
Denmark

Jeffrey L. Cummings
Department of Neurology
UCLA School of Medicine
710 Westwood Plaza
Los Angeles, CA 90024
USA

Dierdre Dawson
Department of Occupational Therapy
Faculty of Medicine
University of Toronto
256 McCaul Street
Toronto, Ontario M5T 1W5
Canada

Heather Dickinson-Anson
The Salk Institute for Biological Studies
Laboratory of Genetics
P.O. Box 85800
10010 North Torrey Pines Road
San Diego, CA 92186–5800
USA

Roger A. Dixon
Department of Psychology
University of Victoria
Victoria, BC V8W 3P5
Canada

Anthony Feinstein
Department of Psychiatry
Sunnybrook Health Science Centre
2075 Bayview Ave
North York, Ontario M4N 3M5
Canada

Zoltan L. Fulop
Department of Neurology
Emory University School of Medicine
Atlanta, GA 30322
USA

Fred H. Gage
The Salk Institute for Biological Studies
Laboratory of Genetics
P.O. Box 85800
10010 North Torrey Pines Road
San Diego, CA 92186–5800
USA

Robbin Gibb
Department of Psychology
University of Lethbridge
4401 University Drive
Lethbridge, Alberta T1K 3M4
Canada

Elizabeth L. Glisky
The Amnesia and Cognition Unit
Department of Psychology
The University of Arizona
Tucson, AZ 85721
USA

Martha L. Glisky
Department of Psychology
The University of Arizona
Tucson, AZ 85721
USA

Cheryl L. Grady
Rotman Research Institute
Baycrest Centre for Geriatric Care
3560 Bathurst Street
Toronto, Ontario M6A 2E1
Canada

Shitij Kapur
PET Centre, Ground Floor
Clarke Institute of Psychiatry
250 College Street
Toronto, Ontario M4T 1R8
Canada

Douglas I. Katz
Division of Neurology
Braintree Hospital
250 Pond Street
P.O. Box 9020
Braintree, MA 02184
USA

Bryan Kolb
Department of Psychology
University of Lethbridge
4401 University Drive
Lethbridge, Alberta T1K 3M4
Canada

Fredda L. Leiter
Department of Psychiatry and Behavioral Sciences
UCLA School of Medicine
710 Westwood Plaza
Los Angeles, CA 90024
USA

Nadina Lincoln
Department of Psychology
University of Nottingham
University Park
Nottingham NG7 2RD
UK

Catherine A. Mateer
Department of Psychology
University of Victoria
P.O. Box 3050
Victoria, British Columbia V8W 3P5
Canada

Virginia M. Mills
Neurorehab Associates of New England
19 Edgewater Drive
Wellesly, MA 02181–1617
USA

Morris Moscovitch
Rotman Research Institute
Baycrest Centre for Geriatric Care
3560 Bathurst Street
Toronto, Ontario M6A 2E1
Canada

George P. Prigatano
Barrow Neurological Institute
Mercy Healthcare Arizona
350 West Thomas Road
Phoenix, AZ 85013–4496
USA

Guy-B. Proulx
Department of Psychology
Baycrest Centre for Geriatric Care
3560 Bathurst Street
Toronto, Ontario M6A 2E1
Canada

Ian H. Robertson
Department of Psychology
Trinity College
Dublin
Ireland

Robin L. Roof
Department of Psychology
Texas Christian University
Fort, Worth, TX
USA

Douglas H. Smith
Division of Neurosurgery
University of Pennsylvania Medical Center
105 Hayden Hall, 3320 Smith Walk
Philadelphia, PA 19104–6316
USA

Donald G. Stein
Emory University
202 Administration Building
Atlanta, GA 30322
USA

Donald T. Stuss
Rotman Research Institute
Baycrest Centre for Geriatric Care
3560 Bathurst Street
Toronto, Ontario M6A 2E1
Canada

Edward Taub
Department of Psychology
University of Alabama
415 Campbell Hall
Birmingham, AL 35294
USA

Gitendra Uswatte
Department of Psychology
University of Alabama
CH 415, 1300 University Blvd
Birmingham, AL 35294–1170
USA

Robert T. Wertz
Audiology and Speech Pathology (126)
VA Medical Center
1310 24th Avenue South
Nashville, TN 37212
USA

Barbara A. Wilson
MRC Applied Psychology Unit
Rehabilitation Research Group
P.O. Box 58, Addenbrooke's Hospital
Cambridge CB2 2QQ
UK

Gordon Winocur
Rotman Research Institute
Baycrest Centre for Geriatric Care
3560 Bathurst Street
Toronto, Ontario M6A 2E1
Canada

Preface

From where

Each year, the Rotman Research Institute of Baycrest Centre for Geriatric Care, an academic centre affiliated with the University of Toronto, holds a conference that focuses on one of the major research thrusts of the institute. The content of past conferences had been on the cognitive functions to which the scientists direct their efforts, such as the functions of the frontal lobes, attention and memory; or on groups of people who may exhibit changes in these functions, such as normal old people, and patients with acute or progressive neurological disorders such as stroke and Alzheimer's disease.

The philosophy of the Rotman Institute has been to develop basic science, theory and methodologies which would then be directed to the development of more applied research. This was exemplified in each conference, in which the organization of the two days started with basic research findings, with the second day dedicated to clinical applications. It seemed appropriate to maintain this organization when the decision was made to have a more applied content for the fifth annual (1995) conference. Sponsored by Baycrest Centre and the Ontario Mental Health Foundation, the conference, entitled 'Cognitive Rehabilitation: Advances in the Rehabilitation of Acute and Age-related Brain Disorders,' was a resounding success. At the termination of the conference, many of the attendees asked if a book would be forthcoming based on the content of the conference. We were hesitant for several reasons. First, we do not make it a practice to ask our presenters to write up their presentations as chapters, and we had not forewarned them that this would be the case. Second, conference proceedings often do not transfer into good editions. Third, we felt that the content of our conference, while excellent, was not sufficiently comprehensive to be the type of book on cognitive rehabilitation we would want to edit.

Why

The urging of the conference attendees did lead us to consider the matter, and several other factors pushed us to initiate the project. There was an absence of a truly comprehensive survey of cognitive rehabilitation which would (1) span the spectrum from basic science related to rehabilitation efforts to functional outcome; (2) consider theoretical and methodological issues related not only to the specific rehabilitation procedures but also to programme organization and management; (3) review the multiple determinants that contribute to the success of cognitive rehabilitation; and (4) present the most scientifically sound methods of cognitive rehabilitation. We agreed on the need for a book that would review the current status of cognitive rehabilitation. While our desire was to fill a void and edit a 'comprehensive' approach to cognitive rehabilitation, we realized that we could only approximate this wish if we were to have a book of reasonable size. We hoped that the book would serve as an update as well as a handy reference for those interested in the science and practice of cognitive rehabilitation. A hope rather than a specified objective was that this book might spur the next surge in cognitive rehabilitation. A final factor that pushed us to produce the book was our own desire to develop the next aspect of the Rotman Institute – a research programme which would lead to the development of directed cognitive rehabilitation procedures. To achieve this objective, we needed to expand our interactions, and Ian Robertson became a part-time scientist of the institute. While remaining a full-time researcher at the Cambridge MRC APU, Ian, through his interactions and visits to the Rotman Institute, expanded his rehabilitation efforts. We also obtained funding from the McDonnell Foundation to develop a cognitive rehabilitation programme, which led to two workshops designed to address the needs of rehabilitation endeavours. Many of the ideas developed in our introductory

sections were discussed in these workshops, and the participants are all acknowledged: (in alphabetical order) C. Alain, M. Alexander, S. Black, P. Burgess, F. Craik, M. Cusimano, D. Dawson, M. Freedman, C. Grady, L. Jacoby, S. Kapur, B. Kolb, M. Kopelman, B. Levine, T. Manly, R. McIntosh, M. Moscovitch, J. Murre, S. O'Mara, T. Picton, G. Pizzamiglio, G.-B. Proulx, I. Robertson, M. Schwartz, T. Shallice, D. Stuss, B.A. Wilson, and G. Winocur.

Reflections

In editing the book, we asked all the authors to make the chapters scientifically solid, readable, and practically useful, with a reasonably comprehensive if selective reference list. In this way our objective was to develop a resource handbook on the current status of cognitive rehabilitation. In each chapter, the reader will find not only summary paragraphs, but also 'bullets' which highlight the main points of different sections in the chapter. Our goal here was for the volume to serve as a handy and easy reference book in addition to being a general resource book.

We think the book is unique in its breadth of information. Most books on rehabilitation deal with one disorder, such as head injury, or one dysfunction, usually memory. Our overall goal was to develop a foundation on which rehabilitation should be formulated. We hope that, if we have achieved our objectives, this edited volume will serve as a seed for the growth and development of basic and applied research into cognitive disorders, and the implementation of this knowledge into the clinical domain.

The book will have value for virtually all health care professionals and scientists working in the field of understanding and/or treating cognitive deficits secondary to altered brain functioning. This includes psychologists, neurologists, psychiatrists, imaging scientists, occupational therapists and physiotherapists. It is also our hope that the book will have value for nurses, social workers, and others who have direct involvement with patients.

D.T. Stuss
G. Winocur
I.H. Robertson

Acknowledgements

This book was possible because of the support of Baycrest Centre for Geriatric Care. We thank all the contributors for their efforts in preparing their chapters, and in responding to the editors.

The preparation of any book is an extremely time-consuming task. The submission of this edition was possible because of the efforts of our excellent staff. We are truly grateful to Carole Copnick and Darlene Floden, with the additional support of Stacey Paterson and Sean Bisschop.

Introduction and overview

Had we chosen to define cognitive rehabilitation when we began to organize this book, we probably would have limited it to the application of behavioural strategies – whether remedial or compensatory – aimed at improving functioning in those realms of mental function normally considered as part of 'cognitive psychology'. In this, we include memory, attention, perception, praxis, executive function, among others. If we had just looked at the cognitive rehabilitation literature, we might well have missed the fact that cognitive psychology has moved on to cognitive neuroscience, and that the artificial – and probably handicapping – distinction between cognition, emotion and motivation has steadily been breaking down. Furthermore, particularly with the advent of functional neuroimaging, it has become increasingly difficult to study cognitive functions without some consideration of their biological substrate.

By stopping ourselves from becoming enmeshed in outdated notions of cognition, we believe that we have brought together some of the world's leading experts to address the issue of cognitive rehabilitation from all of these perspectives – biology, motivation and social context as well as the more traditional aspects of cognition themselves. Furthermore, we have also considered the critical aspects of what rehabilitation of cognitive function means in terms of the whole person in a social context. Finally, and most importantly, we have repeatedly come up against the issue of the theoretical basis for this whole enterprise.

We propose to consider cognitive rehabilitation as a truly integrative discipline which we confidently expect to contribute towards a revolution in theory and clinical practice pertaining to the brain's capacity for plastic reorganization. The theoretical basis for cognitive rehabilitation is the framework for consideration of several important themes: the biological context and limits to cognitive rehabilitation; biologically based interventions and their relationship to behaviourally based interventions; the role of motivation and emotion in cognitive rehabilitation; and whole-person integration and the social context.

The content and structure of the volume derive from our convictions and beliefs about cognitive rehabilitation. The first is that basic science is the foundation of rehabilitation. There are many corollaries to this first principle. Because something is applied does not mean that it is sound or even worthwhile. Rehabilitation without scientific evaluation is probably a waste of money. The most valuable clinical application will probably derive from the knowledge provided by basic science and applied by a sensitive, educated and questioning clinician. A good example of this relationship exists in the history of the development of magnetic resonance imaging. Now considered as a relevant clinical imaging methodology, this technique evolved because of the scientific discovery of the magnetic properties of blood and living tissue. When this was first discovered, however, no one would have considered this basic science finding as clinically relevant. We hope that our conviction about the research base of rehabilitation is reflected in this book, and that it will serve to motivate the scientific study of the development and assessment of rehabilitation techniques.

A second principle we hold is that the successful outcome of cognitive rehabilitation is dependent on the specificity of the rehabilitation. The disorder has to be understood before it can be rehabilitated. You cannot rehabilitate what you do not know. An excellent example of this lies in the work on attention. The dissociation of the attentional disorders has facilitated the development of rehabilitation techniques. The authors we have selected demonstrate how this focus on a specific nature of the disorder facilitates improvement.

The third principle is that, while specificity of rehabilitation is important, recovery is in reality likely to be multidetermined. Many factors may contribute to the actual recovery process, of which cognitive rehabilita-

tion treatment may be only one aspect. The factors include biological issues such as the course of recovery; psychological status such as mood and motivation; social context such as the family environment; and historical matters such as education and age. It will become clear that, while this third principle is stressed by many authors, there is an absence of research data demonstrating the relationship of these factors to outcome.

A fourth principle we stress is that the assessment of outcome must be broadened. Emphasis is placed on how outcome should be assessed. Clearly, this is a challenge for the future. There is a need to demonstrate how improvement in cognitive abilities relates to real-world outcome such as holding down a job, and interacting appropriately in different environments.

Structure of the volume

The book is divided into several parts, each preceded by a brief introduction to serve as an overview and guide. The first part after this introduction is titled 'Mechanisms and principles of recovery'. It outlines the important scientific bases needed to develop and measure rehabilitation efforts. The next part contains three chapters related to 'Pharmacological approaches'. As we are addressing rehabilitation in neurological patients, one important approach may be the combination of cognitive and pharmacological therapy.

In the next part, the multiple factors necessary for successful rehabilitation are reviewed. These include the development of programmes, issues related to the use and development of outcome measures, and the role of factors such as mood, awareness, and psychosocial context. The last major part of the book constitutes what is usually the heart of cognitive rehabilitation books – the specific techniques of cognitive rehabilitation. A selective mix of rehabilitation of identified cognitive processes such as attention and memory is presented, and the rehabilitation of neurological causes of brain dysfunction such as traumatic brain injury is addressed. The approach in each chapter is varied, but each brings a view from experienced rehabilitation clinicians and scientists that will be helpful to the reader. The book ends with an epilogue that looks to the future of cognitive rehabilitation.

PART I

Mechanisms and principles of recovery

Introduction

Gordon Winocur

One of the purposes of this volume is to provide a comprehensive survey of issues related to the complex field of cognitive rehabilitation. A survey of this nature would be incomplete without due attention to the mechanisms by which attenuation of cognitive deficits is achieved. A consideration of mechanisms provides direction in terms of formulating strategies of rehabilitation but, in addition, highlights the complexity of the overall challenge. The chapters in this part illustrate the breadth of operative mechanisms, ranging as they do from the molecular to the psychosocial. They also illustrate the variety of research paradigms (from animal models to clinical trials) that can and have been used to study the mechanisms and principles of recovery. As will become apparent to the reader, not all the mechanisms discussed in the ensuing chapters are incorporated into cognitive rehabilitation programmes and, in some cases, it would be premature to do so. On the other hand, the practical benefits that can be expected from most existing programmes are limited and there is considerable room for improvement. A broader consideration of the research-based issues addressed here might well be a progressive development in achieving this objective. That is one hope in beginning the book with this section.

In the first chapter, Kolb and Gibb remind us that the brain is a far more plastic organ than was long thought to be the case and that, following injury, it is capable of considerable reorganization that could form the basis of functional recovery. In their review of injury-related anatomical changes, the authors stress the importance of regional dendritic arborization that results in increased connections amongst surviving neurons.

What are especially important from the point of view of cognitive rehabilitation are the demonstrated relationships between dendritic growth and the recovery of apparently lost functions. As might be expected, age at the time of injury, extent of damage, and experiential factors can all influence structural–functional changes. Apart from describing the neural changes that occur following brain damage, the challenge is to understand the principles that drive them and, through appropriate intervention, maximize the growth processes to achieve optimal functional recovery. In their concluding section, Kolb and Gibb are optimistic that various techniques, including behavioural therapy, pharmacological treatment, and intracerebral grafting, alone or possibly in combination, have the potential to reinstate function in damaged brain regions.

The controversial procedure of neural grafting is taken up in the chapter by Dickinson-Anson, Aubert and Gage, who extend the application of this technique to the cognitive problems associated with normal ageing and neurodegenerative diseases, including Alzheimer's disease. The authors' optimism regarding the potential benefits of grafting procedures derives from successful demonstrations of nerve fibre regeneration following the implantation of cholinergic-rich tissue in the septo-hippocampal system in various animal models. A consistent finding of several studies is that such procedures attenuate learning and memory deficits reliably associated with impairment to this system and related structures. In discussing possible mechanisms whereby neural transplantation brings about cognitive improvement, Dickinson-Anson et al. refer to evidence that successful transfer of fetal tissue facilitates the release of the neurotrophin nerve growth factor. This is important in that it links with Kolb and Gibb's observation that the enhanced presence of nerve growth factor is a critical factor in promoting brain reorganization following injury.

Dickinson-Anson et al.'s chapter also highlights the potential of gene therapy for reversing cognitive ageing and disease-related deficits at the molecular level. While still in the early stages of development, an impressive body of evidence indicates that gene transfer techniques may be used to target regeneration in specific brain regions. The authors' review of the mechanisms by which transgenic procedures influence damaged tissue reveals a striking similarity to those mechanisms associated with neural tissue transplants, and illustrates an important point of convergence between the two procedures.

If brain damage leads to neuroanatomical and molecular changes that alter the way the brain works, these changes should be reflected in measures of neurophysiological function. Until recently, in-vivo measurements of physiological activity were restricted to relatively insensitive electroencephalogram techniques, but advances in the field of functional neuroimaging have created exciting new potentials in this area. Improvements in the spatial resolution of capabilities of positron emission tomography (PET) scanning allow fine-grained determinations of relationships between specific functions and localized brain regions. Grady and Kapur, in their chapter, draw heavily on research involving normal old people and brain-damaged patients to show the application of PET imaging to cognitive rehabilitation. Comparisons of normal and damaged brains consistently reveal that different regions participate in solving the same cognitive tasks, and Grady's own work has demonstrated parallel effects in normal ageing brains. An important objective is to understand better the mechanisms that underlie this functional reorganization but, as Grady and Kapur point out, one possibility is related to the capacity of the brain to form new structural networks that translate into new functional systems. A hypothesis that follows from the available evidence is that brain-damaged and aged individuals use their reorganized neural systems to create different strategies for per-

forming learning and memory tasks. There is mounting evidence to support this hypothesis and, indeed, at times old people and patients can be very successful in applying these strategies. Grady and Kapur suggest that a fuller understanding of brain reorganization can impact on rehabilitation in at least three ways: (1) by helping to develop alternate cognitive strategies; (2) by identifying promising candidates for rehabilitation; and (3) by monitoring the effectiveness of rehabilitation at various stages of the programme. The authors make a compelling case for the inclusion of functional neuroimaging in developing and assessing cognitive rehabilitation programmes – part of the challenge in this respect is to create and commit sufficient resources to this endeavour.

Dixon and Bäckman are also concerned with plasticity but at a different level. They discuss theoretical and practical issues related to teaching compensatory skills, to promote behavioural and physiological reorganization. The concept of compensation, with its inherent assumptions concerning losses and gains, has always had a special place in the psychological literature but, in their chapter, Dixon and Bäckman underscore its direct relevance to cognitive neurorehabilitation. Drawing heavily on their own work in this area, the authors outline principal components of the compensatory process and show how they apply to overcoming cognitive problems associated with normal ageing, brain injury, and neurodegenerative diseases. Of particular importance is the need to consider the patient's role in rehabilitation, issues related to his or her level of awareness, and the impact of positive and negative consequences of treatment. Dixon and Bäckman's approach is broad in scope and, in line with that of Grady and Kapur, recognizes the benefits of bringing together traditional clinical assessment of outcome with neuroimaging techniques for measuring reorganized brain function. In this regard, they raise an interesting question as to what we are learning from PET evidence that damaged or ageing brains have their own unique operating characteristics. Do these demonstrations provide examples of compensatory mechanisms or are they, in fact, linked to the factors that contribute to the cognitive deficits? Dixon and Bäckman raise another important question. To what extent can the individual, through strategic and deliberate hard work, control compensatory responses at the neuroanatomical level? Answers to these and related questions will undoubtedly factor into comprehensive rehabilitation programmes but, as Dixon and Bäckman point out, these answers can only be attained through concerted and interdisciplinary research efforts.

The chapter by Stein, Roof, and Fulop emphasizes the very important observation that men and women differ in their natural capacity to recover from brain trauma, and identifies hormonal variations as a critical modulator of this difference. In general, women experience a more favourable outcome after traumatic brain injury and some of this effect can be attributed to less localized representation of cognitive function in female brains. However, the results of animal and human research show that sex differences in recovery are greatest when comparisons are made with women who sustained injury when levels of the steroid hormone progesterone were high as part of normal cycling. In an elegant series of experiments involving the rat model, Stein and his group showed that exogenously administered progesterone reduced trauma-induced cerebral oedema, a major cause of structural atrophy, as well as the cognitive impairments associated with such conditions. An important finding of their research was that progesterone was effective for males and females, thereby underscoring the generalized potential of this form of hormonal treatment. Stein et al. close their chapter by reviewing some of the possible mechanisms whereby progesterone exerts its rehabilitative effects. One of the interesting possibilities that resonates with the observations of other contributors to this part of the book (eg. Kolb and Gibb, Dickinson-Anson et al., Grady and Kapur) is that progesterone promotes dendritic growth that results in reconstituted neural systems capable of supporting compensatory cognitive strategies. Stein et al. suggest that this may be the result of direct inhibitory action on microglia that helps sustain

vulnerable neurons, or due to blocking of free radical metabolism and the ensuing neural toxicity that causes further damage to brain cells. These are plausible hypotheses and Stein et al. have rendered a valuable service in guiding future research in these promising directions.

In the final chapter in this part, Dawson, Winocur and Moscovitch review evidence that a variety of nonbiological, lifestyle-related factors can interact with brain dysfunction to affect cognitive performance. Their review draws primarily on the cognitive ageing literature but, as is apparent from other contributions to this volume (e.g. Christensen and Caetano, Katz and Mills, Glisky and Glisky), similar relationships probably exist in cases of brain injury. The message is that the entire person must be considered in cognitive rehabilitation and, to be maximally effective, any such programme must be holistic in nature. The authors review a recently completed longitudinal study in which the relationship between psychosocial status and cognitive function was studied in groups of institutionalized and community dwelling old people. The results showed that, in both populations, fluctuations in cognitive performance over time were accompanied by corresponding changes in psychosocial attributes that included feelings of personal control, optimism, and general activity. The study indicated that cognitive performance, at least in the elderly, is influenced by factors related to psychological well-being, and implies that such factors should be taken into account in cognitive rehabilitation efforts. Accordingly, Dawson et al. conclude by sketching a model for a cognitive rehabilitation programme that would combine cognitive skills training with individual and group psychosocial counselling components. This combined approach has not been attempted previously and needs to be tested in clinical/research trials, but it would appear to hold considerable promise with respect to remediating cognitive problems in various populations.

1

Neuroplasticity and recovery of function after brain injury

Bryan Kolb and Robbin Gibb

Introduction

Perhaps the most significant and perplexing question concerning the clinical neuropsychological investigation of the patient with brain injury relates to the issue of how to repair the injured nervous system in order to restore lost functions. It has long been known that damage to specific regions of cerebral cortex causes a change both in the remaining brain and in behaviour (for a review, see Kolb and Whishaw, 1996). Until recently, it was commonly believed that the adult mammalian cortex was structurally static, providing little opportunity for behavioural recovery following cortical injury. Evidence has begun to accumulate, however, suggesting that at least some cortical circuits might be modifiable following cortical injury. (This property of modifiability of neurons is often referred to as neuroplasticity, or plasticity.) It follows that if neural circuits can be modified after injury, then one might anticipate some type of functional change as well. In principle, there are three ways that the brain could show plastic changes that might support recovery.

Recovery could result from the reorganization of remaining circuits

The general idea is that the nervous system could reorganize in some way to do 'more with less'. It seems unlikely, however, that a complexly integrated structure like the cerebral cortex could undergo a wholesale reorganization of cortical connectivity, at least in the adult. Rather, recovery from cortical injury would be most likely to result from a change in the intrinsic organiza-tion of local cortical circuits in regions directly or indirectly disrupted by the injury. It should be noted, however, that it might be possible to produce significant reorganization of cortical connectivity in the young brain, especially if cortical development were incomplete, and for this potentiated alteration of connectivity to support more recovery than is seen in adults. For example, as the brain of the infant animal develops, it must produce millions of interconnections between brain cells. If the brain is injured during this period of connective growth, it should be possible to reorganize or replace many of the lost connections. A simple analogy might be that if the main trunk of a tree is damaged early in life, the tree can adapt by growing a new trunk. Similar injury in a mature tree will not be as easily repaired.

Cerebral reorganization could be stimulated by the exogenous application of different treatments

This could take the form of some sort of behavioural therapy or it might involve the application of some sort of pharmacological treatment that would influence reparative processes in the remaining brain. Once again, it would seem most likely that the induced neuronal changes would be in the intrinsic organization of the cortex. One might predict that the changes are likely to be more extensive than in the case of endogenous change, in part because the treatment could act upon the whole brain. To pursue the injured-tree metaphor, if the tree were given fertilizer and extra water, the effect of this therapy would be observed over the entire tree.

It should be possible, at least in principle, to replace lost neurons and at least some functions

This logic has led to considerable work on neural transplantation (e.g. Dunnett and Bjorkland, 1994), although the utility of this approach is far from proven. There is, in addition, another and even less developed possibility: it may be possible to stimulate the injured brain to replace its own neurons. This route is far more speculative but recent findings are encouraging. (This topic is also dealt with in some detail in Chapter 2).

The remainder of this chapter summarizes findings from studies that provide evidence that morphological changes in the brain are correlated with behavioural restitution. It begins with consideration of the assumptions that underlie such an approach. Because we presume that mechanisms underlying reparative changes in the injured brain are likely to be observed in response to experience in the normal brain, consideration is then given to the nature of structural changes in the normal brain and their relation to behaviour. This is followed by a summary of endogenous changes in the injured brain, manipulation of these endogenous changes, and, finally, the role of neurotrophins in stimulating regeneration of injured or lost brain circuits. Throughout the chapter, the focus is on studies that have correlated changes in brain and behaviour in the same subjects, usually laboratory rats.

Assumptions

- Restoration of function is possible after brain injury.
- Structural changes in the brain underlie behavioural change.

The authors must admit to three assumptions that strongly influence both their research and their interpretation of the research of others.

At least partial restoration of function can occur naturally after cerebral injury

Note that the assumption is not that there is a return of the original lost behaviour but rather that there is simply some form of restitution of lost function. This distinction is important because there is considerable

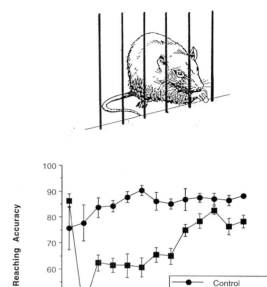

Fig. 1.1 *Top.* Illustration of the Whishaw reaching task. *Bottom.* Example of recovery of forelimb reaching accuracy after small motor cortex lesions.

debate over what constitutes recovery (e.g. Kolb, 1995). For the current purposes, recovery is defined as an improvement in function over time. Consider the following two examples.

Figure 1.1 illustrates the Whishaw reaching task in which rats are trained to reach through bars to obtain small pieces of food. Like people, rats excel in the use of their forelimbs and forepaws to retrieve quite small objects. The Whishaw task therefore allows us to study recovery of a behaviour that is commonly disrupted after cerebral injury in humans. In a typical study, rats were given small motor cortex lesions after training on the Whishaw task and were then retested at different intervals over the following weeks. Typically, such animals showed a slow improvement in their success at retrieving food by reaching with the affected limb. The

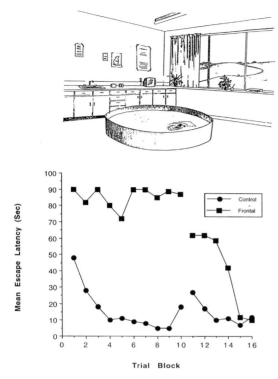

Fig. 1.2 *Top*. Illustration of the Morris water task. *Bottom*. Example of recovery of spatial navigation performance after medial frontal cortex lesions. Animals were first tested two weeks after surgery, given six months' recovery time, then retested. There is a dramatic improvement after six months' recovery.

a large tank of murky water in which there is a small platform hidden just below the water surface. The rats' task is to learn to locate the hidden platform in order to escape from the water. Rats are aquatic animals and learn this task with ease. In contrast, rats with large bilateral frontal lesions are very poor at this task, in large part because their initial strategy of swimming around the perimeter of the pool is completely ineffective in finding the platform, which is located well away from the pool wall. Thus, when rats are trained two weeks after cortical injury they often fail to find the platform and swim around and around the pool until rescued. Even when the animals do locate the platform they appear to learn little about its location in the tank. In contrast, however, when the same animals are retrained six months later they are able to learn the task and can eventually perform surprisingly efficiently, although their navigation is never as accurate as that of control rats. Normal rats learn to swim directly to the platform, whereas rats with large frontal lesions learn a strategy to find the platform by swimming a fixed distance from the wall. With extended training, however, the rats with frontal lesions can learn the platform location. Thus, there is evidence of behavioural improvement in a 'motor task' such as forepaw reaching as well as in a 'cognitive task' such as the performance of a spatial navigation task. In neither case are the animals as proficient as intact control animals, but there is a clear improvement over time. One explanation for the behavioural improvement is that the animals have adapted to the cortical injury by using other, remaining cortical circuitry. The question is whether this circuitry has been modified in order to facilitate this behavioural improvement.

An understanding of the structural changes in the brain after injury is important for understanding how to stimulate functional recovery

Although this assumption is self-evident to most behavioural neuroscientists, it may not be as obvious to those who are preoccupied with the very real practical problems of helping brain-injured patients. Nonetheless, the key point here is that if we can understand which morphological changes are associated with functional recovery, then we can direct our attention to designing

performance of the animals never returned to normal levels, however, and, perhaps more importantly, when similar animals have been examined in other experiments by Whishaw and his colleagues, it has been shown clearly that the animals make markedly different movements (Whishaw et al., 1991). Thus, the apparent recovery in the reaching accuracy reflects not only some functional recovery but also behavioural compensation. Nonetheless, there is a behavioural change over time and this change is presumably associated with some form of neural modification.

Parallel results have been found in the Morris water task performance of rats with frontal cortex removals in adulthood (Fig. 1.2). In the Morris task, rats are placed in treatments that will stimulate such plastic changes. An important corollary of this assumption is that if such plastic changes do not occur after an injury, then there will be an absence of functional recovery.

The mechanisms of cortical plasticity are most likely to be found at the synapse

Synaptic changes can be measured by analysis of either presynaptic or postsynaptic structure but it is the authors' view that the simplest way to correlate synaptic change and behaviour is to focus on the postsynaptic, or dendritic, side. This requires that the complete cell body and dendritic tree be stained, such as in a Golgi-type stain. Because the dendritic surface receives more than 95 per cent of the synapses on a neuron, it is therefore possible to infer changes in synapse number from measurements of dendritic extent and spine density (Fig. 1.3). One clear advantage of this measure is that one need not know a priori where to look because it is possible to stain, and to examine, the structure of cells throughout the entire brain. In addition, analysis requires only a light microscope (and a lot of time!). A strong bias of this review, therefore, will be towards studies that have utilized Golgi-type analyses of postsynaptic structure.

Finally, although the emphasis in most studies of structure–function relationships falls upon the analysis of neurons, there are solid grounds for looking at changes in the structure and number of glial cells. Glial cells play an important role in synaptic modification and thus can be a clue to the location and nature of experience-dependent changes in neurons and their synapses. The plasticity of glia can be analysed by estimating the number and types of glia as well as by measuring morphological characteristics such as soma size and the extent of arm-like protuberances. For example, when laboratory animals such as rats are placed in complex environments filled with novel 'toys' that they have an opportunity to interact with (so-called 'enriched environments'), there is a marked increase in the number and size of glial cells (e.g. Sirevaag and Greenough, 1991; Hawrylak and Greenough, 1995). This change in the glial cells is correlated with the changes in neuronal morphology and it is thought that the glial

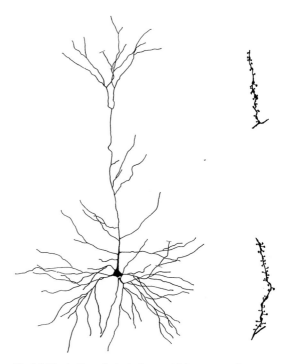

Fig. 1.3 Illustration of a typical pyramidal neuron and enlarged illustrations of spines on dendritic branches selected from different regions of the neuron.

cells may play an important role in stimulating the neuronal changes.

Changes in the normal brain

- Neurons in the normal brain change their morphology during development and ageing.
- Neurons in the normal brain show specific changes in response to specific environmental experiences.

In order to understand the ways in which the injured brain changes, we must first consider the manner in which the uninjured brain changes. The logic here is that the nervous system is conservative, and plastic changes that occur in response to experience in the normal brain are likely to be recruited in the attempt to repair the abnormal brain. There are two principal types of changes in the normal brain (1) changes during brain development; and, (2) experience-dependent changes.

Neuronal changes during development

The mammalian brain follows a general pattern of development, beginning as a hollow tube in which a thin layer of presumptive neural cells surrounds a single ventricle. The development of the brain from the neural tube involves several stages, including: cell birth (mitosis), cell migration, cell differentiation, dendritic and axonal growth, synaptogenesis, and cell and synaptic death. The order of these events is similar across species, but because the gestation time varies dramatically across different mammalian species, the timing of the events relative to birth varies considerably. This can be seen in the common observation that, whereas kittens and puppies are born helpless and blind (their eyes do not open for about two weeks), human babies are born somewhat more mobile and with open eyes, whereas calves at birth are able to stand and walk about and, of course, have their eyes open. It is worth noting that rats, which are the subject of choice in most plasticity and recovery studies, are born even less mature than kittens and their eyes do not open until about postnatal day 15. They are weaned at around 21 days of age, reach adolescence at about 60 days, and can be considered adults by about 90 days. Thus, as we compare the effects of brain injury in infant laboratory rats and human infants, we need to consider the precise nature of the developmental events underway at the time of injury. Figure 1.4 summarizes a tentative timetable for comparing rats and people.

There are two aspects of neural development that are especially important in the current context. First, the cells from which the nervous system is derived are referred to as stem cells. Stem cells give rise to the cells that subsequently form particular body structures. For example, there are stem cells for blood, stem cells for the liver, and stem cells for the nervous system. If we fall and scrape our skin, we generate new cells by a process in which the skin stem cells generate new skin cells. Neural stem cells remain in the adult mammalian brain and thus provide the potential source of new cells to replace those lost to injury or diseases (for a review of the evidence for neural stem cells in adults, see Weiss et al., 1996). The challenge is to find the switch to turn on controlled cell production when it is

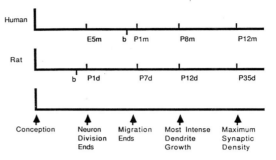

Fig. 1.4 Schematic illustration of the comparable developmental ages of the brain of the rat and human. E, embryonic day; P, postnatal day; b, day of birth. Note that the day of birth in the rat is much earlier in embryonic development than the day of birth in the human. Rhesus monkeys are born even more developed than humans.

needed. The second important aspect of neural development is the development of synapses. As neurons reach their final destination, they begin to develop axons and dendrites that will form synapses. Axons must not only grow but their growth must be directed towards appropriate targets. Dendrites do not have the same 'spatial navigation' problems of axons but they do form characteristic spatial patterns of branching. For instance, pyramidal cells, which are the primary output cells of the brain, have an easily recognizable pattern that is characterized by a vertical stalk (the apical stalk) with lateral branches that are reminiscent of branches off a tree trunk (see Fig. 1.3). In addition, there are basilar branches that grow laterally from the cell body and, like the apical stalk, they also have further branches (see Fig. 1.3). The apical and basilar fields are normally analysed separately because they typically have markedly different connections. Both the apical and basilar branches are covered with spines that form later. Both axons and dendrites grow rapidly during development and can also show remarkable plasticity in adulthood as dendrites can form spines and axons can form new axon terminations in hours and possibly even minutes. Note that the growth of new axonal arborizations does not represent the growth, de novo, of a long fibre from the cell body but is more likely to involve simply the growth of either

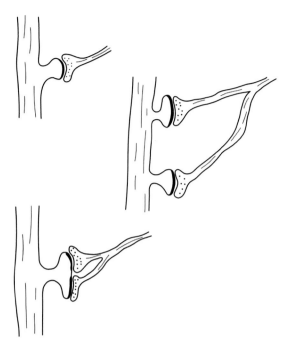

Fig. 1.5 Illustration of probable mechanisms of synapse formation. *Top.* A single synapse from an axon terminal. *Middle.* The axon terminal splits and forms two distinct synapses on two spatially separated spines. *Bottom.* The axon terminal splits and forms two synapses on the same spine.

additional end feet or connections en passant, as illustrated in Fig. 1.5.

Experience-dependent changes

It has long been assumed in the psychological literature that experiences in early childhood have greater effects upon later behaviour than do similar experiences in adulthood. The analysis of dendritic changes following exposure to enriched environments suggests that there is a structural basis to this differential effect of early experience on behaviour (e.g. Kolb et al., 1998). For example, the authors constructed 'rat condominiums', which are large enclosures (1.2 × 1.2 × 2.5 m high) with various runways, sticks, and miscellaneous toys, the latter being changed weekly. Rats were housed in same-sex groups of six for three months, beginning at weaning (21 days of age), at young adulthood (four months of age), or in senescence (two years or older). It was found that the age at which animals were placed in the enriched environments had qualitatively different effects upon dendritic structure. Rats placed into the complex environments versus standard laboratory housing in young adulthood showed effects similar to those reported by others: there was a large increase in dendritic length relative to cage-housed control rats. In addition, there was a small increase in spine density. Together, these dendritic changes would reflect a substantial increase in synapse number, a result that confirmed electron microscope studies by Greenough and his colleagues (e.g. Greenough and Chang, 1988). Parallel results were seen in senescent animals, as they showed significant increases in dendritic length and spine density relative to age-matched control rats. In contrast, when the changes in animals that were placed in the complex environments as juveniles were analysed, there was an increase in dendritic branching but a consistent decrease in spine density. That is, in comparison to older rats, the young rats showed a qualitatively different change in the distribution of synapses on pyramidal neurons. They had longer dendrites with spines placed further apart. Although the synapse number has not actually been counted, it seems likely that the young rats may actually have fewer synapses than the older ones. In contrast, however, these animals have the potential to add new spines quickly because there is space available. This capacity presumably reflects the increased potential for these animals to learn new information later.

The differential effect of enrichment in the young versus older rats led the authors to look at the effects of environmental manipulation even earlier in the rats' lives. It has been shown that tactile stimulation of premature human babies with a brush leads to faster growth and earlier hospital discharge (e.g. Solkoff and Matuszak, 1975; Field et al., 1986; Schanberg and Field, 1987). In addition, studies in infant rats have shown that similar treatment alters the structure of olfactory bulb neurons and has effects on later olfactory-guided behaviour (e.g. Coopersmith and Leon, 1984; Leon, 1992). Infant rats were therefore stroked with a camel-hair paintbrush three times daily from day 7 to day 21 of life.

Animals were subsequently raised in standard laboratory cages and were sacrificed in adulthood. Golgi analysis revealed that the early experience had no effect upon dendritic length in adulthood but there was a significant drop in spine density (Kolb et al., 1997b). Curiously, this anatomical change was correlated with significant improvement in the performance of animals in both the Whishaw reaching task and Morris water task. Thus, we see that experience can alter the brain's structure and function.

These results lead to several conclusions. First, 'enriched' experience can have very different effects upon the brain at different ages. Second, experience not only leads to 'more' but can also lead to 'less'. That is, although there is a temptation to presume that experiences lead to increased numbers of synapses and probably to increases in glia, it appears that there may be either increases or decreases, the details varying with age at experience. Third, changes in dendritic length and dendritic spine density are clearly dissociable. It is not immediately clear what the differences mean in terms of neuronal function but it is clear that experience can alter these two measures independently and in different ways at different ages. Finally, because the changes in neural structure that are associated with experience are correlated with more proficient production of a variety of behaviours, it is reasonable to expect that similar changes might be observed in animals with cerebral injuries. Note, however, that there is not a single change to look for in the injured brain but rather several different types of changes.

Evidence of morphological changes in the human brain

The idea that morphological change is associated with functional change is central to the thrust of this chapter. It is reasonable to ask in the context of the rehabilitation of humans, however, if there is any evidence for anatomical–functional correlations in humans. Such studies are difficult to carry out because they require the availability of postmortem tissue from people whose behaviour was characterized premorbidly. Recently, Scheibel and his colleagues have published a series of papers that are germaine to this question.

For example, Jacobs, Schall and Scheibel (1993) found a relationship between the extent of dendritic arborization in a cortical language area (Wernicke's area) and amount of education. Hence, the cortical neurons from the brains of deceased people with university education had more dendritic arbor than those from people with high school education who, in turn, had more dendritic material than those with less than high school education. Of course, it may have been that people with larger dendritic fields were more likely to go to university but that is not easy to test. In another study, Jacobs et al. (1993) took advantage of the now well-documented observation that females have verbal abilities that are superior to those of males (for a review, see Kolb and Whishaw, 1996). Their hypothesis was that this might be reflected in a sex difference in the structure of cortical neurons, and it was: females have more extensive dendritic arbors than males. Furthermore, this sex difference was present as early as age nine, suggesting that such sex differences emerge within the first decade.

Scheibel et al. (1990) approached the matter in a slightly different way. They began with two hypotheses. First, they suggested that there is a relationship between the complexity of dendritic arbor and the nature of the computational tasks performed by a brain area. To test this hypothesis they examined the dendritic structure of neurons in different cortical regions that they proposed to have functions that varied in computational complexity. For example, when they compared the structure of neurons corresponding to the somatosensory representation of the trunk versus the structure of those for the fingers, they found the latter to have more complex cells. They reasoned that the somesthetic inputs from receptive fields on the chest wall would constitute less of an integrative and interpretive challenge to cortical neurons than those from the fingers and thus the neurons representing the chest were less complex. Similarly, when they compared the cells in the finger area to those in the supramarginal gyrus, a region that is associated with higher cognitive processes, they found the supramarginal gyrus neurons to be more complex.

The second hypothesis was that dendritic trees in all regions are subject to experience-dependent change. As a result, Scheibel et al. hypothesized that predominant life experiences (e.g. occupation) should be reflected in the structure of dendritic trees. Although they did not test this hypothesis directly, they did make an interesting observation. In their study comparing cells in the trunk area, the finger area, and the supramarginal gyrus, they found curious individual differences. For example, especially large differences in trunk and finger neurons were found in the brains of three people – a typist, a machine operator, and an appliance repairman. In each of these, a high level of finger dexterity maintained over long periods of time may be assumed. In contrast, one case with no trunk–finger difference was a salesman in whom one would not expect a good deal of specialized finger use. These results are suggestive, although we would agree with Scheibel et al.'s caution that 'a larger sample size and far more detailed life, occupation, leisure, and retirement histories are necessary' (p. 101). The preliminary findings in this study do suggest that such an investigation would be fruitful. Furthermore, taken together, the Scheibel studies suggest that, just as in laboratory animals, there are structural correlates of behavioural capacities in humans.

Endogenous change in the injured brain

- Cortical injury results in changes in dendritic fields of remaining neurons.
- Dendritic changes vary with age at injury.
- Dendritic changes are correlated with functional outcome.
- During development there are especially 'good' and 'bad' times for injury.

As a general rule of thumb, we can state that when neurons lose connections there is a retraction of dendritic processes and when neurons gain connections there is an extension of dendritic branches and/or an increase in spine density. Thus, when the brain is injured and neurons are lost there will be a decrease in connections for some neurons and, as the brain reorganizes, there will be a subsequent increase. For example, when frontal cortex was removed in adult rats, an initial drop in dendritic arborization in proximal cortical regions such as the parietal cortex was found. This atrophy slowly resolved and four months later there was

a significant increase in dendritic morphology, which was correlated with the partial restitution of function on the Whishaw reaching task and Morris water task (e.g. Kolb, 1995). This type of compensatory change has been described after injury to both the neocortex and hippocampus (e.g. Steward, 1991; Kolb, 1995) and can probably occur after damage to subcortical regions as well.

Even more dramatic evidence of functional recovery correlated with dendritic growth can be seen in brains with injury during development. The first systematic studies showing better recovery from brain injury during infancy than in adulthood were done by Margaret Kennard, who studied the effects of motor cortex lesion in infant monkeys. Her seminal observation was that the animals with early lesions showed better recovery of motor functions than those with injuries in adulthood (e.g. Kennard, 1940). This observation was later termed the Kennard Principle by Teuber. Although Kennard did not study anatomical change, she predicted that there would be some sort of corresponding change in the remaining cortical cells, and the authors have shown this to be the case. Extensive frontal cortex lesions were made in infant rats at seven to ten days of age and it was shown that these animals had dramatic functional recovery in adulthood (e.g. Kolb and Whishaw, 1981), a phenomenon consistent with the Kennard Principle. It was then shown that this functional recovery, which was measured both on neuropsychological learning tasks as well as on motor behaviours, was correlated with a dramatic increase in dendritic length as well as an increase in dendritic spine density (for a review, see Kolb, 1995). Thus, as in adult rats, functional recovery was correlated with dendritic growth. However, in contrast to the effects of injury in adult animals, the changes in the young animals were far more widespread and could be found throughout the neocortex (e.g. Kolb, Gibb and van der Kooy, 1994). For example, anomalous connections were found from the prefrontal and motor regions to the striatum. Similarly, there were abnormal projections from the mesencephalic dopaminergic zones to the parietal cortex. In other words, functional recovery after early brain damage is correlated with more widespread changes in cortical connectivity than after similar injury in adulthood. This young versus old difference in plasticity probably accounts for the Kennard effect. Enhanced dendritic changes are not unique to animals with frontal lesions as similar results have been found in animals with occipital lesions, temporal lesions, motor lesions, and hemidecortications (for a review, see Kolb, 1995).

It was noted earlier that if dendritic growth plays a role in recovery of function, then in the absence of dendritic growth we should not see recovery. Indeed, this is the case. Hebb (1949) postulated that brain injury early in life will, under some circumstances, result in more severe behavioural disruption than similar damage later in life. In other words, Hebb proposed what is essentially the opposite of the Kennard Principle. He based his hypothesis on his observation that children with perinatal injuries to the frontal lobe appeared to fare worse in adulthood than children with injuries later in life or in adulthood. As the authors manipulated the age of their animals with frontal removals in infancy, it was found that when removals were made earlier than seven days, and especially in the first four days of life, animals were produced whose behavioural outcome was dismal relative to that of animals with similar lesions in adulthood and, of course, relative to those with similar injuries just a few days later. Such animals were not capable of learning the Morris task, even with extensive training, and they could not reach for food in the Whishaw reaching task. Dendritic analysis revealed that, in contrast to the increased dendritic growth in the rats with removals on days seven to ten, these animals had a marked atrophy of dendritic arbor and a decrease in spine density (Fig. 1.6). Hence, whereas the animals with lesions around ten days of age had an increase in cortical synapses that was correlated with dramatic recovery, animals with lesions at one to four days of age had a decrease in cortical synapses that was correlated with an absence of recovery. Indeed, such animals performed more poorly on most of the behavioural tests than animals with similar injuries in adulthood. This is reminiscent of the retardation seen after injuries in the third trimester in humans. It is known that children with various forms of retardation show a decrease in the density of dendritic spines, which are the point of synapse of the majority of excitatory synapses on pyramidal neurons. When changes in spine density after the early lesions were analysed, it was found that spine density increased after day ten lesions and, like the retarded children, it decreased after day one lesions. Curiously, it was found that changes in spine density and dendritic growth could be dissociated: frontal lesions at seven days of age resulted in partial functional recovery (Whishaw reaching task and other motor tasks, Morris water task) that was correlated with increased spine density but not with dendritic growth (Kolb, Stewart and Sutherland, 1997c). This is reminiscent of the authors' observations in the normal brain that showed that similar experiences at different ages could alter spine density, dendritic growth, or both. Thus, it appears that the brain recruits mechanisms to sustain learning and memory similar to those recruited to support functional recovery.

An absence of significant functional recovery can also be seen in adult rats with large unilateral devascularizing lesions including portions of motor, parietal, and anterior visual cortex. These animals have a severe and chronic impairment in various motor and cognitive tasks that is correlated with a permanent atrophy of remaining cortical neurons (Kolb et al., 1997a). This result is interesting because the lesion mimics the effects of large middle cerebral artery strokes in humans. Thus, it may be that the reason for such dismal recovery in people with these strokes is that the rest of the hemisphere fails to compensate.

Manipulation of endogenous change

- Behavioural treatments stimulate dendritic growth and potentiate recovery.
- Behavioural treatments provide the greatest benefit for those with the least naturally occurring recovery.
- Pharmacological treatment with neurotrophins stimulates dendritic growth and functional growth.

It has been seen that if a cerebral injury is followed by an increase in dendritic space there is a good functional outcome, whereas if an injury leads to an atrophy of dendritic space there is a poor functional outcome. It follows that if we can potentiate dendritic growth in animals showing poor recovery of function, we should enhance functional recovery. The treatments for the potentiated growth range from behavioural therapy to the application of some sort of pharmacological

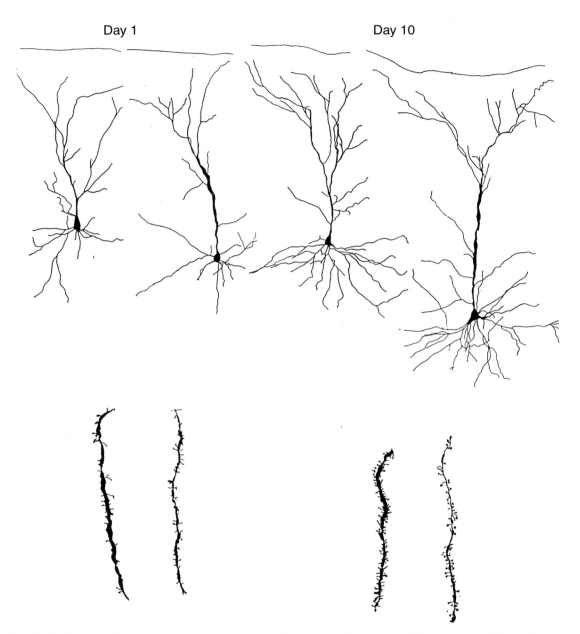

Day 1   Day 10

Fig. 1.6 *Top*. Camera lucida drawings of representative neurons from the parietal cortex of an adult rat with a medial frontal lesion on day one or day ten. The neurons from day ten brains have far more extensive dendritic arborization than neurons from day one brains. *Bottom*. Camera lucida drawings of segments of the terminal dendrites from cells from the same brains as illustrated in the top figure. There is a clear difference in the density of dendritic spines.

treatment. The pharmacological treatments could be of various forms, including growth factors (e.g. nerve growth factor, NGF), hormones (e.g. sex steroids), or chemicals that influence transmitters, especially the neuromodulators such as acetylcholine and noradrenaline. The focus here is on behavioural therapy and growth factors. (The role of sex hormones and neuromodulators is reviewed elsewhere: Kolb, 1995; Kolb et al., 1997a).

Behavioural therapy

Although it is generally assumed that behavioural therapies will improve recovery from cerebral injury in humans, there have been few direct studies of how this might work, when the optimal time for therapy might be, or even whether it actually is effective. Furthermore, as we try to develop animal models of cognitive or motor therapies, we are left with the problem of determining what an appropriate therapy might be. There have been many studies of the effects of various types of experience on functional outcome after cerebral injury in laboratory animals but the results have been inconsistent and generally disappointing (for reviews, see Schulkin, 1989; Will and Kelche, 1992). One difficulty with these studies is that few actually measured neuronal morphology; most focused primarily on functional outcome with different environmental manipulations. The authors' approach has been somewhat different. They have chosen behavioural manipulations that were known to be capable of changing the brain of intact animals and then exposed the brain-injured animals, especially those with poor functional outcomes, to the same experiences. The following illustration is from examples of the authors' work with rats with infant lesions. It was noted earlier that the developing brain is influenced by tactile stimulation during infancy and that the young animal is influenced by housing in enriched environments. Because the animal with a cortical lesion in the first days of life is functionally devastated in adulthood, and because it shows atrophy of cortical neurons, it was anticipated that such animals would benefit most from early experience.

In one series of studies, animals were given frontal or posterior parietal lesions at four days of age, followed by tactile stimulation (stroking) until weaning. The animals were group housed in laboratory cages and then tested on various tasks sensitive to frontal or parietal injury. For example, tests such as the Whishaw and Morris tasks were used to assess frontal injury and tests such as the landmark task (Kolb and Walkey, 1987) and tests of limb dexterity (Kolb and Whishaw, 1983) were used to assess parietal injury. The rats with tactile stimulation showed an unexpectedly large attenuation of the behavioural deficits of cerebral injury as a result of this rather brief 'therapy'. In fact, the rats with frontal lesions on day four showed a nearly complete recovery of performance in the Whishaw reaching task as they performed as well as control rats that had not been given the tactile experience. This was a stunning reversal of a devastating functional loss normally seen in animals with such injuries at this age. Analysis of the brains showed a reversal of the atrophy of the remaining cortical neurons normally associated with such early lesions and, more interestingly, a reversal of the decrease in spine density that is normally associated with the tactile stimulation. In other words, stroking leads to a decrease in spine density in normal animals but to an increase in spine density in the lesion animals. Thus, it is clear that not only can experience alter the brain, it can alter the normal and injured brain in different ways.

In another series of experiments, rats that had lesions on postnatal days one, five or seven were placed in enriched environments for three months, beginning at the time of weaning. It was anticipated that the animals with the earliest injuries would show the greatest functional benefit because the experience would reverse the neuronal atrophy. In contrast, it was expected that the animals with the best recovery would show the least benefit because their neurons had already grown after the injury. This was indeed the case. Rats with day one or day five lesions showed a dramatic reversal of functional impairments that was correlated with a reversal of dendritic atrophy (e.g. Kolb and Elliott, 1987). Animals with day seven lesions showed only a small enhancement of recovery and neural structure. The dramatic improvement in the animals with the earliest injuries carries an important message for it suggests that even the young animal with substantial neural atrophy and behavioural dysfunction is capable of considerable neuroplasticity and functional recovery in response to behavioural therapy. The important remaining therapeutic questions relate to the nature of the most beneficial therapy and the optimal timing for initiating the therapy.

But what about the effects of therapeutic experience in adulthood? There is a considerable literature suggesting that specific training is generally not beneficial to laboratory animals with cerebral injuries, although there are exceptions (e.g. Will and Kelche, 1992). Few studies have actually looked at morphological and behavioural change, however. The authors would predict that behavioural therapies that changed the brain would enhance recovery whereas those treatments that did not change the brain would not influence recovery. They therefore made large frontal lesions in rats and then either placed them in the enriched environments or returned them to their standard laboratory cages (Kolb and Gibb, 1991). After two months of recovery and experience, the animals were tested on various behavioural tasks. The functional results were disappointing as only a limited benefit was found from the special housing in the brain-injured animals. This result made sense, however, when the neuronal morphology of the animals was analysed. Specifically, it was found that the enriched experience interacted with the lesion-induced changes in neuronal morphology. Thus, the frontal lesions stimulated an increase in dendritic arborization in parietal cortex but did not affect visual cortex. Enrichment had no additional effect on the parietal neurons but stimulated growth in the occipital neurons. It therefore appears that neuronal changes induced by the lesion may place limits upon the environment's capacity for further neuronal, and subsequently functional, change. Specifically, once having been altered in response to a frontal injury, adjacent parietal neurons may be unable to change further in response to experience.

Perhaps the best way to proceed at this time is to determine what types of behavioural treatment are most effective in changing the adult brain and then use such treatments to influence recovery. A series of studies by Black, Greenough and their colleagues (e.g. Black et al., 1987, 1990; Black, Polinsky and Greenough,

1989) is germane. These authors trained animals to negotiate a complex obstacle course ('acrobat rats') or placed rats in running wheels where they obtained forced exercise. The animals in the wheels showed increased capillary formation in the cerebellum but no change in cerebellar Purkinje cell synapses, whereas the acrobat rats showed a 30 per cent increase in Purkinje synapses. Thus, merely increasing neuronal support does not change the neurons. The critical feature for neuronal change is presumably increased neuronal processing, which would be facilitated by a complementary increase in metabolic support. A critical experiment would be to train animals in running wheels, which would potentiate capillary growth in brain, and then to give the animals specific training. It could be predicted that animals with the metabolic support in place would show an enhanced benefit from the training and, more speculatively, animals with cerebral injuries would show even more benefit.

In sum, the effects of experience on the injured brain are complex and vary with precise age at injury as well as with the time of onset of experience. Nonetheless, the authors have shown that behavioural therapies do influence functional outcome from cortical injury and that this outcome is associated with changes in the morphology of cortical neurons. Perhaps the most important message is that the infant with the most miserable functional outcome is especially helped by behavioural therapy. This is an important lesson for the treatment of children with perinatal brain injuries.

Growth factors

Basic neurobiological research over the past decade has shown that there are several proteins that have the property of stimulating neuromitosis as well as synaptogenesis both during development and in adulthood. Two classes of such proteins have been identified (Table 1.1). These compounds have generated considerable interest because of their potential for the treatment of dementing diseases (e.g. Hefti et al., 1991) as well as for recovery from injuries (e.g. Hagg, Louis and Varon, 1993). One example of the effect of neurotrophic factors on recovery and dendritic growth is described.

It was mentioned earlier that rats given large

Table 1.1 Molecules exhibiting neurotrophic activities

Proteins initially characterized as neurotrophic factors
  Nerve growth factor (NGF)
  Brain-derived neurotrophic factor (BDNF)
  Neurotrophin-3 (NT-3)
  Ciliary neurotrophic factor (CNTF)
Growth factors with neurotrophic activity
  Fibroblast growth factor, acidic (aFGF or FGF-1)
  Fibroblast growth factor, basic (bFGF or FGF-2)
  Epidermal growth factor (EGF)
  Insulin-like growth factor (ILGF)
  Transforming growth factor (TGF)
  Lymphokines (interleukin 1, 3, 6 or IL-1, IL-3, IL-6)
  Protease nexin I, II
  Cholinergic neuronal differentiation factor

Notes:
For reviews see Hefti and Knusel (1991), and Hagg et al. (1993).

ischaemic lesions of the dorsolateral cortex have poor functional recovery and develop widespread atrophy of the dendritic fields of remaining cortical neurons. Nerve growth factor was administered to such animals via intraventricular cannulae (Kolb et al., 1997a). The major findings were that: (1) NGF stimulated dendritic growth and increased spine density in cortical pyramidal neurons in normal brains; (2) NGF stimulated partial functional recovery measured in the Whishaw reaching task; and, (3) this NGF-stimulated recovery was associated with increased dendritic growth and increased spine density (Fig. 1.7). The authors have now conducted parallel experiments with another neurotrophin, basic fibroblast growth factor (bFGF), which acts to increase the endogenous production of NGF, and have found analogous results (Rowntree and Kolb, 1997). These results are exciting because they imply that treatments with trophic factors can stimulate recovery from cortical injury and that this recovery is supported by morphological change in remaining cortical neurons (see also Chapter 2).

One of the difficulties in the use of trophic factors to treat brain-injured people is that they do not pass the blood–brain barrier easily. There is, therefore, considerable interest in developing compounds that might stim-

ulate the brain to produce trophic factors. Recently, it has become evident that the production of trophic factors may be stimulated by experience. For example, it has been shown that animals placed in an enriched environment have increased bFGF activity if they subsequently have cortical injury (Kolb et al., 1997a). In other words, experience appears to stimulate the brain's endogenous bFGF reaction to an injury. This type of result provides a direct link between behavioural therapy, neuronal growth and trophic factors. Thus, it may be possible to enhance the effects of behavioural therapies by coadministration of trophic factors.

Stimulation of neural regeneration

- The infant rat brain is capable of spontaneous regeneration of lost neurons.
- Stimulation of the adult brain with neurotrophins may stimulate neurogenesis and functional recovery.

The demonstration that there are quiescent stem cells in the adult mammalian brain has important implications for the study of recovery of function (Weiss et al., 1996). Several studies have now shown that these cells can be removed from the adult human brain, placed in culture, and stimulated to divide and to produce both neurons and glia (Kirschenbaum et al., 1994). Furthermore, it now appears that at least two brain regions, the olfactory bulb and hippocampus, produce new neurons throughout the life of mammals, including primates (e.g. Altman and Bayer, 1993; Lois and Alvarez-Buylla, 1994). Thus, the mammalian brain not only has the potential to develop new neurons in adulthood but it actually does. In principle, it therefore should be possible to stimulate these cells to produce new neurons after an injury. There are, however, several practical problems for the nervous system. First, the neurons must get to the site of injury. Second, they must differentiate into the appropriate neuronal types. Third, they must develop the appropriate connections. In other words, the cells must replicate the normal sequence of brain development well after this development is complete. The question that arises is what is it that stimulates the brain to undergo this series of steps in the first place? One possibility is the presence of specific trophic factors. It follows that it might be possible to induce regrowth by

Control   **NGF**

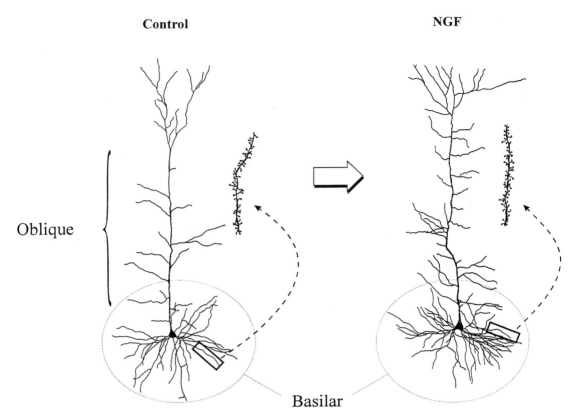

Oblique

Basilar

Fig. 1.7 Examples of layer V pyramidal cells taken from the cingulate cortex of a vehicle control rat (left) and an NGF-treated rat (right). The inset illustrates spine density in a typical terminal tuft from basilar fields. NGF treatment increased dendritic arborization and spine density in the terminal branches.

stimulating the brain with the appropriate growth factors. Of course, the brain is producing these during development so we might predict that the best time to stimulate the brain to regrow is when it is still growing. Recently, it has been demonstrated that this is the case (Kolb et al., 1997b).

In the course of studying rats with restricted lesions of midline frontal region in infancy, the authors noticed that there was no lesion cavity when the brains were examined in adulthood. Although this cavity loss might have been due to a mechanical shifting of the remaining neural tissue, the authors have now shown that the cavity fills with neurons that are born after the injury and that the new neurons develop appropriate connec-

tions with the rest of the brain. Furthermore, animals with this regrowth show virtually complete restitution of function and, if the regrowth process is blocked with a substance that interferes with stem cell activity, the recovery of function is blocked. This is an exciting discovery because it implies that not only is it possible to regrow lost neural regions, but also these neural regions are functional.

The demonstration of neuronal regeneration in the developing brain does not, however, prove that such a process is possible in the adult brain. Indeed, we know that even very small midline frontal lesions in adult brains do not lead to neurogenesis. It is hoped, however, that by providing the adult brain with appropriate trophic factors that might mimic the signals present during development, it might be possible to stimulate cerebral regeneration in adults. The authors' preliminary studies show that by providing the brain with a mixture of trophic factors that might mimic the state during development, it is possible to stimulate the brain to produce new neurons and for these neurons to migrate to the lesion cavity. It has yet to be shown, however, that the newly generated neurons can support functional recovery.

Conclusions

1. At least partial restitution of function (i.e. recovery of function) is possible after cerebral injury. Functional restitution does not necessary imply the return of lost abilities but is more likely to reflect the development of compensatory strategies to cope with the lost neural circuits. The challenge for rehabilitation is to find ways to encourage the brain to develop these compensatory strategies.

2. Functional recovery after cerebral injury usually results from reorganization of remaining cortical circuits. This reorganization can be inferred from changes in the dendritic morphology of cortical neurons. Processes that serve to enhance advantageous morphological changes will lead to enhanced functional recovery, whereas processes that retard or prevent morphological change will interfere with functional recovery. It follows that the absence of recovery of function reflects an absence of sufficient reorganization of cerebral circuitry. Thus, one challenge for rehabilitation is to provide treatments that will stimulate the brain into making the necessary morphological adjustments.

3. The compensatory changes in neuronal morphology that underlie functional recovery are similar in nature to those that the brain uses normally during brain development and during the processes of learning and memory. Because the normal brain uses multiple experience-dependent changes to code experiences, we can expect multiple injury-dependent changes to underlie recovery of function. An understanding of the nature of normal experience-dependent changes is therefore critical to under-

standing the nature of processes underlying recovery of function.

4. Although the processes underlying experience-dependent change and injury-induced change may be similar, there is no guarantee that experience affects the uninjured brain in the same manner as the injured brain. Indeed, the fact that the brain is changing in response to injury means that the same experience may be acting on a fundamentally different neural substrate in the normal and injured brain.

5. The reorganization of remaining cortical circuits can be potentiated by the application of different treatments, including behavioural therapy, trophic factors, and other pharmacological agents. The enhanced reorganization of cortical circuits will lead to enhanced functional recovery. Different treatments may interact to enhance recovery. For example, behavioural therapies may act, in part, via their action in stimulating the endogenous production of trophic factors. Thus, combining behavioural therapies with the pharmacological administration of compounds to increase the availability of trophic factors may lead to enhanced functional outcome.

6. There are times during development when morphological changes, and subsequently functional recovery, are more likely to occur. For humans, the least favourable time is probably at the end of the gestational period and perhaps including the first month or so of life, whereas the most favourable time is likely to be at one to two years of age.

7. There is preliminary evidence to suggest that it may be possible to induce neural regeneration in the injured brain and that the regenerated brain functions to support functional recovery.

References

Altman, J. and Bayer, S. 1993. Are new neurons formed in the brains of adult mammals? A progress report, 1962–1992. In *Neuronal Cell Death and Repair*, ed. A.C. Cuello, pp. 203–25. New York: Elsevier.

Black, J.E., Greenough, W.T., Anderson, B.J. and Isaacs, K.R. 1987. Environment and the ageing brain. *Can J Psychol*, **41**, 111–30.

Black, J.E., Isaacs, K.R., Anderson, B.J., Alcantara, A.A. and Greenough, W.T. 1990. Learning causes synaptogenesis, whereas motor activity causes angiogenesis, in cerebellar cortex of adult rats. *Proc Natl Acad Sci USA* **87**, 5568–72.

Black, J.E., Polinsky, M. and Greenough, W.T. 1989. Progressive failure of cerebral angiogenesis supporting neural plasticity in ageing rats. *Neurobiol Aging* **10**, 353–8.

Coopersmith, R. and Leon, M. 1984. Enhanced neural response to familiar olfactory cues. *Science* **225**, 849–51.

Dunnett, S.B. and Bjorklund, A. (eds.) 1994. *Functional Neural Transplantation*. New York: Raven Press.

Field, T., Schanberg, S.M., Scafidi, F. et al. 1986. Tactile/kinesthetic stimulation effects on preterm neonates. *Pediatrics* **77**, 654–58.

Greenough, W.T. and Chang, F.F. 1988. Plasticity of synapse structure and pattern in the cerebral cortex. In *Cerebral Cortex*, Vol. 7, ed. A. Peters and E.G. Jones, pp. 391–440. New York: Plenum Press.

Hagg, T., Louis, J.-C. and Varon, S. 1993. Neurotrophic factors and CNS regeneration. In *Neuroregeneration*, ed. A. Gorio, pp. 265–88. New York: Raven Press.

Hawrylak, N. and Greenough, W.T. 1995. Monocular deprivation alters the morphology of glial fibrillary acidic protein-immunoreactive astrocytes in the rat visual cortex. *Brain Res* **683**, 187–99.

Hebb, D.O. 1949. *The Organization of Behaviour*, New York: Wiley.

Hefti, F., Brachet, P., Will, B. and Christen, Y. (eds.) 1991. *Growth Factors and Alzheimer's Disease*. Berlin: Springer-Verlag.

Hefti, F. and Knusel, B. 1991. Neurotrophic factors and neurodegenerative diseases. In *Growth Factors and Alzheimer's Disease*, ed. F. Hefti, P. Brachet, B. Will and Y. Christen, pp. 1–14. Berlin: Springer-Verlag.

Jacobs, B., Schall, M. and Scheibel, A.B. 1993. A quantitative dendritic analysis of Wernicke's area. II. Gender, hemispheric, and environmental factors. *J. Comp Neurol* **237**, 97–111.

Kennard, M.A. 1940. Relation of age to motor impairment in man and in subhuman primates. *Arch Neurol Psychiatry* **44**, 377–97.

Kirschenbaum, B., Nedergaard, M., Preuss, A., Barami, K., Fraser, F.A.R. and Goldman, S.A. 1994. In vitro neuronal production and differentiation by precursor cells derived from the adult forebrain. *Cereb Cortex* **4**, 576–89.

Kolb, B. 1995. *Brain Plasticity and Behavior*. Mahwah, NJ: Erlbaum.

Kolb, B., Cote, S., Ribeiro-da-Silva, A. and Cuello, A.C. 1997a. NGF stimulates recovery of function and dendritic growth after unilateral motor cortex lesions in rats. *Neuroscience* **76**, 1139–51.

Kolb, B. and Elliott, W. 1987. Recovery from early cortical damage in rats. II. Effects of experience on anatomy and behavior following frontal lesions at 1 or 5 days of age. *Behav Brain Res* **26**, 47–56.

Kolb, B., Forgie, M., Gibb, R., Gorny, G. and Rowntree, S. 1998. Age, experience and the changing brain. *Neurosci Biobehav Rev*, **22**, 143–59.

Kolb, B. and Gibb, R. 1991. Environmental enrichment and cortical injury: behavioral and anatomical consequences of frontal cortex lesions in rats. *Cereb Cortex*, **1**, 189–98.

Kolb, B., Gibb, R., Gorny, G. and Whishaw, I.Q. 1997b. Possible regeneration of rat medial frontal cortex following neonatal frontal lesions. *Behav Brain Res* **91**, 127–41.

Kolb, B., Gibb, R. and van der Kooy, D. 1994. Neonatal frontal cortical lesions in rats alter cortical structure and connectivity. *Brain Res* **645**, 85–97.

Kolb, B., Stewart, J. and Sutherland, R.J. 1997c. Recovery of function is associated with increased spine density in cortical pyramidal cells after frontal lesions and or noradrenaline depletion in neonatal rats. *Behav Brain Res* **89**, 61–70.

Kolb, B. and Walkey, J. 1987. Behavioural and anatomical studies of the posterior parietal cortex in the rat. *Behav Brain Res*, **23**, 127–45.

Kolb, B. and Whishaw, I.Q. 1981. Neonatal frontal lesions in the rat: sparing of learned but not species-typical behavior in the presence of reduced brain weight and cortical thickness. *J Comp Physiol Psychol* **95**, 863–79.

Kolb, B. and Whishaw, I.Q. 1983. Dissociation of the contributions of the prefrontal, motor, and parietal cortex to the control of movement in the rat: an experimental review. *Can J Psychol* **37**, 211–32.

Kolb, B. and Whishaw, I.Q. 1996. *Fundamentals of Human Neuropsychology*, 4th edn. New York: W.H. Freeman & Co.

Leon, M. 1992. Neuroethology of olfactory preference development. *J Neurobiol* **23**, 1557–73.

Lois, C. and Alvarez-Buylla, A. 1994. Long-distance neuronal migration in the adult mammalian brain. *Science* **264**, 1145–8.

Rowntree, S. and Kolb, B. 1997. Blockade of basic fibroblast growth factor retards recovery from motor cortex injury in rats. *Eur J Neurosci* **9**, 2432–42.

Schanberg, S.M. and Field, T.M. 1987. Sensory deprivation stress and supplemental stimulation in the rat pup and preterm human neonate. *Child Dev* **58**, 1431–47.

Scheibel, A.B., Conrad, T., Perdue, S., Tomiyasu, U. and Wechsler, A. 1990. A quantitative study of dendrite complexity in selected areas of the human cerebral cortex. *Brain Cogn* **12**, 85–101.

Schulkin, J. (ed.) 1989. *Preoperative Events: their Effects on Behavior Following Brain Damage*. Hillsdale, NJ: Erlbaum.

Sirevaag, A.M. and Greenough, W.T. 1991. Plasticity of GFA-immunoreactive astrocyte size and number in visual cortex of rats reared in complex environments. *Brain Res* **540**, 273–8.

Solkoff, N. and Matuszak, D. 1975. Tactile stimulation and behavioral development among low-birthweight infants. *Child Psychiatry Hum Dev* **6**, 33–7.

Steward, O. 1991. Synapse replacement on cortical neurons following denervation. In *Cerebral Cortex*, Vol. 9, ed. A. Peters and E.G. Jones, pp. 81–131. New York: Plenum Press.

Weiss, S., Reynolds, B.A., Vescovi, A.L., Morshead, C., Craig, C.G. and van der Kooy, D. 1996. Is there a neural stem cell in the mammalian forebrain? *Trends Neurosci* **19**, 387–93.

Whishaw, I.Q., Pellis, S.M., Gorny, B.P. and Pellis, V.C. 1991. The impairments in reaching and the movements of compensation in rats with motor cortex lesions: an endpoint, videorecording, and movement notation analysis. *Behav Brain Res* **42**, 77–91.

Will, B. and Kelche, C. 1992. Environmental approaches to recovery of function from brain damage: a review of animal studies (1981 to 1991). In *Recovery from Brain Damage: Reflections and Directions*, ed. F.D. Rose and D.A. Johnson, pp. 79–104. New York: Plenum Press.

2

Intracerebral transplantation and regeneration: practical implications

Heather Dickinson-Anson, Isabelle Aubert and Fred H. Gage

Introduction

Intracerebral transplantation is a powerful tool to study neural development, plasticity and regeneration in the brain, and has emerged as a promising strategy for repairing the damaged central nervous system (Fisher and Gage, 1993). In particular, intracerebral grafts of fetal tissue have been used extensively to examine biological mechanisms underlying neurodegeneration and functional deterioration in age-associated central nervous system disorders such as Parkinson's disease and Alzheimer's disease. As a result, there is now substantial evidence that intracerebral grafting may be a useful technique for re-establishing severed connections and replacing lost cells and pathways in the adult mammalian brain, resulting in functional recovery. For example, results from many studies using cholinergic fetal tissue grafted in animal models of Alzheimer's disease demonstrate that the grafts are capable of innervating host tissue and inducing behavioural restoration (Gage and Chen, 1992). Various tissue-derived factors have been proposed as mediating the anatomical and functional effects observed following fetal tissue implantation. Trophic factors produced by fetal tissue may rescue degenerating neural cells and promote other mechanisms of plasticity such as sprouting and regeneration of disrupted host neuronal circuitry. Alternatively, grafts may deliver depleted neurotransmitters following degeneration (Gage and Buzsaki, 1989; Gage and Fisher, 1991; Dunnett and Björklund, 1994). The role of specific, fetal tissue-derived factors in anatomical and/or functional recovery can be revealed by cells genetically engineered to produce targeted molecules, such as growth factors or neurotransmitters. This chapter summarizes findings from fetal tissue studies which have suggested a role for trophic and neurotransmitter replacement in functional restoration, and discusses the more recent use of engineered cells to clarify the involvement of discrete substances in such recovery.

Basal forebrain cholinergic system and ageing

- The basal forebrain cholinergic system is crucial in memory/attention processes in a variety of species, including humans.
- The basal forebrain cholinergic system is vulnerable during ageing, particularly in cases of Alzheimer's disease in humans, in which cholinergic deficits correlate with decline in cognitive function.
- Treatment strategies for Alzheimer's disease and cognitive dysfunction have aimed at augmenting the function of the basal forebrain cholinergic system.

The basal forebrain cholinergic system is considered to play a crucial role in memory and/or attentional processes (Decker and McGaugh, 1991). Cholinergic neurons within the basal forebrain are located in the medial septum, the diagonal band of Broca, and the nucleus basalis magnocellularis. Cholinergic neurons of the medial septum/diagonal band of Broca project dorsally to the hippocampus, primarily through the fimbria–fornix, and account for approximately 90 per cent of hippocampal cholinergic innervation (Storm-Mathisen, 1974; Amaral and Kruz, 1985). Approximately 80–90 per cent of the neurons in the nucleus basalis magnocellularis are cholinergic and provide the major

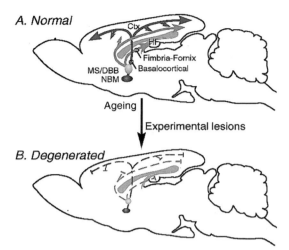

A. Normal

Ctx

HF

Fimbria-Fornix
MS/DBB   Basalocortical
NBM

Ageing

Experimental lesions

B. Degenerated

Fig. 2.1 Septohippocampal and basalocortical cholinergic pathways. A. Normal cholinergic projection pathways of the basal forebrain. Cholinergic neurons in the medial septal and diagonal band nuclei (MS/DBB) project to the hippocampal formation through the fimbria fornix pathway. Nucleus basalis magnocellularis neurons (NBM) send cholinergic fibres throughout the neocortical mantle. B. Age or experimental lesions induce degeneration of these central cholinergic pathways (dashed lines).

source of cholinergic input to the neocortex (Fig. 2.1; Mesulam et al., 1983; Saper, 1984). The integrity of the basal forebrain cholinergic system is closely linked to mnemonic function in a variety of animals, including humans, nonhuman primates and rodents. Lesions or pharmacological manipulations aimed at disrupting the function of this system lead to robust learning and memory deficits that can be ameliorated by the administration of cholinomimetics (Olton, Walker and Gage, 1978; O.G. Nilsson et al., 1987; Brito and Brito, 1990; Decker and McGaugh, 1991).

The basal forebrain cholinergic system appears to be particularly vulnerable during ageing, often showing a progressive deterioration that has been linked to the cognitive dysfunction of Alzheimer's disease. Clinically, Alzheimer's disease is characterized by a progressive deterioration of cognitive functions, including profound perturbations of learning and memory processes. Postmortem examination of Alzheimer's disease brains reveals the presence of senile plaques, β-amyloid

deposits, neurofibrillary tangles, neuronal loss and reduced synaptic density throughout the association areas of the parietal–temporal cortex, hippocampus, entorhinal cortex and the amygdaloid complex (Katzman, 1986). Although several transmitter systems are affected in the Alzheimer's disease brain, the severe deterioration of the cholinergic system is one of the earliest and most consistent pathological changes observed (Bartus et al., 1982; Coyle, Price and DeLong, 1983). A dramatic cholinergic cell loss is observed in the basal forebrain nuclei, especially in the nucleus basalis magnocellularis (Bartus et al., 1982; Coyle et al., 1983; Perry, 1986). In addition, the activity of choline acetyltransferase (ChAT), the synthetic enzyme for acetylcholine (ACh), is reduced by as much as 90 per cent in the cerebral cortex and hippocampal formation of the Alzheimer's disease brain (Davies and Maloney, 1976; Bartus et al., 1982; Coyle et al., 1983; Perry, 1986).

Based on findings that there is a correlation between the decline in the integrity of the basal forebrain cholinergic system and the severity of dementia observed in Alzheimer's disease, the 'cholinergic hypothesis of geriatric memory dysfunction' was postulated by Bartus and colleagues in 1982. This hypothesis has led to therapeutic approaches focused on replacing depleted ACh in animal models of cholinergic dysfunction and in Alzheimer's disease. Strategies aimed at increasing cholinergic activity via the administration of ACh precursors or cholinesterase inhibitors have resulted in temporary improvements at best. This limited success may be due to problems with dose, nonspecific receptor stimulation, pharmacokinetics and inefficient crossing of the blood–brain barrier by the compound. Strategies based on stimulation of cholinergic receptors have recently emphasized targeting specific cholinergic receptor subtypes. Both nicotinic and muscarinic cholinergic receptors are abundant in basal forebrain cholinergic target regions and are involved in the regulation of ACh release (nicotine receptors and M2 muscarinic receptors: Quirion, 1993; Levey, 1996; Vidal, 1996) as well as in postsynaptic activation of cortical and hippocampal areas (nicotinic, M1: Eglen and Watson, 1996; Levey, 1996; Vidal, 1996). Postmortem analyses of Alzheimer's disease brain tissue reveal that up to 40–45 per cent of M2 receptors are still present in the cerebral cortex and hippocampal formation (Mash, Flynn and Potter, 1985; Aubert et al., 1992). Furthermore, it has been shown that postmortem Alzheimer's disease tissue has the capacity to synthesize and release ACh (Rylett, Ball and Colhoun, 1983; L. Nilsson et al., 1987). In rodents, age-induced cognitive impairments are reversed by the blockade of M2 receptors, which increases ACh release (Quirion et al., 1995). Taken together, these data suggest that one appropriate strategy for the treatment of Alzheimer's disease may be inactivation of M2 muscarinic autoreceptors. With regard to the stimulation of postsynaptic cholinergic receptors, the binding parameters of postsynaptic M1 muscarinic receptors are relatively unchanged in postmortem brains of Alzheimer's disease patients (Mash et al., 1985; Aubert et al., 1992). Recent studies have shown that the administration of muscarinic M1/M3 specific agonists reverses cognitive deficits in animal models of Alzheimer's disease (Davis et al., 1993; Dawson et al., 1994). In addition, nicotinic receptor agonists (which can stimulate ACh release presynaptically and activate postsynaptic nicotinic receptors) can reverse age-induced cognitive deficits in laboratory animals and attenuate some aspects of the cognitive deficits observed in Alzheimer's disease, suggesting promise for the therapeutic use of nicotinic ligands for cognitive dysfunction (Levin, 1992; Socci, Sanberg and Arendash, 1995; Vidal, 1996). Taken together, these data suggest that treatment strategies aimed at stimulating cholinergic receptors in Alzheimer's disease merit consideration.

Animal models of Alzheimer's disease

- Animal models of cholinergic dysfunction are essential for the evaluation of the impact of neural transplantation on cell survival, axonal regeneration, target reinnervation and functional recovery. They include the use of:
  (1) aged animals
  (2) animals with experimental transections of cholinergic pathways
  (3) animals with experimental lesions of basal forebrain cholinergic system nuclei using toxic agents.

The 'cholinergic hypothesis' has led to the development of a number of animal models of cholinergic depletion. Such models are essential for evaluating the potential of treatment strategies for reversing Alzheimer's disease-associated cognitive deficits (see Fig. 2.1). To date, animal models of Alzheimer's disease do not reproduce all changes associated with ageing and Alzheimer's disease, but rather mimic a few of the morphological, neurochemical and cognitive deficits. Nevertheless, such models are useful to evaluate the impact of intracerebral grafting as a potential therapy to sustain cell survival, induce neuronal recovery and axonal regeneration, and target reinnervation and the supplementation of depleted neurotransmitters.

Aged animals

Aged animals represent a naturally occurring impairment model showing some of the neurochemical and morphological changes characteristic of aged humans. In aged animals, basal forebrain cholinergic system neurons undergo degenerative changes, as demonstrated by marked decreases in ACh synthesis and release, altered high-affinity choline uptake (which measures functional cholinergic terminals) and decreased ACh receptor binding (Dunnett, 1990). Morphometric analyses show significant atrophy and loss of ChAT-positive neurons in the basal forebrain cholinergic system (Decker, 1987). These age-induced impairments of the system are highlighted by findings that, as is observed in Alzheimer's disease patients, aged laboratory animals show a heightened sensitivity to the cognitively impairing effects of anticholinergic drugs, which has been interpreted as suggesting a compensatory response to loss of endogenous cholinergic function (Sunderland et al., 1985; Nilsson and Gage, 1993).

Behaviourally, aged rats are impaired on a variety of learning and memory tasks, including complex spatial tasks such as the Morris water maze (Gage, Dunnett and Björklund, 1984; Rapp, Rosenberg and Gallagher, 1987; Gallagher and Pelleymounter, 1988; Fischer, Gage and Björklund, 1989; Fischer et al., 1991b; Frick et al., 1995). Aged nonhuman primates also show cognitive deficits, many of which parallel those observed in aged humans (Presty et al., 1987; Bachevalier et al., 1991; Rapp and

Amaral, 1991; Ströessner-Johnson, Rapp and Amaral, 1992). Several of these age-induced cognitive deficits are linked to neurodegenerative changes that occur in the basal forebrain cholinergic system (Bartus et al., 1982; Gallagher and Pelleymounter, 1988; Fischer et al., 1991b; Ströessner-Johnson et al., 1992). Interestingly, as is observed in humans, age-related behavioural deficits in rats and nonhuman primates show marked individual differences (Gage et al., 1984; Presty, et al., 1987; Bachevalier et al., 1991). In general, neuronal loss and cell atrophy in the basal forebrain cholinergic system correlate with poor performance on behavioural tasks geared to assess the function of the system (Fischer et al., 1991b). It should be noted, however, that ChAT activity and other cholinergic parameters, especially in the cerebral cortex and hippocampal formation of age-impaired animals, are affected less, or differently, than is observed in Alzheimer's disease patients (Fischer et al., 1989; Fischer, Nilsson and Björklund, 1991c; Aubert et al., 1995; Quirion et al., 1995). Additionally, other transmitter systems show age-induced deficits. Aged rats and primates exhibit declines in levels of dopamine and noradrenalin, as well as deterioration of serotonergic cells in the dorsal raphe and noradrenergic neurons in the locus ceruleus (Dunnett, 1990; Chen and Gage, 1994).

Lesion models

To address cholinergic cell rescue, axonal regeneration and target reinnervation, experimental approaches consisting of lesioning specific cholinergic pathways in rodents and nonhuman primates have been used extensively (Smith, 1988; Dunnett and Barth, 1991). Such strategies mimic a few specific, age-induced anatomical and/or cognitive deficits. Most common are lesions of the (1) septo-hippocampal and nucleus basalis magnocellularis–cortical cholinergic pathways; (2) basal forebrain cholinergic system nuclei (i.e. medial septum/diagonal band of Broca or nucleus basalis magnocellularis: Armstrong et al., 1987) efferent targets (i.e. hippocampus or cerebral cortex). One model of cholinergic degeneration consists of transecting the fimbria–fornix, thereby axotomizing the septo-hippocampal projections. This procedure induces ret-

rograde and anterograde degeneration of the cholinergic neurons in the medial septum and virtually eliminates cholinergic input to the dorsal hippocampal formation (Gage et al., 1986; Armstrong et al., 1987). Behaviourally, lesions of the fimbria–fornix often produce robust deficits on a variety of learning and memory tasks (Dunnett, 1990; Sinden, Gray and Hodges, 1994; Devan, Goad and Petri, 1996). Both anterograde and retrograde degeneration strategies are used to disrupt the nucleus basalis magnocellularis–cortical (basalocortical) cholinergic projection and produce performance deficits on a variety of learning and memory tasks (Connor, Langlais and Thal, 1991; Dekker, Connor and Thal, 1991; Dunnett and Barth, 1991; Chen and Gage, 1994; Mallet et al., 1995). Intranucleus basalis magnocellularis infusions of excitotoxins result in a loss of cholinergic neurons and anterograde degeneration of the basalocortical innervation (Winkler and Thal, 1995). Devascularization of cortical target regions of the nucleus basalis magnocellularis results in retrograde degeneration of the basalocortical pathways (Maysinger et al., 1992; Piccardo, Maysinger and Cuello, 1992).

The lesion strategies described thus far do not exclusively damage cholinergic systems. For example, fimbria–fornix lesions disrupt GABAergic, galanin, and substance P septo-hippocampal projections (Wainer et al., 1993), as well as serotonergic afferents from the dorsal raphé and noradrenergic afferents from the locus ceruleus (Decker and McGaugh, 1991). Similarly, excitotoxic lesions of the nucleus basalis magnocellularis damage cholinergic and GABAergic neurons at the site of injection (Rossner, Schliebs and Bigl, 1994) and decrease monoamine levels in several brain regions (Lindefors et al., 1992).The fact that multiple neurotransmitter systems are affected in all of these animal models offers a closer representation of Alzheimer's disease and thus offers an appropriate model to address experimental questions related to cholinergic cell saving, axonal regeneration, target reinnervation and the sufficiency of cholinergic replacement strategies for recovery of function (Emson and Lindvall, 1986; Rossor and Iversen, 1986; Reinikainen, Soininen and Riekkinen, 1990; Francis et al., 1993).

The recent development of an immunotoxin (192

IgG-saporin), which targets cholinergic neurons expressing the low-affinity nerve growth factor receptor (p75), allows for specific lesions of basal forebrain cholinergic system nuclei (Wiley, 1992). In rats, either intraventricular or local infusions of IgG-saporin in these nuclei result in a near-complete and selective loss of cholinergic neurons throughout the basal forebrain cholinergic system without affecting other neurotransmitter systems or producing nonspecific tissue damage (Heckers et al., 1994, Torres et al., 1994). Behaviourally, IgG-saporin-induced lesions of these nuclei induce varying degrees of performance deficits in a variety of learning and memory tasks (Berger-Sweeney et al., 1994; Torres et al., 1994; Waite et al., 1995). Because the functional and anatomical effects of IgG-saporin are still being characterized, there are very few studies examining the impact of intracerebral grafts on lesion-induced deficits (Leanza et al., 1996; Rossner et al., 1996).

Grafting strategies: embryonic tissue

- Cholinergic-rich embryonic tissues (basal forebrain cholinergic system grafts) are efficacious in the re-innervation of deafferented basal forebrain cholinergic system target regions and ameliorate a variety of functional deficits.
- Such tissue grafts attenuate cognitive deficits in all cholinergic depletion models. This recovery has been correlated with indices of cholinergic activity.
- Fetal tissue grafts may mediate recovery through a release of trophic factors, neurotransmitters and/or replacement of lost neural cells.

Fetal tissue implants

Cholinergic-rich fetal tissue has been grafted into the hippocampus and cortex of aged animals, or of young animals with lesions of either the basal forebrain cholinergic system nuclei or their efferent pathways. It is now well established that grafts of cholinergic-rich fetal tissue survive, innervate host tissue and establish functional connections that influence targeted neuronal populations in animal models of Alzheimer's disease (Fine et al., 1985; Dunnett, 1990; Sinden et al.,

1994; Tarricone et al., 1996). Extensive evidence indicates that embryonic transplants in deafferented basal forebrain cholinergic system target areas are capable of reversing a variety of lesion-induced perturbations in anatomical, electrophysiological, neurochemical, and histochemical functions (Gage, et al., 1987; Fisher and Gage, 1993; Sinden et al., 1994; Tarricone et al., 1996).

Cell savings and fibre regeneration

Grafts of fetal tissue can function as a substrate for the regeneration of denervated septo-hippocampal projection neurons. One recent study demonstrated a very robust regeneration of the septo-hippocampal cholinergic projection. Leanza and colleagues (1996) grafted fetal cholinergic tissue in the septum of neonatal rats following immunotoxic (IgG-saporin) lesions of cholinergic septal cells. Analyses using a combination of retrograde tracing, biochemical, histochemical and immunocytochemical techniques showed that the fetal grafts survived and integrated into the host tissue up to six months after grafting. The grafts extended cholinergic axons along the original septo-hippocampal pathway, innervated the appropriate dorso-hippocampal terminal fields and induced recovery of cholinergic activity in the reinnervated targets. There are reports of limited fetal tissue-induced septo-hippocampal regeneration in the adult rat (Kromer, Björklund and Stenevi, 1980, 1981; Segal, Stenevi and Björklund, 1981). For example, in a study conducted by Kromer and colleagues (1981), fetal hippocampal tissue was grafted into the lesion cavity of fimbria–fornix-lesioned rats. The results showed that some transected septal cholinergic neurons could traverse the graft and reinnervate the hippocampus. However, the majority of studies using adult rats reveal only limited host regeneration across fetal bridges into the hippocampus, and most of the cholinergic neurons in the medial septum/diagonal band of Broca undergo retrograde degeneration and die (Kromer et al., 1980, 1981; Tuszynski, Buzsaki and Gage, 1990; Tuszynski and Gage, 1995). It is encouraging to note that recent findings suggest that fetal grafts may be more successful in regenerating the damaged septo-hippocampal circuitry if they are transiently combined with infusions of trophic factors. Tuszynski and Gage (1995) demonstrated that rescue of axotomized cholinergic septal cells, as well as reinnervation of the host hippocampus by embryonic transplants, were significantly enhanced in the presence of concurrent infusions of the neurotrophin nerve growth factor.

Results from embryonic grafts in the damaged basalocortical projection system indicate that cortical cell suspensions grafted in the damaged cortex can prevent retrograde degeneration of nucleus basalis magnocellularis cholinergic neurons, suggesting the implants released trophic factors that rescued the damaged neural cells (Sofroniew, Isacson and Björklund, 1986). In rats with excitotoxic lesions of the nucleus basalis magnocellularis, basal forebrain cholinergic system fetal tissue grafts induce dense acetylcholinesterase (AChE)-positive and ChAT-positive fibre reinnervation of the host neocortex (Welner et al., 1988; Lescaudron, Sutton and Stein, 1993). Additionally, basal forebrain cholinergic system tissue grafted into the nucleus basalis magnocellularis of aged rats produces hypertrophy of the host cholinergic cells (Chen et al., 1989), suggesting either that the grafts are capable of replacing host cholinergic neurons, or that they have a trophic effect on the surviving host cells.

Functional recovery

Transplantation of cholinergic-rich fetal tissue in the hippocampus or nucleus basalis magnocellularis cortical targets has been shown to attenuate a variety of learning and memory deficits in animal models of Alzheimer's disease. Findings that the administration of cholinergic receptor antagonists can reverse the functional recovery produced by cholinergic-rich transplants suggest that such recovery is mediated, at least in part, by cholinergic mechanisms (Gage and Björklund, 1986; O.G. Nilsson et al., 1987; Li, Simon and Low, 1992). In a number of cases, the graft-induced functional restoration is significantly correlated with both fibre ingrowth from the grafts and restoration of cholinergic status, as measured by AChE staining and high-affinity choline uptake (Table 2.1). For example, several studies have shown that graft-derived AChE-positive fibre innervation of the denervated hippocampus (Dunnet et al., 1982; Daniloff et al., 1985; Arendt et al., 1989), as well

as graft-induced increases of high-affinity choline uptake activity (Low et al., 1982; Daniloff et al., 1985; Tarricone et al., 1991), correlate with functional recovery on learning and memory tasks. Similar results are reported using nonhuman primates. Ridley and colleagues (1991, 1992) grafted fetal basal forebrain cholinergic system tissue into the hippocampus of fibria–fornix-lesioned monkeys and examined learning performance on a variety of tasks. Grafted animals showed significant reversal of lesion-induced learning deficits as well as a normalization of AChE staining in the host hippocampus and AChE-positive outgrowth extending from the graft into host tissue (Ridley et al., 1991). Significant correlations have also been reported between behavioural recovery and graft-induced restoration of hippocampal ACh levels (Arendt et al., 1989). Finally, indices of cholinergic neurochemical, receptor and behavioural recovery have been correlated. In a series of experiments using fimbria–fornix-lesioned rats with intrahippocampal fetal septal tissue grafts, Tarricone and colleagues (1991, 1993) reported positive correlations between graft-induced increases in high-affinity choline uptake and ChAT activity and stabilization of muscarinic receptor binding with recovery of spatial performance.

Despite the large number of studies demonstrating a positive correlation between behavioural recovery and indices of cholinergic restoration, the functional and morphological impact of embryonic basal forebrain cholinergic system grafts into the central nervous system of Alzheimer's disease animal models is quite variable. For example, functional restoration is not always correlated with indices of cholinergic recovery and/or graft innervation of host tissue. Tarricone and colleagues (1991, 1993) reported that graft-induced increases in hippocampal high-affinity choline uptake levels in fibria–fornix-lesioned rats were not always indicative of recovery of spatial performance. Moreover, Dunnett et al. (1984) reported behavioural impairments in fibria–fornix-lesioned rats with robust graft innervation of host, and functional improvement in some rats with poor fibre ingrowth. Behaviourally, cholinergic-rich grafts transplanted in the cortex or hippocampus of animal models of Alzheimer's disease induce varying degrees of functional recovery, from robust improve-

Table 2.1 Functional and anatomical impact of grafts in animal models of cholinergic hypofunction

AD animal model	Tissue/graft site	Structural impact	Functional impact
FF lesion/rat	Fetal septal/ hippocampus	Graft AChE-positive fibres innervate host Hippocampal HACU improved	T maze improved/correlated with graft innervation HACU correlates with T and water maze improvements
FF lesion/rat	Fetal hippocampal/ lesion cavity plus ICV NGF infusion	Rescue ChAT-positive cells; AChE fibre re-innervation	Behaviour-dependent theta restored
FF lesion/primate	Fetal BFC/ hippocampus	Graft AChE-positive fibres innervate host	Discrimination learning improved
Cortex lesion/rat	Fetal cortex grafts/ neocortex	Halted retrograde degeneration of host NBM neurons; grafts innervated by host cholinergic neurons	
NBM lesion/rat	Fetal BFC graft/ neocortex	AChE-positive fibre innervation of host cortex	T maze alternation improved
Aged rat	Fetal septal grafts/ hippocampus	AChE-positive fibre innervation	Water maze improvements correlated with graft-derived innervation
Aged rat	Fetal septal grafts/ hippocampus	Formed synaptic connections in dentate gyrus	Behaviour improved
Aged rat	Fetal BFC grafts/NBM	Hypertrophy NBM cholinergic neurons	Water maze improved
FF lesion/rat	NGF cells/lesion cavity	Rescue septal cholinergic neurons; induce host AChE-positive septal sprouting, innervated graft	
FF lesion/rat	NGF cells + collagen/ lesion cavity	Rescue septal cholinergic neurons; Septal axons reinnervate hippocampus	Limited habituation recovery; no water maze impact
FF lesion/rat	ACh cells/hippocampus		Improved water maze
FF lesion/aged primate	NGF cells/ICV	Rescue septal cholinergic neurons; induced host sprouting	
NBM lesion/rat	NGF cells/cavity	Hypertrophy NBM cholinergic neurons; cholinergic fibre innervation neocortex	Partial water maze recovery
NBM lesion/rat	NGF cells + BFC fetal tissue/neocortex	Robust increase in cortical cholinergic cell survival	
NBM lesion/rat	ACh cells/NBM		Water maze improved
Aged rat	NGF cells/NBM	Hypertrophy cholinergic cells	Water maze improved
Aged rat	NGF progenitors/ NBM and/or septum	Rescue cholinergic NBM and/or septal cells	Partial water maze recovery

Notes:
FF, fimbria–fornix; HACU, high-affinity choline uptake; NGF, nerve growth factor; ICV, intracerebral ventricular; BFC, basal forebrain cholinergic system; NBM, nucleus basalis magnocellularis.

A. Grafting of Embryonic Tissue

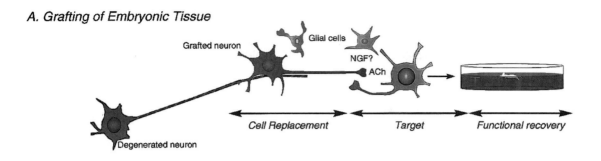

B. Grafting of Genetically Engineered Cells

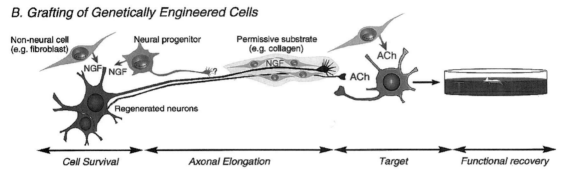

Fig. 2.2 Strategies of intracerebral transplantation for regeneration and functional recovery. A. Fetal grafts comprised of many cell types, including neurons and glial cells, may induce varied functional recovery via reciprocal innervation between graft and host tissue, supply of trophic factors or replacement of depleted neurotransmitters. B. Grafts comprised of genetically engineered cells can be tailored to provide trophic support for cell survival (NGF fibroblasts) and axonal elongation through permissive substrate (NGF cells) leading to target innervation (neuron). Additionally, grafts of ACh-producing fibroblasts can replace lost neurotransmitter to the target. These grafts individually have led to variable functional recovery.

ments to no recovery, or even detrimental effects (Dunnett, 1990; Dunnett and Björklund, 1994; Chen and Gage, 1994; Tarricone et al., 1996). The partial recovery produced by grafts of cholinergic-rich tissue is perhaps not surprising given the fact that most animal models of Alzheimer's disease disrupt a variety of neurotransmitter systems. Indeed, cholinergic fetal grafts are more efficacious in inducing functional recovery in rats with specific lesions of cholinergic projection neurons as opposed to rats with lesions that disrupt multiple systems (e.g. septal or cholinergic neurotoxin lesions versus fimbria-fornix lesion: Chan and Gage, 1994). Moreover, cografts of cholinergic and serotonergic tissue in rats with combined septal and raphe lesions are more effective in inducing functional recovery than septal or raphe grafts alone (Nilsson, Brundin and Björklund, 1990). These results suggest that replacement

of multiple neurotransmitter systems may be required to achieve optimal cognitive recovery in models that disrupt a number of brain transmitter systems.

Because embryonic basal forebrain cholinergic system tissue contains a mixture of cell types, including noncholinergic neuronal and glial cells, factors mediating graft-induced morphological and functional recovery are poorly understood. Such grafts may influence the function of the system in a variety of ways, including graft-induced upregulation of ACh levels, graft release of trophic factors that support surviving host neurons, reciprocated synaptic innervation between graft and host neurons, as well as providing bridging material for sprouting fibres from damaged host neurons (see Fig. 2.2A; Gage and Buzsaki, 1989; Gage and Fisher, 1991). Gene transfer to the central nervous system has been used with increasing frequency to examine the contribution and efficacy of individual factors in regeneration, cell rescue and functional recovery.

Gene transfer

- Gene transfer techniques allow punctate temporal delivery of discrete targeted molecules to the brain.
- In lesioned and aged animal models of basal forebrain cholinergic system degeneration, intracerebral transplantation of cells genetically modified to produce and release nerve growth factor can:
  - (a) mediate basal forebrain cholinergic system cell survival and regeneration of cholinergic axons,
  - (b) induce limited functional recovery.
- Intracerebral grafting of cells genetically engineered to produce and release ACh in basal forebrain cholinergic system lesioned rats is sufficient to mediate cognitive recovery in the absence of regeneration or rescue of the system's circuitry.
- Neural progenitors offer many advantages as cell types to be used for gene transfer and intracerebral grafting.

Gene therapy for neurodegenerative diseases

Gene therapy offers one of the most promising avenues by which to intervene in neural disease processes. Gene transfer techniques involve introducing a new gene (transgene) in cells which then deliver specific molecules in selected brain regions (Fig. 2.2B). This strategy is advantageous because discrete molecules can be delivered in a temporal and punctate manner (Fig. 2.2B). Such flexibility expands the window of opportunity for intervening in disease processes. Thus, gene transfer can be used: (1) prophylactically to protect a target population of neurons that are known to degenerate in certain diseases (such as the GABAergic neurons in Huntington's disease); (2) to halt and/or repair neuronal and fibre damage once a disease is underway; (3) as a vehicle to replace and augment depleted neurotransmitter, once irreparable damage has occurred (Fisher, 1995). There are two primary approaches used to deliver transgenes to the brain. Ex-vivo gene transfer consists of introducing a transgene in cultures of neural or nonneural cells. The genetically

modified cells are then selected and characterized for transgene expression in vitro and finally grafted intracerebrally in animals. In-vivo gene transfer is performed by direct intracerebral injections of chemical and viral transgene carriers. In this case, the endogenous neural cells will incorporate and express the transgene of interest. To date, the majority of studies focusing on repair of the damaged basal forebrain cholinergic system have used ex-vivo gene transfer because the methodology underlying this approach has generally been developed further than in-vivo techniques.

Cell savings and regeneration

In animal models of Alzheimer's disease, infusion of the neurotrophin nerve growth factor is known to rescue basal forebrain cholinergic system neurons, induce axonal regrowth towards appropriate target areas, and reverse age-related cognitive deficits (Hagg et al., 1990; Fischer et al., 1991a). These findings, together with evidence that fetal basal forebrain cholinergic system tissue grafts can induce limited reinnervation of host cholinergic neurons in lesioned animals, have led to the hypothesis that one of the contributing factors of fetal graft-induced improvements is the release and/or stimulation of trophic factors from host tissue (Dunnett and Björklund, 1987; Gage and Fisher, 1991). Indeed, chronic intraventricular infusions of nerve growth-factor can induce anatomical and behavioural recovery that is comparable to that observed following fetal tissue grafts (Barone et al., 1991; Lucidi-Phillipi and Gage, 1993), and augments septal cholinergic cell rescue when combined with fetal grafts (Tuszynski et al., 1990; Tuszynski and Gage, 1995). However, various problems are associated with long-term intracerebral ventricular administration of nerve growth factor. For example, miniosmotic pumps require periodic replenishment of nerve growth factor; and cannulae induce tissue damage and are a focal point of infection. Cells genetically modified to produce and release nerve growth factor offer an alternative strategy to examine the role of this neurotrophin in the rescue and regeneration of lesioned cholinergic neurons, and to explore its therapeutic potential for reversing cognitive deficits produced by damage or age-induced neurodegeneration.

Cell savings

The first step in the regeneration in the central nervous system is the rescue and maintenance of surviving cells. Cells genetically modified to deliver trophic factors have been used in an attempt to rescue basal forebrain cholinergic system degenerating cells (see Fig. 2.2B). Rosenberg et al. (1988) injected nerve growth factor-secreting 208F rat fibroblasts in the lesion cavity and the lateral ventricle of fimbria-fornix-lesioned rats. Two weeks postsurgery, 92 per cent of ChAT-positive septal cells were rescued. In contrast, fibria-fornix-lesioned rats grafted with control cells showed only a 49 per cent survival of cholinergic septal cells. The nerve growth factor grafts also induced robust sprouting of AChE-positive fibres in the septum, with the highest density proximal to the graft (Rosenberg et al., 1988). This sprouting was not observed in control grafted animals (Rosenberg et al., 1988). Similarly, Strömberg and colleagues (1990) reported that nerve growth factor-producing mouse 3T3 fibroblasts grafted into the cavity of fimbria-fornix-lesioned rats rescued 92 per cent of AChE-positive septal cells and induced AChE-positive fibre innervation of the graft from host tissue.

The use of rat 208F and mouse 3T3 fibroblasts for intracerebral grafting can lead to tumour formation. Because safety is a major concern with regard to using engineered cells to treat human neurodegenerative disease, efforts have been made to reduce the risk of tumour formation. The use of polymer encapsulation of immortalized cell lines or grafting of primary cells circumvents the problem of tumour formation. Polymer encapsulation consists of engineered cells embedded in a permeable material which allows delivery of desired products while restricting cellular growth. For example, in animals with fimbria-fornix lesions, encapsulated cells modified to produce nerve growth factor were shown to rescue ChAT-positive cells of the septum without causing tumour formation (Hoffman et al., 1993; Chen and Gage, 1994; Emerich et al., 1994; Schinstine et al., 1995; Winn et al., 1994, 1996). However, most studies of ex-vivo gene transfer and its application for septo-hippocampal regeneration have used primary fibroblasts genetically modified to produce nerve growth factor. Autologous and isologous grafts of primary skin fibroblasts can survive up to 12 months following implantation, maintain a constant volume and express transgenes in vivo (Kawaja et al., 1991; Kawaja and Gage, 1992; Chen and Gage, 1995; Eagle et al., 1995; Tuszynski et al., 1994). Nerve growth-factor-producing primary skin fibroblasts grafted into the septum of fimbria-fornix-lesioned rats have been shown to rescue 75 per cent of nerve growth factor-positive (Kawaja et al., 1992) and 80 per cent of ChAT immunoreactive cells (Lucidi-Phillipi et al., 1995) in the ipsilateral septum. Similarly, primary adult monkey fibroblasts transduced to secrete nerve growth factor and grafted into the medial septum increased cholinergic cell survival by as much as 92 per cent and induced AChE-positive sprouting (Tuszynski et al., 1996). Although grafts of nerve growth factor-producing fibroblasts produce robust savings of septal cholinergic cells, there is no reconstruction of the septo-hippocampal projections. When the engineered cells are grafted in the axotomized septum, the deafferented cells do not generate fibres that traverse the lesion cavity and reinnervate the hippocampus.

Ex-vivo gene transfer of trophic factors has also been used to mediate cell savings in rat nucleus basalis magnocellularis lesion models. Following excitotoxic lesions of the nucleus basalis magnocellularis, nerve growth factor-producing 3T3 cells alone or mixed with fetal basal forebrain cholinergic system tissue were implanted in the denervated frontal and parietal cortices (Ernfors et al., 1989). Four weeks later, cholinergic cortical cell survival was increased five-fold in rats with nerve growth factor-producing 3T3 fibroblasts and ten-fold by the nerve growth factor-producing 3T3 fibroblasts plus fetal basal forebrain tissue transplants. Following unilateral cortical devascularizing lesions, fibroblasts (cell line Rat 1) modified to secrete nerve growth factor were embedded in Gelfoam and placed over the lesioned area (Maysinger et al., 1992; Piccardo et al., 1992). After four weeks, ChAT activity was increased by 38 per cent (Piccardo et al., 1992), and stimulated ACh release in the cortex of lesioned nerve growth factor-grafted was restored to the levels of un-lesioned controls (Maysinger et al., 1992). In the ipsilateral nucleus basalis magnocellularis, 88 per cent of ChAT-positive neurons were rescued (Piccardo et al., 1992) and ChAT activity was not decreased (Maysinger et al., 1992) after grafting of nerve growth-factor-secreting fibroblasts into the lesioned cortex. In addition, the average cross-sectional areas of cholinergic neurons in the nucleus basalis magnocellularis were equivalent between controls and lesioned animals treated with nerve growth factor-producing fibroblasts (Maysinger et al., 1992). Two weeks following excitotoxic lesions of the nucleus basalis magnocellularis in rats, Dekker et al. (1994) grafted primary rat fibroblasts engineered to produce nerve growth factor in the lesioned area. The grafts increased the size of remaining nerve growth factor-receptor (p75) immunoreactive neurons in the nucleus basalis magnocellularis by 25 per cent. Although the transplants did not restore ChAT activity in the dorsal neocortex, ChAT-positive fibre staining was restored to 86 per cent of control values in the ventral neocortex.

Rossner and colleagues (1996) examined the effect of intraventricular grafts of nerve growth factor-secreting cells on basal forebrain cholinergic system neurons after IgG-saporin-induced lesions of nucleus basalis magnocellularis and medial septum/diagonal band of Broca cholinergic neurons in rats. Transplants of nerve growth factor-producing mouse fibroblasts normalized both ChAT and high-affinity choline uptake in the hippocampus and cortex of lesioned rats. Moreover, AChE-positive fibres in both the cerebral cortex and hippocampus were restored to control levels.

In a recent study, cognitively impaired aged rats received bilateral ventricular grafts of baby hamster kidney (BHK) cells genetically modified to produce nerve growth factor (Lindner et al., 1996). Forty days after transplantation, the size of ChAT/p75 nerve growth factor receptor-positive neurons was equivalent to that found in young controls. Similarly, primary fibroblasts genetically modified to produce nerve growth factor and grafted in the nucleus basalis magnocellularis of the aged rat can increase the size and number of nucleus basalis magnocellularis cells immunoreactive for p75 nerve growth factor receptor (Chen and Gage, 1995). Nerve growth factor-mediated rescue of cholinergic septal cells was examined using aged Rhesus monkeys that received unilateral fimbria-fornix lesions and intraventricular transplants of polymer-encapsulated BHK fibroblasts genetically modified to secrete human nerve growth factor (Kordower et al., 1994). Three to four weeks after lesion and transplantation, monkeys that received nerve growth factor-producing grafts displayed only a modest loss of ChAT (0–36 per cent) and p75 nerve growth factor receptor (7–22 per cent) immunoreactivity in the septal neurons compared to animals that received control grafts (immunoreactivity decreased by 57–75 per cent and 53 per cent for ChAT and p75 nerve growth factor receptor, respectively). In addition, a robust sprouting was observed in the septum ipsilateral to nerve growth factor transplant. Similar results are reported by Tuszynski and colleagues (1996). These data demonstrate that human nerve growth factor can provide trophic and tropic influences on cholinergic neurons of the basal forebrain undergoing lesion-induced degeneration in aged nonhuman primates.

Only two studies have used ex-vivo gene transfer to examine the impact of trophic factors, other than nerve growth factor, on basal forebrain cholinergic cell rescue. Brain-derived neurotrophic factor (BDNF), like nerve growth factor, is present in the adult hippocampus and can promote survival of septal cholinergic neurons following lesions of the fimbria–fornix (Knusel et al., 1992; Morse et al., 1993). One study grafted BDNF-producing primary fibroblasts in the rat deafferented septum (Lucidi-Phillipi et al., 1995). Analysis of cholinergic septal cell survival showed that the BDNF-producing grafts failed to protect the ChAT-positive and p75-positive cells from lesion-induced death. Although gene transfer of other trophic factors has not been studied using either the basalocortical or aged animal models of basal forebrain cholinergic system dysfunction, a recent study examined the impact of BDNF on cholinergic neurons in intact rats. Martínez-Serrano, Hantzopoulos and Björklund (1996) grafted BDNF-producing progenitor cells into the nucleus basalis magnocellularis of intact rats. Immunocytochemical analysis four weeks later showed that the BDNF-producing grafts induced a hypertrophic response of ChAT-immunoreactive and p75-nerve growth factor receptor-immunoreactive nucleus basalis magnocellularis cells.

Regeneration of pathways

To examine the efficacy of supplying structural support through which regenerating septo-hippocampal axons may traverse and therefore reinnervate the hippocampus, nerve growth factor-producing primary fibroblasts have been embedded into collagen for grafting (see Fig. 2.2B). Gage and collaborators grafted nerve growth factor-producing primary fibroblasts embedded in collagen into the fimbria-fornix lesion cavity of rats and examined the extent of axonal septo-hippocampal regeneration. Ultrastructural and confocal microscopic examination showed cholinergic axons traversed the grafts and entered the host hippocampus (Kawaja et al., 1992; Eagle et al., 1995). Furthermore, analysis seven months posttransplantation showed a robust reinnervation of the deafferented dentate gyrus by AChE-positive axons. Kawaja and colleagues (1992) also reported several cases in which topographically organized AChE-positive axons formed synaptic contacts in the deafferented dentate gyrus and extended laterally into the CA2-3 fields, in a distribution similar to that found in the normal hippocampal formation. Retrograde labelling analysis indicated that axons that entered the nerve growth factor-producing grafts and entered the denervated hippocampus originated predominantly in the ipsilateral medial septum/diagonal band of Broca (Kawaja et al., 1992). Thus, nerve growth factor-producing cells embedded in collagen bridging material rescue medial septal cells and guide them to reinnervate the deafferented hippocampus. In contrast, administration of nerve growth factor in the absence of bridging material (e.g. intracerebral ventricular nerve growth factor infusions or nerve growth factor-producing suspension grafts) can mediate septal cell survival following axotomy but does not induce host hippocampal reinnervation, whereas fetal grafts can reinnervate the host when proximal to, or within, the hippocampus but do not rescue axotomized septal cells.

The results of several studies indicate that cholinergic nucleus basalis magnocellularis neurons have the capacity to sprout in response to ex-vivo nerve growth factor delivery (Emson and Lindvall, 1986; Kawaja and Gage, 1991; Martinez-Serrano et al., 1995b; Chalmers, Peterson and Gage, 1996). Dekker et al. (1994) have

shown that following bilateral excitotoxic lesions of the nucleus basalis magnocellularis, grafts of nerve growth factor-producing fibroblasts in the lesioned site increased the size of remaining p75-immunoreactive nucleus basalis magnocellularis neurons by 25 per cent. Additionally, ChAT-positive fibre staining was restored to 86 per cent of unoperated control values in the ventral neocortex, compared to the 46 per cent observed in the lesioned-only group (Decker et al., 1994). These findings suggest that nerve growth factor-producing fibroblasts grafted in the lesioned nucleus basalis magnocellularis may induce partial restoration of the basalocortical pathway. However, based on the evidence that the remaining nucleus basalis magnocellularis neurons are hypertrophic, this restoration probably represents sprouting of undamaged nucleus basalis magnocellularis neurons, rather than axonal regeneration, as is observed in the septo-hippocampal lesion model following nerve growth factor-producing grafts.

Nerve growth factor has been shown to induce sprouting in the nonhuman primate. BHK fibroblasts engineered to secrete human nerve growth factor were grafted intraventricularly in aged Rhesus monkeys with unilateral fimbria–fornix lesions (Kordower et al., 1994). The nerve growth factor grafts produced robust sprouting in the ipsilateral septum adjacent to the graft and these fibres extended towards the ependymal lining of the ventricle. Thus, human nerve growth factor can have a tropic influence on basal forebrain cholinergic neurons undergoing degeneration in aged nonhuman primates.

Functional recovery

It is well known that fimbria–fornix lesions produce performance deficits in a variety of behavioural tasks, including spatial water maze, habituation and locomotor activity. Only one study has examined the impact of ex-vivo nerve growth factor gene transfer on the behavioural performance of fimbria–fornix-lesioned rats. Eagle and colleagues (1995) grafted nerve growth factor-producing fibroblasts into the lesioned cavity of fimbria–fornix-lesioned rats. Seven months later, learning and memory performance were tested on spatial water maze and habituation tasks. The habituation task entails placing rats in a novel environment. Initially, the rats show active exploratory behaviour, which decreases over time, reflecting habituation to the new surroundings. During subsequent reintroductions to the same setting, activity levels are typically lower than those during the initial exposure, and are thus used as an index of memory for the environment. Eagle et al. (1995) report that grafts of nerve growth factor-producing fibroblasts embedded in collagen and placed in the fimbria–fornix lesion cavity of rats resulted in significant cholinergic cell savings and axonal regeneration seven months postsurgery. The grafts also induced a limited functional recovery as measured by the simple habituation memory task. Nerve growth factor-grafted rats performed significantly better than either fimbria–fornix lesion only or fimbria–fornix lesion plus control cell grafted groups, but were still significantly worse than unoperated controls. However, the grafts did not impact fimbria–fornix lesion-induced water maze deficits. The performances of both lesion-only and lesion-plus graft groups were equally impaired compared to that of unoperated controls. Thus, the partial hippocampal reinnervation improved performance on a simple memory task, but not on one requiring more complex associative processing.

Several studies have also investigated the cognitive impact of ex-vivo nerve growth factor delivery in the basalocortical lesion model. In a study by Dekker et al. (1994), rats received bilateral excitotoxic nucleus basalis magnocellularis lesions and grafts of nerve growth factor-producing fibroblasts in the lesioned nucleus. Two weeks later, spatial learning and memory were assessed in a water maze task. Compared to unoperated controls, the performance of rats with nucleus basalis magnocellularis lesions alone was significantly impaired on both acquisition and spatial acuity measures. Lesioned rats with nerve growth factor-producing grafts performed significantly better than lesion-only and control cell-grafted rats; however, the recovery was partial. The performance of nerve growth factor-grafted rats was still significantly worse than that of unoperated controls (Decker et al., 1994).

Recently, the functional impact of nerve growth factor-producing cells grafted in the aged brain has been examined. Aged cognitively impaired rats received bilateral ventricular grafts of BHK cells genetically modified to produce nerve growth factor (Lindner et al., 1996). Forty days after transplantation, the water maze performance of the grafted rats did not differ from that of young controls and was significantly better than that of age-impaired rats with control cell grafts. Similar findings are reported by Chen and Gage (1995). Primary fibroblasts genetically modified to produce nerve growth factor and grafted in the nucleus basalis magnocellularis of aged rats reversed age-induced water maze performance deficits (Chen and Gage, 1995).

Interestingly, as is observed using grafts of fetal tissue, nerve growth factor-producing cell lines often produce only a partial recovery of complex cognitive function. Perhaps, grafts that combine trophic factor delivery with neural connectivity may be more efficacious in mediating full functional recovery. Progenitor cells, engineered to produce nerve growth factor, can be used to address this issue.

Use of progenitors for cell savings and functional recovery

The isolation and use of neural precursor cells for transplantation and gene transfer are currently the objects of intense research due to a number of factors. Cells of non-neural origin, such as fibroblasts, do not integrate into the host brain tissue but remain relatively isolated as a tissue mass at the site of implantation, and do not form synapses with host cells. Because neural progenitors have the capacity to migrate, differentiate and integrate into the cellular architecture of the host, they are interesting candidates for ex-vivo gene transfer (see Fig. 2.2B). The efficacy of progenitors to mediate cell rescue has been examined in both fimbria–fornix-lesioned and aged animal models of basal forebrain cholinergic dysfunction. Hippocampus-derived, conditionally immortalized, temperature-sensitive neural progenitor (CINP) cells have been modified to secrete nerve growth factor (Martínez-Serrano, Fischer and Björklund, 1995a). Intraseptal grafts of these nerve growth factor-secreting progenitor cells into fimbria–fornix-lesioned rats have been shown to rescue 93 per cent of cholinergic medial septal cells (Martínez-Serrano et al., 1995b). These cells were also grafted in the nucleus basalis magnocellularis or in the nucleus basalis magnocellularis plus the medial septum/diagonal band of Broca of aged cognitively impaired rats. The CINP–nerve growth factor transplants reversed age-induced atrophy of p75-nerve growth factor receptor-immunopositive neurons in the grafted areas. Behaviourally, placement of the nerve growth factor-producing grafts in either the nucleus basalis magnocellularis or the nucleus basalis magnocellularis plus septum reversed spatial water maze deficits up to one month postgrafting (Martínez-Serrano et al., 1995a).

Neurotransmitter replacement

To date, the only strategies of neurotransmitter replacement in animal models of Alzheimer's disease have used primary fibroblasts genetically modified to produce ACh (see Fig. 2.2B). Primary fibroblasts were transduced with *Drosophila* ChAT and were found to secrete ACh in vitro and in vivo (Fisher et al., 1993b). dChAT-producing fibroblasts have a high-affinity choline uptake system (Fisher, Raymon and Gage, 1993a) that insures the transport of choline, a precursor of ACh, into the fibroblasts. Once in the fibroblasts, choline and acetyl-coenzyme A are converted to ACh by ChAT. In addition, fibroblasts have intrinsic mechanisms for packaging ACh and releasing it in a quantal fashion (Morimoto et al., 1995).

ACh-producing fibroblasts have been implanted into several target regions of the basal forebrain cholinergic system. Results indicate that ACh-producing fibroblasts survive in a well-delineated area in both the hippocampus and the neocortex (Fisher et al., 1993b; Winkler et al., 1995). In both areas, engineered cells have been shown to deliver ACh successfully to the host brain (Fisher et al., 1993b; Winkler et al., 1995) for at least four weeks postgrafting (Winkler et al., 1995). In two different lesion models of cholinergic dysfunction, ACh-producing fibroblasts have successfully reversed learning and memory deficits when implanted into target regions of the damaged basal forebrain cholinergic nuclei. Specifically, neocortical grafts attenuate

deficits produced by excitotoxic lesions of the nucleus basalis magnocellularis (Winkler et al., 1995), and hippocampal grafts ameliorate cognitive impairments produced by lesions of the septo-hippocampal pathway (Dickinson-Anson et al., 1998). These results indicate that augmentation of ACh in the neocortex or hippocampus of basal forebrain cholinergic system-lesioned rats is sufficient to mediate functional recovery in the absence of cell rescue or regeneration of deafferented fibres. Moreover, the finding that ACh-producing fibroblasts had a functional impact in the presence (Winkler et al., 1995) or absence (Dickinson-Anson et al., 1998) of cholinergic circuitry indicates that ACh replacement is efficacious through a range of cholinergic depletions.

In-vivo gene transfer

Only one report examines the potential of in-vivo gene transfer in animal models of basal forebrain cholinergic dysfunction (Castel-Barthe et al., 1996). A replication-defective adenovirus expressing nerve growth factor (Ad-NGF) was injected unilaterally in the nucleus basalis magnocellularis of aged rats. Three weeks postinjection, the Ad-NGF resulted in a 16 per cent increase of ipsilateral nucleus basalis magnocellularis cholinergic (AChE-positive) cell soma relative to the contralateral side. Control injections of Ad-*LacZ* did not produce a similar hypertrophic response in AChE-positive cells. No behavioural testing was reported in this study.

Conclusions

The therapeutic aim of intracerebral transplantation is to halt the neurodegenerative processes, re-establish disrupted circuitries and mediate complete functional recovery. Although these goals are not yet realized in human therapies, the results from animal studies using fetal tissue and gene transfer strategies are quite encouraging. Intracerebral grafting in animal models of neural degeneration has proven to be effective in promoting survival and/or replacing damaged neural cells, promoting axonal growth and extension to re-establish severed pathways, and inducing functional recovery.

Embryonic basal forebrain cholinergic tissue grafts can replace lost neural cells, provide trophic and structural support to damaged host cholinergic neurons, induce reciprocal innervation of host tissue, supplement depleted ACh, and induce some recovery on complex cognitive tasks. Fetal grafts can influence host tissue in a variety of ways but the mechanisms by which grafts exert their functional effects are still unknown. Thus, behavioural recovery may be the result of grafts innervating and re-establishing synaptic contact with the deafferented host and/or due to the grafted cells secreting ACh into depleted host tissue (see Fig. 2.2A).

Genetically modified cells offer an approach to examine the capacity of individual molecules to induce anatomical and/or functional recovery. Because trophic factors promote neuronal survival, nerve growth factor-producing cells have been grafted following basal forebrain cholinergic system damage. Such grafts can rescue degenerating cholinergic neurons, promote axonal elongation and induce various levels of functional recovery. Although such findings suggest that synaptic connectivity and neuronal regulation are important for the functional recovery observed following fetal tissue grafts, findings that cells engineered to produce ACh also induce positive behavioural effects indicate that replacement of depleted ACh is sufficient to induce equivalent levels of behavioural recovery (see Fig. 2.2B).

The functional recovery observed after either fetal tissue or engineered cell grafts is often partial. This is not surprising given the diffuse damage observed in cholinergic degeneration models. A strategy that combines the transplantation of cells that replace lost transmitters and/or establish neural connections with the denervated target may be optimal for the induction of complete and long-lasting functional recovery. One approach is to combine the implantation of a mixture of cells genetically engineered to produce trophic factors, permissive substrates and/or transmitters. For successful regeneration to occur in the central nervous system, not only the availability of trophic factors is required but the presence of a permissive substrate is also crucial for the axons to regrow. Intracerebral grafting of Schwann cells in animal models of cholinergic degeneration has been shown to promote axonal regeneration

(Montero-Menei et al., 1992; Neuberger, Cornbrooks and Kromer, 1992). Recent studies have shown that Schwann cells normally expressing the neurite outgrowth-promoting cell surface molecule L1 (Zhang et al., 1995), as well as genetically modified L1-producing fibroblasts (Kobayashi et al., 1995) and astrocytes (Mohajeri et al., 1996), can encourage central nervous system axons to regrow. Although the precise role of L1 and other axonal growth-promoting molecules in the regeneration of the central cholinergic pathway still needs to be evaluated, these molecules are viable candidates to augment the 'repair' of central nervous system circuitry. Ultimately, cografts may be able to impact degenerative processes on several levels. Trophic factors with survival-promoting effects and permissive factors can support host and fetal neural cells and promote the regrowth of projection fibres, resulting in improved integration and survival of grafted tissue. Tonic and diffuse release of depleted transmitters offers functional support until the reconstruction of damaged neuronal circuits is complete (see Fig. 2.2B). Such transplantation strategies are promising for a range of cognitively debilitating processes from the slow neurodegenerative decline in Alzheimer's disease to acute insults. The goals are the same: to protect surviving neurons; and to replace lost cells and promote the regeneration of injured pathways.

Finally, delivery of neural progenitors genetically modified to produce lost neurotransmitter offers a great deal of potential for the reconstruction of the damaged basal forebrain cholinergic system. Such cells have the capacity to differentiate into neurons and glia, and to migrate and integrate into host architecture. Such attributes suggest that these cells can contribute to the reconstruction of the damaged central nervous system as well as induce immediate amelioration of functional deficits produced by lost transmitter.

Progress over the last 15 years has been dramatic: from the initial hypothesis of cholinergic linkage to cognitive dysfunction, to the demonstration that fetal cholinergic tissue can restore lost function, and finally, to the development of gene transfer methods to prove the importance of cholinergic replacement in functional recovery. In addition, progress continues to be made in the realm of behavioural tasks which more specifically assess age-induced and injury-induced basal forebrain cholinergic dysfunction. For example, Winocur and colleagues have developed a nonspatial learning and memory paradigm which is sensitive to basal forebrain-injured and aged rats (Winocur, 1992). This task dissociates memory deficits produced by prefrontal cortex damage from those produced by hippocampal damage. Importantly, aged rats show deficits consistent with both structures, suggesting that age-induced degeneration of both structures may contribute to the observed cognitive decline. Graft-induced functional recovery on a variety of behavioural tasks which are sensitive to basal forebrain cholinergic dysfunction would strengthen the use of transplantation as a therapeutic technique. Technological advances continue that will clearly provide new strategies for functional and structural repair of the damaged cholinergic system, and new tools to understand the details of the mechanisms by which ACh relates to cognitive performance.

Acknowledgements

The authors would like to thank Dr Lisa J. Fisher and Mary Lynn Gage for critical reading of the manuscript. They gratefully acknowledge the support of the Medical Research Council of Canada (I.A), NIH, NIA.

References

Amaral, D.G. and Kruz, J.M. 1985. An analysis of the origins of the cholinergic and noncholinergic septal projections to the hippocampal formation of the rat. *J Comp Neurol* **281**, 337–61.

Arendt, T., Allen, J., Marchbanks, R.M. et al. 1989. Cholinergic system and memory in the rat: effects of chronic ethanol, embryonic basal forebrain transplants and excitotoxic lesions of the basal forebrain projection system. *Neuroscience* **33**, 435–62.

Armstrong, D.M., Terry, R.D., Deteresa, R.M., Bruce, G., Hersh, L.B. and Gage, F.H. 1987. Response of septal cholinergic neurons to axotomy. *J. Comp Neurol* **264**, 421–36.

Aubert, I., Araujo, D.M., Cécyre, D., Robitaille, Y., Gauthier, S. and Quirion, R. 1992. Comparative alterations of nicotinic and muscarinic binding sites in Alzheimer's and Parkinson's diseases. *J Neurochem* **58**, 529–41.

Aubert, I., Rowe, W., Meaney, M.J., Gauthier, S. and Quirion, R. 1995. Cholinergic markers in aged cognitively impaired Long–Evans rats. *Neuroscience* **67**, 277–92.

Bachevalier, J., Landis, L.S., Walker, L.C. et al. 1991. Aged monkeys exhibit behavioral deficits indicative of widespread cerebral dysfunction. *Neurobiol Aging* **12**, 99–111.

Barone, S. Jr, Tandon, P., McGinty, J.F. and Tilson, H.A. 1991. The effects of NGF and fetal cell transplants on spatial learning after intradentate administration of colchicine. *Exp Neurol* **114**, 351–63.

Bartus, R.T., Dean, R.L. III, Beer, B. and Lippa, A.S. 1982. The cholinergic hypothesis of geriatric memory dysfunction. *Science* **217**, 408–17.

Berger-Sweeney, J.S.H., Mesulam, M.M., Wiley, R.G., Lappi, D.A. and Sharma, M. 1994. Differential effects on spatial navigation of immunotoxin-induced cholinergic lesions of the medial septal area and nucleus basalis magnocellularis. *J Neurosci* **14**, 4507–19.

Brito, L.S. and Brito, G.N. 1990. Locomotor activity and one-way active avoidance after intrahippocampal injection of neurotransmitter antagonist. *Braz J Med Biol Res* **23**, 1015–19.

Castel-Barthe, M.N., Jazat-Poindessous, F., Barneoud, P. et al., 1996. Direct intracerebral nerve growth factor gene transfer using a recombinant adenovirus: effect on basal forebrain cholinergic neurons during ageing. *Neurobiol Dis* **3**, 76–86.

Chalmers, G.R., Peterson, D.A. and Gage, F.H. 1996. Sprouting adult CNS cholinergic axons express NILE and associate with astrocytic surfaces expressing neural cell adhesion molecule. *J Comp Neurol* **371**, 287–99.

Chen, K.S., Buzsaki, G., Benoualid, M. and Gage, F.H. 1989. Fetal cholinergic grafts to the basal forebrain in the aged rat. *Soc Neurosci Abstr* **15**, 1095.

Chen, K.S. and Gage, F.H. 1994. Transplantation, aging, and memory. In *Functional Neural Transplantation*, S.B. Dunnett and A. Björklund, pp. 295–315. New York: Raven Press.

Chen, K.S. and Gage, F.H. 1995. Somatic gene transfer of NGF to the aged brain: behavioral and morphological amelioration. *J Neurosci* **15**, 2819–25.

Connor, D.J., Langlais, P.J. and Thal, L.J. 1991. Behavioral impairments after lesions of the nucleus basalis by ibotenic acid and quisqualic acid. *Brain Res* **555**, 84–90.

Coyle, J.T., Price, D.L. and DeLong, M.R. 1983. Alzheimer's disease: a disorder of cortical cholinergic innervation. *Science* **219**, 1184–90.

Daniloff, J.K., Bodony, R.P., Low, W.C. and Wells, J. 1985. Cross-species embryonic septal transplants: restoration of conditioned learning behavior. *Brain Res* **346**, 176–80.

Davies, P. and Maloney, A.J.F. 1976. Selective loss of central cholinergic neurons in Alzheimer's disease. *Lancet* **2**, 1403.

Davis, R., Raby, C., Callahan, M.J. et al. 1993. Subtype selective muscarinic agonists: potential therapeutic agents for Alzheimer's disease. In *Progress in Brain Research*, Vol. 98, ed. A.C. Cuello, pp. 439–45. Elsevier Science Publishers.

Dawson, G.R., Bayley, P., Channell, S. and Iversen, S.D. 1994. A comparison of the effects of the novel muscarinic receptor agonists L-689,660 and AF102B in tests of reference and working memory. *Psychopharmacology* 113, 361–8.

Decker, M.W. 1987. The effects of ageing on hippocampal and cortical projections of the forebrain cholinergic system. *Brain Res Rev* 12, 423–38.

Decker, M.W. and McGaugh, J.L. 1991. The role of interactions between the cholinergic system and other neuromodulatory systems in learning and memory. *Synapse* 7, 151–68.

Dekker, A., Connor, D.J. and Thal, L.J. 1991. The role of cholinergic projections from the nucleus basalis in memory. *Neurosci and Biobehav Rev* 15, 299–317.

Dekker, A.J., Winkler, J., Ray, J., Thal, L.J. and Gage, F.H. 1994. Grafting of nerve growth factor-producing fibroblasts reduces behavioral deficits in rats with lesions of the nucleus basalis magnocellularis. *Neuroscience* 60, 299–309.

Devan, B.D., Goad, E.H. and Petri, H.L. 1996. Dissociation of hippocampal and striatal contributions to spatial navigation in the water maze. *Neurobiol Learn Mem* 66, 305–23.

Dickinson-Anson, H., Aubert, I., Gage, F.H. and Fisher, L.J. 1998. Hippocampal grafts of acetylcholine-producing cells are sufficient to improve behavioural performance following a unilateral fimbria–fornix lesion. *Neuroscience* 84, 771–81.

Dunnett, S.B. 1990. Neural transplantation in animal models of dementia. *Eur J Neurosci* 2, 567–87.

Dunnett, S.B. and Barth, T.W. 1991. Animal models of dementia (with an emphasis on cortical cholinergic systems). In *Behavioural Models in Psychopharmacology*, ed. P. Willner, pp. 359–418. Cambridge: Cambridge University Press.

Dunnett, S.B. and Björklund, A. 1987. Mechanisms of function of neural grafts in the adult mammalian brain. *J Exp Biol* 132, 265–89.

Dunnett, S.B. and Björklund, A. 1994. Mechanisms of function of neural grafts in the injured brain. In *Functional Neural Transplantation*, ed. S.B. Dunnett and A. Bjorkulund, pp. 531–67. New York: Raven Press.

Dunnett, S.B., Gage, F.H., Björklund, A., Stenevi, U., Low, W.C. and Iversen, S.D. 1984. Hippocampal deafferentation: transplant-derived reinnervation and functional recovery. *Acta Psychiatr Scand* Suppl. 331, 46–56.

Dunnett, S.B., Low, W.C., Iversen, S.D., Stenevi, U. and Björklund, A. 1982. Septal transplants restore maze learning in rats with fimbria-fornix lesions. *Brain Res* 251, 335–48.

Eagle, K.S., Chalmers, G.R., Clary, D.O. and Gage, F.H. 1995. Axonal regeneration and limited functional recovery following hippocampal deafferentation. *J Comp Neurol* 363, 377–88.

Eglen, R.M. and Watson, N. 1996. Selective muscarinic receptor agonists and antagonists. *Pharmacol Toxicol* 78, 59–68.

Emerich, D.F., Winn, S.R., Harper, J., Hammang, J.P., Baetge, E.E. and Kordower, J.H. 1994. Implants of polymer-encapsulated human NGF-secreting cells in the nonhuman primate: rescue and sprouting of degenerating cholinergic basal forebrain neurons. *J Comp Neurol* 349, 148–64.

Emson, P.C. and Lindvall, O. 1986. Neuroanatomical aspects of neurotransmitters affected in Alzheimer's disease. *Br Med Bull* 42, 57–62.

Enfors, P., Ebendal, T., Olson, L., Mouton, P., Strömberg, I. and Persson, H. 1989. A cell line producing recombinant nerve growth factor evokes growth responses in intrinsic and grafted central cholinergic neurons. *Proc Natl Acad Sci USA* 86, 4756–60.

Fine, A., Dunnett, S.B., Björklund, A., Clarke, D. and Iversen, S.D. 1985. Transplantation of embryonic ventral forebrain neurons to the neocortex of rats with lesions of nucleus basalis magnocellularis. I. Biochemical and anatomical observations. *Neuroscience* 16, 769–86.

Fischer, W., Björklund, A., Chen, K. and Gage, F.H. 1991a. NGF improves spatial memory in aged rodents as a function of age. *J Neurosci* 11, 1889–906.

Fischer, W., Chen, K.S., Gage, F.H. and Björklund, A. 1991b. Progressive decline in spatial learning and integrity of forebrain cholinergic neurons in rats during ageing. *Neurobiol Aging* 13, 9–23.

Fischer, W., Gage, F.H. and Björklund, A. 1989. Degenerative changes in forebrain cholinergic nuclei correlate with cognitive impairments in aged rats. *Eur J Neurosci* 1, 34–45.

Fischer, W., Nilsson, O.G. and Björklund, A. 1991c. *In vivo* acetylcholine release as measured by microdialysis is unaltered in the hippocampus of cognitively impaired aged rats with degenerative changes in the basal forebrain. *Brain Res* 556, 44–52.

Fisher, L.J. 1995. Engineered cells: a promising therapeutic approach for neural disease. *Restor Neurol Neurosci* 8, 49–57.

Fisher, L.J. and Gage, F.H. 1993. Grafting in the mammalian central nervous system. *Physiol Rev* 73, 583–616.

Fisher, L.J., Raymon, H.K. and Gage, F.H. 1993a. Cells engineered to produce acetylcholine: therapeutic potential for Alzheimer's disease. *Ann NY Acad Sci* 695, 278–84.

Fisher, L.J., Schinstine, M., Salvaterra, P., Dekker, A.J., Thal, L. and Gage, F.H. 1993b. *In vivo* production and release of acetylcholine from primary fibroblasts genetically modified to express choline acetyltransferase. *J Neurochem* **61**, 1323–32.

Francis, P.T., Sims, N.R., Procter, A.W. and Bowen, D.M. 1993. Cortical pyramidal neurone loss may cause glutamatergic hypoactivity and cognitive impairment in Alzheimer's disease: investigative and therapeutic perspectives. *J Neurochem* **60**, 1589–604.

Frick, K.M., Baxter, M.G., Markowska, A.L., Olton, D.S. and Price, D.L. 1995. Age-related spatial reference and working memory deficits assessed in the water maze. *Neurobiol Aging* **16**, 149–60.

Gage, F.H. and Björklund, A. 1986. Cholinergic septal grafts into the hippocamal formation improve spatial learning and memory in aged rats by an atropine sensitive mechanism. *J Neurosci* **6**, 2837–47.

Gage, F.H. and Buzsaki, G. 1989. CNS grafting: mechanisms of action. In *Neural Regeneration and Transplantation*, ed. F.J. Seil, pp. 211–26. New York: Alan R. Liss.

Gage, F.H., Buzsaki, G., Nilsson, O. and Björklund, A. 1987. Grafts of fetal cholinergic neurons to the deafferented hippocampus. *Prog Brain Res* **71**, 335–47.

Gage, F.H. and Chen, K.S. 1992. Neural transplants: prospects for Alzheimer's disease. *Curr Opin Neurol Neurosurg* **5**, 94–9.

Gage, F.H., Dunnett, S.B. and Björklund, A. 1984. Spatial learning and motor deficits in aged rats. *Neurobiol Aging* **5**, 43–8.

Gage, F.H. and Fisher, L.J. 1991. Intracerebral grafting: a tool for the neurobiologist. *Neuron* **6**, 1–12.

Gage, F.H., Wictorin, K., Fischer, W., Williams, L.R. Varon, S. and Björklund, A. 1986. Retrograde cell changes in medial septum and diagonal band following fimbria-fornix transection: quantitative temporal analysis. *Neuroscience* **19**, 241–55.

Gallagher, M. and Pelleymounter, M.A. 1988. An age-related spatial learning deficit: choline uptake distinguishes 'impaired' and 'unimpaired' rats. *Neurobiol Aging* **9**, 363–9.

Hagg, T., Manthorpe, M., Vahlsing, H.L. and Varon, S. 1990. Nerve growth factor roles for cholinergic axonal regeneration in the adult mammalian central nervous system. *Comments Dev Neurobiol* **1**, 157–75.

Heckers, S., Ohtake, T., Wiley, R.G., Lappi, D.A., Geula, C. and Mesulam, M.M. 1994. Complete and selective cholinergic denervation of rat neocortex and hippocampus but not amygdala by an immunotoxin against the p75 NGF receptor. *J Neurosci* **14**, 1271–89.

Hoffman, D., Breakefield, X.O., Short, M.P. and Aebischer, P. 1993. Transplantation of a polymer-encapsulated cell line genetically engineered to release NGF. *Exp Neurol* **122**, 100–6.

Katzman, R. 1986. Alzheimer's disease. *N Engl J Med* **314**, 964–73.

Kawaja, M.D., Fagan, A.M., Firestein, B.L. and Gage, F.H. 1991. Intracerebral grafting of cultured autologous skin fibroblasts into the rat striatum: an assessment of graft size and ultrastructure. *J Comp Neurol* **307**, 695–706.

Kawaja, M.D. and Gage, F.H. 1991. Reactive astrocytes are substrates for the growth of adult CNS axons in the presence of elevated levels of nerve growth factor. *Neuron* **7**, 1019–30.

Kawaja, M.D. and Gage, F.H. 1992. Morphological and neurochemical features of cultured primary skin fibroblasts of Fischer 344 rats following striatal implantation. *J Comp Neurol* **317**, 102–16.

Kawaja, M.D., Rosenberg, M.B., Yoshida, K. and Gage, F.H. 1992. Somatic gene transfer of nerve growth factor promotes the survival of axotomized septal neurons and the regeneration of their axons in adult rats. *J Neurosci* **12**, 2849–64.

Knusel, B., Beck, K.D., Winslow, J.W. et al. 1992. Brain-derived neurotrophic factor administration protects basal forebrain cholinergic but not nigral dopaminergic neurons from degenerative changes following axotomy in the adult rat brain. *J. Neurosci* **12**, 4391–402.

Kobayashi, S., Miura, M., Asou, H., Inoue, H.K., Ohye, C. and Uyemura, K. 1995. Grafts of genetically modified fibroblasts expressing neural cell adhesion molecule L1 into transected spinal cord of adult rats. *Neurosci Lett* **188**, 191–4.

Kordower, J.H., Winn, S.R., Liu, Y.T. et al. 1994. The aged monkey basal forebrain: rescue and sprouting of axotomized basal forebrain neurons after grafts of encapsulated cells secreting human nerve growth factor. *Proc Natl Acad Sci USA* **91**, 10898–902.

Kromer, L.F., Björklund, A. and Stenevi, U. 1980. Innervation of embryonic hippocampal implants by regenerating axons of cholinergic septal neurons in the adult rat. *Brain Res* **210**, 153–71.

Kromer, L.F., Björklund, A. and Stenevi, U. 1981. Regeneration of the septo-hippocampal pathways in adult rats is promoted by utilizing embryonic hippocampal implants as bridges. *Brain Res* **210**, 173–200.

Leanza, G., Nikkhah, G., Nilsson, O.G., Wiley, R.G. and Björklund, A. 1996. Extensive reinnervation of the hippocampus by embryonic basal forebrain cholinergic neurons grafted into the septum of neonatal rats with selective cholinergic lesions. *J Comp Neurol* **373**, 355–72.

Lescaudron, L., Sutton, R.L. and Stein, D.G. 1993. Effects of fetal forebrain transplants in ibotenic-injured nucleus basalis: an anatomical investigation. *Int J Neurosci* **69**, 97–104.

Levey, A.I. 1996. Muscarinic acetylcholine receptor expression in memory circuits: implications for treatment of Alzheimer disease. *Proc Natl Acad Sci USA* **93**, 13541–6.

Levin, E.D. 1992. Nicotinic systems and cognitive function. *Psychopharmacology* **108**, 417–31.

Li, Y.J., Simon J.R. and Low, W.C. 1992. Intrahippocampal grafts of cholinergic-rich striatal tissue ameliorate spatial memory deficits in rats with fornix lesions. *Brain Res Bull*, **29**, 147–55.

Lindefors, N., Boatell, M.L., Mahy, N. and Persson, H. 1992. Widespread neuronal degeneration after ibotenic acid lesioning of cholinergic neurons in the nucleus basalis revealed by in situ hybridization. *Neurosci Lett* **135**, 262–4.

Lindner, M.D., Kearns, C.E., Winn, S.R., Frydel, B. and Emerich, D.F. 1996. Effects of intraventricular encapsulated hNGF-secreting fibroblasts in aged rats. *Cell Transplant* **5**, 205–23.

Low, W.C., Lewis, P.R., Bunch, S.T. et al. 1982. Function recovery following neural transplantation of embryonic septal nuclei in adult rats with septohippocampal lesions. *Nature* **300**, 260–336.

Lucidi-Phillipi, C.A. and Gage, F.H. 1993. Functions and applications of neurotrophic molecules in the adult central nervous system. *Semin Neurosci* **5**, 269–77.

Lucidi-Phillipi, C.A., Gage, F.H., Shults, C.W., Jones, K.R., Reichardt, L.F. and Kang, U.J. 1995. Brain-derived neurotrophic factor-transduced fibroblasts: production of BDNF and effects of grafting to the adult rat brain. *J Comp Neurol* **354**, 361–76.

Mallet, P.E., Beninger, R.J., Flesher, S.N., Jhamandas, K. and Boegman, R.J. 1995. Nucleus basalis lesions: implication of basoamygdaloid cholinergic pathways in memory. *Brain Res Bull* **36**, 51–6.

Martínez-Serrano, A., Fischer, W. and Björklund, A. 1995a. Reversal of age-dependent cognitive impairments and cholinergic neuron atrophy by NGF-secreting neural progenitors grafted to the basal forebrain. *Neuron* **15**, 473–84.

Martínez-Serrano, A., Hantzopoulos, P.A. and Björklund, A. 1996. Ex vivo gene transfer of brain-derived neurotrophic factor to the intact rat forebrain: neurotrophic effects on cholinergic neurons. *Eur J Neurosci* **8**, 727–35.

Martínez-Serrano, A., Lundberg, C., Horellou, P. et al. 1995b. CNS-derived neural progenitor cells for gene transfer of nerve growth factor to the adult rat brain: complete rescue of axotomized cholinergic neurons after transplantation into the septum. *J Neurosci* **15**, 5668–80.

Mash, D.C., Flynn, D.D. and Potter, L.T. 1985. Loss of M2 muscarine receptors in the cerebral cortex in Alzheimer's disease and experimental cholinergic denervation. *Science* **228**, 1115–17.

Maysinger, D., Piccardo, P., Goiny, M. and Cuello, A.C. 1992. Grafting of genetically modified cells: effects of acetylcholine release in vivo. *Neurochem Int* **21**, 543–8.

Mesulam, M.M., Mufson, E.J., Levey, A.I. and Wainer, B.H. 1983. Cholinergic innervation of cortex by the basal forebrain: cytochemistry and cortical connections of the septal area, diagonal band nuclei, nucleus basalis (substantia innominata), and hypothalamus in the rhesus monkey. *J Comp Neurol* **214**, 170–97.

Mohajeri, M.H., Bartsch, U., van der Putten, H., Sansig, G., Mucke, L. and Schachner, M. 1996. Neurite outgrowth on non-permissive substrates in vitro is enhanced by ectopic expression of the neural adhesion molecule L1 by mouse astrocytes. *Eur J Neurosci* **8**, 1085–97.

Montero-Menei, C.N., Pouplard-Barthelaix, A., Gumpel, M. and Baron-Van Evercooren, A. 1992. Pure Schwann cell suspension grafts promote regeneration of the lesioned septo-hippocampal cholinergic pathway. *Brain Res* **570**, 198–208.

Morimoto, T., Popov, S., Buckley, K.M. and Poo, M.M. 1995. Calcium-dependent transmitter secretion from fibroblasts: modulation by synaptotagmin I. *Neuron* **15**, 689–96.

Morse, J.K., Wiegand, S.J., Anderson, K. et al. 1993. Brain-derived neurotrophic factor (BDNF) prevents the degeneration of medial septal cholinergic neurons following fimbria transection. *J Neurosci* **13**, 4146–56.

Neuberger, T.J., Cornbrooks, C.J. and Kromer, L.F. 1992. Effects of delayed transplantation of cultured Schwann cells on axonal regeneration from central nervous system cholinergic neurons. *J Comp Neurol* **315**, 16–33.

Nilsson, L., Adem, A., Hardy, J., Winblad, B. and Nordberg, A. 1987. Do tetrahydroaminoacridine (THA) and physostigmine restore acetylcholine release in Alzheimer brains via nicotinic receptors? *J Neural Transm* **70**, 357–68.

Nilsson, O.G., Brundin, P. and Björklund, A. 1990. Amelioration of spatial memory impairment by intrahippocampal grafts of mixed septal and raphe tissue in rats with combined cholinergic and serotonergic denervation of the forebrain. *Brain Res* **515**, 193–206.

Nilsson, O.G. and Gage, F.H. 1993. Anticholinergic sensitivity in the ageing rat septo-hippocampal system as assessed in a spatial memory task. *Neurobiol Aging* **14**, 487–97.

Nilsson, O.G., Shapiro, M.L., Gage, F.H., Olton, D.S. and Björklund, A. 1987. Spatial learning and memory following fimbria-fornix transection and grafting of fetal septal neurons to the hippocampus. *Exp Brain Res* **67**, 195–215.

Olton, D.S., Walker, J.A. and Gage, F.H. 1978. Hippocampal connections and spatial discrimination. *Brain Res* **139**, 295–308.

Perry, E.K. 1986. The cholinergic hypothesis – ten years on. *Br Med Bull* **42**, 63–9.

Piccardo, P., Maysinger, D. and Cuello, A.D. 1992. Recovery of nucleus basalis cholinergic neurons by grafting NGF secretor fibroblasts. *Neuroreport* **3**, 353–6.

Presty, S.K., Bachevalier, J., Walker, L.C. et al. 1987. Age differences in recognition memory of the rhesus monkey (*Macaca mulatta*). *Neurobiol Aging* **8**, 435–40.

Quirion, R. 1993. Cholinergic markers in Alzheimer's disease and the autoregulation of acetylcholine release. *J Psychiatry Neurosci*, **18**, 226–34.

Quirion, R., Wilson, A., Rowe, W. et al. 1995. Facilitation of acetylcholine release and cognitive performance by an M2-muscarinic receptor antagonist in aged memory-impaired rats. *J Neurosci* **15**, 1455–62.

Rapp, P.R. and Amaral, D.G. 1991. Recognition memory deficits in a sub-population of aged monkeys resemble the effects of medial temporal lobe damage. *Neurobiol Aging* **12**, 481–6.

Rapp, P.R., Rosenberg, R.A. and Gallagher, M. 1987. An evaluation of spatial information processing in aged rats. *Behav Neurosci* **101**, 3–12.

Reinikainen, K.J., Soininen, H. and Riekkinen, P.J. 1990. Neurotransmitter changes in Alzheimer's disease: implications to diagnostics and therapy. *J Neurosci Res* **27**, 576–86.

Ridley, R.M., Gribble, S., Clark, B., Baker, H.F. and Fine, A. 1992. Restoration of learning ability in fornix-transected monkeys after fetal basal forebrain but not fetal hippocampal tissue transplantation. *Neuroscience* **48**, 779–92.

Ridley, R.M., Thornley, H.D., Baker, H.F. and Fine, A. 1991. Cholinergic neural transplants into the hippocampus restore learning ability in monkeys with fornix transections. *Exp Brain Res* **83**, 533–8.

Rosenberg, M.B., Friedmann, T., Robertson, R.C. et al. 1988. Grafting genetically modified cells to the damaged brain: restorative effects of NGF expression. *Science* **242**, 1575–8.

Rossner, S., Schliebs, R. and Bigl, V. 1994. Ibotenic acid lesion of nucleus basalis magnocellularis differentially affects cholinergic, glutamatergic and GABAergic markers in cortical rat brain regions. *Brain Res* **668**, 85–99.

Rossner, S., Yu, J., Pizzo, D. et al. 1996. Effects of intraventricular transplantation of NGF-secreting cells on cholinergic basal forebrain neurons after partial immunolesion. *J Neurosci Res* **45**, 40–56.

Rossor, M. and Iversen, L.L. 1986. Non-cholinergic neurotransmitter abnormalities in Alzheimer's disease. *Br Med Bull* **42**, 70–4.

Rylett, R.J., Ball, M.J. and Colhoun, E.H. 1983. Evidence for high affinity choline transport in synaptosomes prepared from hippocampus and neocortex of patients with Alzheimer's disease. *Brain Res* **289**, 169–75.

Saper, C.B. 1984. Organization of cerebral cortical afferent systems in the rat: I. Magnocellular basal nucleus. *J Comp Neurol* **222**, 313–42.

Schinstine, M., Fiore, D.M., Winn, S.R. and Emerich, D.F. 1995. Polymer-encapsulated Schwannoma cells expressing human nerve growth factor promote the survival of cholinergic neurons after a fimbria-fornix transection. *Cell Transplant* **4**, 93–102.

Segal, M., Stenevi, U. and Björklund, A. 1981. Reformation in adult rats of functional septo-hippocampal connections by septal neurons regenerating across an embryonic hippocampal tissue bridge. *Neurosci Lett*, **27**, 7–12.

Sinden, J.D., Gray, J.A. and Hodges, H. 1994. Cholinergic grafts and cognitive function. In *Functional Neural Transplantation*, ed. S.B. Dunnett and A. Björklund, pp. 253–93. New York: Raven Press.

Smith, G. 1988. Animal models of Alzheimer's disease: experimental cholinergic denervation. *Brain Res Rev* **13**, 103–18.

Socci, D.J., Sanberg, P.R. and Arendash, G.W. 1995. Nicotine enhances Morris water maze performance of young and aged rats. *Neurobiol Aging* **16**, 857–60.

Sofroniew, M.U., Isacson, O. and Björklund, A. 1986. Cortical grafts prevent atrophy of cholinergic basal nucleus neurons induced by excitotoxic cortical damage. *Brain Res* **378**, 409–15.

Storm-Mathisen, J. 1974. Choline acetyltransferase and acetylcholinesterase in fascia dentata following lesions of the entorhinal afferent. *J Brain Res* **80**, 119–81.

Ströessner-Johnson, H.M., Rapp, P.R. and Amaral, D.G. 1992. Cholinergic cell loss and hypertrophy in the medial septal nucleus of the behaviorally characterized aged rhesus monkey. *J Neurosci* **12**, 1936–44.

Strömberg, I., Wetmore, C.J., Ebendal, T., Ernfors, P., Persson, H. and Olson, L. 1990. Rescue of basal forebrain cholinergic neurons after implantation of genetically modified cells producing recombinant NGF. *J Neurosci Res* **25**, 405–11.

Sunderland, T., Tariot, P., Murphy, D.L., Weingartner, H., Mueller, E.A. and Cohen, R.N. 1985. Scopolamine challenges in Alzheimer disease. *Psychopharmacology* **87**, 247–9.

Tarricone, B.J., Keim, S.R., Simon, J.R. and Low, W.C. 1991. Intrahippocampal transplants of septal cholinergic neurons: high affinity choline uptake and spatial memory function. *Brain Res* **548**, 55–62.

Tarricone, B.J., Simon, J.R., Li, Y.J. and Low, W.C. 1996. Neural grafting of cholinergic neurons in the hippocampal formation. *Behav Brain Res* **74**, 25–44.

Tarricone, B.J., Simon, J.R. and Low, W.C. 1993. Intrahippocampal transplants of septal cholinergic neurons: choline acetyltransferase activity, muscarinic receptor binding and spatial memory function. *Brain Res* **632**, 41–7.

Torres, E.M., Perry, T.A., Blokland, A. et al. 1994. Behavioural, histochemical and biochemical consequences of selective immunolesions in discrete regions of the basal forebrain cholinergic system. *Neuroscience* **63**, 95–122.

Tuszynski, M.H., Buzsaki, G. and Gage, F.H. 1990. Nerve growth factor infusions combined with fetal hippocampal grafts enhance reconstruction of the lesioned septo-hippocampal projection. *Neuroscience* **36**, 33–44.

Tuszynski, M.H. and Gage, F.H. 1995. Bridging grafts and transient nerve growth factor infusions promote long-term central nervous system neuronal rescue and partial functional recovery. *Proc Natl Acad Sci USA* **92**, 4621–5.

Tuszynski, M.H., Peterson, D.A., Ray, J., Baird, A., Nakahara, Y. and Gage, F.H. 1994. Fibroblasts genetically modified to produce nerve growth factor induce robust neuritic ingrowth after grafting to the spinal cord. *Exp Neurol* **126**, 1–14.

Tuszynski, M.H., Roberts, J., Senut, M-C., U, H-S. and Gage, F.H. 1996. Gene therapy in the adult primate brain: intraparenchymal grafts of cells genetically modified to produce nerve growth factor prevent cholinergic neuronal degeneration. *Gene Ther* **3**, 305–14.

Vidal, C. 1996. Nicotinic receptors in the brain. *Mol Biol Funct Ther* **28**, 3–11.

Wainer, B.H., Steininger, T.L., Roback, J.D., Burke-Watson, M.A., Mufson, E.J. and Kordower, J. 1993. Ascending cholinergic pathways: functional organization and implications for disease models. *Prog Brain Res* **98**, 9–30.

Waite, J.J., Chen, A.D., Wardlow, M.L., Wiley, R.G., Lappi, A.D. and Thal, L.J. 1995. 192 immunoglobulin G-saporin produces graded behavioral and biochemical changes accompanying the loss of cholinergic neurons of the basal forebrain and cerebellar Purkinje cells. *Neuroscience* **65**, 463–76.

Welner, S.A., Dunnett, S.B., Salamone, J.D., Maclean, B. and Iverson, S.D. 1988. Transplantation of embryonic ventral forebrain grafts to the neocortex of rats with bilateral lesions of nucleus basalis magnocellularis ameliorates a lesion-induced deficit in spatial memory. *Brain Res* **463**, 192–7.

Wiley, R.G. 1992. Neural lesioning with ribosome-inactivating proteins: suicide transport and immunolesioning. *Trends Neurosci* **15**, 285–90.

Winkler, J., Suhr, S.T., Gage, F.H., Thal, L.J. and Fisher, L.J. 1995. Essential role of neocortical acetylcholine in spatial memory [see comments]. *Nature* **375**, 484–7.

Winkler, J. and Thal, L.J. 1995. Effects of nerve growth factor treatment on rats with lesions of the nucleus basalis magnocellularis produced by ibotenic acid, quisqualic acid, and AMPA. *Exp Neurol* **136**, 234–50.

Winn, S.R., Hammang, J.P., Emerich, D.F., Lee, A., Palmiter, R.D. and Baetge, E.E. 1994. Polymer-encapsulated cells genetically modified to secrete human nerve growth factor promote the survival of axotomized septal cholinergic neurons. *Proc Natl Acad Sci USA* **91**, 2324–8.

Winn, S.R., Lindner, M.D., Lee, A., Haggett, G., Francis, J.M. and Emerich, D.F. 1996. Polymer-encapsulated genetically modified cells continue to secrete human nerve growth factor for over one year in rat ventricles: behavioral and anatomical consequences. *Exp Neurol* **140**, 126–38.

Winocur, G. 1992. A comparison of normal old rats and young adult rats with lesions to the hippocampus or prefrontal cortex on a test of matching-to-sample. *Neuropsychologia* **30**, 769–81.

Zhang, Y., Campbell, G., Anderson, P.N., Martini, R., Schachner, M. and Lieberman, A.R. 1995. Molecular basis of interactions between regenerating adult rat thalamic axons and Schwann cells in peripheral nerve grafts I. Neural cell adhesion molecules. *J Comp Neurol* **361**, 193–209.

3

The use of neuroimaging in neurorehabilitative research

Cheryl L. Grady and Shitij Kapur

Introduction

The fact that some functions may recover after brain injury while others do not is well known, and has been studied for many years (e.g. Twitchell, 1951; Stein, Rosen and Butters, 1974). For example, in the early 1940s Kennard carried out a series of experiments examining recovery of motor function after lesions in monkeys of various ages (e.g. Kennard, 1942). Shortly thereafter, Twitchell (1951) reported on a large series of hemiplegic patients and documented the stages and extent of their recovery. A much later study documented the time course of recovery of both motor and speech function and found that most recovery occurs in the first three months after the stroke (Skilbeck et al., 1983), although some recovery can be found up to several years after the insult (Katz et al., 1966). Although both Twitchell (1951) and Skilbeck et al. (1983) documented a series of steps that occur during recovery in which low-level functions return before more complex functions, the brain mechanisms that underlie this recovery of function are as yet unknown.

With the application of functional neuroimaging techniques to this problem, one can begin to measure in vivo the specific changes occurring in the brain that accompany the re-emergence of previously lost abilities, at least at a macroscopic level. In addition, the ability to measure activity in multiple brain areas facilitates the assessment of recovery in the context of brain networks. In recent years, neuroscientists have increasingly moved beyond the strict localizationist approach to brain function and have begun to think of both sensorimotor and cognitive processing as the product of activity in functional networks (McIntosh and Gonzalez-Lima, 1994; Bressler, 1995; Vaadia et al., 1995). This system-level approach has allowed researchers to examine the interactions among brain areas during specific types of cognitive or motor function and how these interactions change as behaviour changes. In the context of this network-based analysis, recovery of function after brain damage could take several forms. One possibility would be a reorganization or reweighting of functional interactions within an existing network of brain regions. An example of this might be increased utilization of the supplementary motor area or some other motor-related brain region after damage to primary motor cortex. A second possibility would be recruitment of new areas into the network or use of an alternate network not normally used for task performance. This type of alteration in brain function would imply that the task is being carried out differently compared to the way it was done prior to the injury, perhaps through the use of new strategies. A third potential mechanism for recovery of function is plasticity in regions of cortex surrounding the damaged area, e.g. a change in sensorimotor field representation, that would result in these areas taking over the functions previously represented in the damaged area.

All three of these potential mechanisms for recovery have been demonstrated in humans or nonhuman primates. The purposes of this chapter are to review the evidence for plasticity of brain areas and networks after damage, presenting evidence primarily from neuroimaging studies, and to discuss the relevance of this work to rehabilitation. The use of this kind of information in the design and monitoring of rehabilitation programmes is also addressed.

Reorganization within an existing network and/or recruitment of new networks

- Neuroimaging has shown changes in the brain after recovery from stroke that suggest a reorganization of function to compensate for damaged areas.
- Recovery seems to depend in part on increased participation of related functional systems in the undamaged hemisphere after unilateral stroke.
- Ageing can be used as a model to study functional reorganization and compensation.

One example of reorganization of activity within a known network of brain regions has been reported in a monkey lesion experiment. Recordings of electrical activity in the supplementary motor area have shown increased activity in this region just prior to a monkey's performance of a learned motor movement (i.e. anticipatory activity; Tanji, Okano and Sato, 1987). When the monkey underwent 12 months of practice on this task, thus becoming overtrained, there was no longer any increased activity in the supplementary motor area prior to the learned movements (Aizawa et al., 1991). At this point, a lesion to the primary motor region was made and activity in the supplementary motor area was again recorded. After the lesion, markedly increased activity was seen in the supplementary motor area prior to the learned movement, marking the return of the anticipatory response. This finding was interpreted as a reorganization of activity within the cortical motor network in response to the lesion, which served to compensate for the loss of one of the nodes in the network. That is, removal of primary motor cortex resulted in a modification of the role played by the supplementary motor area in the motor network responsible for task completion. Given the role attributed to the supplementary motor area in the planning and coordination of motor behaviours (Tanji and Kelsetsu, 1994), this result suggests that this reorganization reflects a greater need for these functions after damage to the motor cortex.

Similar results have been found in humans with strokes to different parts of the motor system who later showed motor recovery. In the first such experiment (Chollet et al., 1991), a group of patients with unilateral infarcts was studied, most of whom had subcortical infarcts in the middle cerebral artery territory. The patients were scanned using positron emission tomography (PET) to measure cerebral blood flow while they were engaged in sequential finger-to-thumb opposition with their unaffected hand and with the recovered hand. During movement of the unaffected hand, cerebral blood flow activation was found in the motor areas of the contralateral hemisphere, i.e. in sensorimotor and premotor cortex, putamen and insula, and in the ipsilateral cerebellum. Bilateral activation was seen in supplementary motor cortex and inferior parietal cortex. In contrast, when subjects moved the hand that had recovered from paralysis, bilateral activation was seen in all of these regions, with the exception of the putamen, which was not significantly activated in either hemisphere. The results of this study showed that recovery of motor function was associated with increased utilization of ipsilateral motor pathways, presumably to compensate for dysfunction of the contralateral pathway that is normally used. Although the finding suggested that there was increased synaptic efficiency of these ipsilateral pathways or increased input into these pathways, the mechanism for this alteration remains unknown.

In a later experiment, Weiller and colleagues (1992) studied reorganization in patients with left hemisphere lesions limited to the striatum or internal capsule to avoid any artifacts caused by direct cortical damage per se. Patients were scanned at least three months after the stroke, and all were able to perform a finger opposition task at a rate of three oppositions every two seconds. A control group was also scanned to examine the possibility that cerebral blood flow activation during movement of the unaffected hand in the stroke patients might also be altered. Blood flow at rest was lower in the patient group in a number of cortical regions ipsilateral to the lesion that did not appear to be infarcted, including prefrontal, sensorimotor and insular cortices. During finger opposition, control subjects had increased cerebral blood flow in the contralateral primary sensorimotor cortex, striatum and insula, ipsilateral cerebellum, and bilateral premotor, supplementary motor and inferior parietal cortices. When patients moved their recovered (right) hand, greater cerebral blood flow activation was seen, compared to control subjects, in bilateral premotor, prefrontal, insular and inferior parietal cortices, contralateral cerebellum and anterior cingulate. Even when patients moved their unaffected (left) hand, they showed greater activity in contralateral premotor, insular and prefrontal cortices, bilateral parietal cortices, and anterior cingulate. For the present purposes, there are three important findings in this experiment. First, the study confirmed the earlier report that recovery of motor function after damage to one part of the motor network can be accomplished by increased use of other regions within the network, such as ipsilateral premotor cortex, again suggesting a reorganization of the motor network to compensate for damage. Second, the results showed that other areas, not directly related to the motor system, such as prefrontal and cingulate cortices, were recruited during motor behaviour. These areas are thought to be related to attentional processing (Mesulam, 1981; Posner and Dehaene, 1994), and their recruitment may reflect the increased need for other processes, such as attention, in carrying out this task, which has been rendered more difficult due to the stroke. Third, this experiment also showed that contralateral cerebral blood flow activity during motor function of the unaffected hand was also altered in the patients. This 'hyperactivity' might be due to a functional disinhibition of contralateral motor-related regions due to the stroke or to other remote effects of the lesion, and indicates that the motor network is altered in a general way and not just when attempting movements directly affected by the lesion. Thus, even though the behaviour is quantitatively the same in patients and controls, the means by which the patients perform the behaviour is quite different and utilizes different brain areas.

Reorganization within the language network also has been found with PET (Weiller et al., 1995) in patients after recovery from aphasia due to damage to the left posterior perisylvian region (Wernicke's area). These patients, as well as control subjects, were studied while engaged in two tasks, generating verbs that corresponded to presented nouns and repeating pronounce-

able pseudowords. Controls were found to have activity primarily in the left hemisphere areas known to be important for language (Petersen et al., 1989; Demonet et al., 1992; Bookheimer et al., 1995), i.e. left posterior temporal cortex in both tasks and left inferior prefrontal cortex, including Broca's area, during the verb generation task. There was some activity in homologous right hemisphere areas in the controls, but this was much less than the activation seen in the left hemisphere. The patients were lacking activation in the left posterior region due to their strokes, but had increased activation in left inferior prefrontal cortex during repetition and greater activity than controls in right hemisphere areas, both anterior and posterior, during both tasks. This result suggests that recovery of language function after posterior left hemisphere lesions is made possible by changes within the left anterior portion of the language network as well as recruitment of homologous right hemisphere regions that play only rudimentary roles during normal language function. There was no activation of any area outside the normal language network, indicating that a reweighting of interactions among the remaining nodes in the network was responsible for the recovered function. This result was not surprising, given that we have known for some time that the right hemisphere is capable of mediating language development in children with left hemisphere lesions (Milner, 1973), yet it indicates that a qualitatively similar plasticity also exists in the adult brain. Interestingly, increased activity in right hemisphere language areas during language tasks has also been reported in stutterers (Braun and Ludlow, 1995; Kroll et al., 1998), raising the possibility that this finding represents a reorganization due to left hemisphere dysfunction in this disorder.

Another interesting example was reported by Buckner et al. (1996) of a single patient with a left inferior frontal infarct who had deficits in some aspect of speech production, with others preserved. A word-stem completion task was found on which the patient performed well, and the patient underwent a series of PET scans while performing this task. A control group of subjects was also scanned and found to have increased blood flow in the area of left inferior prefrontal cortex that was damaged in the patient. In contrast, the patient showed activation of the homologous region of right

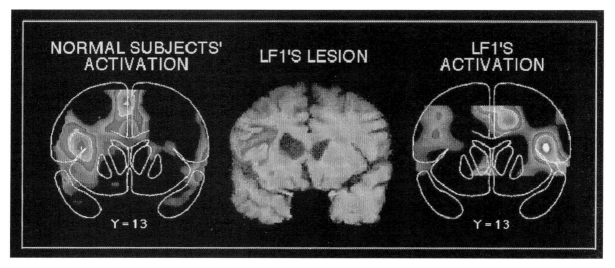

Fig. 3.1 Positron emission tomography data from Buckner et al. (1996) showing cerebral blood flow activation during a semantic retrieval task in normal subjects and in a patient with a left frontal lesion (LF1). Activation is displayed on coronal schematics of the brain where the left hemisphere is shown on the left side of the images. Increased cerebral blood flow in normals is seen in left prefrontal cortex, whereas in patient LF1, activation is found in right prefrontal cortex. The centre image is a coronal slice from the patient's magnetic resonance imaging scan showing the location of the lesion.

prefrontal cortex (Fig. 3.1). Although the authors interpreted this as recruitment of a new region into the language network because normal subjects showed no increase in flow in this area during the word-stem completion task, the above experiment by Weiller et al. showed that normal subjects can have activity in this area in some language tasks. The best interpretation of this finding may be a reorganization within the language network, rather than recruitment of a new area, but only direct examination of this network in both hemispheres will determine between these alternatives.

A final example of bilateral representation of function after recovery from stroke can be found in a case study reported by Engelien et al. (1995) of a patient with bilateral perisylvian strokes. This patient had complete destruction of auditory cortex in the left hemisphere and partial destruction of this area in the right hemisphere. Initially, the patient had a profound auditory agnosia and was unable to recognize either speech or environmental sounds. Eight years after the insult, the patient recovered much of his ability to recognize environmental sounds, but was still markedly impaired in

speech recognition. The patient and a group of control subjects underwent a series of PET scans during passive listening to sounds and during a categorization task. During the categorization task a variety of sounds was presented and the subjects had to indicate to which category the sound belonged, e.g. an animal vocalization vs. a musical instrument. The patient was able to perform this task at near-normal levels at the time of the scan (80 per cent). Controls showed increased cerebral blood flow during passive listening to sounds in bilateral auditory cortex and right inferior parietal cortex. The patient had activation of spared auditory cortex in the right hemisphere and bilateral inferior parietal cortex during passive listening. During the categorization task, compared to passive listening, controls had increased activity only in left hemisphere regions, primarily in prefrontal and temporoparietal cortices, a result that has been reported previously in subjects performing semantic processing of visual information (Tulving et al., 1994; Grady, 1999). The patient, in contrast, showed bilateral activation of these regions. This finding after partial recovery from auditory agnosia is

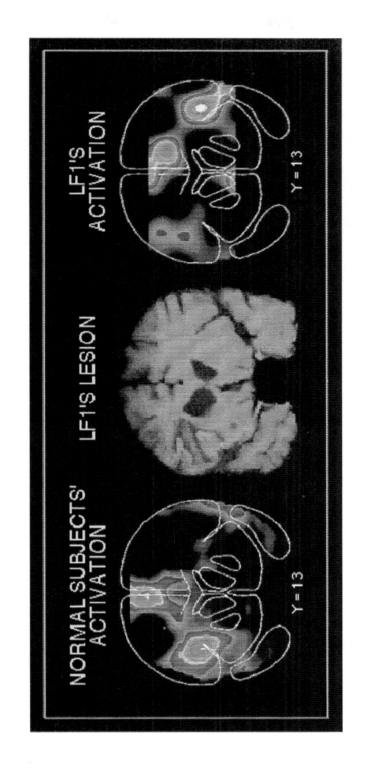

quite similar to those that were reported after recovery from strokes to motor and language areas, discussed above, and suggests a recruitment of right hemisphere areas to accomplish a task that in controls is carried out primarily by the left hemisphere. In this case, however, the effect of increased task difficulty in the patient must also be considered because his categorization performance was not entirely normal, and there is other evidence of right frontal lobe recruitment when task difficulty increases (Grady et al., 1996).

The only other disorder to be examined for brain changes after recovery from stroke is unilateral neglect. Perani and colleagues (1993) carried out a resting metabolic PET scan on a patient with a stroke to the right basal ganglia and a subsequent unilateral neglect. The patient was rescanned eight months later, after complete recovery from neglect. The first scan showed reduced metabolism in both hemispheres, with a greater deficit in the right hemisphere. The second scan showed almost complete return to normal metabolic values in the left hemisphere, but right hemisphere values remained lower in some areas, particularly in the frontal lobes. This finding suggested that recovery of neglect might depend on the resumption of normal metabolic function in the undamaged hemisphere, similar to the results reviewed above in patients who recovered from motor or language deficits. Another study was reported by Pantano et al. (1992), who examined patients with visual neglect of left hemispace as a result of right hemisphere strokes that included cortical areas in some patients. This study also demonstrated that changes could be seen in the brain as a result of a specific rehabilitation programme. Patients were studied before and after participation in a training programme involving visual scanning, reading, copying drawings and verbal description of pictures. During the scans, both before and after treatment, the patients were performing a visual scanning task. After treatment there were increases of cerebral blood flow in left anterior and right posterior portions of the brain, but only the left anterior increase was correlated with improvements in an index of neglect severity. This left anterior increase, attributed to increased activity of the frontal eye field, may represent compensatory reweighting of activity in the eye movement network following the

rehabilitation training, thus facilitating exploration of the previously neglected part of space.

In addition to the study of stroke patients, a useful model for examining reorganizational changes in the brain is to study the phenomenon in older, healthy subjects. Older individuals undergo various changes in the structure and function of the brain as a consequence of normal ageing, including cell loss and dendritic changes (Kemper, 1984; Creasey and Rapoport, 1985; Masliah et al., 1993), although some investigators believe that age-related cell loss is not as widespread as originally thought (Peters et al., 1994). Some cognitive functions are accordingly diminished with age (Bayles, Tomoeda and Boone, 1985; McCrae, Arenberg and Costa, 1987; Craik, Morris and Gick, 1990), but many remain unaffected (Borod, Goodlgass and Kaplan, 1980; LaBarge, Edwards and Knesevich, 1986; Nebes, Boller and Holland, 1986). This phenomenon provides an opportunity to study functional reorganization in the brain as it occurs in response to these gradual age-related changes. Although there have been very few studies that have examined cerebral blood flow during cognitive tasks in older subjects, these examples provide evidence for situations in which old subjects show functional reorganization as well as for situations in which they do not. The first evidence that functional reorganization can take place in the aged brain was demonstrated in a study of visual perception (Grady et al., 1994). This experiment was designed to demonstrate in humans the ventral and dorsal visual processing streams that had been identified in the monkey (Ungerleider and Mishkin, 1982; Desimone and Ungerleider, 1989). Subjects underwent PET scans while engaged in face matching, a task involving the ventral object recognition stream, and spatial location matching, which utilizes the dorsal spatial processing stream. In that study, both young and old subjects showed activation of occipital and inferior temporal regions, i.e. the ventral visual processing stream, during the face-matching task, and dorsal occipital and parietal areas during location matching. However, during both tasks, the old subjects also had activation in areas in which young subjects did not, including areas in prefrontal cortex. An analysis of the functional interactions among ventral stream regions during face matching

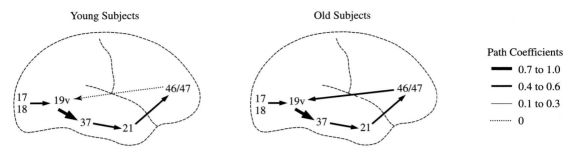

Fig. 3.2 Cortical networks for face perception in young and old subjects (from McIntosh et al., 1994, and Horwitz et al., 1995). Both groups show strong functional interactions among the ventral stream regions, i.e. striate, extrastriate, inferior temporal and inferior frontal. However, the old subjects also show feedback from frontal cortex to occipital cortex, indicating an age-related alteration in the network.

(Fig. 3.2) showed that both young and old subjects had similar interactions among ventral occipitotemporal and anterior temporal regions (McIntosh et al., 1994; Horwitz et al., 1995). However, the old subjects had a strong feedback influence from frontal cortex to occipital cortex, not seen in young subjects. This indicated that, although the old subjects utilized the same ventral visual network for face perception, they had altered functional interactions among the regions in this network. In addition, because their performance accuracy was equivalent to that of young subjects, this reorganization of brain function may have been responsible for their maintained perceptual function, although at a cost of reduced response speed.

Another example of reorganization can be found using the model of memory in the healthy elderly, in this case involving recruitment of new areas into the task network. Episodic memory, or memory for specific events, is reduced in older individuals to varying degrees, depending on the type of item to be remembered and the conditions under which memory is tested (e.g. Smith and Winograd, 1978; Moscovitch, 1982; Park, Puglisi and Smith, 1986; Craik and Jennings, 1992). Prefrontal cortex is one of the brain regions that has been shown to be differentially activated during memory, with activation of left prefrontal cortex during encoding of new material and activation of right prefrontal cortex during retrieval, whether recall or recognition (Tulving et al., 1994; Nyberg, Cabeza and Tulving, 1996). A recent study of encoding and recognition of faces in old and young subjects (Grady et al., 1995)

showed that not only were the old subjects impaired on this task, but they also had markedly different blood flow patterns, particularly during encoding. Whereas young subjects had increased activity during encoding in a number of areas, including left prefrontal and right medial temporal cortices, old subjects showed no additional activations above what was seen during perception of faces prior to the encoding condition. During the retrieval phase both groups showed activation of right prefrontal cortex, but there was no evidence of functional reorganization in the old subjects. Quite different results were obtained in a later experiment (Cabeza et al., 1997), in which subjects encoded and retrieved lists of word pairs. Unlike the study of face memory, older subjects were not impaired on memory for these word pairs. During encoding, old subjects showed less activation in the areas that were active in young subjects, i.e. left prefrontal and temporal cortex, but activated bilateral insula and right occipital cortex to a greater extent than young subjects. During both recognition and recall, old subjects had increased activity in right prefrontal cortex, as did young subjects, but again had additional activation in other areas, such as precuneus during recognition and left prefrontal during recall. Thus, the old subjects in this study had less activity in the encoding network utilized by young subjects, but showed evidence of a reorganization of function during both encoding and retrieval. These results suggest that old subjects do not utilize as effectively the encoding network used by younger individuals, but that, if they are able to engage other areas during both encoding and retrieval, their performance will not suffer. Thus, in both visual perception and memory, functional reorganization has been shown in the brains of older people, and this reorganization occurs in the context of relatively preserved task performance. This reorganization may thus be serving as a compensatory mechanism in the same way as it does in patients with recovery after stroke.

Changes in sensorimotor representations within specific regions

- Another mechanism for recovery of function after brain damage is a reorganization of sensorimotor fields resulting in re-representation of lost functions in new areas of cortex.
- This may reflect inherent plasticity of cortical cells and connections.

It has been known for some time that lesions in sensory or motor areas of the nonhuman primate brain can result in reorganization of the representational maps in cortex. For example, a lesion in the hand area of sensory cortex results in a reorganization of the topographic map such that the areas of the hand that originally were represented in the lesioned area are now represented in adjacent areas of cortex, causing other receptive fields to be displaced to make room for the new representation (Jenkins and Merzenich, 1987). In one study (Nudo et al., 1996), monkeys were retrained in a skilled hand movement after a lesion was made in the hand area of motor cortex. In some monkeys, the hand area expanded into areas formerly occupied by other body parts. That is, stimulation of areas that formerly resulted in movement of other parts of the body resulted in hand movement after the lesion. In addition, those monkeys that participated in the rehabilitation training showed an increase in the representational area of the wrist and forearm compared to control monkeys that received the lesions but not the training. This suggests that the rehabilitation, and hence recovery, resulted in specific plastic changes in parts of motor cortex not damaged by the lesion that allowed hand movement to resume normally.

A similar finding was reported in an imaging study of patients who showed recovered finger opposition movements after capsular infarcts (Weiller et al., 1993). In this experiment (also discussed above) half of the studied patients showed increased activation in contralateral motor cortex compared to controls, but inferior to the area normally activated by finger movement. This finding suggested that the remaining motor field associated with finger movement had expanded into the area normally responsible for the face. In addition, this occurred primarily in patients with lesions in the posterior limb of the internal capsule, indicating that this plasticity might be dependent to some extent on the location of the lesion. This is evidence of plasticity of sensorimotor representations in human cortex, similar to that which has been seen in the monkey. The opposite finding, i.e. the face area enlarging to include the arm and hand area, has been shown using functional magnetic resonance imaging in human somatosensory cortex after amputation of the arm (Yang et al., 1994). Thus, plasticity of representations in adult sensory and motor cortex has been demonstrated in humans as well as monkeys, and may well underlie recovery of function in some patients.

The neural mechanism that is responsible for the reorganization of topographical maps in cortex is unknown, although it has been shown in reorganized cells in striate cortex that function is essentially normal (Chino et al., 1995). Some have suggested that cortical reorganization is due to changes that occur in subcortical areas, such as the brainstem or thalamus, that are relayed back up to the cortex (Pons et al., 1991). However, a series of studies (Darian-Smith and Gilbert, 1994, 1995) has shown that these changes that occur in striate cortex are not the result of concomitant changes in the lateral geniculate nucleus, but are intrinsic to the cortex itself. That is, the reorganization is related to sprouting of laterally projecting cortical neurons rather than to any remodelling imposed by subcortical structures, suggesting inherent plasticity in cortex. Similarly, the cellular mechanisms underlying the reorganization of brain networks discussed above may be intrinsic to the cortex itself, such as increased efficacy of existing connections (Merzenich et al., 1983; Donoghue, Suner and Sanes, 1990), or rearrangements of dendritic trees, known to occur even in the brains of older individuals (Flood et al., 1985).

Implications for rehabilitation

- Examples have been presented of specific brain changes after therapeutic intervention.
- Neuroimaging could be useful both in designing rehabilitation programmes and in monitoring the effectiveness of such programmes.

Although neuroimaging tools have not been widely used to examine recovery of function after brain damage, the application of this method holds great potential for expanding our knowledge in this field. There are several ways in which measurement of brain reorganization with neuroimaging can aid rehabilitation efforts. It provides insight into alternate ways a particular cognitive or motor task can be accomplished. For example, if one could determine that patients with lesions to brain region A have greater utilization of area B when functional recovery has taken place, regardless of whether area B is a part of the normal network or recruited de novo, then one could design a training programme that makes use of strategies or processes in which area B plays a role. A behavioural study that examined visual function in a patient with a frontal lobe lesion can be seen as an example of the kind of alternate strategy that one might want to access during rehabilitation. Kosslyn and colleagues (1993) reported a series of experiments carried out on a patient with a lesion to subcortical regions of the left inferior frontal lobe. The investigators theorized that the lesion would disrupt the functional interactions between inferior temporal areas important for object perception and the frontal structures to which they are connected, thus affecting the ventral visual stream for object identification. This lesion would not be expected to disrupt the function of the dorsal visual stream responsible for spatial location due to the more dorsal location of the frontal projections of this visual stream. Using a series of perceptual tasks, it was hypothesized that the patient encoded objects as filled locations rather than as shapes, thus utilizing the dorsal stream to perform what would normally be a ventral stream task. The addition of neuroimaging data during task performance in this patient would have been very useful in helping to confirm this hypothesis, which if it were confirmed could aid in the development of specific strategies for cognitive rehabilitation.

In addition, imaging studies that determine which brain areas are necessary for recovery to occur could aid in identifying those patients most likely to benefit from rehabilitation. For example, a study by Binkofski et al. (1996) has shown that motor recovery in patients with strokes in the middle cerebral artery territory is dependent on functional integrity of the thalamus and the amount of damage to the pyramidal tract. In their sample, the thalamus was not damaged by the stroke, but was probably hypometabolic due to damage to its connections with lesioned cortex. This finding suggests that the thalamus, and by implication its connections with motor cortex, is critical for any reorganization of motor areas that occurs after the stroke, and that without its participation, recovery is unlikely. The absence of cerebellar metabolic asymmetry after stroke also may be an indicator of good recovery of neurological function (Serrati et al., 1994). These studies indicate that those patients with relative functional preservation of certain motor-related areas will recover with standard physiotherapy, whereas patients without such preservation might be candidates for rehabilitative measures that focused on other brain regions, if such could be designed.

Finally, another use of neuroimaging would be to monitor the effectiveness of rehabilitation procedures as training progresses or after training is complete. The degree to which the new network or modified network is engaged during task performance could be determined as well as whether any unexpected changes have occurred. Correlation of specific brain patterns with recovered or nonrecovered behaviours would be a very powerful way of determining whether the goals of the rehabilitation effort have been achieved, and how the recovered function has been implemented via altered brain responses. Examples of demonstrable changes in the brain after drug or cognitive therapy that are specific to those patients who respond to treatment can be found in obsessive–compulsive disorder and stuttering. Both orbitofrontal cortex and the caudate nucleus have been implicated in the pathophysiology of obsessive–compulsive disorder (Rapoport, 1989) and have been found to be abnormally hypermetabolic on PET scans (Swedo et al., 1989; Baxter et al., 1990). After treatment with various medications, it was found that orbitofrontal metabolism was decreased in patients with obsessive–compulsive disorder and that this decrease was correlated with clinical improvement (Swedo et al., 1992). Similarly, Schwartz et al. (1996) found that caudate metabolism decreased after successful treatment with behaviour modification in patients with obsessive–compulsive disorder. In addition, the intercorrelations among orbitofrontal cortex, caudate and thalamus decreased in those patients who responded to therapy. In the case of stuttering, successful treatment does not change the abnormally increased activity seen in the right hemisphere during reading, but does result in increased activation of left hemisphere speech areas compared to untreated stutterers (Kroll et al., 1998).

The results of all of these studies suggest that successful intervention, whether it be cognitive or pharmacological, can directly affect the brain mechanisms that are responsible for a behavioural deficit and that these alterations can be quantitated with imaging.

Conclusions

- Neuroimaging has proven to be useful in demonstrating changes in the brain that are related to recovery of function after brain damage.
- These studies suggest, albeit indirectly, that undamaged brain areas and functional systems are capable of supporting recovery via a reorganization of functional networks.
- Future work should focus on the use of these techniques to aid in the design and evaluation of rehabilitation strategies, as well as a more direct assessment of neural networks.

The experiments reviewed here lend considerable support to the idea that neuroimaging has the potential to be a powerful tool in the quest to understand how the brain can adapt to damage either spontaneously or with the aid of rehabilitation. Clearly, defining the neural substrates of improvement after cognitive procedures and/or drug adjuncts will improve our ability to design effective rehabilitation strategies. However, one should keep in mind that, although this review has been placed in the context of functional brain networks, in none of the experiments reviewed here were the actual functional networks examined explicitly. Rather, the networks were inferred from the patterns of cerebral blood flow activation that were observed in the patient groups compared to controls. A better approach would be to identify directly the network involved in recovery, rather than focusing on individual regions, using techniques newly developed for this purpose (McIntosh and Gonzalez-Lima, 1994; McIntosh et al., 1996). The reason for this is that cerebral blood flow activation per se, or lack of it, does not necessarily indicate whether or not a particular brain area participates in the functional network. For example, a network analysis of data from the face perception experiment described above, in which cerebral flood flow activation in visual cortex was bilateral, revealed that only in the right hemisphere was there a demonstrable and significant set of functional interactions among the regions thought to be responsible for task performance (Horwitz et al., 1993; McIntosh et al., 1994). Despite the fact that such analyses are as yet lacking in the search for the brain mechanisms underlying recovery of function, the evidence presented here indicates that the neuroimaging approach is a valid one and holds promise both for our understanding of the brain and for our ability to rehabilitate those who suffer from brain damage.

References

Aizawa, H., Inase, M., Mushiake, H., Shima, K. and Tanji, J. 1991. Reorganization of activity in the supplementary motor area associated with motor learning and functional recovery. *Exp Brain Res* **84**, 668–71.

Baxter, L.R., Schwartz, J.M., Guze, B.H., Bergman, K. and Szuba, M.P. 1990. PET imaging in obsessive compulsive disorder with and without depression. *J Clin Psychiatry* **51** [4, Suppl.], 61–9.

Bayles, K.A., Tomoeda, C.K. and Boone, D.R. 1985. A view of age-related changes in language function. *Dev Neuropsychol* **1**, 231–64.

Binkofski, F., Seitz, R.J., Arnold, S., Classen, J., Benecke, R. and Freund, H.-J. 1996. Thalamic metabolism and corticospinal tract integrity determine motor recovery in stroke. *Ann Neurol* **39**, 460–70.

Bookheimer, S.Y., Zeffiro, T.A., Blaxton, T., Gaillard, W. and Theodore, W. 1995. Regional cerebral blood flow during object naming and word reading. *Hum Brain Map* **3**, 93–106.

Borod, J.D., Goodlgass, H. and Kaplan, E. 1980. Normative data on the Boston Diagnostic Aphasia Examination, Parietal Lobe Battery, and the Boston Naming Test. *J Clin Neuropsychol* **2**, 209–15.

Braun, H.G. and Ludlow, C. 1995. Advances in stuttering research using positron emission tomography brain imaging. *ASHA* **37**, 89.

Bressler, S.L. 1995. Large-scale cortical networks and cognition. *Brain Res Rev* **20**, 288–304.

Buckner, R.L., Corbetta, M., Schatz, J., Raichle, M.E. and Petersen, S.E. 1996. Preserved speech abilities and compensation following prefrontal damage. *Proc Natl Acad Sci USA* **93**, 1249–53.

Cabeza, R., Grady, C.L., Nyberg, L. et al. 1997. Age-related differences in neural activity during memory encoding and retrieval: a positron emission tomography study. *J Neurosci* **17**, 391–400.

Chino, Y.M., Smith, E.L., Kaas, J.H., Sasaki, Y. and Cheng, H. 1995. Receptive-field properties of deafferentated visual cortical neurons after topographic map reorganization. *J Neurosci* **15**, 2417–33.

Chollet, F., DiPiero, V., Wise, R.J.S., Brooks, D.J., Dolan, R.J. and Frackowiak, R.S.J. 1991. The functional anatomy of motor recovery after stroke in humans: a study with positron emission tomography. *Ann Neurol* **29**, 63–71.

Craik, F.I.M. and Jennings, J.M. 1992. Human memory. In *The Handbook of Aging and Cognition*, ed. F.I.M. Craik and T.A. Salthouse, pp. 51–110. Hillsdale, NJ: Lawrence Erlbaum.

Craik, F.I.M., Morris, R.G. and Gick, M.L. 1990. Adult age differences in working memory. In *Neuropsychological Impairments of Short-term Memory*, ed. G. Vallar and T. Shallice, pp. 247–67. Cambridge: Cambridge University Press.

Creasey, H. and Rapoport, S.I. 1985. The aging human brain. *Ann Neurol* **17**, 2–10.

Darian-Smith, C. and Gilbert, Cc.D. 1994. Axonal sprouting accompanies functional reorganization in adult cat striate cortex. *Nature* **368**, 737–40.

Darian-Smith, C. and Gilbert, C.D. 1995. Topographic reorganization in the striate cortex of the adult cat and monkey is cortically mediated. *J Neurosci* **15**, 1631–47.

Demonet, J.-F., Chollet, F., Ramsay, S. et al. 1992. The anatomy of phonological and semantic processing in normal subjects. *Brain* **115**, 1753–68.

Desimone, R. and Ungerleider, L.G. 1989. Neural mechanisms of visual processing in monkeys. In *Handbook of Neuropsychology*, ed. H. Goodglass and A.R. Damasio, pp. 267–300. Amsterdam: Elsevier.

Donoghue, J.P., Suner, S. and Sanes, J.N. 1990. Dynamic organization of primary motor cortex output to target muscles in adult rats. II. Rapid reorganization following motor nerve lesions. *Exp Brain Res* **79**, 492–503.

Engelien, A., Silbersweig, D., Stern, E. et al. 1995. The functional anatomy of recovery from auditory agnosia. A PET study of sound categorization in a neurological patient and normal controls. *Brain* **118**, 1395–409.

Flood, D.G., Buell, S.J., DeFiore, C.H., Horwitz, G.J. and Coleman, P.D. 1985. Age-related dendritic growth in dentate gyrus of human brain is followed by regression in the 'oldest old'. *Brain Res* **345**, 366–8.

Grady, C.L. 1999. Neuroimaging and activation of the frontal lobes. In *The Human Frontal Lobes: Function and Disorders*, ed. B.L. Miller and J.L. Cummings, pp. 196–230. New York: Guilford Press.

Grady, C.L., Horwitz, B., Pietrini, P. et al. 1996. The effect of task difficulty on cerebral blood flow during perceptual matching of faces. *Hum Brain Map* **4**, 227–39.

Grady, C.L., Maisog, J.M., Horwitz, B. et al. 1994. Age-related changes in cortical blood flow activation during visual processing of faces and location. *J Neurosci* **14**, 1450–62.

Grady, C.L., McIntosh, A.R., Horwitz, B. et al. 1995. Age-related reductions in human recognition memory due to impaired encoding. *Science* **269**, 218–21.

Horwitz, B., Maisog, J., Kirschner, P. et al. 1993. Functional pathways in the brain during object and spatial visual processing: An rCBF PET/correlation analysis. *J Cereb Blood Flow Metab* **13** (Suppl. 1), S527.

Horwitz, B., McIntosh, A.R., Haxby, J.V. et al. 1995. Network analysis of PET-mapped visual pathways in Alzheimer type dementia. *Neuroreport* **6**, 2287–92.

Jenkins, W.M. and Merzenich, M.M. 1987. Reorganization of neocortical representations after brain injury: a neurophysiological model of the bases of recovery from stroke. *Prog Brain Res* **71**, 249–66.

Katz, S., Ford, A.B., Chinn, A.B. and Newill, V.A. 1966. Prognosis after strokes. Part II. Long term course of 159 patients. *Medicine (Baltimore)* **45**, 236–46.

Kemper, T. 1984. Neuroanatomical and neuropathological changes in normal ageing and in dementia. In *Clinical Neurology of Aging*, ed. M. Albert, pp. 9–52. New York: Oxford University Press.

Kennard, M.A. 1942. Cortical reorganization of motor function. Studies on series of monkeys of various ages from infancy to maturity. *AMA Arch Neurol Psychiatry* **48**, 227–40.

Kosslyn, S.M., Daly, P.F., McPeek, R.M., Alpert, N.M., Kennedy, D.N. and Caviness, V.S. 1993. Using locations to store shape: an indirect effect of a lesion. *Cereb Cortex* **3**, 567–82.

Kroll, R.M., De Nil, L.F., Kapur, S. and Houle, S. 1998. A positron emission tomography investigation of post-treatment brain activation in stutterers. In *Speech Motor Control, Brain Research Production: and Fluency Disorders*, ed. H.F.M. Peters, W. Hulstijn and P. Van Lieshout, pp. 307–20. Amsterdam: Elsevier Science Publishers.

LaBarge, E., Edwards, D. and Knesevich, J.W. 1986. Performance of normal elderly on the Boston Naming Test. *Brain Lang* 27, 380–4.

Masliah, E., Mallory, M., Hansen, L., DeTeresa, R. and Terry, R.D. 1993. Quantitative synaptic alterations in the human neocortex during normal aging. *Neurology* 43, 192–7.

McCrae, R.R., Arenberg, D. and Costa, P.T. 1987. Decline in divergent thinking with age: cross-sectional, longitudinal and cross-sequential analyses. *Psychol Aging* 2, 130–2.

McIntosh, A.R., Bookstein, F.L., Haxby, J.V. and Grady, C.L. 1996. Spatial pattern analysis of functional brain images using Partial Least Squares. *Neuroimage* 3, 143–57.

McIntosh, A.R. and Gonzalez-Lima, F. 1994. Structural equation modeling and its application to network analysis in functional brain imaging. *Hum Brain Map* 2, 2–22.

McIntosh, A.R., Grady, C.L., Ungerleider, L.G., Haxby, J.V., Rapoport, S.I. and Horwitz, B. 1994. Network analysis of cortical visual pathways mapped with PET. *J Neurosci* 14, 655–66.

Merzenich, M.M., Kaas, J.H., Wall, J.T., Sur, M., Nelson, R.J. and Felleman, D.J. 1983. Progression of change following median nerve section in the cortical representation of the hand in areas 3b and 1 in adult owl and squirrel monkeys. *Neuroscience* 10, 639–65.

Mesulam, M.M. 1981. A cortical network for directed attention and unilateral neglect. *Ann Neurol* 10, 309–25.

Milner, B. 1973. Hemispheric specialization: scope and limits. In *The Neurosciences: Third Study Program*, ed. F.O. Schmitt and F.G. Worden, pp. 75–89. Cambridge, MA: MIT Press.

Moscovitch, M. 1982. A neuropsychological approach to perception and memory in normal and pathological aging. In *Aging and Cognitive Processes*, ed. F.I.M. Craik and S. Trehub, pp. 55–78. New York: Plenum Press.

Nebes, R.D., Boller, F. and Holland, A. 1986. Use of semantic context by patients with Alzheimer's disease. *Psychol Aging* 1, 261–9.

Nudo, R.J., Wise, B.M., SiFuentes, F. and Milliken, G.W. 1996. Neural substrates for the effects of rehabilitative training on motor recovery after ischemic infarct. *Science* 272, 1791–4.

Nyberg, L., Cabeza, R. and Tulving, E. 1996. PET studies of encoding and retrieval: the HERA model. *Psychonom Bull Rev* 3, 135–48.

Pantano, P., De Piero, V., Fieschi, C., Judica, A., Guariglia, C. and Pizzamiglio, L. 1992. Pattern of CBF in the rehabilitation of visuospatial neglect. *Int J Neurosci* 66, 153–61.

Park, D.C., Puglisi, J.T. and Smith, A.D. 1986. Memory for pictures: does an age-related decline exist? *Psychol Aging* 1, 11–17.

Perani, D., Vallar, G., Paulesu, E., Alberoni, M. and Fazio, F. 1993. Left and right hemisphere contribution to recovery from neglect after right hemisphere damage – an [18F]FDG PET study of two cases. *Neuropsychologia* 31, 115–25.

Peters, A., Leahu, D., Moss, M.B. and McNally, K.J. 1994. The effects of aging on area 46 of the frontal cortex of the rhesus monkey. *Cereb Cortex* 6, 621–35.

Petersen, S.E., Fox, P.T., Posner, M.I., Mintun, M. and Raichle, M.E. 1989. Positron emission tomographic studies of the processing of single words. *J. Cogn Neurosci* 1, 153–70.

Pons, T., Garraghty, P.E., Ommaya, A.K., Kaas, J.H., Taub, E. and Mishkin, M. 1991. Massive cortical reorganization after sensory deafferentation in adult macaques. *Science* 252, 1857–60.

Posner, M. and Dehaene, S. 1994. Attentional networks. *Trends Neurosci* 17, 75–9.

Rapoport, J.L. 1989. The biology of obsessions and compulsions. *Sci Am* 260, 82–9.

Schwartz, J.M., Stoessel, P.W., Baxter, L.R., Martin, K.M. and Phelps, M.E. 1996. Systematic changes in cerebral glucose metabolic rate after successful behavior modification treatment of obsessive–compulsive disorder. *Arch Gen Psychiatry* 53, 109–13.

Serrati, C., Marchal, G., Rioux, P. et al. 1994. Contralateral cerebellar hypometabolism: a predictor for stroke outcome? *J Neurol Neurosurg Psychiatry* 57, 174–9.

Skilbeck, C.E., Wade, D.T., Hewer, R.L. and Wood, V.A. 1983. Recovery after stroke. *J Neurol Neurosurg Psychiatry* 46, 5–8.

Smith, A.D. and Winograd, E. 1978. Adult age differences in remembering faces. *Dev Psychol* 14, 443–4.

Stein, D.G., Rosen, J.J. and Butters, N. (1974). *Plasticity and Recovery of Function in the Central Nervous System*. New York: Academic Press.

Swedo, S.E., Pietrini, P., Leonard, H.L. et al. 1992. Cerebral glucose metabolism in childhood-onset obsessive–compulsive disorder. Revisualization during pharmacotherapy. *Arch Gen Psychiatry* 49, 690–4.

Swedo, S.E., Schapiro, M.B., Grady, C.L. et al. 1989. Cerebral glucose metabolism in childhood-onset obsessive–compulsive disorder. *Arch Gen Psychiatry* 46, 518–23.

Tanji, J. and Kelsetsu, S. 1994. Role for supplementary motor area cells in planning several movements ahead. *Nature* 371, 413–16.

Tanji, J., Okano, K. and Sato, K.C. 1987. Relation of neurones in the non-primary motor cortex to bilateral hand movements. *Nature* 327, 618–20.

Tulving, E., Kapur, S., Craik, F.I.M., Moscovitch, M. and Houle, S.

1994. Hemispheric encoding/retrieval asymmetry in episodic memory: positron emission tomography findings. *Proc Natl Acad Sci USA* **91**, 2016–20.

Twitchell, T.E. 1951. The restoration of motor function following hemiplegia in man. *Brain* **74**, 443–80.

Ungerleider, L.G. and Mishkin, M. 1982. Two cortical visual systems. In *Analysis of Visual Behavior*, ed. D.J. Ingle, M.A. Goodale and R.J.W. Mansfield, pp. 549–86. Cambridge, MA: MIT Press.

Vaadia, E., Haalman, I., Abeles, M. et al. 1995. Dynamics of neuronal interactions in monkey cortex in relation to behavioral events. *Nature* **373**, 515–18.

Weiller, C., Chollet, F., Friston, K.J., Wise, R.J.S. and Frackowiak, R.S.J. 1992. Functional reorganization of the brain in recovery from striatocapsular infarction in man. *Ann Neurol* **31**, 463–72.

Weiller, C., Isenee, C., Rijntjes, M. et al. 1995. Recovery from Wernicke's aphasia: a positron emission tomography study. *Ann Neurol* **37**, 723–32.

Weiller, C., Ramsay, S.C., Wise, R.J.S., Friston, K.J. and Frackowiak, R.S.J. 1993. Individual patterns of functional reorganization in the human cerebral cortex after capsular infarction. *Ann Neurol* **33**, 181–9.

Yang, T.T., Gallen, C.C., Ramachandran, V.S., Cobb, S., Schwartz, B.J. and Bloom, F.E. 1994. Noninvasive detection of cerebral plasticity in adult human somatosensory cortex. *Neuroreport* **5**, 701–4.

4

Principles of compensation in cognitive neurorehabilitation

Roger A. Dixon and Lars Bäckman

Every excess causes a defect; every defect an excess ... For everything you have missed, you have gained something else; and for everything you gain, you lose something. Ralph Waldo Emerson (1900).

Introduction

In some areas of psychology there is a perspective from which compensation is believed to be almost as common and simple as the above poetic quotation by Emerson might indicate. From this perspective, compensation is presented as an elegant, hovering principle of balance, a natural 'sublime law' (Emerson's term) of regression or egression to the norm, a tendency to return to normalcy. Note the intrinsic and dynamic balance suggested in Emerson's passage: for every loss there is a corresponding gain and for every gain there is a corresponding loss. For every defect or deficit there is some way to recover. It represents the human organism, the human brain, and human lifespan development as a dynamic, variable, adaptive and self-correcting system. How well does Emerson's view represent contemporary perspectives of compensation across a broad range of disciplines in psychology? How well does it represent the empirically based theoretical views of compensation emerging in such specialty areas of psychology as cognitive ageing, cognitive neuropsychology, and cognitive neurorehabilitation?

To preview, there is indeed a sense in which the elegant simplicity of Emerson's view continues to apply to contemporary scholarship in psychological compensation. Nevertheless, numerous intriguing general and specific questions about the scope and depth of Emerson's relevance must be posed. For example, does Emerson's 'sublime law' work as effectively and as comprehensively as implied in the quotation? Does it operate similarly for all deficits, regardless of type, severity or duration? What are the specific mechanisms of compensation and how do they operate? Is compensation enacted spontaneously or automatically, or as the result of effort or training? What constitutes a 'defect' in cognitive psychology and cognitive neuropsychology? How is variability from the norm – the origin of compensation – portrayed? These are issues explored in this chapter.

The chapter begins with a definition and principles of compensation as they apply to selected domains within contemporary psychology. The framework is then applied to the related areas of cognitive neuropsychology (compensation for organic memory impairment) and cognitive neuroscience (compensatory brain activation).

Concept of compensation in psychology

- The term *compensation* is used by a wide range of literatures in psychology. Principal literatures include neurosciences, neurological disorders, acquired speech and language disorders, sensory injuries or deficits, cognitive ageing, and others.
- Common to these literatures is the notion that compensation refers to a process of overcoming losses or deficits through one of several identifiable mechanisms.

In psychology, the term compensation refers to a process through which deficits or losses are moderated. The term enjoys wide usage in psychology and, although there are some differences across areas, it converges upon several identifiable themes. For an earlier review (Bäckman and Dixon, 1992), scores of articles pertaining to compensation in psychology were collected. The use of the term in psychology was traced back to Emerson in the early part of this century, into the 1920s and 1930s, and through a rapid acceleration in the 1960s and 1970s. Brandtstädter and Wentura (1995) located even earlier homologous usages of compensation in eighteenth-century philosophy. For example, they quoted Formey (1759) as remarking that, 'for man, there is never gain without loss, and no loss without gain . . . compensation everywhere' (Brandtstädter and Wentura, 1995, p. 83). Examples of early literature in psychology include Adler's (1927) view of compensation in personality as a crucial defence mechanism. More pertinent, perhaps, was the early optimistic notion that a deficit in sensitivity in one sensory system could be counterbalanced by a gain in sensitivity in an intact modality (e.g. Hartmann, 1933; Hayes, 1933; see Rönnberg, 1995, for a review). Although the empirical evidence in both cases – as well as other early examples of compensation research – was somewhat mixed, the concept spread and proliferated. As noted elsewhere, among the reasons for the resilience and power of the concept of compensation in twentieth-century psychology are the related facts that (a) it is nearly as intuitively attractive as Emerson makes it sound; (b) it possesses potential theoretical importance of considerable magnitude; and (c) it has immediate and compelling practical implications for several applied areas of psychological scholarship (Dixon and Bäckman, 1995b).

Selected areas of compensation research

In the authors' initial and subsequent reviews (Bäckman and Dixon, 1992; Dixon and Bäckman, 1995b), the concept and empirical deployment of compensation were surveyed in a wide range of psychological literatures. The goal was to develop a comprehensive model of compensation, one that was derived from research in a wide range of psychological domains. The following principal literatures – presented with sample citations and an illustrative compensatory idea – were consulted in these reviews.

1. Neurosciences (e.g. Gehring et al., 1993; Woodruff-Pak and Hanson, 1995) in which behavioural, electrophysiological, neuroimaging, and morphological evidence suggests that the human brain displays plasticity, including reorganization and substitution of function, as a response to impairment, damage and fallibility (errors).

2. Neurological disorders (e.g. Grady and Parasuraman, 1995; Wilson, 1995; Becker et al., 1996a, 1996b; Buckner et al., 1996; Mateer, 1996; Wilson and Watson, 1996) in which deficits associated with either organic diseases (e.g. Alzheimer's disease) or other neurological injuries may be compensated by a variety of strategies for improving cognitive performance (e.g. utilization of preserved skills).

3. Acquired speech and language disorders (e.g. Rothi and Horner, 1983; Ahlsén, 1991; Towne, 1994; Gonzalez Rothi, 1995; Buckner et al., 1996) in which a deficit resulting from an injury or stroke may be compensated through the use of an alternative communication mechanism or through physiological restitution.

4. Sensory injuries or deficits (e.g. Ohlsson, 1986; Smith and Curthoys, 1989; Neville, 1990; Rönnberg, 1995; Szlyk, Seiple and Viana, 1995; Stevens, Foulke and Patterson, 1996) in which an impairment in one modality of the visual or auditory system could be compensated by increased sensitivity in an alternative system.

5. Cognitive ageing and decline (e.g. Salthouse, 1984, 1987, 1990; Bäckman, 1985, 1989; Dixon and Bäckman, 1993) in which ageing-related declines in molecular components (such as speed of processing) of skills may be compensated by the development of alternative mechanisms.

6. Reading deficits (e.g. Stanovich, 1984; West, Stanovich and Cunningham, 1995) in which deficiencies at a particular level in the processing hierarchy can be compensated for by greater use of information from different contexts.

7. Social and personal developmental losses (e.g. Brandtstädter and Wentura, 1995; Carstensen, Hanson and Freund, 1995; Marsiske et al., 1995) in which declining personal resources may be accommodated by adjusting goals, reducing criteria of success, rearranging priorities, or constructing palliative meanings.

These literatures are too extensive to review in this context (see Dixon and Bäckman, 1995a), but they support a set of principles, definitions and implications for both theoretical (e.g. experimental cognitive neuropsychology) and applied (e.g. rehabilitation and clinical neuropsychology) work. These implications are discussed in the following sections.

Working definition

The authors' analysis of the concept and principles of compensation has benefited substantially from many scholars contributing to the domains listed above. Several reviews covering different substantive areas, as well as the authors' continuing effort to clarify the concept of compensation, have led them to offer the following working definition (see Dixon and Bäckman, 1995b). This definition is designed to cut across the principal literatures listed above and provoke integrative empirical and theoretical activities. Little previous cross-fertilization has occurred in research on compensation, despite the fact that there is both common ground and unique perspectives.

Overall, compensation is a process of overcoming losses or deficits through one of several recognizable mechanisms. These compensatory mechanisms include: (a) investing more time and effort through training, practice or trying harder in performing a task reflective of the loss or deficit (remediation); (b) substituting a latent skill for a declining or defective one (substitution with latent process); (c) developing a new skill to take over the performance of an absent, lost or declining skill (substitution with novel process); (d) adjusting one's goals, expectations, priorities and criteria to be more concordant with the match between the demands of one's current context and the skills one currently possesses (accommodation); and (e) modifying the environment or adjusting the expectations of others (assimilation). These mechanisms are dealt with below.

The principal features of the process of compensation

- Compensation refers to the moderation of psychological (e.g. sensory, neurological) deficits or losses.
- Psychological literatures in which compensation has been a prominent concern include neurosciences, neurological disorders, acquired speech and language disorders, sensory injuries or deficits, cognitive ageing and decline, reading deficits, and social and personal developmental losses.
- Several mechanisms of compensation have been identified from a broad review of the literature. These include remediation, substitution with latent process, and substitution with novel process, accommodation, assimilation.
- The four principal issues in the process of compensation are origins, mechanisms, awareness and consequences.

The authors have identified four leading issues in compensation, each of which is more or less relevant to specific literatures. For example, in a recent review, Wilson and Watson (1996) analysed the application of these four issues to promoting and understanding compensatory behaviour in adults with organic memory impairment. The four principles identified are origins, mechanisms, awareness and consequences. In one sense these may be viewed as 'steps' in the process of compensation, for they roughly represent the chronological progress of compensatory behaviour from the moment a need or opportunity is presented. That is, compensation must originate in a deficit, which provides an opportunity (although not an automatic necessity) for restitution. A variety of mechanisms may be available, depending on the nature and extent of the deficit as well as on the resources of individual. In addition, it is often important to consider the role that awareness of the deficit or of compensatory opportunities and efforts may play, as well as the impact or consequences the compensatory effort and results may have. These principles as they pertain to the process of compensation are shown in Figure 4.1. The model is elaborated in the following sections.

Origin

The authors have proposed that compensation, broadly conceived, must have its origin in a mismatch between the skills a person possesses and the actual demands of the environment. Put simply, when one's skills match the demands of the environment there is no need or rationale for compensation. Most commonly, the mismatch is objectively observable. As can be seen in Fig. 4.1, it may develop as a result of a reduced skill level relative to the environmental demands and expected

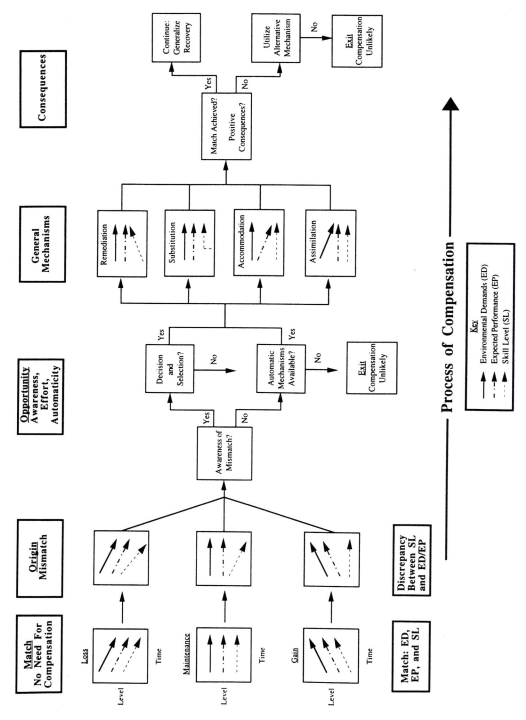

Fig. 4.1 Model representing the process of compensation. (Adapted from Bäckman and Dixon, 1992).

performance or as result of a stable skill level relative to increasing environmental demands or expected performance.

The former is of most interest in the context of applied sciences such as clinical rehabilitation. Consider the vast array of well-documented psychologically relevant deficits, defects, injuries or declines. Deficits result from head injuries, progressive diseases, acute illnesses, neurological ageing, congenital birth defects, genetic disorders, and so forth. The deficits are manifest in a mismatch between the skills individuals possess and the extent to which they are able to adapt to or perform in specific contexts. In such situations, this key premise of compensation is fulfilled. The general purpose of compensation is to close the gap between expected or required performance and actual level of skill. The challenge is to identify effective strategies, mechanisms, accommodations, or perhaps even prostheses that can render the deficit less problematic, acute, comprehensive or debilitating.

Notably, compensation does not always occur for every mismatch (Bäckman and Dixon, 1992). For both theoretical and applied perspectives, there are two important reasons for this. First, if there is a high degree of performance support in the individual's environment – such as caregivers taking over the cognitive load – there may be no need for the affected individual to develop new compensatory skills, whether as a result of self-initiated effort or other-trained experience (as in a rehabilitation setting). Second, if the deficit is too severe, compensation may not be possible at all, or at least not until after some delay. For example, the profound cognitive deficits associated with late stages of Alzheimer's disease may be difficult, if not impossible, to compensate (Herlitz et al., 1991; Herlitz, Lipinska and Bäckman, 1992). On the other hand, severe language deficits associated with stroke may, in some instances, be subject to both self-initiated and other-trained compensation following a delay (Ahlsén, 1991).

Mechanisms

Compensatory mechanisms refer to the means through which an alleviation, remediation or attenuation of the mismatch is effected. The mechanisms identified above include remediation (increasing time, effort or training

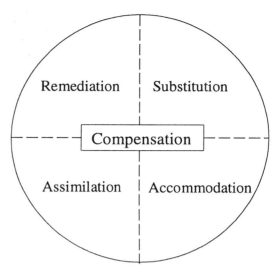

Fig. 4.2 Conceptual domain of compensation. (Adapted from Dixon and Bäckman, 1995b.)

to maintain or recover the affected skill), substitution of latent skill (from the individual's present repertoire of skills), substitution of new skill (developed such that it replaces a declining or defective skill), accommodation (adjusting priorities or criteria, selecting new goals) and assimilation (adjusting the expectations of others, constructing forgiving environments).

The typical mechanism of compensation in cognitive neurorehabilitation is the development of latent skills to substitute for those affected by the injury or disease. However, it is also useful to incorporate other mechanisms of compensation. For example, both accommodation and assimilation may be useful mechanisms in specific instances (Wilson and Watson, 1996). Although the mechanisms of compensation are conceptually different, they can be portrayed as contributing to a unified conceptual space of compensation (Fig. 4.2). Each of the mechanisms works to accomplish the goal of reducing the gap between skill level, on the one hand, and expected performance or environmental demands, on the other.

Awareness and self-regulation

To what extent is awareness of the deficit (the origin of compensation) and of mechanisms for overcoming the mismatch a requirement for an inference of compensation? This is a theoretical question about which there may be some disagreement (e.g. Dixon and Bäckman, 1995b; Salthouse, 1995). The authors' position is that compensatory mechanisms may be enacted and effective in some cases with varying degrees of awareness. They view awareness as a continuum along which compensatory mechanisms may be associated with more-or-less effortful or automatic metacognitive processes, such as self-monitoring, self-initiation and cognitive self-efficacy. This is consistent with a broad range of literature (see Bäckman and Dixon, 1992), in which one can locate examples of the phenomena that occur with full awareness of the deficit and deliberate compensatory efforts (e.g. at the social and behavioural levels), as well as examples in which little or no awareness of either the deficit or the compensatory mechanism is displayed (e.g. at the organic, sensory or biological level).

It is possible that changes in awareness can occur during the process of compensation. Like skills (Ericsson and Charness, 1994), compensatory efforts may become relatively automatized and less effortful to execute across time (Ohlsson, 1986). As one learns and practises mnemonic skills, applying them to suitable memory tasks becomes less effortful and more automatic. This gradual transition from effortful to automatic processing occurs whether an individual is shifting from normal towards expert memory (e.g. Kliegl and Baltes, 1987) or from impaired memory towards normal memory (Wilson and Watson, 1996). Indeed, it may be that one indicator of improvement is a diminishment of effortful requirements.

In recovery from brain injury, automatic and effortful processes may complement one another. These processes may complement one another sequentially, as may happen if relatively automatic reconstitution (e.g. morphological changes, recruitment of alternative activation sites) occurs early and is followed by deliberate efforts on the part of the recovering individual (Bach-y-Rita, 1990; Bach-y-Rita and Bach-y-Rita, 1990; Kolb and Whishaw, 1996). They may also complement one another in a more overlapping or even opposite sequence (e.g. Ahlsén, 1991). If the nature and severity of the injury – and the prognosis for recovery – is such that the principal source of compensation is automatic, organic or pharmacological, then initially awareness may not play a role. If, however, behavioural training, monitoring or rehabilitation is involved, then awareness may very well play a crucial role in recovery from the effects of decline or injury.

To date, very little systematic data on awareness of compensation exists, but such data could be valuable for both theoretical and applied purposes (Dixon and Bäckman, 1993). Means of collecting such information are well established in cognitive psychology. For example, the authors have suggested that verbal information be collected during training, practice and task performance. Information pertaining to awareness issues could be collected during individual sessions (as think-aloud protocols: Ericsson and Simon, 1984), dyadic collaborative sessions (e.g. psychologist–patient, caregiver–patient, between injured and uninjured spouses: Dixon, 1996; Fox, 1997), or via questionnaire or interviews (e.g. the Compensation Questionnaire: Dixon and Bäckman, 1993). Such procedures may be related to metacognitive training and rehabilitation approaches, which may address issues of insight and verbal self-regulation (Mateer, 1996). Other techniques of examining monitoring and compensatory processes have been suggested by Gehring et al. (1993). Their work uses event-related brain potentials to generate evidence for neural-based monitoring and compensatory processes as a function of normal errors (in the absence of impairment or pathology) committed during complex cognitive activity. A convergence of metacognitive, self-report and observable indicators of awareness or monitoring in compensation could be in order.

Consequences

The implicit expectation of many scholars has been that compensation results in an improvement in functioning, a restoration of some level of performance in an impaired domain. That compensation may lead to negative consequences has been surprising to some observers, with some even suggesting that a positive outcome should be incorporated into the definition of compensation. The pertinent literature and arguments for including both positive and negative consequences are described in some detail elsewhere (Dixon and Bäckman, 1995b). One basis of the argument can be found in the Emerson quotation with which this chapter began: it is not only that there is a balancing gain for every loss, there is also a balancing loss for every gain. This principle has found empirical and theoretical support in some areas of cognitive and social ageing. Given ageing-related diminishing resources, compounded by injuries or other losses, maintaining specific resource-demanding skills may result in losses in other skills or domains (Brandtstädter and Wentura, 1995). Maintaining and managing a highly valued skill (skill X) may become ever more difficult as basic resources (e.g. sensory, neurological) decline with ageing. Downward pressure on skill X may be relieved, if only temporarily, by relaxing the requirement of simultaneously maintaining (at a high level) skills Y and Z. Thus, there are losses involved (in skills Y and Z) in compensating for declines in a more valued skill (skill X).

Other examples of negative consequences of compensation are more concrete. Masterton and Biederman (1983) noted that some behaviours of autistic children (such as reliance on proximal sensory input) were initially viewed as compensatory but, from a long-term perspective, were recognized as limiting adaptation, if not being actually maladaptive. Occasionally, well-meaning parents of children with injuries or losses may attempt to buffer or substitute for the child's behavioural deficit. Although this may have the transitory desired effect of helping the child negotiate selected daily activities or tasks, the long-term effect may be one of hindering the child's development of his or her own compensatory mechanisms (Wasserman, Allen and Solomon, 1985). Such a phenomenon may very well extend to caregivers of cognitively impaired adults (e.g. older dementia patients). In fact, Wilson and Watson (1996) noted that this phenomenon could occur for parents of brain-injured adult children, as the following poignant vignette illustrates.

The father of one head-injured young woman with memory problems became very protective after the accident. He had already lost a son in another accident and felt he had to do everything for his daughter. He tried to anticipate her every wish and meet her every need. She, in turn, relied on her father to tell her what to do, when to do it, and how to do it. It is likely that without such intense supervision from her father, the young woman would have learned to use her own compensatory strategies and become more independent (Wilson and Watson, 1996, p. 475).

There are numerous examples of compensation resulting in (a) initial gains but overall long-term losses, (b) losses in overall potential for recovery, or (c) gains for the individual but losses for others in the context. For this reason, researchers and rehabilitation specialists may wish to consider the consequences dimension in theory development or applied pursuits.

Compensation in cognitive neurorehabilitation

- The principles of compensation were derived from reviews of several neighbouring literatures, including the neurosciences and neuropsychology, and are therefore represented in recent literature in neurorehabilitation.
- Neuropsychologists have explicitly evaluated the model of compensation and its application to issues of rehabilitation for memory impairment resulting from brain injury.
- Prominent strategic or behavioural mechanisms of compensation for neuropathological conditions include substitution, remediation and accommodation.
- New research techniques (e.g. neuroimaging) have vast potential for unlocking the mysteries of compensation occurring at the neuroanatomical level.
- New examples of compensation via the activation of latent or novel mechanisms in the brain include distribution or recruitment of alternative pathways or activation sites. Evidence for such compensatory hyperactivation has been found for mild Alzheimer's disease and aphasia.
- It is possible that automatic neuroanatomical compensation can be boosted through deliberate behavioural compensation. Such a linkage between levels of analysis and mechanisms of compensation deserves further attention in cognitive neurorehabilitation.

Thus far, the main purpose in this chapter has been to present the principles of compensation, as the authors have understood and derived them from a broad spectrum of literature. Featuring prominently in this review have been the neighbouring research areas of neurosciences, neurological disorders, and cognitive development. In addition to the theoretical analysis, the authors' own research in compensation has been in the area of cognitive ageing (e.g. Bäckman, 1985, 1989; Dixon and Bäckman, 1993, 1995b; Dixon, 1996; Dixon and Gould, 1996), as well as cognitive neuropsychology and dementia (e.g. Bäckman, Mäntylä and Hertlitz, 1990; Herlitz et al., 1992). We turn now to selected brief illustrations of recent work in compensation and neurorehabilitation. The goal is not to review this literature comprehensively, but rather to illustrate how the principles of compensation – some of which were derived from seemingly distant literatures – may find a voice and an application in cognitive neurorehabilitation. Therefore, only selected projects are briefly dealt with.

Behavioural compensation for organic cognitive impairment

Several recent reviews of cognitive rehabilitation strategies for adult brain injury have attended to issues of compensation, including the principles of mechanisms, awareness and consequences (e.g. Mateer, 1996). One perspective is especially consonant with the model sketched above. In her recent work, Wilson (1995; Wilson and Watson, 1996) has evaluated a model of compensation and its application to issues of rehabilitation for memory impairment resulting from brain injury. To the authors' knowledge, this is one of the most comprehensive efforts to apply compensation theory to clinical neuropsychological settings. For example, Wilson and Watson review three of the principles of compensation as they apply to rehabilitation for organic memory impairment. With respect to *origins*, they confirm that the principal origin of interest in this field is that of a decrease in skill as a function of brain injury. Furthermore, although the resultant mismatch is the occasion for compensation, there are circumstances in which compensatory behaviours are not developed. These include circumstances in which a

high degree of contextual support (or environmental adaptations) obviates the need for compensatory mechanisms operating through or in the recovering individual. In addition, Wilson and Watson consider the important role of severity of deficit (Bäckman and Dixon, 1992).They report that for brain injuries our predicted inverse relationship between the severity of the deficit and the probability of self-initiated behavioural compensation is likely to depend in part on whether executive functioning is implicated. Specifically, when executive deficits are prominent, even people who are only mildly impaired in the criterion skill may not readily or effectively initiate compensatory behaviour. Conversely, people with unimpaired executive functioning may develop compensatory strategies even though they show more pronounced deficits in the criterion skill.

Wilson and Watson (1996) reported that, not only were *remediation* and *substitution* employed as mechanisms of compensating for organic memory impairment, but so was *accommodation*. They reported examples of injured patients investing more effort in the cognitively demanding tasks of their everyday lives (Wilson, 1995). They also reported substitutable strategies, such as teaching the use of external aids, as being effective (see also Mateer, 1996). Wilson (1995) described the case of a young adult law student who, following a cerebral haemorrhage and period of rehabilitation, accommodated to his residual cognitive deficit by rearranging his priorities, devaluing blocked goals, and possibly constructing palliative meanings. Finally, as noted above, Wilson and Watson reported several examples of negative consequences of compensatory behaviour in organic memory impairment. The one of most concern to the rehabilitation specialist may well be when a brain-injured person engages in compensatory behaviour that is successful in overcoming at least some of the deficit (i.e. positive consequences) but this same behaviour has negative consequences for others in close proximity. Their example is 'the amnesic patient who is constantly interrupting to record something on a tape recorder or in a diary is acting sensibly on the one hand, but disruptively on the other' (Wilson and Watson, 1996, p. 475).

Compensatory brain activation

Whereas the previous section briefly reviewed selected literature pertaining to neurorehabilitation at the behavioural or strategic level, there is another body of research indicating the possibility of compensation occurring also at the neuroanatomical level. In previous work (e.g. Bäckman and Dixon, 1992) the authors have noted several examples of compensatory mechanisms operating at the neuroanatomical level. These include collateral sprouting and regeneration, which are two of the dozen neural mechanisms listed in the Kolb and Whishaw (1996) taxonomy. Two features of this taxonomy could be noted at this juncture. First, it (appropriately) emphasizes neural mechanisms of recovery from brain damage. The richness of Kolb and Whishaw's conceptual analysis complements other observers' analyses of behavioural compensation per se, as well as those instances in which behavioural and neural mechanisms may operate serially or interactively (e.g. Bach-y-Rita and Bach-y-Rita, 1990; Ahlsén, 1991; Bäckman and Dixon, 1992; Wilson and Watson, 1996). Second, one mechanism identified by Kolb and Whishaw represents a general form of compensation and is pertinent to a variety of literatures. Specifically, as used by Kolb and Whishaw (1996, p. 554), substitution operates at the neuroanatomical level when an otherwise 'underused area of the brain . . . assume[s] functions of a damaged area'. Although the authors caution that substitution is not presently 'in vogue' in this literature, some recent advances in neuroimaging (see Chapter 3) are promising.

An interesting question for compensation theory is whether neurological compensatory mechanisms are under the deliberate control of the injured individual (e.g. LeVere and LeVere, 1982; Bäckman and Dixon, 1992). As compared to some behavioural mechanisms, neurological mechanisms are unlikely to be the product of self-initiated and deliberate effort. Indeed, they may not even be available to awareness or monitoring. To the extent that the overall process of recovery involves both behavioural and neurological mechanisms, some degree of awareness and control could be involved. Another theoretical question concerns the con-

sequences, which are likely to be gains (rather than losses). The implication is one of recovery of function following brain damage. In general, this notion of compensatory brain activation has a long and durable history (e.g. Munk, 1881; Lashley, 1924; Luria, 1963, 1966). More recent work has continued this tradition, with rapid advancements due to powerful new technologies (e.g. Scheff, 1984; Grady and Parasuraman, 1995; Woodruff-Pak and Hanson, 1995). The following are some brief examples of this recent work, especially as it is pertinent to compensation theory.

Two recent studies using neuroimaging techniques are especially noteworthy. Becker et al. (1996a, 1996b) examined patterns of regional cerebral blood flow (acquired via positron emission tomography, PET) during episodic retrieval performance in mildly impaired Alzheimer's disease patients, as well as in normal, older, adult controls. There is much research – both longitudinal and cross-sectional – demonstrating both ageing-related and Alzheimer's disease-related decrements in episodic memory performance (e.g. Bäckman, 1992; Craik and Jennings, 1992; Hultsch et al., 1998). Consistent with this vast research, Becker et al. found moderate deficits in episodic memory performance on the part of the Alzheimer's disease patients. Becker et al. observed an intriguing discrepancy in patterns of brain activation between the Alzheimer's disease patients and the normal controls. In comparing PET-obtained functional activity during memory performance and rest, the Alzheimer's disease patients showed activations in the same regions as the controls, but also in a broader range of regions not typically activated during verbal retrieval. Specifically, although both groups showed the typical prefrontal activation during retrieval, the Alzheimer's disease patients (unlike the controls) also showed activation in several posterior brain regions. The authors speculated that this hyperactivation in regions not typically associated with verbal memory performance could reflect altered cortical connections in Alzheimer's disease patients, who have experienced neuropathological changes. They refer to this phenomenon as compensatory hyperactivation, or compensatory reallocation of brain resources. The phenomenon is consistent with the interpretation that automatic substitution is occurring at this stage of Alzheimer's disease, perhaps as a 'response' to neurodegeneration.

Three instructive caveats should be mentioned. First, and perhaps most important, in several of the brain regions in which the Alzheimer's disease patients, as opposed to the controls, showed increased activity during retrieval (e.g. precuneus, anterior cingulate gyrus), increased activity is typically seen in young adults as well (see Cabeza and Nyberg, 1997, for an overview). Obviously, such a parallel pattern of brain activation in young adults and Alzheimer's disease patients raises questions concerning the inference that the activation pattern of these patients is a compensatory response to the neurodegenerative process. Second, the presumed compensatory hyperactivation is not entirely successful, in that the Alzheimer's disease patients did not perform the memory tasks at the level of normal older adults. However, given present knowledge on the neurodegeneration associated with Alzheimer's disease and the well-established patterns of declining cognitive performance, it is not surprising that normal levels would not be achieved. Possibly – but not yet certainly – the consequence of the apparent compensatory reallocation is that retrieval performance in Alzheimer's disease patients may be less affected than if the reallocation had not occurred.

A third caveat is that it is not clear from these data that: (a) the between-group differences in patterns of blood flow reflect changes in Alzheimer's disease patients as a function of neuropathological loss; or (b) the consequences of these presumed changes are in fact gains for these patients. Attention to such issues is inspired in part by compensation research in neighbouring domains, as discussed earlier. Further research on the mechanisms and consequences of such reallocation are being pursued, and will be required before definitive conclusions can be made about compensation. One means of determining empirically the functional significance of the altered pattern of brain activation in the Alzheimer's disease group would be to examine the relationship between breadth and degree of brain activation and actual memory performance (cf. Nyberg et al., 1996).

Buckner et al. (1996) focused also on the intriguing question of the mechanisms and extent of recovery following injury in the human brain. They presented data from a 72-year-old stroke patient (LF1), who experienced damage in portions of the left inferior frontal cortex, with no other lesions evident from magnetic resonance imaging (MRI) evidence. They codified their approach to investigating compensation following brain injury in the following manner.

The unique feature of this approach is to determine which brain area is damaged in a patient and identify tasks that are known to activate that area in neuroimaging studies of normal subjects. By testing the patient on these tasks, preserved performance can be used as a predictor of tasks likely being accomplished by compensatory brain pathways. Then, neuroimaging can be used to determine these compensatory pathways. As a final step, additional behavioral testing can be conducted to determine task capabilities potentially using the compensatory pathways. (Buckner et al., 1996, p. 1249)

Using PET techniques, Buckner et al. found that during a semantic retrieval task (word-stem completion), LF1 activated a pathway similar to normal subjects, except that it was in the right prefrontal cortex rather than in the typical left prefrontal cortex (see Frith et al., 1991; Buckner et al., 1995). (Activation in the right prefrontal cortex in normal control subjects was virtually nonexistent.) The authors are appropriately cautious and hopeful. They offer their approach for future researchers, and suggest that if the results are replicable in other aphasic patients, it may indicate one important basis for (automatic) partial recovery in aphasia.

Interactions between brain and behavioural compensation

The two forms of compensation discussed in this section occur at different levels of analysis and involve different compensatory mechanisms. Nevertheless, the concept of compensation occurring in both literatures may be incorporated into the model sketched here and presented elsewhere. Accordingly, this section closes with reference to a feature of this model (see especially Bäckman and Dixon, 1992) that has not been specifically mentioned in this chapter. In brief, the notion is that, under some conditions, these two levels of compensatory mechanisms may be profitably linked – and linked on the basis of the principles of compensation.

Although both are empirical questions, we begin with two assumptions. First, it is assumed that the consequences of both compensatory brain activation and strategic efforts are positive, that they represent functional gains for the injured person. Second, it is assumed that the degree of awareness of active compensatory mechanisms is less (and low) in the case of compensatory brain activation than it is (or could be) in the case of behavioural compensation for organic cognitive impairment. That is, people with brain injuries are unlikely to be able to initiate compensatory hyperactivation or reallocation of brain resources. They may, however, with training and deliberate effort, be able to initiate and effect some strategic compensatory behaviours. The question posed in the past is the extent to which these two processes may interact or compound one another. For example, in the process of compensation for a brain injury, it is conceivable that the initial compensation is automatic and at the neuroanatomical level. Following this, it is possible that, with guidance in neurorehabilitation or self-initiation, some patients may boost the overall functional effectiveness of their compensation through deliberate behavioural efforts. Furthermore, it is possible that eventually the two compensatory processes can continue simultaneously, resulting in even greater levels of recovery of function. As the authors reported in 1992, this linkage between the biological (neuroanatomical) and behavioural (strategic, mnemonic) levels has been supported by both animal and human data. They recommend that further interdisciplinary research be conducted explicitly linking these mechanisms in cognitive neurorehabilitation.

Conclusions

To describe compensation as a 'sublime' law of nature would require more poetic licence than the authors are willing to claim. Although compensation may not be as common, simple and poetic as portrayed by Emerson in the opening quotation, it is a process that is: (a) surprisingly common, in that it is frequently observed and studied as it operates on several levels of analysis in a wide range of psychological literature; (b) elegantly simple, in that a multifaceted appearance is belied by a coherent underlying conceptual structure; and (c) scientifically intriguing and useful to a broad swath of contemporary experimental, theoretical and applied psychologists. This chapter began with the focus on the concept of compensation, and presentation of a sketch of the authors' working definition and model. In whatever literature and through whatever mechanism, compensation involves losses and gains. Whether as a result of injury, disease, degeneration, congenital condition or decline, compensation originates in a deficit – a mismatch between skills, expectations and demands. Through the various mechanisms of substitution, remediation, accommodation or assimilation, compensation involves closing one or more gaps between skills, expectations and demands.

There are several principles through which observers may evaluate and categorize exemplars of psychological compensation. These include origins, mechanisms, awareness and consequences (for more details, see Dixon and Bäckman, 1995b; Wilson and Watson, 1996). In the field of cognitive neurorehabilitation, compensation is an important and growing concept. The chapter illustrates the application of the concept of compensation to two general areas of research, namely: (a) behavioural compensation for organic cognitive impairment, and (b) compensatory brain activation. Although different in level of analysis – as well as in other respects – compensation is an integrative concept in these two areas. In the first, the emphasis is at the behavioural or strategic level: compensation is often the product of self-initiated or other-initiated behaviour. As emphasized earlier, such compensatory behaviour may be deliberate, automatic, or both (whether sequentially or interactively). In the second, compensation may be examined in terms of plasticity at the neuroanatomical level. Although perhaps not exclusively automatic responses, numerous examples of compensatory mechanisms following brain damage (e.g. collateral sprouting) are unlikely to be under deliberate control.

In any event, rich and promising theoretical and applied research is being conducted in these areas. Further empirical linkages between these levels of analysis should be pursued. Stitching these levels together – using perhaps the thread of compensation – may serve to advance both theoretical and practical goals.

Acknowledgements

RAD acknowledges grant support from both the Natural Sciences and Engineering Research Council of Canada and the US National Institute on Ageing (AG08235). LB acknowledges support from both the Swedish Council for Social Research and the Swedish Council for Research in the Humanities and the Social Sciences. The authors appreciate the helpful comments of Ian Robertson and the technical assistance of Maria Larsson.

References

Adler, A.A. 1927. *Practice and Theory of Individual Psychology*, tr. P. Radin. New York: Harcourt, Brace. (Original work published 1920.)

Ahlsén, E. 1991. Body communication as compensation for speech in a Wernicke's aphasic: a longitudinal study. *J Commun Dis* 24, 1–12.

Bach-y-Rita, P. 1990. Brain plasticity as a basis for recovery of function in humans. *Neuropsychologia* 28, 547–54.

Bach-y-Rita, P. and Bach-y-Rita, E.W. 1990. Biological and psychosocial factors in recovery from brain damage in humans. *Can J Psychol* 44, 148–65.

Bäckman, L. 1985. Compensation and recoding: a framework for ageing and memory research. *Scand J Psychol* 26, 193–207.

Bäckman, L. 1989. Varieties of memory compensation by older adults in episodic remembering. In *Everyday Cognition in Adulthood and Late Life*, ed. L.W. Poon, D.C. Rubin and B.A. Wilson, pp. 509–44. Cambridge: Cambridge University Press.

Bäckman, L., ed. 1992. *Memory Functioning in Dementia*. Amsterdam: North-Holland.

Bäckman, L. and Dixon, R.A. 1992. Psychological compensation: a theoretical framework. *Psychol Bull* 112, 259–83.

Bäckman, L., Mäntylä, T. and Herlitz, A. 1990. The optimization of episodic remembering in old age. In *Successful Ageing: Perspective from the Behavioral Sciences*, ed. P.B. Baltes and M.M. Baltes, pp. 118–63. Cambridge: Cambridge University Press.

Becker, J.T., Mintun, M.A., Aleva, K., Wiseman, M.B., Nichols, T. and DeKosky, S.T. 1996a. Alterations in functional neuroanatomical connectivity in Alzheimer's disease: positron emission tomography of auditory verbal short-term memory. *Ann NY Acad Sci* 777, 239–42.

Becker, J.T., Mintun, M.A., Aleva, K., Wiseman, M.B., Nichols, T. and DeKosky, S.T. 1996b. Compensatory reallocation of brain resources supporting verbal episodic memory in Alzheimer's disease. *Neurology* 16, 692–700.

Brandtstädter, J. and Wentura, D. 1995. Adjustment to shifting possibility frontiers in later life: complementary adaptive modes. In *Compensating for Psychological Deficits and Declines: Managing Losses and Promoting Gains*, ed. R.A. Dixon and L. Bäckman, pp. 83–106. Mahwah, NJ: Erlbaum.

Buckner, R.L., Corbetta, M., Schatz, J., Raichle, M.E. and Petersen, S.E. 1996. Preserved speech abilities and compensation following prefrontal damage. *Proc Natl Acad Sci* 93, 1249–53.

Buckner, R.L., Petersen, S.E., Ojemann, J.G., Miezin, F.M., Squire, L.R. and Raichle, M.E. 1995. Functional anatomical studies of explicit and implicit retrieval tasks. *J Neurosci* 15, 12–29.

Cabeza, R. and Nyberg, L. 1997. Imaging cognition: an empirical review of PET studies with normal subjects. *J Cogn Neurosci* 9, 1–26.

Carstensen, L.L., Hanson, K.A. and Freund, A.M. 1995. Selection and compensation in adulthood. In *Compensating for Psychological Deficits and Declines: Managing Losses and Promoting Gains*, ed. R.A. Dixon and L. Bäckman, pp. 107–26. Mahwah, NJ: Erlbaum.

Craik, F.I.M. and Jennings, J.M. 1992. Human memory. In *The Handbook of Aging and Cognition*, ed. F.I.M. Craik and T.A. Salthouse, pp. 51–110. Hillsdale, NJ: Erlbaum.

Dixon, R.A. 1996. Collaborative memory and ageing. In *Basic and Applied Memory Research: Theory in Context*, ed. D. Herrmann, C. McEvoy, C. Hertzog, P. Hertel and M.K. Johnson, pp. 359–83. Mahwah, NJ: Erlbaum.

Dixon, R.A. and L. Bäckman, L. 1993. The concept of compensation in cognitive ageing: the case of prose processing in adulthood. *Int J Aging Hum Dev* 36, 199–217.

Dixon, R.A. and Bäckman, L. (ed.) 1995a. *Compensating for Psychological Deficits and Declines: Managing Losses and Promoting Gains*. Mahway, NJ: Erlbaum.

Dixon, R.A. and Bäckman, L. 1995b. Concepts of compensation: integrated, differentiated, and Janus-faced. In *Compensating for Psychological Deficits and Declines: Managing Losses and Promoting Gains*, ed. R.A. Dixon and L. Bäckman, pp. 3–20. Mahwah, NJ: Erlbaum.

Dixon, R.A. and Gould, O.N. 1996. Adults telling and retelling stories collaboratively. In *Interactive Minds: Life-span Perspectives on the Social Foundation of Cognition*, ed. P.B. Baltes and U.M. Staudinger, pp. 221–41. Cambridge: Cambridge University Press.

Emerson, R.W. 1900. *Compensation*. New York: Caldwell.

Ericsson, K.A. and Charness, N. 1994. Expert performance: its structure and acquisition. *Am Psychol* **49**, 725–47.

Ericsson, K.A. and Simon, H.A. 1984. *Protocol Analysis: Verbal Reports as Data*. Cambridge, MA: MIT Press.

Fox, D.P. 1997. Effects of collaboration on problem solving performance in healthy elderly couples and Parkinsonian–caregiver dyads. Unpublished doctoral dissertation, University of Victoria, Victoria, BC, Canada.

Frith, C.D., Friston, K.J., Liddle, P.S. and Frackowiak, R. 1991. A PET study of word finding. *Neuropsychologia* **29**, 1137–48.

Gehring, W.J., Goss, B., Coles, M.G.H., Meyer, D.E. and Donchin, E. 1993. A neural system for error detection and compensation. *Psychol Sci* **4**, 385–90.

Gonzalez Rothi, L.J. 1995. Behavioral compensation in the case of treatment of acquired language disorders resulting from brain damage. In *Compensating for Psychological Deficits and Declines: Managing Losses and Promoting Gains*, ed. R.A. Dixon and L. Bäckman, pp. 219–30. Mahwah, NJ: Erlbaum.

Grady, C.L. and Parasuraman, R. 1995. Functional compensation in Alzheimer's disease. In *Compensating for Psychological Deficits and Declines: Managing Losses and Promoting Gains*, ed. R.A. Dixon and L. Bäckman, pp. 231–48. Mahwah, NJ: Erlbaum.

Hartmann, G.W. 1933. Changes in visual acuity through simultaneous stimulation of other sense organs. *J Exp Psychol* **16**, 393–407.

Hayes, S.P. 1933. New experimental data on the old problem of sensory compensation. *Teachers Forum* **5**, 22–6.

Herlitz, A., Adolfsson, R., Bäckman, L. and Nilsson, L.-G. 1991. Cue utilization following different forms of encoding in mildly, moderately, and severely demented patients with Alzheimer's disease. *Brain Cogn* **15**, 119–30.

Herlitz, A., Lipsinska, B. and Bäckman, L. 1992. Utilization of cognitive support for episodic remembering in Alzheimer's disease. In *Memory Functioning in Dementia*, ed. L. Bäckman, pp. 73–96. Amsterdam: North-Holland.

Hultsch, D.F., Hertzog, C., Dixon, R.A. and Small, B. 1998. *Memory Change in the Aged*. New York: Cambridge University Press.

Kliegl, R. and Baltes, P.B. 1987. Theory-guided analysis of development and aging mechanisms through testing-the-limits and research on expertise. In *Cognitive Functioning and Social Structure over the Life Course*, ed. C. Schooler and K.W. Schaie, pp. 95–119. Norwood, NJ: Erlbaum.

Kolb, B. and Whishaw, I.Q. 1996. *Fundamentals of Human Neuropsychology*, 4th edn. New York: Freeman.

Lashley, K.S. 1924. Studies of cerebral functioning in learning: V. The retention of motor habits after destruction of the so-called motor areas in primates. *Arch Neurol Psychiatry* **12**, 249–76.

LeVere, N.D. and LeVere, T.E. 1982. Recovery of function after brain damage: support for the compensation theory of the behavioural deficit. *Physiol Psychol* **10**, 165–74.

Luria, A.R. 1963. *Restoration of Function after Brain Injury*. New York: MacMillan.

Luria, A.R. 1966. *Higher Cortical Functions in Man*. New York: Basic Books.

Marsiske, M., Lang, F.R., Baltes, P.B. and Baltes, M.M. 1995. Selective optimization with compensation: life-span perspectives on successful human develoment. In *Compensating for Psychological Deficits and Declines: Managing Losses and Promoting Gains*, ed. R.A. Dixon and L. Bäckman, pp. 35–79. Mahwah, NJ: Erlbaum.

Masterton, B.A. and Biederman, G.B. 1983. Proprioceptive versus visual control in autistic children. *J Autism Dev Disord* **13**, 141–52.

Mateer, C.A. 1996. Rehabilitation of individuals with frontal lobe impairment. In *Neuropsychological Rehabilitation and Treatment of Brain Injury*, ed. J. Leon-Carrion, pp. 285–300. Delory Beach, FL: St Lucie Press.

Munk, H.M. 1881. *Über die Funktion der Grosshirnrinde: Gesammelte Mittheilungen aus den Jahren 1877–80* [On the function of the cerebral cortex: collected works from the years 1877–80]. Berlin: Hirschwald.

Neville, H.J. 1990. Intermodal competition and compensation in development: evidence from studies of the visual system in congenitally deaf adults. In *The Development and Neural Bases of Higher Cognitive Functions*, ed. A. Diamond, pp. 71–91. New York: New York Academy of Sciences.

Nyberg, L., McIntosh, A.R., Houle, S., Nilsson, L.-G. and Tulving, E. 1996. Activation of medial temporal structures during episodic memory retrieval. *Nature* **380**, 715–17.

Ohlsson, K. 1986. Compensation as skill. In *Communication and Handicap: Aspects of Psychological Compensation and Technical Aids*, ed. E. Hjelmquist and L.-G. Nilsson, pp. 85–101. Amsterdam: North-Holland.

Rönnberg, J. 1995. Perceptual compensation in the deaf and blind: myth or reality? In *Compensating for Psychological Deficits and Declines: Managing Losses and Promoting Gains*, ed. R.A. Dixon and L. Bäckman, pp. 251–74. Mahwah, NJ: Erlbaum.

Rothi, L.J. and Horner, J. 1983. Restitution and substitution: two theories of recovery with applications to neurobehavioral treatment. *J Clin Neuropsychol* **5**, 73–81.

Salthouse, T.A. 1984. Effects of age and skill in typing. *Exp Psychol Gen* **113**, 345–71.

Salthouse, T.A. 1987. Age, experience, and compensation. In *Cognitive Functioning and Social Structure over the Life Course*, ed. C. Schooler and K.W. Schaie, pp. 142–50. New York: Ablex.

Salthouse, T.A. 1990. Cognitive competence and expertise in aging. In *Handbook of the Psychology of Aging*, 3rd edn, ed. J.E. Birren and K.W. Schaie, pp. 310–19. San Diego, CA: Academic Press.

Salthouse, T.A. 1995. Refining the concept of psychological compensation. In *Compensating for Psychological Deficits and Declines: Managing Losses and Promoting Gains* ed. R.A. Dixon and L. Bäckman, pp. 21–34. Mahwah, NJ: Erlbaum.

Scheff, S.W. (ed.) 1984. *Aging and Recovery of Function in the Central Nervous System*. New York: Plenum Press.

Smith, P.F. and Curthoys, I.S. 1989. Mechanisms of recovery following unilateral labyrinthectomy: a review. *Brain Res Rev* **14**, 155–80.

Stanovich, K.E. 1984. The interactive–compensatory model of reading: a confluence of developmental, experimental, and educational psychology. *Rem Spec Educ* **5**, 11–19.

Stevens, J.C., Foulke, E. and Patterson, M.Q. 1996. Tactile acuity, ageing and Braille reading in long-term blindness. *J Exp Psychol* **2**, 91–106.

Szlyk, J.P., Seiple, W. and Viana, M. 1995. Relative effects of age and compromised vision on driving performance. *Hum Factors* **37**, 430–6.

Towne, R.L. 1994. Effect of mandibular stabilization on the diadochokinetic performance of children with phonological disorder. *J Phonetics*, **22**, 317–32.

Wasserman, G.A., Allen, R. and Solomon, C.R. 1985. At-risk toddlers and their mothers: the special case of physical handicaps. *Child Dev* **56**, 73–83.

West, R.F., Stanovich, K.E. and Cunningham, A.E. 1995. Compensatory processes in reading. In *Compensating for Psychological Deficits and Declines: Managing Losses and Promoting Gains* ed. R.A. Dixon and L. Bäckman, pp. 275–96. Mahwah, NJ: Erlbaum.

Wilson, B.A. 1995. Memory rehabilitation: compensating for memory problems. In *Compensating for Psychological Deficits and Declines: Managing Losses and Promoting Gains*, ed. R.A. Dixon and L. Bäckman, pp. 171–90. Mahwah, NJ: Erlbaum.

Wilson, B.A. and Watson, P.C. 1996. A practical framework for understanding compensatory behaviour in people with organic memory impairment. *Memory* **4**, 456–86.

Woodruff-Pak, D.S. and Hanson, C. 1995. Plasticity and compensation in brain memory systems in aging. In *Compensating for Psychological Deficits and Declines: Managing Losses and Promoting Gains*, ed. R.A. Dixon and L. Bäckman, pp. 191–218. Mahwah, NJ: Erlbaum.

5

Brain damage, sex hormones and recovery

Donald G. Stein, Robin L. Roof and Zoltan L. Fulop

Introduction

- Brain injury is a complex cascade of events that unfolds over relatively long periods of time.
- Sex differences in response to brain injury have not been given much attention for social, political, economic and methodological reasons.

Traumatic brain injury afflicts almost 500 000 people per year in the USA alone and 50 000 of these patients will die of their injuries (Greenberg and Brawanski, 1994). Of those individuals with moderate to severe brain damage, only about 15 per cent will be able to return to regular employment similar to that which they had prior to their accident (Sakata and Leung, 1991). This poor prognosis for brain-injury victims is primarily due to the lack of safe and effective treatments. The focus of research in developing such treatments has, until recently, been limited by the long-standing belief that repair of damage in the central nervous system was not possible. With the recent surge in neurotrauma research, however, our knowledge of the complex nature of brain injury has improved. The severity of damage sustained by the brain at the time of the trauma is now known to be only the beginning of events determining the final outcome for the victim. Of equal importance is the complex cascade of biochemical processes which is triggered by the initial injury and which may last for days or weeks. These 'secondary injury processes', which include cerebral oedema, excitotoxic cell death, calcium overload and lipid peroxidation, to list just a few, can greatly exacerbate the extent of tissue loss and functional impairment. A number of potential treatments for brain injury are aimed at modifying these secondary consequences and limiting the extent of neuronal loss.

Despite the recent advances in neurotrauma research, there is still very little known about how the different sexes respond to traumatic brain injury and whether there are any sex differences in the mechanisms of brain injury and repair. This is primarily because the overwhelming majority of studies of brain injury have included only males as subjects. One reason for this is because laboratory researchers are reluctant to include females in their studies because of the added complications produced by hormone fluctuations associated with the female menstrual cycle. The common assumption is that results from studies of brain injury in males will apply to females as well. Furthermore, the increased time and cost involved in comparing males and females, while at the same time controlling for hormonal cycles, discourages the addressing of the issue of sex differences in these studies.

The prevalence of this inattention to sex differences in brain injury outcome is demonstrated by the authors' informal survey of 210 articles in five neuroscience journals (*Brain Research, Experimental Neurology, Journal of Neuroscience, Neuroscience*, and *Restorative Neurology and Neuroscience*) covering a span of 24 months. It was observed that 86 papers specifically identified males as the subjects, whereas 76 did not trouble to specify which sex was used in the experiments (it can be assumed that the subjects were males). Of the 210 papers, only three studied sex differences on any of the outcome measures. Avoidance of female subjects in research is not limited to animal studies. Until the recently initiated changes at the National Institutes of Health mandated new drug development protocols, human female subjects were rarely tested because of the potential risk of affecting their childbearing, even though their hormonal fluctuations could have a significant influence on drug kinetics, metabolism and central nervous system activity. In fact, the US General Accounting Office took the National Institutes of Health[1] to task for not implementing its own, as well as the Food and Drug Administration's, guidelines requiring women to be included in biomedical research and Phase 1 and Phase 2 drug testing (Jensvold, Heilbreich and Hamilton, 1996).

In spite of the lack of attention to sex differences in neurotrauma research, substantial evidence from other areas of neuroscience supports the idea that such differences may be an important factor in the brain's response to injury. The well-known dimorphisms between male and female brains emphasize the importance that the sex hormones may have on brain function and structures throughout the lifespan.

Sexual dimorphism of the brain

- There are brain structures that differ in shape and size in males and females of a number of different species, including humans.
- Some structures are said to be larger in females, such as the corpus callosum and posterior temporal cortex.
- Dendritic branching and synaptic contacts may be influenced by fluctuations in gonadal hormones such as oestrogen.

Early work on sexual dimorphism focused on describing the anatomical differences in brain structures that were thought to mediate mating and reproductive behaviours. Some of these differences are easy to observe, whereas others are more subtle. One of the most striking examples of sexually dimorphic brains is seen in the canary. Fernando Nottebohm and his students (Nottebohm and Arnold, 1976; Nottebohm, 1985) have shown that the differences in song behaviour of male and female canaries are sexually 'dimorphic' and depend upon the presence of testosterone. Male canaries have neural centres involved in singing that are four times larger than the homologous structures in females,

which do not sing – unless they are treated with testosterone. The hormone treatments given to adult females practically double the size of the nuclei that mediate song behaviour and their songs mimic those of the males. As the hormone is metabolized, the size of the nuclei shrink back to female size and the canaries stop singing.

Some studies indicate that the human male brain volume is, on average, 10 per cent larger than that of the female (Allen and Gorski, 1990), whereas others suggest that females have larger brains in relation to body size (Juraska, 1986; Peters, 1991). Some specific brain areas, such as the corpus callosum and anterior commissures, are said to be larger in females (deLacoste, Adesanya and Woodward, 1990; Witelson and Kigar, 1993); other studies report a dramatic sex difference in the shape of these structures (Allen et al., 1991; Allen and Gorski, 1991). Simon LeVay (LeVay, 1994) has claimed that hemispheric lateralization is not the same for human males and females. Recently, Witelson, Glezer and Kigar (1995) examined the posterior temporal cortex in cognitively normal human males and females who were all right handed. Neuron counts were taken in both hemispheres and through each of the six layers comprising the cortex. The number of neurons per unit volume (cell packing density) was 11 per cent greater in females and was particularly obvious in layers II and IV of this cortical region. The authors point out that these neuromorphological differences could account for the known sex differences in cognitive functions such as verbal fluency and visuospatial perception that are seen when men and women are tested on these tasks. Witelson et al. point out that in most anatomical studies, very little attention is paid to sex differences in the microscopic structure of the human cortex. They refer to an 'influential' article by Rockel, Horns and Powell (1980) which concluded that, with respect to the number of neurons in cortical columns, there is a basic uniformity in the cortex across and within mammalian species. Witelson et al. noted that these conclusions were drawn from the study of only two human brains – both of which were male.

In the rodent hippocampus, a part of the brain implicated in memory storage and retrieval, females show changes in dendritic branching and densities of synaptic contacts depending upon in what stage of the oestrus cycle they are. For example, McEwen and Wooley (1994) have shown that dendritic spine density can be increased in the CA1 area by giving oestradiol and can be decreased by giving progesterone. Similar fluctuations in dendritic spine density and synaptogenesis take place over a 24-hour period between pro-oestrus and oestrus. Females also show greater dendritic branching than males in response to enriched environments (Juraska, 1986).

Sex differences in brain functions

- Although the performance of intact laboratory rats on cognitive and spatial tasks may be the same, the behavioural response to traumatic brain injury may differ dramatically in male and female animals.
- Cognitive performance in healthy human females can vary with the phases of their menstrual cycle.
- Males with left hemisphere lesions appear to be more impaired in speech and praxis than females with the same injury.
- Male and female human subjects appear to use different brain areas to process information and perform cognitive tasks.

Lesion experiments coupled with behavioural testing have also been used to describe 'dimorphic' cognitive responses to brain injury. Patricia Goldman (1974) was one of the first to demonstrate sex differences in the cognitive behaviour of rhesus monkeys which had been brain damaged in early life. Male and female monkeys received bilateral orbitofrontal cortex lesions at 50 days of age and testing then began for object discrimination learning. The males with this injury were impaired in object reversal learning when they were tested at 2.5 months of age, but females with the same surgery did not differ in performance from their intact counterparts. In other experiments, Goldman examined male and female monkeys which had orbitofrontal surgery at 50 days of age and were then retested a year later on delayed response performance to determine if they had persistent deficits. Goldman reported that the females were much less impaired in their cognitive performance than the males when tested as 'toddlers', but the differences disappeared when the animals were tested

again at 18 months of age. She suggested that males were worse because their orbitofrontal cortex developed and became functional more rapidly, so that its removal at an early stage of life led to greater cognitive deficits than would be seen in the less developed female orbital region.

Sex differences in recovery from brain injury have also been observed in rats when lesions are inflicted at maturity. In one recent experiment (Roof, Duvdevani and Stein, 1993), unilateral lesions of the entorhinal cortex were produced in adult male and female Sprague–Dawley rats and testing began seven days later for learning and retention on a spatial navigation task in the Morris water maze. This task requires the rats to find a submerged platform in milky water by using distal cues situated around the circular tank, and therefore it is considered to be a spatial reference memory task. During each test period, animals are placed individually into the tank at different starting points (N, S, E, W). This experimental paradigm was used because unilateral lesions of the entorhinal cortex have been shown to produce substantial impairments on this task, which depends on an intact working memory (Glasier et al., 1995). It was found that normal, uninjured male and female controls had the same ability to learn quickly the shortest route to the platform, indicating that there were no differences in normal cognitive performance of the two sexes. After injury to the entorhinal cortex, a different picture emerged. The brain-injured male rats were significantly more impaired in the retention of the spatial learning task than the brain-injured females, whose performance did not differ from their normal counterparts, despite the fact that the extent of the entorhinal cortex damage was the same for males and females.

In humans, Doreen Kimura (1994) has shown that cognitive performance can vary with the phases of the menstrual cycle in healthy females and with longer-term, seasonal variations in testosterone in males. In one study, Hampson and Kimura (1988; Kimura, 1987) found that normal, young adult women fluctuated in their intellectual performance according to where they were in their menstrual cycle at the time that they were tested. During the midluteal phase, performance was better on motor coordination tasks (finger tapping,

Purdue pegboard, sequencing tasks) and worse on visual perceptual–spatial tasks (Witkin rod and frame test) as compared to performance during menstruation. During the midluteal phase, the women were less accurate in their ability to align a rod to a true vertical position than they were during menstruation. The authors suggested that high levels of female hormones enhanced performance on tasks at which females excel but made them worse on tasks at which men excel, speculating that sex differences on cognitive tasks may have a substantial hormonal basis.

There is also a growing number of neuropsychological and metabolic studies showing that there are sex differences in the cerebral organization of speech and praxis. For example, Lansdell (1973) found that men with left hemisphere lesions to treat parkinsonism or with temporal lobe epilepsy had more difficulty in making popular word associations than females with the same injury. When tested years later to determine the extent of recovery (Lansdell, 1989), the women showed better recovery than the men regardless of the type of surgery performed initially. Kimura (1983) examined the incidence of aphasia and apraxia in 143 male and 73 female right-handed patients who had suffered unilateral lesions of the left hemisphere and in another group of 81 patients who had damage to the anterior or posterior cortical regions. Aphasia was more frequent in the males and there were differences in the areas representing speech between the sexes. The females had speech and apraxic disorders more often from damage to the anterior part of the left hemisphere than to the posterior region, whereas this was not true for the males. Kimura also notes that there are sex differences in parietal lobe function: 'Both brain lesions and cortical stimulation in the left parietal region produce speech disorders less frequently in women than in men; however, lesions of the left anterior hemisphere produce a high incidence of apraxia in women' (Kimura, 1983, p. 1084).

More recent studies have used sophisticated scanning techniques to demonstrate that human male and female subjects use different brain areas to process information and perform cognitive tasks. For example, Shaywitz et al. (1995) used functional magnetic resonance imaging (fMRI) to study sex differences in cerebral blood flow during the performance of letter recognition, rhyming and semantic categorization tasks in healthy male and female volunteers. During the performance of these tasks, the cerebral activation (as indicated by increased blood flow to the region) in males was lateralized to the left frontal cortex, whereas in women the pattern of cerebral activation was much more diffuse and was seen in both left and right hemispheres. Murphy et al. (1996) recently also used MRI, and positron emission tomography (PET) to look at sex differences in brain structures and glucose metabolism as a function of ageing. They undertook this study because postmortem examinations have found, among other morphological changes, that brain weights decrease earlier in females than in males, whereas ventricular enlargements occur earlier in males than in females. All of the subjects were participants in a clinical programme on brain ageing conducted at the National Institute on Ageing, Bethesda, Maryland. All were right handed, medication free, and did not differ significantly in age or intelligence. The subjects were divided into young (20–35 years) or old (60–85 years) groups and all were tested on the Wechsler Adult Intelligence Scale (WAIS). On MRI, women had a significantly larger volume of thalamic and caudate nuclei than men, but there was greater right–left asymmetry of the lateral ventricles in men. Men had a greater age-related decrease in the total volume of the cerebral hemispheres than women, who in turn had more loss of volume in the parietal lobes and hippocampus.

With respect to metabolic activity (PET), there was significantly less right–left metabolic asymmetry in females than in males, but women had a greater age-related metabolic decline in the hippocampus and thalamus than males. In general, age-related declines in metabolism in men were greater in the left than in the right hemisphere; whereas in women the ageing effect was more or less equal in both hemispheres. These sex differences in the locations of increased cerebral blood flow could explain why drugs affecting central nervous system function could have differential effects in males and females. This especially could be the case in younger subjects, in whom fluctuations in the hormonal milieu are more likely to play a larger role than in later life.

Sex hormones have a direct influence on central nervous system organization and response to brain injury

- Some cerebral function(s) in females may be more bilaterally distributed than in males, who show more lateralized functions.
- Differences in anatomical organization may be *one* reason why females have a more favourable outcome after traumatic brain injury than males.
- Traumatic brain injury timed to coincide with pro-oestrus affects the functional outcome of the injury in laboratory animals.
- Female rats injured when progesterone levels are high compared to oestrogen are much *less* impaired than females injured when their progesterone levels are low relative to oestrogen.

Differences in the anatomical organization of male and female brains during development and at maturity can be used to explain why females may have more favourable (or at least different) outcomes following cerebral stroke or trauma than males. The reasoning behind this idea is that if cortical information processing or cerebral function in females is bilaterally distributed, whereas in males it is unilateral, then damage to the dominant hemisphere of the male is likely to result in more disruption of cognitive behaviours than if the 'functions' are more diffuse, as is reported to be the case for females. Kimura (1987) also provides additional hypotheses to account for sex differences in brain organization which, in turn, could account for the *functional* differences that are observed after brain injury.

1. Differential specialization of the two hemispheres in males and females: for example, language function may be localized to the left hemisphere in males, whereas it is represented in both hemispheres in females.
2. Differential 'allotment' of total brain space to various traits or abilities, regardless of hemisphere: thus, spatial ability might require more neurons in males,

whereas language might take up more neural space in females.
3. Within hemispheres, cortical and subcortical functions could be organized differently.
4. Given the organizational and morphological differences, the same hormones and other neurochemicals could exert different effects.
5. All of the above could account for sex differences in the outcome of brain injury.

Although the differences in lateralization of function and cerebral organization could be employed to explain why females with certain types of brain injury recover better than males, there might be another explanation related to the presence of specific sex hormones at the time of injury. In other words, for females especially, the timing of brain damage with respect to hormonal fluctuations could be as important as the locus of the injury in determining the severity of deficits and functional outcomes.

To examine this idea, in one of the authors' earlier experiments with laboratory rats (Attella, Nattinville and Stein, 1987), it was decided to determine whether brain surgery timed to coincide with pro-oestrus would affect the functional outcome of bilateral removals of the medial frontal cortex. Lesions were made of the frontal cortex because extensive injury to this brain area results in severe and long-lasting deficits in the ability to solve spatial learning tasks in both rats and humans. There is also clinical evidence suggesting that female patients with injury of the frontal cortex are less impaired on cognitive tasks than males with the same locus of injury (Basso, Capitani and Moraschini, 1983). Female rats were used which were 90 days of age at the start of the experiment. Normal cycling rats had surgery on the day of their pro-oestrus when oestrogen levels were at their peak. Surgery for the pseudopregnant rats was done on the sixth day of pseudopregnancy when progesterone was at its peak. Pseudopregnancy was induced by mild cervical stimulation, which produces a surge in progesterone levels that lasts eight to ten days after induction. In pro-oestrus, oestrogen is high while progesterone is relatively low.

When the intact, normal cycling and pseudopregnant rats were tested on their ability to learn a delayed spatial learning task in a T-maze, there were no differences in performance between the two groups. Unlike the human results mentioned above (Hampson and Kimura, 1988), hormonal state at the time of testing in intact, healthy female rats did not appear to have any effect on cognitive performance on this task. Once the animals learned the spatial alternation problem, they were subjected to bilateral removals of the medial frontal cortex or to sham surgery with no damage to brain tissue. When tested, all of the rats with lesions were worse than intact controls, as might be expected after such substantial damage. However, when postoperative performance of the pseudopregnant and normal cycling females was examined, some interesting differences emerged. On each of three measures of relearning, the pseudopregnant rats showed better retention than those which suffered the same extent of damage during their normal cycling. In other words, when progesterone[2] levels were high relative to oestrogen, bilateral removals of the frontal cortex produced less cognitive impairment than the same injury inflicted when oestrogen levels were higher relative to progesterone.

When the brain tissue was examined for histological verification of the lesions, there were no significant differences in the extent of the lesions between the normal cycling and pseudopregnant rats. However, it was noted that there was substantially less ventricular dilatation in pseudopregnant rats compared to what was observed in the normal cycling females. It is interesting to note that higher levels of oestradiol at the time of injury are accompanied by higher levels of antidiuretic hormone released by oestrogen-sensitive neurons in the hypothalamus (Pfaff and McEwen, 1983). Increased water retention caused by the circulation of antidiuretic hormone could lead to increased blood and intracranial pressure and thus to the ventricular dilatation observed in the normal cycling, brain-injured rats. Rats injured during pseudopregnancy would have decreased plasma levels of antidiuretic hormones and therefore less oedema-induced intracranial pressure. The authors hypothesized that the enlarged ventricles could be taken to reflect the neuronal loss caused by the initial oedema and that progesterone may have prevented or reduced the oedema caused by the initial lesions.

Progesterone plays an important role in determining the outcome of brain injury

- Bilateral contusions of medial frontal cortex lead to profound cognitive and learning deficits in humans, nonhuman primates and laboratory animals.
- Contusions will cause extensive necrosis and extensive cerebral oedema in the lesion area as well as apoptosis and diffuse axonal injury in remote structures.
- There are very few, if any, effective clinically approved treatments for severe traumatic brain injury.
- Males have significantly more cerebral oedema following traumatic brain injury than females with the same extent and locus of injury.
- Glucocorticoids such as methylprednisolone are specifically *not* recommended for the treatment of severe head trauma.

The areas of the human brain that are most likely to be damaged by contusion are the anteroinferior, frontotemporal lobes and the parasagittal convexities (Gean, Kates and Lee, 1995). To model this type of injury, the frontal cortex was exposed in anaesthetized rats and then a pneumatic piston device was used (Hoffman, Fulop and Stein, 1994) to create a contusion of the medial frontal cortex in both males and females.

Contusion injury, in addition to necrosis and cell death, produces substantial oedema, haematomas, and diffuse axonal injury typical of what is also seen in human patients (Gean et al., 1995). Cerebral oedema, often occurring after brain contusion, is one of the most common and serious complications of head injury, leading to additional neuronal loss and even death of the patient; however, there is currently no completely effective (and safe) clinical treatment to control it. Recently, the American Association of Neurological Surgeons and the Brain Trauma Foundation published guidelines for the management of severe head injury (Bullock et al., 1996). The guidelines note that the osmotic diuretic drug mannitol has been used to reduce cerebral perfusion pressure and blood viscosity, although its use has never been subjected to a controlled clinical trial against placebo. Mannitol can also produce acute renal failure if administered in large doses and therefore may not be suitable as a prolonged therapy for postinjury oedema. Similarly, etomidate in

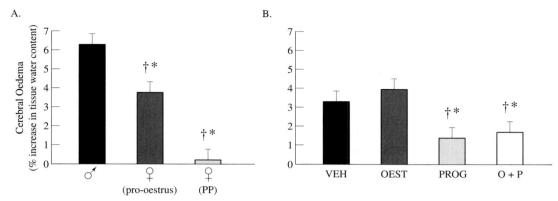

Fig. 5.1 The percentage increase in the water content of brain tissue samples from injured areas compared to noninjured distal areas taken 24 hours after a medial frontal cortical contusion injury. A. Samples from male, pro-oestrus female, and pseudopregnant (PP) female rats. B. Samples from ovariectomized female rats given no hormones (VEH), oestrogen implants (OEST), progesterone alone (PROG), or oestrogen implants and progesterone injections (O + P). Asterisks indicate significant differences ($p<0.05$) from shams. Crosses indicate significant difference ($p<0.05$) from the oil-treated group.

propylene glycol vehicle has sometimes been used for the control of refractory cerebral oedema (Levy et al., 1995; McConnell et al., 1996), but it appeared to cause lactic acidosis, haemolysis and renal complications. In another approach, the long-term administration of high colloid oncotics has also been tried as a treatment for vasogenic oedema caused by brain contusion in human patients (Tomita et al., 1994). The treatment group received 25% albumin solution administered intravenously for two weeks postinjury. Maintaining high oncotic pressure (26–30 mmHg) for the 14-day duration resulted in significantly less oedema, no renal failure and fewer neurological deficits than were observed in the untreated patients, of whom 30 per cent remained in poor condition. Similar results were obtained in a gerbil model of ischaemia by Hakamata et al. (1995), but in work by Tomita et al. (1994), no cognitive testing was done to determine if functional recovery resulted from the reduced oedema. For more detailed information concerning brain oedema after head injury and its possible treatments, readers are referred to the following review papers: Kimelberg (1992), Shapira and Shohami (1993) and Kempski and Volk (1994). Glucocorticoids such as methylprednisolone have also been used in patients undergoing surgery for tumours and for the treatment of severe head injuries (Gobiet et al., 1976; Dearden et al., 1986;

Hall, 1992), but most clinical trials studying methylprednisolone treatment for severe head injury did not reveal any beneficial effects (Kelly, 1995). In fact, the guidelines specifically do *not* recommend glucocorticoids for improving brain injury outcome or for reducing intracranial pressure.

Because the effects of gender and the role of gonadal hormones in the cascade of events that follow brain damage are relatively unexplored, the authors decided to examine the effects of cerebral contusions on the formation of postinjury oedema in male and female rats (Roof et al., 1993). In the first part of the study, three groups of mature rats were used: males, pseudopregnant females, and normal cycling females in pro-oestrus. The animals received bilateral contusions of the medial frontal cortex while under deep anaesthesia. For the females, the contusions were produced on the sixth day of pseudopregnancy or on the day of pro-oestrus in the normal cycling group. Control groups received the same anaesthesia and placement in a stereotaxic apparatus, but no further surgery.

As can be seen in Fig. 5.1A, the brain-injured males had much more cerebral oedema than females with the same brain injury. The males showed more than a 6 per cent increase in water content compared to control tissue taken from the posterior cortex. Although the normally cycling females showed a significant increase in postinjury oedema (3.5 per cent), they remained well below the levels evidenced by the males. The pseudo-pregnant females showed *no evidence of cerebral oedema in the lesion area* (0.3 per cent water content), indicating that the hormonal state at the time of brain injury played a determining role in the functional outcome of the trauma. It is important to note that in this study, endogenous levels of progesterone sufficient to sustain pregnancy were enough to reduce cerebral oedema almost to levels seen in nonbrain-injured animals.

Targeting progesterone as the key factor in reducing the effects of brain injury

- It is the presence of progesterone and *not* oestrogen which is the critical factor in reducing cerebral oedema caused by traumatic brain injury.
- Exogenous administration of progesterone also reduces cerebral oedema in males with traumatic brain injury.
- Both male and female rats treated with progesterone injections show evidence of better *functional* recovery on a cognitive, spatial learning task.
- In addition to reducing oedema, progesterone treatment rescues neurons that would die during retrograde degeneration.

To rule out the possibility that, in the females, the observed effects were due to the oestrogen rather than to the progesterone, it was decided to add additional groups of rats that had been ovariectomized prior to brain injury in order to eliminate the endogenous sources of oestrogen and progesterone. One week after this surgery, five groups were formed, of which one group received oestrogen implants (5-mm silastic capsules filled with crystalline 17-b E_2) followed by injections of progesterone (4 mg/kg for six days), one group received oestrogen and progesterone injections, one group received progesterone injections alone, and one group was given only oestrogen treatment and the last group was given only the oil vehicle. Following cortical contusions, tissue samples were taken and analysed as described above. In the ovariectomized animals with no treatment or just oestrogen implants, there was about a 4 per cent increase in water content, whereas the females given progesterone treatment

alone or combined with oestrogen had less than a 2 per cent increase following the same injury. These data are presented graphically in Fig. 5.1B.

The authors take these findings to indicate that the presence of progesterone and not oestrogen was the critical factor in reducing the levels of cerebral oedema following severe contusions of the frontal cortex. In fact, ovariectomized rats given the oestrogen implants had levels of oedema equivalent to those of the ovariectomized rats with no treatments, indicating that the removal of circulating oestrogen does not have any effect on the formation of oedema after brain damage. As circulating oestrogen was surgically eliminated in some animals and positive effects of the progesterone injections were still obtained, it might be the case that progesterone does not act to reduce oedema via the oestrogen-mediated progesterone receptor (McLuskey and McEwen, 1978). Recent studies have shown that progesterone receptors can be found in the plasma membrane of nerve tissue of both sexes and that locus may account for the rapid effects of steroid hormones in the central nervous system because it can act by nongenomic mechanisms (Ke and Ramirez, 1990). Some authors have suggested that, because of its rapid metabolism, progesterone may not be acting as progesterone per se but rather exerts its effects through reduced metabolites that could activate other neuroendocrine functions (Karavolas et al., 1984). Although the authors cannot describe a specific, neuronal receptor mechanism to explain the beneficial effects of progesterone, several potential pathways by which the hormone might act to enhance recovery from brain damage are discussed in the latter part of this chapter.

Because the progesterone appeared to have such salutary effects in females with brain injury, it became reasonable to ask whether brain-injured males could also benefit from the exogenous administration of progesterone. Would progesterone be likely to have effects in male subjects, and how might it act on damaged nerve tissue? One potentially negative side-effect of the hormone is that, over the course of prolonged treatment, progesterone or its metabolites can reduce sexual activity in males (Connolly, Handa and Resko, 1988; Zumpe et al., 1996); however, in the face of massive brain damage, the potentially beneficial effects of acute progesterone treatment would probably outweigh the disadvantage of temporarily reduced sexual potency. The authors decided to proceed with an experiment designed to determine if progesterone treatment in males could attenuate cerebral oedema after contusion injury. They were also encouraged by the results and conclusions of a study conducted by Betz and Coester (1990) who examined the effects of steroids on oedema and sodium uptake during focal ischaemia in rats. These investigators *pretreated* adult male rats with progesterone one hour before the rats received four hours of middle cerebral artery occlusion. Betz and Coester reported that the rats given either progesterone or dexamethasone had significantly reduced postischaemic oedema, although the dexamethasone was more effective in reducing the size of the ischaemic zone. They stated that 'the fact that progesterone has any effect at all on ischaemic brain oedema and blood–brain-barrier permeability suggests that its effect is not mediated through corticosteroid receptors since progesterone has a negligible interaction with these receptors' (Betz and Coester, 1990, p. 1203).

Progesterone (4 mg/kg) was administered by subcutaneous injection to male and female rats beginning one hour *after* bilateral contusion injury to the medial frontal cortex and then at 6, 24, and 48 hours after surgery (Roof et al., 1992). The females received their contusions during the pro-oestrus phase of their cycle. Seventy-two hours after injury the rats were anaesthetized and their brains were exposed for the tissue-punch assay described earlier. Both groups of untreated animals with the same lesions showed significant oedema in tissue taken from the injured area (males 4.42 per cent increase, females 3.28 per cent increase). However, both the males and the females given progesterone treatments showed a dramatic decline in postinjury oedema, indicating that the treatment is equally effective in both sexes (Fig. 5.2).[3]

Progesterone enhances cognitive and behavioural recovery from brain damage in both male and female rats

- Most treatment for traumatic brain injury *must* be given within the first few hours after the injury if there is to be any hope of recovery.
- Progesterone treatments can be delayed for as long as

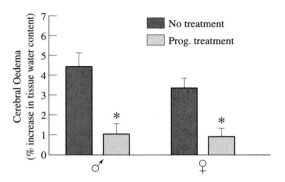

Fig. 5.2 The percentage increase in the water content of brain tissue samples from the lesion area compared to noninjured, distal control areas taken 72 hours after cortical contusion injury in male and female rats treated with progesterone (Prog. treatment) or oil vehicle. Asterisks indicate significant differences ($p < 0.05$) compared to oil-treated rats.

24 hours after traumatic brain injury and *still* have a dramatic effect on cerebral oedema.

- Progesterone treatments reduce oedema in three days to levels not seen until seven days in untreated animals.

The fact that progesterone has been shown to reduce postinjury cerebral oedema is a significant finding relevant to the search for an effective treatment for traumatic brain injury, but in order to determine its clinical effectiveness, it is important to know whether the reduction in cerebral oedema is accompanied by improved functional outcome. For example if focal cerebral oedema is reduced, one could expect that the neuropil in the area surrounding the contusion and more distal regions would be restored to a more normal state, with consequent improvement in sensory, motor and cognitive performance.

Accordingly, adult male rats were given either sham surgery or bilateral contusions of the medial frontal cortex (Roof et al., 1994). Progesterone injections (4 mg/kg) began one hour after the contusion, with the first injection being given intraperitoneally and then all remaining injections being given subcutaneously at six hours postinjury and again at 24, 48, 72, 96 and 120 hours postinjury. Control subjects received the same surgery followed by injections of peanut oil. The lesion groups were then compared to the sham operated rats given the same regime of progesterone or peanut oil

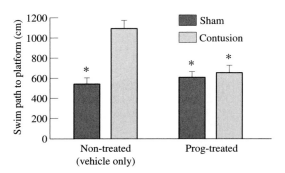

Fig. 5.3 Water maze performance on Trial 1: the overall mean length of path to platform in centimetres for oil-treated or progesterone-treated male rats after cortical contusion or sham surgery. Asterisks indicate significant differences ($p < 0.05$) compared to oil-treated, contused rats.

injections. Behavioural testing in the Morris water maze began seven days after surgery and continued for ten days.

It was observed that rats given progesterone treatments for cortical contusions were able to learn the spatial navigation task more rapidly than the lesion-alone counterparts (Fig. 5.3). Whereas all of the lesion rats were worse than unoperated controls on the performance of this task, the animals with progesterone treatment performed consistently better than those rats without treatment. Thus, in addition to resolving oedema much more rapidly, the progesterone treatments also led to improved recovery of cognitive performance in a spatial learning task even though the lesion size remained the same in treated and untreated animals.

When the number of surviving neurons in the dorsomedial nucleus of the thalamus (a structure with afferent projections to the medial frontal cortex) was counted, it was noted that progesterone-treated male rats had a significantly higher neuronal count than those left untreated. These data can be taken to suggest that the progesterone is 'neuroprotective' because fewer neurons are lost to lesion-induced retrograde degeneration (Fig. 5.4). In a recent confirming experiment, Chopp and his coworkers (Jiang et al., 1996) created a transient, middle cerebral artery occlusion model of stroke and then used progesterone to attenu-ate the effects of the occlusion in male adult rats. In this study the right middle cerebral artery was occluded for two hours. Progesterone treatment began 30 minutes before the occlusion and then 6 and 24 hours later. Infarct volume was significantly decreased in treated animals and their subsequent neurological deficits were less severe when measured 24 and 48 hours after reperfusion.

With respect to the potential for clinical treatment, there are two additional and important questions. First, how rapidly will progesterone reduce cerebral oedema? If cerebral oedema can kill injured nerve cells, then it is critically important to eliminate it as soon as possible to prevent further neuronal loss. Second, if progesterone treatment is delayed for some reason, how long after the injury will it still be effective? These two questions were addressed in both male and female rats with contusions of the medial frontal cortex using the same doses and oedema assay methods as described previously (Roof et al., 1996). In the first phase of the experiment, groups of contused, male and female rats were given injections of progesterone or peanut oil vehicle beginning one hour after contusion. Additional subcutaneous injections were given at 6 and 24 hours postinjury and then repeated once every 24 hours until the rats were killed. Oedema assessments were carried out at two and six hours, and one, three and seven days after the contusion. The results (Fig. 5.5) showed that oedema formation is evident within two hours after the injury, peaks at 24 hours and drops off significantly by seven days. Consistent with the authors' previous findings, oedema was higher at one day postinjury in males compared to females. Both males and females benefited when progesterone treatments began one hour after injury. Rats of both sexes given progesterone showed reduced oedema at six hours, one day and three days after injury. Clearly, the hormone dramatically reduced the levels of oedema so that at three days after injury they were equivalent to those in untreated rats seen only by seven days. This suggests that the progesterone can reduce the duration of oedema by nearly half, and that this may be a key aspect of its neuroprotective effects.

In the second experiment, surgery and treatment were the same as in the first experiment, except for the time of treatment initiation. One quarter of the rats

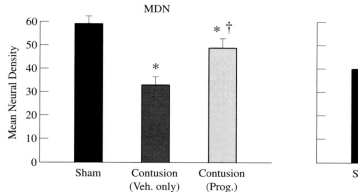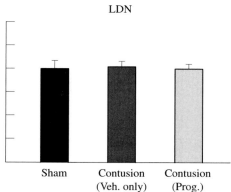

Fig. 5.4 Mean neuronal counts in the mediodorsal thalamic nucleus (MDN) and the lateral dorsal thalamic nucleus (LDN). All healthy neurons within 9 to 25 squares of a 5×5 ocular square grid were counted. The grid was placed over the left then the right nuclei at three rostrocaudal levels (-2.3, -2.8 and -3.3 from Bregma (Paxinos and Watson, 1986) at a magnification of $40 \times$. Means represent average total grid count. Asterisks indicate significant differences ($p < 0.05$) from sham counts. Cross indicates significant difference ($p < 0.05$) from counts of the oil-treated group. Veh. = vehicle, Prog. = progesterone.

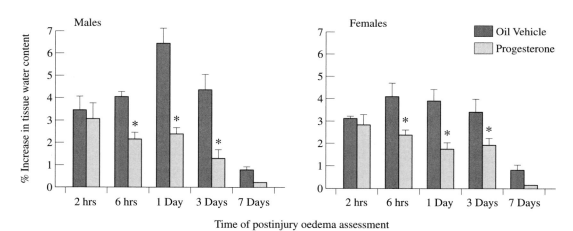

Fig. 5.5 Progression of oedema over time in the brain tissue of cortically contused male and female rats treated with progesterone or oil after contusion. Asterisks indicate significant differences ($p < 0.05$) from oil-treated rats at that particular time point.

were given injections beginning at 2 hours postinjury, one quarter at six hours postinjury, one quarter at 24 hours postinjury and one quarter at 48 hours postinjury. Three days postinjury, the rats were killed and assessed for oedema. The results (Fig. 5.6) showed that progesterone treatment can be delayed up to 24 hours after injury and still remain effective in reducing cerebral oedema in male and female rats. In fact, the treatments

given at one and six hours after surgery were not more effective than those given at 24 hours in reducing cerebral water content. These data show that progesterone can reduce cerebral oedema, even when the first injection is given 24 hours after the injury has occurred. These findings stand in contrast to those obtained with methylprednisolone, which must be administered within eight hours to be effective in treating spinal cord

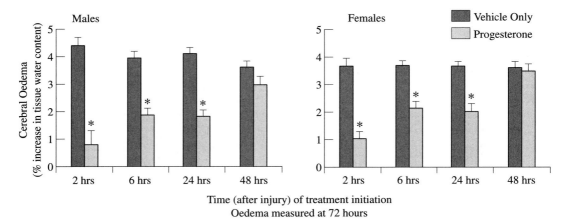

Fig. 5.6 The percentage increase in the water content of brain tissue samples from the lesion area compared to noninjured, distal control areas taken 72 hours after cortical contusion injury in male and female rats treated with progesterone or oil vehicle when treatment was delayed for 24 and 48 hours. Asterisks indicate significant differences ($p<0.05$) from oil-treated rats at that time point.

damage, but which is not indicated for the treatment of traumatic *brain* damage. To the best of the authors' knowledge, progesterone may have the largest window of opportunity for the treatment of the secondary consequences of brain injury of any putative agent currently available.

Progesterone and posttraumatic epilepsy

- Progesterone administration can prevent or reduce the formation of epilepsy and may serve as an anxiolytic agent.
- Reduction of injury-induced seizures may attenuate the excitotoxicity caused by the initial trauma and thereby slow the further loss of neurons.

In some females, catemenial epilepsy has been traced to the withdrawal of progesterone. For example, Herzog (1991) has reported that topical or intravenous application of oestradiol in rabbits significantly increases spontaneous paroxysmal spike discharges in the cortex, whereas the administration of progesterone lessens them. Thus, oestrogen would seem to *lower* the threshold for seizures and other forms of abnormal, neural activity and this is especially the case in animals with pre-existing brain damage (Herzog, 1991). In human females, intravenous infusions of progesterone

'sufficient to produce luteal phase serum levels' significantly reduced interictal spiking in about 60 per cent of women diagnosed with partial epilepsy (Backstrom et al., 1984). Similarly, Swanson and Phillis (1987) showed that intravenous administration of progesterone can potentiate the effects of adenosine, an endogenous anticonvulsant. In their model, progesterone plus adenosine produced a marked depression of spontaneous neural activity in cortical cholinergic neurons. Related to its anticonvulsant properties, progesterone may also serve as an anxiolytic drug and, as such, could have important consequences in brain-injured subjects, in whom increased emotionality, stress response and hyperactivity are often observed. Thus, progesterone administration to either males or females can have effects on heart rate, EKG, blood pressure and respiration that are similar to the effects of the benzodiazepines (Carter-Little, Matta and Jahn, 1974; Gavish et al., 1987; Bitran, Shiekh and McLeod, 1995).

These studies, taken together, suggest that in addition to reducing cerebral oedema, one additional mechanism by which progesterone administration can improve functional outcome after brain injury is by preventing or reducing the formation of epileptogenic spiking in vulnerable or injured neurons associated with the area of tissue destruction. Preventing abnormal spiking activity immediately after brain damage may provide a sufficient opportunity for 'stabilization' of affected neurons. By reducing seizure activity, progesterone could also prevent additional excitotoxicity and further loss of neurons, and thus slow or prevent the injury cascade.

Effects of progesterone on glia and other immune responsive cells

- Schwann cells in the peripheral nervous system are a potent source of progesterone.
- Activation of Schwann cells leads to release of progesterone which, in turn, enhances neurite outgrowth and formation of new myelin sheaths.
- Application of progesterone in cultured nerve segments also stimulates significant neurite outgrowth.
- Progesterone may also be synthesized directly in the central nervous system by male and female glial cells and will stimulate the differentiation of these cells.
- Progesterone can also inhibit inflammatory monocytes and other 'immune' cells, leading to less swelling and oedema.

Some recent experiments also point to a role for progesterone in the direct repair of damaged peripheral neurons and the findings may have relevance in explaining how progesterone can exert beneficial effects in the damaged brain. Koenig et al. (1995) examined the effects of progesterone administration on the repair and remyelination of damaged sciatic nerve and dorsal root ganglia. The researchers found that in castrated and adrenalectomized male mice, the levels of progesterone remained high in the sciatic nerve although it was cleared from the plasma. They took this finding to indicate that the progesterone was synthesized locally in the sciatic nerve itself. Koenig et al. found that the Schwann cells surrounding the sciatic nerve were a potent source of progesterone, whereas oligodendrocytes synthesized the hormone in the central nervous system (Jung-Testas et al., 1992). Koenig et al. (1995) damaged the sciatic nerve in adult male mice by cryogenic freezing to cause Wallerian degeneration. This response triggers the formation of new myelin sheaths and increased concentrations of pregnenolone and progesterone in the area of the

lesion. Inhibiting the conversion of pregnenolone to progesterone significantly decreased the thickness of the remyelination as measured by electron microscopy. However, reapplication of progesterone significantly increased the thickness of the myelin sheaths.

In their dorsal root ganglion cultures, daily application of progesterone (20 nM) for four weeks led to significant neurite outgrowth and a much higher number of myelinated nerve segments than was observed in control tissue. These data can be taken to suggest that progesterone may also play a role in the regenerative repair of damaged brain as well as peripheral nerve cells, although further work would need to be done to clarify this issue. Because neuronal retrograde degeneration is reduced in male and female rats treated with progesterone following cortical contusions, we can speculate that some of the benefits may be due to progesterone's effects on oligodendrocytes (or astrocytes), providing a matrix for axonal repair and regeneration. This possibility, coupled with reduced inflammatory response caused by progesterone's putative ability to suppress microglia and other immunoreactive cells, may help to preserve neurons that would have ordinarily died as a result of the injury. The surviving cells would then be able to put out growth cones, increase terminal sprouting and maintain more synaptic contacts than would be found in untreated controls. This is a provocative idea but it needs to be tested empirically before we can draw any definitive conclusions.

There is now literature to suggest that progesterone, synthesized from cholesterol and pregnenolone by glial cells within the central nervous system (Robel and Baulieu, 1994), can play a role in affecting neurotransmission. Using cultured, neonatal rat glial cells, Jung-Testas et al. (1992) have shown that progesterone can be synthesized in both male and female glia and that, in turn, these cells have receptors for progesterone, glucocorticoids, oestrogen and androgens. What was particularly interesting to note was that application of progesterone *inhibited* glial cell proliferation but at the same time the progesterone *increased* the differentiation of processes in both oligodendrocytes and astrocytes. Especially in oligodendrocytes, the processes were 'longer, straighter and more numerous' in the presence of progesterone. Levels of glial fibrillary acidic protein were also much higher in astrocytes exposed to progesterone. This would indicate that the resident astrocytes were activated by the progesterone even though the hormone did not increase their proliferation. Activated astrocytes can take up excitotoxins and at the same time release neurotrophic factors into the zone of injury (Schwartz et al., 1993), which can then prevent additional neurodegeneration.

Although the effects of these hormones on microglia – which can release neurotoxins and inflammatory cytokines into the area of injury (Giulian and Vaca, 1993) – were not examined, it is believed that the inhibition of microglial activity might reduce some of the inflammatory reactions leading to the formation of oedema. Support for this idea can be drawn from a report by Ganter et al. (1992). These investigators showed that progesterone could inhibit microglial proliferation in isolated cultures, although not as effectively as the corticosteroids hydrocortisone and aldosterone. Similarly, Sherblom et al. (1985) showed that serum taken from cows treated with progesterone could significantly suppress the stimulation of lymphocytes compared to serum taken from control cows, and these effects were seen within eight days after the start of treatment. Stites, Bugbee and Siiteri (1983) also showed that progesterone could prevent the proliferation of cytotoxic T-cells by immunosuppression. If the production of inflammatory monocytes, lymphocytes T-cells and cytokines were inhibited in the presence of progesterone, it might explain why this hormone has the capacity to reduce the 'brain swelling' caused by the inflammatory reaction to the contusion seen in the early stages of the injury process.

Effects of progesterone on excitatory amino acid and free radical metabolism

- Progesterone can upregulate GABA or GABA-receptors and thereby alter the cascade of excitatory and excitotoxic activity.
- Progesterone administration can reduce excitation in Purkinje cells.
- Progesterone also reduces the lipid peroxidation that often accompanies traumatic brain injury and this prevents the formation of cerebral oedema.

In both traumatic brain injury and ischaemic stroke, large amounts of excitatory amino acids such as glutamate are released from dying and injured neurons and glia. These excitatory amino acids can in turn cause additional neurotoxicity, leading to more cell death or to dysfunctional neuronal activity. One way to prevent the cascade of excitotoxicity is to block receptors to excitatory amino acids or to inhibit additional excitatory activity by upregulating GABA or GABA receptors. Smith (1991), for example, has shown that progesterone can dramatically inhibit excitation of rat cerebellar Purkinje cells caused by the application of excitatory amino acid agonists such as quisqualate, kainate and N-methyl-D-aspartate. At physiological levels, progesterone has also been shown to affect GABA-induced inhibition of abnormal neuronal firing (Smith, 1994).

There is also some evidence that progesterone may help to stem some of the free-radical-induced lipid peroxidation caused by the destruction of central nervous system tissue. Free radicals are reactive oxygen metabolites produced during the synthesis of prostaglandins. They attack cell membranes and the microvasculature because the latter contains high levels of phospholipid-containing unsaturated fatty acids. It is very likely that some of the vasogenic oedema produced by contusion injury to the brain is due to lipid peroxidation caused by free radical attack (Kontos and Povlishock, 1986; Braughler and Hall, 1992). Because it is a steroid, the authors speculated that progesterone may have the capacity to reduce the detrimental effects of free radicals by its ability to stabilize phospholipids in cell membranes (Roof, Hoffman and Stein, 1997). The hypothesis was tested in male rats given contusion injuries of the frontal cortex followed by progesterone or control injections at five minutes after contusion and again at 6 and 24 hours postinjury. The rats were killed at 24, 48 or 72 hours after surgery to evaluate the extent to which progesterone treatments could attenuate lipid peroxidation. An indirect enzyme immunoassay was used (Hoffman, Roof and Stein, 1996) for levels of 8-iso-prostaglandin $F_{2\alpha}$ (8-isoPGF$_{2\alpha}$). This prostaglandin is a byproduct of the oxidation of tissue phospholipids caused by oxygen free radicals.

At 24 hours after injury, 8-isoPGF$_{2\alpha}$ levels were almost three times greater in oil-treated rats than in those

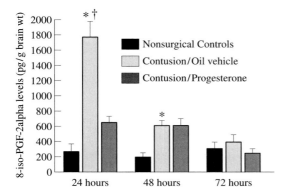

Fig. 5.7 Levels of 8-isoPGF$_{2\alpha}$ (pg/g brain tissue) in male rats 24, 48 or 72 hours after cortical contusion and sham surgery when treated with progesterone or oil after contusion. Asterisks indicate significant differences ($p<0.05$) from shams. Cross indicates significant difference ($p<0.05$) from progesterone-treated rats.

treated with progesterone (Fig. 5.7). By 48 hours after injury, the free-radical levels had declined in both groups of brain-damaged rats. These data can be taken to suggest that early progesterone treatment can reduce additional injury to the brain by reducing free-radical lipid peroxidation of vulnerable nerve cell membranes. The largest effects of lipid peroxidation are seen within the first 24 hours after contusion injury but even though free-radical activity may be reduced by 48 hours, lipid peroxidation is still occurring in nontreated animals, in whom it can continue to kill injured or vulnerable neurons. The reduced oedema also seen in progesterone-treated animals may be due to the decreases in lipid peroxidation-induced damage to neurons and glia; it is not hard to imagine that less neurotoxicity would lead to less accumulation of inflammatory tissue byproducts and therefore less brain swelling.

Conclusions

- Progesterone has more complex effects in the central nervous system than previously imagined; it may be an effective treatment in a wide range of neuropathological disorders.
- Progesterone may reduce the physiological consequences associated with high-altitude sickness.

- There is mounting evidence to show that the timing of mastectomy surgery to coincide with high levels of progesterone may reduce the reoccurrence of breast cancer and increase the rate of survival in patients.
- Sex hormones and hormonal cycling play an important role in the organism's response to injury and disease.

The ability of progesterone to influence a number of physiological events in both males and females that are not directly associated with pregnancy is no longer seriously questioned. The research summarized in this chapter clearly shows that progesterone can have dramatic effects on the outcome of brain injury in both sexes. In addition, the hormone can affect neuronal excitability by modulating receptors sensitive to excitatory amino acids as well as other transmitters in the central nervous system. In turn, these alterations can affect stress, mood and memory (Robel and Baulieu, 1994). There is recent evidence to suggest that exogenous progesterone can stimulate the glial cell production of trophic factors, which in turn can enhance regenerative responses in damaged nerve cells (see Koenig et al., 1995).

It now appears that sex hormones can play a critical role in the modulation of other diseases as diverse as mountain sickness and breast cancer. With respect to the first, Ou et al. (1994) exposed male and female rats to chronic hypoxia in a model designed to mimic the effects of high-altitude sickness in humans. After chronic exposure to a simulated altitude of 5500 m for 40 days, the animals were examined on a number of physiological parameters. The male rats suffered a much higher mortality rate than the females, although both sexes showed signs of chronic mountain sickness. Both sexes showed severe pulmonary hypertension, cardiac hypertrophy and heart failure; females even more so than the males. Yet the females survived and the males died. As with the effects of progesterone on brain injury, the specific mechanisms by which females are more protected from mountain sickness than males is not yet known. Ou et al. speculate that progesterone is a potent ventilatory stimulant and in the absence of progesterone (the males) the 'ventilatory response to hypoxia could be depressed and hypoxemia could be enhanced' (Ou et al., 1994, p. 432).

With respect to breast cancer, there is now mounting, although still controversial, evidence that where a woman is in her menstrual cycle at the time she has a mastectomy for tumour removal will determine the subsequent outcome. In one study, Badwe et al. (1991) examined several hundred premenopausal women who were to receive surgery for operable breast tumours. The researchers compared one group of women who had their mastectomy 3–12 days after their last menstrual period to another group with surgery at 0–2 or 13–32 days after their last menstrual period. Survival ten years later was 54 per cent in the first group versus 84 per cent for the second. These authors claim that 'patients who underwent tumor excision during a phase of unopposed estrogen stimulation had a much poorer outlook than those operated during other phases of the menstrual cycle' (Badwe et al., 1991, p. 1263). Furthermore, they also noted that 'malignant cells shed under conditions of unopposed estrogen might be more able to proliferate and to become established as micro-metastases than at other times. In contrast, the addition of progesterone to estrogen may inhibit the growth-promoting effect of estrogen alone' (p. 1264). Other studies by Senie et al. (1991), Saad et al. (1994) and Veronesi et al. (1994) obtained similar results in that at five to ten or more years after surgery for operable breast carcinoma, women whose initial surgery was during the follicular phase of the cycle had significantly poorer survival rates than those who underwent operations during the luteal phase (42 per cent versus 72 per cent survival respectively). It is important to note that others have taken issue with these findings (e.g. McGuire, Hilsenbeck and Clark, 1992; Sauerbrei, Baster and Schmoor, 1994) with regard to statistical methodology and sampling.

Nonetheless, given all of the data presented in this chapter, there is good reason to think that sex hormones and hormonal cycling do indeed play an important role in mediating the organism's response to injury and disease. It is also clear that much more research needs to be done to examine and determine the specific mechanisms by which progesterone acts to promote its effects. Progesterone and its related substances may act at the level of the genome or at the level of the cell membrane or by indirect pathways that still remain to be found. In terms of brain-injury repair, we need to be aware that if appropriate pharmacological agents are to be found, we will have to be much more concerned about the role of gender in determining the right therapy. This decision may also have to include not only the sex of the subject but also the timing of treatment designed to coincide with the appropriate hormonal and biochemical milieux (Hrushesky, 1993).

This chapter may raise questions in the minds of readers concerning the potential benefits of progesterone treatments for the human victims of brain injury, the current state of clinical research using progesterone as a potential therapy for brain injury and what benefits have been reported, whether progesterone treatment improves cognitive performance in a clinical setting. Because this chapter suggests that progesterone appears to be more effective than oestrogen in the treatment of brain injury, what are the clinical benefits of progesterone in relation to the current interest in oestrogen therapy in Alzheimer's disease, for example?

These are all very legitimate questions and the authors wish they had the answer, and that it were possible to indicate here that progesterone has proven to be highly effective in treating human stroke or traumatic brain damage. Unfortunately, a thorough review of recent clinical literature failed to reveal any indication that progesterone is currently being applied as a treatment for central nervous system injury. However, oestrogen therapy *is* being tested in elderly women with Alzheimer's disease because there is some indication that this hormone may slow the progression of this affliction (Cohen et al., 1993; Henderson et al., 1994). Readers are referred to several recent papers for a more through review of these investigations (Brenner et al., 1994; Gibbs, 1994; Hamilton, 1994; Paganini-Hill and Henderson, 1994; Behl et al., 1995; Fillit, 1995; Mortel and Meyer, 1995; Samsioe, 1995; Henderson, Watt and Buckwalter, et al., 1996; Schneider et al., 1996; Simpkins, Singh and Bishop, et al., 1996; Smalheiser and Swanson, 1996; Birge, 1997; Henderson, 1997; Kawas et al., 1997; Reiss, 1997). There is no indication, however, that progesterone is also being examined in the same context.

Given the relative safety of acute, systemic progesterone administration used in the authors' animal model of head trauma (two to four injections postinjury, 4.0

mg/kg), they believe that the time is ripe for the design of a comprehensive, multicentre, clinical study to gauge the hormone's effectiveness in treating brain damage. To the best of the authors' knowledge, there are, as yet, no therapeutic drugs that have proven to be safe and effective in reducing the physiological and behavioural consequences of moderate to severe brain traumas. Progesterone is a good candidate, partly because it is inexpensive and nonproprietary. It could be a major benefit in emergency treatment, but its availability and very low cost may also be a potential problem when it comes to generating large profits for patent attorneys, pharmaceutical companies and health-care providers. The authors are currently working with colleagues in neurosurgery, neurology and emergency medicine to design protocols for testing progesterone in human brain-injury patients, but there are no data to report at this time.

Acknowledgements

The research reported in this Chapter was carried out at Rutgers, Emory and Texas Christian University and was supported by grants from the Centers for Disease Control (CDC) (R49/CCR208836) and GenRe Corp. to DGS. The contents of this paper are solely the responsibility of the authors and do not necessarily represent the official views of the CDC or GenRe Corp.

Endnotes

1 *Guideline for the Study and Evaluation of Gender Differences in the Clinical Evaluation of Drugs*. 1994. NIH Guide 23, No. 11. Federal Register (58FR 39406). NIH guidelines on the inclusion of women and minorities as subjects in clinical research.

2 Progesterone is a representative of *progestins*, a group of steroid hormones that aid in maintaining pregnancy in placental mammals. Progesterone was isolated first in 1934 and named so because it promotes gestation or pregnancy. Because the major producer of progesterone is the corpus luteum in the ovary, the cycle in which progesterone is produced is referred to as the luteal stage. Steroids are synthesized from cholesterol. Cholesterol can be converted to progesterone through four chemical reactions; progesterone then can be converted to a glucocorticoid (corticosterone),

which in turn can be converted to a mineralocorticoid (aldosterone). Alternatively, progesterone can be transformed to testosterone. Normal males also secrete progesterone but in small quantities (only about 0.75 mg/day, whereas women produce 20–40 mg progesterone a day in their midluteal stage). Thus, the idea that androgens and progestins are 'male' hormones while oestrogens are 'female' hormones is overly simplistic; both sexes make both classes of hormones although in quite different proportions, which vary with the species (Becker and Breedlove, 1992). The corpus luteum lasts for two weeks in women and continuously secretes progesterone. If implantation of a fertilized egg does not take place, the corpus luteum decreases in function, and there will be a measurable drop in both progesterone and oestrogen secretion. If pregnancy does occur, the corpus luteum will produce large amounts of progesterone for up to two months. At two months the placenta takes over the function of the corpus luteum. The placenta makes an increasing amount of oestrogen and progesterone as pregnancy progresses, with peak levels found just before birth. In the central nervous system, progesterone seems to act: (1) as a depressant in humans; (2) in combination with an appropriate amount of oestrogen to cause oestrus behaviour in animals; (3) to inhibit ovulation (via decreased luteinizing hormone secretion); and (4) to cause the appearance of maternal behaviour (in some species).

3 One question that has arisen with respect to the use of progesterone as a treatment for head injury is whether the dose (4 mg/kg) might be too high for use in human patients. For example, translating this to a human patient, a 60-kg female (approximately 130 lb) would receive 240 mg. Interestingly, progesterone has been used in the USA for the treatment of premenstrual syndrome but has not been beneficial, according to some authors *because of the relatively low doses used in this country* (100–400 mg daily, compared with Europe where 800 mg and higher doses are employed: Jensvold, 1996). One study (Rickels et al., 1994) used 1700 mg/day to treat premenstrual syndrome and found no symptom relief for this disorder; however, there were no dramatic side-effects noted at this dose, which is considerably higher than the authors employed to reduce cerebral oedema following brain contusions.

References

Allen, L.S. and Gorski, R.A. 1990. Sex differences in the bed nucleus of the stria terminalis of the human brain. *J Comp Neurol* **302**(4), 697–706.

Allen, L.S. and Gorski, R.A. 1991. Sexual dimorphism of the anterior commissure and massa intermedia of the human brain. *J Comp Neurol* **312**(1), 97–104.

Allen, L.S., Richey, M.F., Chai, Y.M. et al. 1991. Sex differences in the corpus callosum of the living human being. *J Neurosci* **11**(4), 933–42.

Attella, M.J., Nattinville, A. and Stein, D.G. 1987. Hormonal state affects recovery from frontal cortex lesions in adult female rats. *Behav Neural Biol* **48**, 352–67.

Backstrom, T., Zetterlund, B., Blom, S. and Romano, M. 1984. Effects of intravenous progesterone infusions on the epileptic discharge frequency in women with partial epilepsy. *Acta Neurol Scand* **69**, 240–8.

Badwe, R.A., Gregory, W.M., Chaudry, M.A. et al. 1991. Timing of surgery during menstrual cycle and survival of premenopausal women with operable breast cancer. *Lancet* **337**, 1261–4.

Basso, A., Capitani, E. and Moraschini, S. 1983. Sex differences in recovery from aphasia. *Cortex* **18**, 469–75.

Becker, J.B. and Breedlove, S.M. 1992. Introduction to behavioral endocrinology. In *Behavioral Endocrinology*, ed. J.B. Becker, S.M. Breedlove and D. Crews, pp. 3–37. Cambridge, MA: MIT Press.

Behl, C., Widmann, D., Trapp, T. and Holsboer, F. 1995. 17-beta estradiol protects neurons from oxidative stress-induced cell death in vitro. *Biochem Biophys Res Commun* **216**, 473–82.

Betz, A.L. and Coester, H.C. 1990. Effects of steroids on edema and sodium uptake of the brain during focal ischemia in rats. *Stroke* **21**, 1199–204.

Birge, S.J. 1997. The role of progesterone in the treatment of Alzheimer's disease. *Neurology* **48**, 536–41.

Bitran, D., Shiekh, M. and McLeod, M. 1995. Anxiolytic effect of progesterone is mediated by the neurosteroid allopregnanolone at brain GABAa receptors. *J Neuroendocrinol* **7**, 171–7.

Braughler, J.M. and Hall, E.D. 1992. Involvement of lipid peroxidation in CNS injury. *J Neurotrauma* **9** (Suppl.), S1–7.

Brenner, D.L., Kukull, W.A., Stergachis, A. et al. 1994. Postmenopausal estrogen replacement therapy and the risk of Alzheimer's disease: a population-based case-control study. *Am J Epidemiol* **140**, 262–7.

Bullock, R., Chesnut, R.M., Clifton, G., Ghajar, J., Marion, D.W. and Narayan, R.K. 1996. Guidelines for the management of severe head injury. *J Neurotrauma* **13**(11), 639–731.

Carter-Little, B., Matta, R.J. and Jahn, T.P. 1974. Physiological and psychological effects of progesterone in man. *J Nerv Ment Dis* **159**, 256–62.

Cohen, D., Eisdorfer, C., Gorelick, P. et al. 1993. Sex differences in the psychiatric manifestations of Alzheimer's disease. *J Am Geriatr Soc* **41**, 229–32.

Connolly, P.B., Handa, R.J. and Resko, J.A. 1988. Progesterone

modulation of androgen receptors in the brain and pituitary of male guinea pigs. *Endocrinology* **126**(6), 2547–53.

Dearden, N.M., Gibson, J.S., McDowell, D.G., Gibson, R.M. and Cameron, M.M. 1986. Effect of high-dose dexamethazone on outcome from severe head injury. *J Neurosurg* **51**, 307–16.

deLacoste, M.C., Adesanya, T. and Woodward, D.J. 1990. Measures of gender differences in the human brain and their relationship to brain weight. *Biol Psychiatry* **28**, 931–42.

Fillit, H. 1995. Future therapeutic developments of estrogen use. *J Clin Pharmacol* **35**, 25S–28S.

Ganter, S., Northoff, D., Mannel, P.J. and Gebicke-Harter, P.J. 1992. Growth control of cultured microglia. *J Neurosci Res* **33**, 218–30.

Gavish, M., Weizman, A., Youdin, M.B.H. and Okun, F. 1987. Regulation of central and peripheral benzodiazepine receptors in progesterone treated rats. *Brain Res* **409**, 386–90.

Gean, A.D., Kates, R.S. and Lee, S. 1995. Neuroimaging in head injury. *New Horizons* **3**, 549–61.

Gibbs, R.B. 1994. Estrogen and nerve growth factor-related systems in the brain. Effects on basal forebrain cholinergic neurons and implications for learning and memory processes and aging. *Ann NY Acad Sci* **743**, 165–99.

Giulian, D. and Vaca, K. 1993. Inflammatory glia mediate delayed neuronal damage after ischemia in the central nervous system. *Stroke* **24**, 84–90.

Glasier, M.M., Sutton, R.L. and Stein, D.G. 1995. Effects of unilateral entorhinal cortex lesion and ganglioside GM1 treatment on performance in a novel water task. *Neurobiol Learn Mem* **64**, 203–14.

Gobiet, W., Bock, W.S., Liesegang, J. et al. 1976. Treatment of acute cerebral edema with high dose of dexamethasone. In *Intracranial Pressure III*, ed. J.W.F. Beks, D.A. Bosch and M. Brock, pp. 231–5. New York: Springer-Verlag.

Goldman, P. 1974. An alternative to development plasticity: heterology of CNS structures in infants and adults. In *Plasticity and Recovery of Function in the Central Nervous System*, ed. D.G. Stein, J.J. Rosen and N. Butters, pp. 149–74. New York: Academic Press.

Greenberg, J. and Brawanski, A. 1994. Cranial trauma. In *Neurocritical Care*, ed. W. Hacke, D.F. Hanley, K.M. Einhaupl et al., pp. 679–707. Berlin: Springer-Verlag.

Hakamata, Y., Ito, U., Hanyu, S. and Yoshida, M. 1995. Long-term high-colloid oncotic therapy for ischemic brain edema in gerbils. *Stroke* **26**, 2149–53.

Hall, E. 1992. The neuroprotective pharmacology of methylprednisolone. *J Neurosurg* **76**, 13–22.

Hamilton, J. 1994. Estrogen, memory and Alzheimer's disease. *Can Med Assoc J* **151**, 1465–7.

Hampson, E. and Kimura, D. 1988. Reciprocal effects of hormonal fluctuations on human motor and perceptual–spatial skills. *Behav Neurosci* **102**, 456–9.

Henderson, V.W. 1997. The epidemiology of estrogen replacement therapy and Alzheimer's disease. *Neurology* **48**, S27–35.

Henderson, V.W., Paganini-Hill, A., Emanuael, C.K., Dunn, M.E., Buckwalter, J.G. 1994. Oestrogen replacement therapy in older women: comparisons between Alzheimer's disease and non demented controls. *Arch Neurol* **51**, 896–900.

Henderson, V.W., Watt, L. and Buckwalter, J.G. 1996. Cognitive skills associated with estrogen replacement in women with Alzheimer's disease. *Psychoneuroendocrinology* **21**, 421–30.

Herzog, A. 1991. Progesterone therapy in women with complex partial and secondary generalized seizures. *Neurology* **45**, 1660–2.

Hoffman, S.W., Fulop, Z. and Stein, D.G. 1994. Bilateral medial prefrontal cortical contusion in the male rat: behavioral deficits and brain histopathology. *J Neurotrauma* **11**, 417–31.

Hoffman, S.W., Roof, R.L. and Stein, D.G. 1996. A reliable and sensitive enzyme immunoassay method for measuring 8-isoprostaglandin F2α: a marker for lipid peroxidation after experimental brain injury. *J Neurosci Methods* **68**, 133–6.

Hrushesky, W.J. 1993. Breast cancer and the menstrual cycle [editorial comment]. *J Surg Oncol* **53**(1), 1–3.

Jensvold, M.F. 1996. Nonpregnant reproductive-age women. Part II. Exogenous sex steroid hormones and psychopharmacology. In *Psychopharmacology and Women: Sex, Gender and Hormones*, ed. M.F. Jensvold, U. Halbriech and J.A. Hamilton, pp. 171–90. Washington, DC: American Psychiatric Press.

Jensvold, M.F., Halbreich, U. and Hamilton, J.A. 1996. *Psychopharmacology and Women: Sex, Gender and Hormones*. Washington, DC: American Psychiatric Press.

Jiang, N., Chopp, M., Stein, D.G. and Feit, H. 1996. Progesterone is neuroprotective after transient middle cerebral artery occlusion in male rats. *Brain Res* **735**, 101–7.

Jung-Testas, I., Renoir, M., Bugnard, H., Greene, G.L. and Baulieu, E.E. 1992. Demonstration of steroid hormone receptors and steroid action in primary cultures of glial cells. *J Steroid Biochem Mol Biol* **41**, 621–31.

Juraska, J.M. 1986. Sex differences in developmental plasticity of behavior and the brain. In *Developmental Neuropsychobiology*, ed. W.T. Greenough and J.M. Juraska, pp. 409–22. New York: Academic Press.

Karavolas, H.J., Bertics, P.J., Hodges, D. and Rudie, N. 1984. Progesterone processing by neuroendocrine structures. In *Metabolism of Hormonal Steroids in the Neuroendocrine Structures*, ed. F. Cellotti, et al. pp. 149–70. New York: Raven Press.

Kawas, C., Resnick, S., Morrison, A. et al. 1997. A prospective study of estrogen replacement therapy and the risk of developing Alzheimer's disease: the Baltimore Longitudinal Study of Aging. *Neurology* **48**, 1517–21.

Ke, F.C. and Ramirez, V.D. 1990. Binding of progesterone to nerve cell membranes of rat brain using progesterone conjugated to ^{125}I-bovine serum albumin. *J Neurochem* **54**, 467–72.

Kelly, D.F. 1995. Steroids in head injury [Review]. *New Horizons* **3**(3), 453–5.

Kempski, O.S. and Volk, C. 1994. Neuron-glia interaction during injury and edema of CNS. *Acta Neurochir* **60** (Suppl. 7), 7–11.

Kimelberg, H.K. 1992. Astrocytic edema in CNS trauma. *J Neurotrauma* **9** (Suppl. 1), 571–81.

Kimura, D. 1983. Sex differences in cerebral organization for speech and praxic functions. *Can J Psychol* **37**, 19–35.

Kimura, D. 1987. Are men's and women's brains really different? *Can Psychol* **28**, 133–47.

Kimura, D. 1994. Cognitive pattern in men and women is influenced by fluctuations in sex hormones. *Curr Dir Psychol Sci* **3**, 57–61.

Koenig, H.L., Schumacher, M., Ferzaz, B. et al. 1995. Progesterone synthesis and myelin formation by Schwann cells. *Science* **268**, 1500–3.

Kontos, H.A. and Povlishock, J.T. 1986. Oxygen radicals in brain injury. *CNS Trauma* **3**, 257–63.

Lansdell, H. 1973. Effect of neurosurgery on the ability to identify popular word associations. *J Abnorm Psychol* **81**, 255–8.

Lansdell, H. 1989. Sex differences in brain and personality correlates of the ability to identify popular word associations. *Behav Neurosci* **103**, 893–7.

LeVay, S. 1994. Evidence for a biological influence in male homosexuality. *Sci Am* **270**(5), 44–9.

Levy, M.L., Aranda, M., Zelman, V. and Giannotta, S.L. 1995. Propylene glycol toxicity following continuous etomidate infusion for the control of refractory cerebral edema. *Neurosurgery* **37**, 363–71.

McConnell, J.R., Ong, C.S., McAllister, J.L. and Gross, T.G. 1996. Propylene glycol toxicity following continuous etomidate infusion for the control of refractory cerebral edema (letter). *Neurosurgery* **38**, 232–3.

McEwen, B.S. and Wooley, C.S. 1994. Estradiol and progesterone regulate neuronal structure and synaptic connectivity in adult as well as developing brain. *Exp Gerontol* **29**, 431–6.

McGuine, W.L., Hilsenbeck, S. and Clark, G.M. 1992. Optimal mastectomy timing. *J Natl Cancer Inst* **84**(5), 346–8.

McLuskey, N.J. and McEwen, B.S. 1978. Oestrogen modulates progestin receptor concentration in some rat brain regions but not others. *Nature* **274**, 276.

Mortel, K.F. and Meyer, J.S. 1995. Lack of postmenopausal estrogen replacement therapy and the risk of dementia. *J Neuropsychiatry Clin Neurosci* **7**, 334–7.

Murphy, D.G., DeCarli, C., McIntosh, A.R. et al. 1996. Sex differences in human brain morphometry and metabolism: an in vivo quantitative magnetic resonance imaging and positron emission tomography study on the effect of aging. *Arch Gen Psychiatry* **53**(7), 585–94.

Nottebohm, F. 1985. Neuronal replacement in adulthood. *Ann NY Acad Sci* **457**, 143–61.

Nottebohm, F. and Arnold, A.P. 1976. Sexual dimorphism in vocal control areas of the songbird brain. *Science* **194**, 211–13.

Ou, L.C., Sardella, G.L., Leiter, J.C., Brinck-Johnsen, T. and Smith, R.P. 1994. Role of sex hormones in development of chronic mountain sickness. *J Appl Physiol* **77**, 427–33.

Paganini-Hill, A. and Henderson, V.W. 1994. Estrogen deficiency and risk of Alzheimer's disease in women. *Am J Epidemiol* **14**, 256–61.

Paxinos, G. and Watson, C. 1986. *The Rat Brain in Stereotaxic Coordinates.* New York: Academic Press.

Peters, M. 1991. Sex differences in human brain size and the general meaning of differences in brain size. *Can J Psychol* **45**, 507–22.

Pfaff, D.W. and McEwen, B.S. 1983. Actions of estrogens and progestins on nerve cells. *Science* **219**, 808–14.

Reiss, J. 1997. [Does estrogen replacement prevent Alzheimer's disease?]. [German]. *Fortschr Med* **115**, 6.

Rickels, K., Schweizer, E., Clary, C., Fox, I. and Weise, C. 1994. Nefazodone and imipramine in major depression: a placebo controlled trial. *Br J Psychiatry* **164**, 802–5.

Robel, P. and Baulieu, E.E. 1994. Neurosteroids: biosynthesis and function. *TEM* **5**, 1–7.

Rockel, R.L., Horns, R.W. and Powell, T.P.S. 1980. The basic uniformity in structure of the neocortex. *Brain* **103**, 221–44.

Roof, R.L., Duvdevani, R., Braswell, L. and Stein, D.G. 1992. Progesterone treatment attenuates brain edema following contusion injury in male and female rats. *Restorative Neurol Neurosci* **4**, 425–7.

Roof, R.L., Duvdevani, R., Braswell, L. and Stein, D.G. 1994. Progesterone facilitates cognitive recovery and reduces secondary neuronal loss caused by cortical contusion injury in male rats. *Exp Neurol* **129**, 64–9.

Roof, R.L., Duvdevani, R., Heyburn, J.W. and Stein, D.G. 1996. Progesterone rapidly decreases brain edema: treatment delayed up to 24 hours is still effective. *Exp Neurol* **138**, 246–51.

Roof, R.L., Duvdevani, R. and Stein, D.G. 1993. Gender influences outcome of brain injury: progesterone plays a protective role. *Brain Res* **607**, 333–6.

Roof, R.L., Hoffman, S.W. and Stein, D.G. 1997. Progesterone protects against lipid peroxidation following traumatic brain injury in rats. *Mol Chem Neuropathol* **31**(1), 1–11.

Saad, Z., Bramwell, J.D., Girott, M. et al. 1994. Timing of surgery in relation to the menstrual cycle in premenopausal women with operable breast cancer. *Br J Surg* **81**, 217–20.

Sakata, R. and Leung, P. 1991. Functional status, referral and cost of treatment for persons with traumatic head injury. *Brain Inj* **5**, 411–19.

Samsioe, G. 1995. The menopause revisited. [Review.] *Int J Gyneacol Obstet* **51**, 1–13.

Sauerbrei, W., Baster, G. and Schmoor, C. 1994. Prognostic effect of timing of surgery during menstrual cycle in premenopausal breast-cancer patients. *Int J Cancer* **59**, 149–50.

Schneider, L.S., Farlow, M.R., Henderson, V.W. and Pogoda, J.M. 1996. Effects of estrogen replacement therapy on response to tacrine in patients with Alzheimer's disease. *Neurology* **46**, 1580–4.

Schwartz, J.P., Sheng, J.G., Mitsuo, K., Shirabe, S. and Nishiyama, N. 1993. Trophic factor production by reactive astrocytes in injured brain. *Ann NY Acad Sci* **679**, 226–34.

Senie, R.T., Rosen, P.P., Rhodes, P. and Lesser, M.L. 1991. Timing of breast cancer excision during the menstrual cycle influences duration of disease-free survival. *Ann Intern Med* **115**, 337–42.

Shapira, Y. and Shohami, E. 1993. Experimental studies on brain oedema after blunt head injury: experimental approaches from animal experimentation to actual or possible clinical application. *Eur J Anaesthesiol* **10**(3), 155–73.

Shaywitz, B.A., Shaywitz, S.E., Pugh, K.R. et al. 1995. Sex differences in the functional organization of the brain for language. *Nature* **373**, 607–9.

Sherblom, A.P., Smagula, R.M., Moody, C.E. and Anderson, G.W. 1985. Immunosuppression, sialic acid and sialyltransferase of bovine serum as a function of progesterone concentration. *J Reprod Fertil* **74**, 509–17.

Simpkins, J.W., Singh, M. and Bishop, J. 1996. The potential role for estrogen replacement therapy in the treatment of the cognitive decline and neurodegeneration associated with Alzheimer's disease. *Neurobiology* **15** (Suppl.) S195–7.

Smalheiser, N.R. and Swanson, D.R. 1996. Linking estrogen to Alzheimer's disease: an informatics approach. *Neurology* **47**, 809–10.

Smith, S.S. 1991. Progesterone administration attenuates excitatory amino acid responses of cerebellar Purkinje cells. *Neuroscience* **42**, 309–20.

Smith, S.S. 1994. Female sex steroid hormones: from receptors to networks to performance actions on the sensorimotor system. *Prog Neurobiol* **44**, 55–88.

Stites, D.P., Bugbee, S. and Siiteri, P.K. 1983. Differential actions of progesterone and cortisol on lymphocyte and monocyte interaction during lymphocyte activation – relevance to immunosuppression in pregnancy. *J Reprod Immunol* 5, 215–28.

Swanson, T.H. and Phillis, J.W. 1987. Progesterone in seizure therapy (letter). *Neurology* 37(8), 1433.

Tomita, H., Ito, U., Tone, H., Masaoka, H. and Tominaga, B. 1994. High colloid oncotic therapy for contusional brain edema. *Acta Neurochirur* 60, 547–9.

Veronesi, V., Luini, A., Mariani, L. et al. 1994. Effect of menstrual phase on surgical treatment of breast cancer. *Lancet* 343, 1545–7.

Witelson, S.F., Glezer, I. and Kigar, D.L. 1995. Women have greater density of neurons in posterior temporal cortex. *J Neurosci* 15, 3418–28.

Witelson, S. and Kigar, D.L. 1993. Anterior commissure in relation to corpus callosum anatomy, hand preference and sex. *Soc Neurosci Abstracts* 19, 232.6.

Zumpe, D., Clancy, A.N., Bonsall, R.W. and Michael, R.P. 1996. Behavioral responses to depo-provera, fadrozole and estradiol in castrated, testosterone-treated cynomolgus monkeys (*Macaca fascicularis*): the involvement of progestin receptors. *Physiol Behav* 60, 531–40.

6

The psychosocial environment and cognitive rehabilitation in the elderly

Deirdre Dawson, Gordon Winocur and Morris Moscovitch

Introduction

Normal ageing typically involves some decline in cognitive abilities which can result in a loss of independence and, in some cases, institutionalization. As the population in most western countries ages, interest in these changing abilities has grown among researchers, clinicians and health policy makers. The high economic and social costs of increasing dependence create large incentives for maintaining and promoting independence in this population. Thus, two questions are of particular interest. Can we slow the rate of cognitive decline in older people? Can we improve cognitive functioning in the normal ageing population?

This chapter addresses these questions in the following manner. The first part reviews the cognitive changes associated with normal ageing, focusing on those related to biological change. The next section considers the impact of nonbiological changes on cognitive function. Developmental changes in the brain occur within a broader psychosocial context and researchers are increasingly noting the importance of this context for cognitive function. The third section reports the results of a major research study that investigated the relationship between cognitive performance and psychosocial adjustment in both community-dwelling and institutionalized elderly.

Whereas the first three sections of the chapter discuss multiple factors involved in cognitive status in the elderly, the last two consider what can be done about cognitive decline. The penultimate section reviews research into cognitive rehabilitation in the elderly. Unfortunately, the techniques used have met with limited success. This may be due in part to the failure of most research to take into account the total environment within which ageing occurs. The final section sketches a broader approach for promoting and maintaining a high level of cognitive function in the elderly, one that assumes the fundamental importance of psychosocial influences.

Cognitive changes in normal ageing

- Cognitive decline with advancing age is related to progressive deterioration within the frontal and medial temporal lobe regions of the brain.
- Explicit memory, working memory, high-level attentional tasks, and executive functions are especially vulnerable to ageing.
- Implicit and procedural memory, overlearned intellectual skills, and sustained attention are relatively well preserved.

Although age-related cognitive decline is highly variable, there is no question that some cognitive abilities are particularly susceptible to the effects of ageing. Indeed, an important distinction can be made between cognitive skills, such as certain types of procedural learning and implicit memory, that are relatively immune to the ageing process, and those that are more vulnerable, such as the ability to form associations between unrelated events or solve new problems. Not surprisingly, the more vulnerable functions are identified with areas of the brain that experience considerable structural and physiological change in old age, specifically the frontal lobes and the medial temporal lobes.

Although the entire brain decreases in size and weight with age (Waxman and deGroot, 1995), changes at the histological and biochemical levels are greatest in the medial temporal lobe system and the frontal lobes. These changes include reductions in the number of neurons and in synaptic density, changes in dendritic structure, development of neurofibrillary tangles and senile plaques, changes in neurotransmitter systems, and reductions in functional interactions with other brain areas (Azari et al., 1992; Golomb et al., 1993; West, 1993; Grady et al., 1995; Moeller et al., 1996; Scheibel, 1996). To gain an understanding of the impact of these changes, the cognitive abilities of patients with frontal lobe or medial temporal lobe lesions have been compared to those of older and younger adults.

Patients with lesions to the medial temporal lobe, including the hippocampus, experience severe memory loss for personal experiences (explicit memory) and when tested in the laboratory perform poorly on tests of recall and recognition. Although not as severe, normal old people exhibit a very similar type of memory loss (Craik, 1991; Huppert, 1991; Moscovitch and Winocur, 1992), while other cognitive abilities including attention span, general intelligence, and remote memory are relatively preserved. In a recent meta-analysis of age differences in memory function, Verhaeghen, Marcoen and Goossens (1993) examined over 100 effect sizes between older and younger subjects and found that all but two were significant. In general, age differences are largest for free recall, less for cued recall, and less again for recognition (Craik, 1991). Interestingly, these effects appear to be more related to acquisition and retrieval difficulties than to reduction in storage capacity (Moscovitch and Winocur, 1992; Zec, 1995). This suggests that age differences in memory performance may be substantially reduced if older adults have the opportunity to learn material to the same level as younger adults. This can often be achieved simply through additional instructions and may be an important factor in developing cognitive rehabilitation programmes for older adults.

Frontal lobe lesions also result in a number of cognitive impairments that are experienced by older adults, including difficulty with working memory (Moscovitch and Winocur, 1992, 1995) and source memory (Shimamura, Janowsky and Squire, 1991), as well as impairments in effortful forms of attention (Stuss et al., 1995) and problem solving (Albert and Moss, 1996). Working memory refers to the ability to retain information for a relatively short period of time while performing other cognitive operations, as is often required in tasks that involve comparisons or the updating of information. Source memory refers to memory for the contextual information surrounding target events such as where and when the event occurred, as well as situational characteristics associated with the event. (See Shimamura et al., 1991; Moscovitch and Winocur, 1992, 1995, for a fuller discussion of specific working and source memory tasks that are sensitive to ageing effects.) Working and source memory require 'online' manipulation of information, a feature that also characterizes effortful attention and problem solving. It is not surprising then that tasks that require divided, alternating or selective attention also result in slower and more errorful performance in older subjects than in younger ones (McDowd and Birren, 1990; Zec, 1995).

Effortful attention is thought to be part of the executive control system, as are problem-solving skills that require abstract thought and the ability to generate and execute plans. Deficits in tasks that utilize these cognitive abilities are consistently found in older adults (Albert and Moss, 1996) and in patients with frontal lobe lesions (Stuss, Eskes and Foster, 1994). For example, series completion tasks, the WAIS-R similarities subtest, and some tests of higher level attentional processes fall within the broad category of age-sensitive tests of executive function (Albert and Moss, 1996).

In contrast to the well-documented decline in the functions described above, others do not typically reveal age differences. For example, memory for stored knowledge is relatively well preserved across the lifespan (Albert and Moss, 1996) as are subtle and indirect types of (implicit) memory that reveal the unconscious effects of past experience. Examples of tests of implicit memory on which the elderly perform normally include most tests of repetition priming (e.g. word-fragment completion, lexical decision), as well as various non-timed procedural learning tasks (Moscovitch and Winocur, 1992). Patients with frontal and medial temporal lobe lesions also perform well on these tasks

(Butters and Stuss, 1989; Shimamura et al., 1991), which suggests that other brain structures mediate implicit memory. An exception to this pattern of spared implicit memory in old age is found in word-stem completion tests of repetition priming. In stem completion, subjects are presented with the first few letters of previously primed and nonprimed words. Implicit memory is reflected in a greater probability of identifying the primed words. Unlike other tests of repetition priming, age differences have been reported on this task (Meiran and Jelicic, 1995; Winocur, Moscovitch and Stuss, 1996). Of particular note is that these differences have been related to variability in frontal lobe function as measured by neuropsychological tests (Winocur et al., 1996; Nyberg et al., 1997). Nevertheless, the fact that critical cognitive functions remain relatively intact in normal old age has important implications for designing cognitive rehabilitation strategies that compensate for impaired abilities.

Psychosocial well-being and cognitive functioning

- Psychosocial status can impact positively on the developmental process of ageing.
- Psychosocial and related factors that affect cognitive status in older adults include education, life-style, locus of control, self-efficacy beliefs, and affect.
- Many psychosocial/environmental factors are amenable to change, thus providing a possible avenue for influencing cognitive status.

Successful ageing is influenced not only through biological processes but also by psychosocial and environmental factors, including the physical environment, lifestyle, and various personal and social variables. Evidence is now accumulating which shows how these factors can affect the general health status of older adults, including their ability to function effectively at the cognitive level. This section reviews this evidence, highlighting those factors that contribute to or protect against cognitive decline.

Few researchers have attempted to model the complex interaction between the variables that make up an individual's psychosocial and cognitive profile (Albert et al., 1995; Uchiyama et al., 1996). Rather, work in this area has focused on individual or select groups of variables. Given the multitude of variables involved, it is notable that several are consistently identified in studies that have attempted to investigate psychosocial and environmental influences on cognitive change in the elderly. These include external factors such as education, living situation, lifestyle, and nutritional status, and internal influences such as locus of control, self-efficacy beliefs, and affect. Other factors have been identified, such as the personality variable, introversion, but for the most part their influence appears to be smaller (Gold and Arbuckle, 1990; Arbuckle et al., 1992).

Of the demographic factors, education may be the most powerful, as its influence on cognitive status remains consistently significant when other psychosocial variables are covaried (Hultsch, Hammer and Small, 1993). Lower levels of education have been found to be predictive of cognitive decline in old age (Arbuckle et al., 1992; Evans et al., 1993). Interestingly, education is most strongly associated with performance on tasks that involve abstract thought processes (Inouye et al., 1993). Of course, early educational experience is not amenable to change and, consequently, from the point of view of enhancing cognitive function in a practical sense, other psychosocial variables are of more interest.

Unlike education, living environment, which contributes significantly to overall functional status, is potentially modifiable. An extensive literature documents the deleterious effects of relocation in the elderly, although most of these studies emphasize health and measures of well-being (Ferraro, 1982). However, there is some evidence that directly relates environmental factors to cognitive function in the elderly. For example, Winocur and Moscovitch (1990) found that high-functioning, institutionalized old people performed worse on standard cognitive tests than closely matched community-dwelling counterparts. As most elderly people must change their living situations at one time or another, and because of the known impact of relocation on well-being, it is important that we identify the specific environmentally related variables that may affect cognitive performance. The next section, which reports findings of the authors' recent work in this area, addresses this issue.

Lifestyle variables that impact on cognition in the

ageing population include nutrition, exercise and mental activity. Older people with deficiencies in specific vitamins and minerals (e.g. folate, vitamin C etc.) tend to perform poorly on cognitive tests, particularly memory and abstract thinking tests (Goodwin, Goodwin & Garry, 1983; Wenk, 1989; Penland, 1994). In contrast, older people who are physically active and enjoy mental stimulation in various forms perform at a higher level on tests of cognitive performance than do less active older people (Chodzko-Zajko et al., 1992; Hultsch et al., 1993; Albert et al., 1995; Goldberg, Dengel and Hagberg, 1996).

Although relatively little is known about the effect of varying nutritional status across the lifespan, increasing physical activity can produce substantial benefits. Several studies provide evidence that elderly people who engage in regular, strenuous activity suffer less cognitive decline than less active individuals (Chodzko-Zajko et al., 1992; Hultsch et al., 1993; Albert et al., 1995, Goldberg et al., 1996; but see Emery, Huppert and Schein, 1995). If, as the bulk of the available evidence suggests, physical activity does have a positive influence on cognitive function, this can be taken into account in designing supportive environments for the elderly.

Internal psychological variables, such as locus of control, self-efficacy beliefs and affect, are all closely related to functional status in the elderly. Furthermore, they appear to be responsive to change and, like lifestyle factors, may provide another avenue for interventions directed at optimizing cognitive function. Of these three variables, locus of control, that is the extent to which we believe we control the external environment, has been the focus of most of the research. Nevertheless, the impact of this variable on cognitive status in the elderly has been and remains controversial. For example, Arbuckle et al. (1992) found that older people with higher levels of internal control performed better on one of four memory measures, although earlier research indicated that perceived control was not predictive of memory (Arbuckle, Gold and Andres, 1986).

One possibility is that the diverse findings with respect to locus of control are related to the complexity of the construct. For example, the impact of locus of control on cognitive status may be mediated through

perceptions of social support (Buschmann and Hollinger, 1994), the individual's coping style (Shaw, 1992; Ruth and Coleman, 1996) and general affect (Hyer, Matteson and Siegler, 1982). Notwithstanding the controversy and complexity, perceived control emerges consistently as a predictor of cognitive status. Furthermore, it also covaries with cognitive status over time (Winocur, Moscovitch and Freedman, 1987a). Thus, interventions targeted at changing perceptions of control may tap into a mechanism for enhancing cognitive function in the elderly. The study described below provides further insight into the relationship between control and cognitive function.

Self-efficacy beliefs, that is, beliefs about one's ability to perform or be effective in various situations, are also linked to both coping and cognition in the elderly (Seeman, Rodin and Albert, 1993; Garfein and Herzog, 1995; Ruth and Coleman, 1996). Such beliefs have been shown to predict metamemory scores (McDougall, 1994) and to protect against cognitive decline (Albert et al., 1995). As with feelings of control, self-efficacy beliefs are closely related to affect (Cavanaugh and Green, 1990) and are amenable to change, even in older adults (McAvay, Seeman and Rodin, 1996). Of particular interest is the finding that these beliefs vary across domains. For example, beliefs about instrumental activities of daily living (e.g. arranging transportation) are better predictors of cognitive performance than beliefs about other life areas (Seeman et al., 1993). Thus, self-efficacy beliefs may be another target for interventions designed to enhance cognitive function.

The relationship between affect and cognitive function in the elderly has been investigated with a particular emphasis on depression, which is prevalent among older adults (Riley, 1994b). Even in samples of healthy older adults, those who score higher on measures of depression have lower cognitive scores, particularly on memory tasks (Perlmutter and Nyquist, 1990; West, Barron and Crook, 1992). A similar relationship is seen between those who report being sad, withdrawn and tense as opposed to happy, gregarious and relaxed (Deptula, Singh and Pomara, 1993). There is also evidence of a direct relationship between clinical depression and cognitive function. It is well known that cognitive performance is adversely affected in old people suffering from depression. In light of evidence that older people who are successfully treated for depression also improve in terms of cognitive function (Zarit, Gallagher, and Kramer, 1981; Beats, 1996), it is reasonable to speculate that manipulations aimed at improving affect in normal older adults may also have beneficial effects on cognitive function.

Clearly, age-related cognitive decline is not purely a biological function. Research demonstrating the influence of psychosocial and environmental variables on cognitive function suggests a means for enhancing and supporting cognitive function that has rarely been explored. However, a first step in developing appropriate interventions is the identification of those variables that reliably correlate with age-related cognitive performance. The next section reports data from what appears to be the first major investigation of these relationships.

The Canadian Aging Research Network (CARNET) Study of Psychosocial Influences on Cognitive Function in Normal Old People

- Institutionalized, healthy old people consistently performed at a lower level on cognitive tests than matched community-dwelling old people.
- Difficulties with psychosocial adjustment affected cognitive function in institutionalized and community-dwelling old people.
- Optimism, activity, locus of control and general happiness emerged as important psychosocial predictors of cognitive status.

It is only recently that research has addressed the possibility that difficulties at the psychosocial level contribute to cognitive decline. This is somewhat surprising in view of the concern often expressed by the elderly over declining mental capacity and the potential link between (real or imagined) cognitive loss and overall functional status.

As a first step in addressing psychosocial adjustment, Winocur and Moscovitch reviewed data from several experiments that revealed age differences in tests of learning and memory (Winocur and Moscovitch, 1983; Moscovitch and Winocur, 1983; Winocur, Moscovitch and Witherspoon, 1987b). In each study, subjects were

elderly individuals living in their own homes in the community or in various institutional settings. All subjects were carefully selected on the same criteria and there were no differences between community and institutional groups in terms of potentially confounding variables (e.g. age, IQ, health status, education). The institutions all had facilities to accommodate highly functioning individuals, with the following features in common: a central dining room that served at least one main meal each day, health care staff, a social programme, and a supervised activity programme.

When organized in terms of living environments, the data consistently showed that community-dwelling older adults significantly outperformed those living in institutions. Subsequently, in an independent study, Winocur and Moscovitch (1990) confirmed the generally superior performance of community-dwelling subjects, especially on cognitive tests that assessed functions associated with the prefrontal cortex and hippocampus. In other words, environmental factors seem to exacerbate the process of decline in those abilities most vulnerable to the ageing process.

An interesting finding of the Winocur and Moscovitch (1990) study was that the institutionalized elderly's cognitive performance was much more variable than that of the community-dwelling group. Closer examination revealed that 30 per cent of the institutionalized group were high functioning, with scores comparable to the community group. The other 70 per cent were low functioning, with performance on several tests reminiscent of the performance of brain-damaged amnesic patients similarly tested in other experiments (Winocur and Weiskrantz, 1976; Winocur et al., 1987a; Winocur, Kinsbourne and Moscovitch, 1989).

Just as there were no apparent differentiating features between the community-dwelling and institutionalized subjects, there were no obvious differences between the higher and lower functioning institutionalized groups that could account for the observed variability. One possibility was that residents differed in their psychosocial adjustment to institutional life, and that this affected cognitive abilities and overall functional status. This hypothesis was explored in another study in which a new group of institutionalized elderly was administered a series of cognitive tests together with psychosocial tests that assessed perceived control, general activity and stress level (Winocur et al., 1987a). As indicated in the previous section, these variables, which contribute significantly to overall well-being, have been linked to cognitive status in the elderly. The results of this study showed a positive correlation between perceived control, activity and cognitive test performance. Moreover, follow-up testing indicated that variations in the psychosocial domain over time were accompanied by corresponding changes in cognitive function. These results pointed to a striking interaction involving ageing effects, environmental factors, psychosocial adjustment, and cognitive function. Furthermore, as many of the cognitive tests used in these experiments were common neuropsychological measures of brain–behavioural relationships, brain function can be included as a variable in this interaction.

These data suggest that older people living in institutions may experience difficulties in relation to their environments. However, it was not clear whether the results reflected a unique effect of institutionalization or a more universal expression of how well older adults in general interact with environments that differ dramatically in terms of support, stimulation and enrichment. To explore this further, a longitudinal study (the CARNET study) was conducted to determine more precisely the relationship between cognitive function and psychosocial adjustment in community-dwelling or institutionalized older people.

The participants in this study were administered cognitive tests together with tests that assessed various aspects of psychological well-being (Table 6.1). Testing was conducted on three occasions, each separated by eight to ten months. Despite the fact that all participants were carefully screened according to the same inclusion and exclusion criteria, community-dwelling older people generally displayed higher levels of cognitive function than those in institutions. Of particular interest was the finding that various psychosocial measures correlated significantly and similarly with cognitive test performance in *both* groups. This indicates that, while level of cognitive performance is affected by living environment, the general relationship between psychosocial status and cognitive function is character-

Table 6.1 Tests to assess cognitive function and psychosocial adjustment

Cognitive tests	Psychosocial tests
Wisconsin Card Sorting Test	Locus of Control
Word Recognition	Hassles Scale – Elderly Form
Face Recognition	Perceived Well Being Scale
Delayed Recall	Health Promoting Lifestyle
Corsi	Profile
Negative Transfer	Memorial University of
Verbal Fluency (FAS)	Newfoundland Scale of
Rey–Osterrieth Complex	Happiness (Munsh)
Figure Test (Recall)	Life Attitude Profile – Revised
California Verbal Learning	Everyday Activities Scale
Test	Future Orientation
	Questionnaire

istic of the normal elderly population at large. The psychosocial variables that correlated most consistently with cognitive function were locus of control, activity, general happiness, optimism and satisfaction with lifestyle. Table 6.2 provides the complete list of psychosocial variables that correlated significantly with cognitive function. Cognitive performance is reflected by a 'cognitive index' that is a composite measure of performance on all the cognitive tests.

An examination of the data over the three test periods revealed that variations in psychosocial status between test sessions were accompanied by parallel changes in the cognitive index. That is, decline or improvement in certain areas of psychosocial function, for whatever reason, was accompanied by changes in cognitive performance in the same direction. This pattern was reflected most clearly in comparisons involving the following psychosocial measures: locus of control, activity, optimism and happiness.

Although the CARNET study provides evidence that psychological well-being and cognitive function are closely related in elderly populations, it was not designed to specify causal relations. Nevertheless, it was possible to determine if performance on the psychosocial and cognitive tests in a particular session predicted performance in the other functional domain on subsequent sessions. In this analysis, optimism,

Table 6.2 Psychosocial variables that correlated significantly with cognitive index in community and institutionalized groups

	Session 1	Session 2	Session 3
Institutionalized	Personal control	Personal control	Personal control
	Activity	Activity	Optimism
	Optimism	Optimism	
	Lifestyle	Lifestyle	
Community	Personal control	Personal control	Personal control
	Activity	Activity	Optimism
	Optimism	Optimism	Lifestyle
	Meaningfulness	Lifestyle	Happiness
	Happiness	Happiness	
	Well-being		

activity and happiness emerged as fairly reliable predictors of subsequent cognitive performance in the combined groups. Interestingly, overall cognitive function proved to be a predictor of activity, optimism and satisfaction with lifestyle. To some extent at least, these results indicate a complementary relationship whereby both types of variables are capable of influencing each other.

In summary, the results of this longitudinal study provide further evidence that age-related cognitive decline is not a linear process governed exclusively by biological change. It was known that psychosocial factors had an influence on cognitive performance. However, this study indicates that the impact may be greater than previously thought. The data also address the plasticity of the underlying mechanisms that mediate cognitive abilities. It is clear that poor performance by older people at a particular point in time does not necessarily reflect an irreversible loss of brain function. Rather, what appears to be age-related cognitive impairment may, in reality, be an inability to perform to potential as a result of mitigating factors. As the influence of these factors is reduced, cognitive function can recover dramatically. These results provide further data suggesting that cognitive function in the elderly is

closely tied to the psychosocial environment. Thus, interventions that focus on vulnerable areas in the psychosocial domain may have the indirect effect of improving cognitive function.

Cognitive rehabilitation

- Interest in applying rehabilitation techniques to cognitive decline in the elderly has increased with a growing understanding of brain–behaviour relationships, neural plasticity, and the impact of impairment on day-to-day function.
- Considerable research has explored the effects of mnemonic training on recall.
- The effects of teaching mnemonics are task specific and generally limited to the immediate posttraining time period.
- Multifaceted training which targets psychosocial skills appears to have some benefit in maintaining a higher level of cognitive function over time.

Interest in developing techniques for limiting age-related cognitive decline has been stimulated in the last 15 years as more has been learned about brain–behaviour relationships, neural plasticity, and the relationship between cognitive impairment and loss of independence in day-to-day function (Poon et al., 1992; Riley, 1994a; Zarit, Johannsson and Malmberg, 1995). Although we now know that this decline is related both to the biological process of ageing and to psychosocial factors, cognitive rehabilitation research has been directed exclusively at improving specific cognitive processes, and the bulk of this work has focused on memory function.

In general, approaches to cognitive rehabilitation are based on the premise that the adult brain has a natural ability to recover and reorganize and that this is, to some extent, activity dependent. For example, Cotman and Neeper (1996) reported that exercise increases neurotropin levels in rats' brains, and others (e.g. Diamond et al., 1985) have shown that enriched environments can promote cortical development in older rats. Generalizing from the animal research, it follows that physical activity can promote neural plasticity in the ageing brain by influencing the expression of particular neurotrophic factors that facilitate structural change associated with behavioural function. Thus, some cognitive rehabilitation efforts have been directed at restoring or reactivating the neural mechanisms responsible for functional decline, whereas others attempt to teach alternative strategies to compensate for lost abilities.

Whereas influencing neural plasticity provides a broad objective of cognitive rehabilitation, specific impairments have led to the design of particular interventions. Thus, as older people are less likely to use effective organizational schemes when encoding information (Yesavage and Rose, 1983), considerable research has been directed at improving memory through teaching organizational strategies (mnemonics). Although there is a variety of mnemonic strategies, three have been especially influential – the method of loci, the use of imagery, and techniques for processing new information more deeply.

The method of loci technique has been employed in various forms for more than 20 years. The basic technique requires subjects to name several locations within a familiar environment and form an association between the locations and the items to be remembered. Several studies indicate that older subjects can effectively use this strategy to improve recall of list items in both experimental and certain practical situations (Robertson-Tchabo, Hausman and Arenberg, 1976; Anschutz et al., 1985; Yesavage, 1985; McCauley, Eskes and Moscovitch, 1996). Similarly, there are reports that encouraging elderly individuals to use visual imagery as a learning aid results in improved memory performance. These techniques have been shown to be helpful with a variety of stimulus material, including faces, names, environmental objects and word lists (West, 1995). On the other hand, the practical use of both techniques seems to be limited, in view of evidence that benefits are often small and that older people do not spontaneously use them in real-world situations (Robertson-Tchabo et al., 1976; Anschutz et al., 1987; Wood and Pratt, 1987; Scogin and Bienias, 1988; Kotler-Cope and Camp, 1990; West, 1995).

It is well known that accurate memory is directly related to the depth to which information is processed at the time of encoding. Information that is encoded together with meaningful associations is more likely to be remembered accurately than the same information superficially encoded (Craik and Lockhart, 1972). Older people do not typically process information as deeply as young adults, and this appears to be an important factor underlying age-related decline in memory function (Craik, 1977). On the other hand, investigators (Craik and Simon, 1980; Moscovitch, 1982) have shown that instructions to encode more deeply can improve memory performance in old people. Some studies found that young people may also benefit from such instructions, and so it is not clear that this technique reliably reduces age differences in tests of memory. Moreover, there is no indication that, following laboratory instruction, old people process information more deeply in their daily lives, once again raising questions about the practical utility of this approach.

There are a number of critical questions about the use of mnemonics that are difficult to answer with single studies. However, a recent meta-analysis allows some general conclusions about mnemonic training (Verhaeghen, Marcoen and Goossens, 1992). First, this meta-analysis confirmed that training older people to use mnemonics to learn and remember highly specific information does result in improved performance relative to nonintervention and placebo-treatment control procedures. Interestingly, there were no significant differences in effects related to the type of mnemonic taught. However, a critical finding of this analysis was that, although posttraining improvement was noted for targeted tasks, improvement did not generalize to other memory tasks. Nor was there evidence of much transfer outside the laboratory setting. In other words, learning mnemonic strategies in highly specific situations, while useful, did not lead to improved memory ability in a practical sense.

The limited success of singular approaches is somewhat offset by evidence that multifaceted training methods have produced more encouraging results. For example, Bäckman and his colleagues (Stigsdotter and Bäckman, 1989; Neely and Bäckman, 1993) showed that a comprehensive training procedure designed to relax older adults, focus their attention, and teach them to encode information-to-be-remembered more deeply resulted in improved memory for that material over a three-year period. Elderly subjects also do better when cues are available to remind them to use previously trained strategies (Hayslip, Maloy and Kohl, 1995). In addition, Flynn and Storandt (1990) found that including an intervention that provided counselling and support with respect to anxiety associated with memory decline contributed significantly to improved performance. Taken together, these results build on the premise that multiple factors contribute to the overall cognitive status of older adults and indicate, therefore, that a multidimensional approach may be most efficacious.

The limitations inherent in training programmes that target specific abilities have led to new approaches for improving cognitive function in patients with brain damage. These techniques frequently capitalize on processes that resist the effects of neurological impairment, such as those that support implicit and procedural memory. Glisky and her colleagues (Glisky, Schacter and Tulving, 1986; Glisky, 1995) were able to teach computer and business-related skills to patients with severe memory impairments by providing them with cues necessary to ensure accurate completion of the tasks, and then gradually removing the cues. Similarly, Wilson and her colleagues used an error-less learning strategy to teach brain-damaged patients with memory disorders to programme an electronic memory aid (Wilson, Baddeley and Evans, 1994). These techniques may also be useful in older adults (see Chapters 21 and 22).

Another avenue for intervention is suggested by reports, including the CARNET study described above, that psychosocial and cognitive function are closely related. Some psychosocial factors appear amenable to change through targeted interventions but, surprisingly, little work has been done in this area. Nevertheless, the available evidence is promising. For example, participants in a rehabilitation programme that included memory training and self-management training scored better on both cognitive and psychosocial measures than a control group (Bach et al., 1995). Implicit in the findings of Bach et al. is the concept that training programmes designed to optimize the 'fit' between environmental demands and the older person's resources and personal needs tend to result in overall enhancement of functional status (see also Kahana and Kahana, 1996). The Bach et al. study showed that cognitive performance is one aspect of functional status that benefits from interventions that take into account the entire individual.

Improving the fit between individuals and their environments has been attempted in a variety of ways – by maximizing individuals' resources or by manipulating psychosocial aspects of the environment. With respect to influencing cognitive function, the former approach entails teaching specific strategies. As we have seen, that approach, on its own, is limited in terms of effectiveness. However, combining it with a broader approach that takes into account psychosocial factors may prove to be more promising. In the next section, suggestions are presented for promoting cognitive abilities by working with various psychosocial variables.

Conclusions

- Preventing and reversing age-related cognitive decline may be possible through a multifaceted rehabilitation programme.
- A cognitive rehabilitation programme is proposed that takes into account research on psychosocial issues and targeted cognitive rehabilitation approaches.
- The proposed programme includes: (1) a psychosocial component to enhance dimensions of psychological well-being (self-efficacy beliefs, feelings of control, optimism); (2) cognitive training to teach practical strategies and promote their use in everyday life; and (3) a physical activity regimen for overall health benefits.

This chapter began with two primary questions: can we slow the rate of cognitive decline in older persons? Can we improve cognitive functioning in the normal ageing population? Although a resounding 'yes' would be an overstatement, the evidence reviewed makes us cautiously optimistic about answering these questions in the affirmative. The authors do not propose that age-related cognitive decline can be entirely prevented or reversed. Structural changes in the brain, particularly in the frontal and medial temporal lobes, seem an unavoidable part of the ageing process. Nevertheless, research on the determinants and covariates of cognitive status in older people suggests that cognitive decline to some extent, at least, may be reversible.

As discussed, much of the research in this area has demonstrated limited success in terms of improving the day-to-day functioning of older adults through cognitive rehabilitation. However, some findings are encouraging. In addition to those already mentioned, it is worth noting that recent research demonstrates that a psychosocial rehabilitation approach does improve or maintain day-to-day functioning in older adults (Clark et al., 1997). It is these findings that the authors draw upon to provide the groundwork for the proposed programme. (See other chapters in this volume, e.g. Chapters 21 and 22, that discuss training techniques that improve cognitive function in neurological populations and have potential for use with relatively healthy, older adults.) The present proposal is based on the premise that a multifaceted approach promises the greatest benefits for achieving enhanced cognitive performance in the elderly. Given the number of factors associated with cognitive status in older people and the considerable variation in cognitive performance, a multifaceted programme indeed, does, seem reasonable.

Available evidence suggests that affect and specific psychosocial attributes, such as perceived control and optimism, influence cognitive status in the elderly. Although a definitive causal relationship has not been established, the CARNET study as well as other research have shown that individuals who are vulnerable to cognitive decline also have difficulties in terms of psychological well-being. Thus, an important component of the authors' programme is the early assessment of psychosocial status to detect particular areas of strengths and weakness. Having identified problem areas that could affect cognitive function, a targeted counselling programme would attempt to change negative attitudes and beliefs which, apart from their impact on other functional areas, are harmful in and of themselves.

There is also compelling evidence that individuals who engage in little physical activity are vulnerable in a variety of health-related areas and experience disproportionate cognitive decline. Thus, for example, the proposed programme incorporates a relatively strenuous physical exercise regimen, both for its overall health benefits as well as for the known effect on cerebral perfusion which can only benefit cognitive function. This programme will be individually designed so that it is meaningful to each person as meaningful activity has been shown to have a positive effect on older adults' functioning (Clark et al., 1997).

Finally, it is important to develop interventions with the aim of providing individuals with practical strategies that compensate for declining cognitive abilities. Research to date has focused largely on strategies whose effectiveness is limited primarily to the training contexts. The authors propose to build on positive results in laboratory situations while modifying training techniques so that they are relevant to 'real-life' situations.

In general, a shift in emphasis is proposed such that rehabilitation efforts encompass what is known about the psychosocial variables associated with cognitive status. The purposes of the overall programme are to maximize cognitive potential, slow down the rate of decline and, in the process, contribute to a higher quality of life and a positive sense of well-being in older adults. The programme is based on empirical evidence, but future research will be necessary to determine the merit of the authors' recommendations. Indeed, the authors hesitate to put their recommendations forward in detail without initial pilot testing. However, the framework of their approach is laid out in the hope that it will be useful for others interested in developing cognitive rehabilitation programmes for the elderly.

The proposed programme combines three relatively diverse strands of therapy: a form of counselling/behavioural therapy to target psychosocial variables, cognitive training to target cognitive function, and complementary physical activity. In setting up this programme, it is proposed that each of these foci would form a module which would be graded to allow maximum individualization of programming. Each module would include pretesting and posttesting that are specific to its focus. Also, quality of life, cognitive function, and psychosocial status would be assessed before and after the programme.

The counselling/behavioural therapy module is guided by evidence that cognitive function in old age is related directly to psychosocial status. The programme would be designed around psychometric assessment that identified specific psychosocial areas in which individuals are at risk. Thus, appropriate testing would look for difficulties in such areas as personal control, optimism, social activity, that is, areas of psychosocial function that have been found to correlate with cognitive performance in normal old people. People's beliefs with regard to psychosocial status would also be assessed to identify any discrepancy between perceived function and objectively determined measures. Rehabilitation strategies, following principles of behavioural therapy practice, would be individually designed to reduce and compensate for difficulties in identified areas. The programme would also be designed to promote self-awareness to help people monitor their progress and encourage personal initiatives that would usefully complement formal intervention (see Chapter 15 for a review of the benefits of promoting self-awareness). The authors think that this approach can enhance psychological well-being and self-efficacy beliefs which, in combination with appropriate cognitive-skills training, will help individuals to make optimal use of learned cognitive strategies in practical settings.

Cognitive-skills training would build on evidence that the elderly do respond, at least to a limited extent, to interventions aimed at improving cognitive function in specific areas. For example, we know that teaching mnemonics has a positive short-term effect on specific memory tasks but that, unless specifically targeted, there is little transfer to the real world. Thus, at the beginning of this module the authors propose asking participants to identify everyday incidents in which they experience difficulty (e.g. forgetting names, appointments, and/or scheduled activities). As research to date has demonstrated little generalization beyond the task on which training occurred, it is proposed to teach strategies appropriate to the class of events or activities represented by the specific tasks. For example, visual imagery mnemonics, typically taught in relation to laboratory tasks, could be taught in relation to remembering names, grocery lists, specific commitments, and so on. It is also proposed that participants be encouraged to keep a diary of planned events and to note when learned strategies are to be employed. These diaries should provide some indication of the individ-

ual's success in applying learned strategies, and should also provide direction for additional cognitive interventions. Proulx and his colleagues (see Chapter 16) have had considerable success using diaries or memory books for this purpose in their programme for improving cognitive performance in brain-damaged patients with severe cognitive disorders.

Finally, part of each training session would include some physical activity individually graded from simple group exercise programmes to much more strenuous fitness activities (see Dean, 1994; Kauffman, 1994). Participants would be encouraged to engage in a form of activity that they could continue on their own and the diary could also be used to track the individual's level of activity. Related to this is the fact that older people are notoriously neglectful of diet and often suffer from inadequate nutrition. In view of growing evidence of a relationship between nutritional status and cognitive function in the elderly, it may well prove desirable to include a nutritional counselling component into this aspect of the programme.

How might such a programme be implemented? Who would participate? Based on the results of previous research, including those of the CARNET study, individuals in institutions are especially at risk for age-related cognitive decline. New residents in institutions might provide the first sample for assessing such a programme. Participants in programmes at seniors' centres would provide a community-dwelling group for comparisons.

The model proposed has, in a sense, moved beyond the available research. However, as demonstrated by Clark and her colleagues (1997), such a programme is feasible and the authors believe that once appropriate modules are developed, it could be run with minimal professional support. A major advantage of this approach over previous cognitive rehabilitation efforts is that it incorporates psychosocial variables that have been shown to be closely related to cognitive status in the older population. It is suggested that this multifaceted, individualized approach has the potential to make meaningful changes in cognitive functioning among older adults that will not only enable them to maintain independence longer, but will also promote a sense of well-being and an enriched quality of life.

Acknowledgements

The CARNET study and preparation of this chapter were supported by research grants to GW and MM from the Government of Canada's Centres for Excellence Research Program and the Medical Research Council of Canada, and by a Halbert Research fellowship to GW. Data analysis of the CARNET study as well as much of the background research for this chapter were accomplished while GW was a research fellow at the Hebrew University in Jerusalem. He wishes to acknowledge the support and hospitality provided by the faculty and staff of the Institute for Canadian Studies and the Department of Psychology at the Hebrew University. DD held an Ontario Ministry of Health Fellowship Award during the preparation of this manuscript.

References

Albert, M., Jones, K., Savage, C. et al. 1995. Predictors of cognitive change in older persons: MacArthur studies of successful ageing. *Psychol Aging* **10**, 578–89.

Albert, M. and Moss, M. 1996. Neuropsychology of ageing: findings in humans and monkeys. In *Handbook of the Biology of Aging*, 4th edn, ed. E. Schneider and J. Rowe, pp. 217–33. Toronto: Academic Press.

Anschutz, L., Camp, C., Markley, R. and Kramer, J. 1985. Maintenance and generalization of mnemonics for grocery shopping by older adults. *Exp Ageing Res* **11**, 157–60.

Anschutz, L., Camp, C., Markley, R. and Kramer, J. 1987. Remembering mnemonics: a three-year follow-up on the effects of mnemonics training in elderly adults. *Exp Aging Res* **13**, 141–4.

Arbuckle, T., Gold, D. and Andres, D. 1986. Cognitive functioning of older people in relation to social and personality variables. *Psychol Aging* **1**, 55–62.

Arbuckle, T., Gold, D., Andres, D., Schwartzman, A. and Chaikelson, J. 1992. The role of psychosocial context, age, and intelligence in memory performance of older men. *Psychol Aging* **7**, 25–36.

Azari, N., Rapoport, S., Salerno, J. et al. 1992. Interregional correlations of resting cerebral metabolism in old and young women. *Brain Res* **589**, 279–90.

Bach, D., Bach, M., Bohmer, F., Fruhwald, T. and Grilc, B. 1995. Reactivating occupational therapy: a method to improve cognitive performance in geriatric patients. *Aging* **24**, 222–6.

Beats, B. 1996. Biological origin of depression in later life. *Int J Geriatric Psychiatry* **11**, 349–54.

Buschmann, M. and Hollinger, L. 1994. Influence of social support and control on depression in the elderly. *Clin Gerontol* **14**, 13–28.

Butters, N. and Stuss, D. 1989. Diencephalic amnesia. In *Handbook of Neuropsychology*, Vol. ed. F. Boller and J. Grafman, pp. 107–48. Amsterdam: Elsevier Science.

Cavanaugh, J. and Green, E. 1990. I believe, therefore I can: self-efficacy beliefs in memory and ageing. In *Ageing and Cognition: Mental Processes, Self-awareness, and Interventions*, ed. E. Lovelace, pp. 189–230. Amsterdam: Elsevier Science.

Chodzko-Zajko, W., Schuler, P., Solomon, J., Heinl, B. and Ellis, N. 1992. The influence of physical fitness on automatic and effortful memory changes in aging. *Int J Aging Hum Dev* **35**, 265–85.

Clark, F., Azen, S.P., Zemke, R. et al. 1997. Occupational therapy for independent-living older adults: a randomized controlled trial. *J Am Med Assoc* **278**, 1321–6.

Cotman, C. and Neeper, S. 1996. Activity-dependent plasticity and the ageing brain. In *Handbook of the Biology of Aging*, 4th edn, ed. E. Schneider and J. Rowe, pp. 283–99. Toronto: Academic Press.

Craik, F.I.M. 1977. Age differences in human memory. In *Handbook of the Psychology of Aging*, ed. J.E. Birren and W.K. Schaie, pp. 384–420. New York: Van Nostrand.

Craik, F.I.M. 1991. Memory functions in normal aging. In *Memory Disorders: Research and Clinical Practice*, ed. T. Yanagihara and R. Peterson, pp. 347–67. New York: Marcel Dekker Inc.

Craik, F. and Lockhart, R. 1972. Levels of processing: a framework for memory research. *J Verb Learning Verbal Behav* **11**, 671–84.

Craik, F.I.M. and E. Simon 1980. Age differences in memory: the roles of attention and depth of processing. In *New Directions in Memory and Aging*, ed. L.W. Poon and J.L. Fozard, pp. 95–110. Hillsdale, NJ: Erlbaum.

Dean, E. 1994. Cardiopulmonary development. In *Functional Performance in Older Adults*, ed. B. Bonder, and M. Wagner, pp. 62–92. Toronto: F.A. Davis.

Deptula, D., Singh, R. and Pomara, N. 1993. Aging, emotional states, and memory. *Am J Psychiatry* **150**, 429–34.

Diamond, M., Johnson, R., Protti, A., Ott, C. and Kajisa, L. 1985. Plasticity in the 904-day-old rat cerebral cortex. *Exp Neurol* **87**, 309–17.

Emery, C. Huppert, F. and Schein, R. 1995. Relationships among age, exercise, health, and cognitive function in a British sample. *The Gerontologist* **35**, 378–85.

Evans, D., Beckett, L., Albert, M. et al. 1993. Level of education and change in cognitive function in a community population of older persons. *Ann of Epidemiol* **3**, 71–7.

Ferraro, K. 1982. The health consequences of relocation among the aged in the community. *J Gerontol* **38**, 90-6.

Flynn, T. and Storandt, M. 1990. Supplemental group discussions in memory training for older adults. *Psychol Aging* **5**, 178–81.

Garfein, A. and Herzog, R. 1995. Robust aging among the young–old, old–old, and oldest–old. *J Gerontol B Psychol Sci Soc Sci* **50**, S77–S87.

Glisky, E.L. 1995. Computers in memory rehabilitation. In *Handbook of Memory Disorders*, ed. A. Baddeley, B. Wilson and F. Watts, pp. 557–75. Toronto: John Wiley & Sons.

Glisky, E.L., Schacter, D. and Tulving, E. 1986. Computer learning by memory-impaired patients: acquisition and retention of complex knowledge. *Neuropsychologia* **24**, 313–28.

Gold, D. and Arbuckle, T. 1990. Interactions between personality and cognition and their implications for theories of ageing. In *Ageing and Cognition: Mental Processes, Self-awareness and Interventions*, ed. E. Lovelace, pp. 351–78. Amsterdam: Elsevier.

Goldberg, A., Dengel, D. and Hagberg, J. 1996. Exercise physiology and aging. In *Handbook of the Biology of Aging*, 4th edn, ed. E. Schneider and J. Rowe, pp. 331–54. Toronto: Academic Press.

Golomb, J., de Leon, M., Kluger, A., George, A., Tarshish, G. and Ferris, S. 1993. Hippocampal atrophy in normal ageing: an association with recent memory impairments. *Arch Neurol* **50**, 967–73.

Goodwin, J.S., Goodwin, J.M. and Garry, P. 1983. Association between nutritional status and cognitive functioning in a healthy, elderly population. *J Am Med Assoc* **249**, 2917–21.

Grady, C., McIntosh, A., Horwitz, B. et al. 1995. Age-related reduction in human recognition memory due to impaired encoding. *Science* **269**, 218–21.

Hayslip, B., Maloy, R. and Kohl, R. 1995. Long-term efficacy of fluid ability interventions with older adults. *J Gerontol B Psychol Sci Soc Sci* **50**, P141–9.

Hultsch, D., Hammer, M. and Small, B. 1993. Age differences in cognitive performance in later life: relationships to self-reported health and activity life style. *J Gerontol Psychol Sci* **48**, P1–P11.

Huppert, F. 1991. Age-related changes in memory: learning and remembering new information. In *Handbook of Neuropsychology*, Vol. 5, ed. F. Boller and J. Grafman, pp. 123–47. Amsterdam: Elsevier Science.

Hyer, L., Matteson, M. and Siegler, I. 1982. Locus of control and long term care. *J Appl Gerontol* **1**, 147–60.

Inouye, S., Albert, M., Mohs, R., Sun, K. and Berkman, L. 1993.

Cognitive performance in a high-functioning community-dwelling elderly population. *J Gerontol Med Sci* **48**, M146–M151.

Kahana, E. and Kahana, B. 1996. Conceptual and empirical advances in understanding aging well through proactive adaptation. In *Adulthood and Aging: Research on Continuities and Discontinuities*, ed. V. Bengtson, pp. 18–40. New York: Springer-Verlag.

Kauffman, T. 1994. Mobility. In *Functional Performance in Older Adults*, ed. B. Bonder and M. Wagner, pp. 42–61. Toronto: F.A. Davis.

Kotler-Cope, S. and Camp, C. 1990. Memory interventions in ageing populations. In *Ageing and Cognition: Mental Processes, Self-awareness, and Interventions*, ed. E. Lovelace, pp. 231–61. Amsterdam: Elsevier Science.

McAvay, G., Seeman, T. and Rodin, J. 1996. A longitudinal study of change in domain-specific self-efficacy among older adults. *J Gerontol Psychol Sci* **51B**, P243–53.

McCauley, M.E., Eskes, G. and Moscovitch, M. 1996. The effect of imagery on explicit and implicit tests of memory in young and old people: a double association. *Can J Exp Psychol* **50**, 34–41.

McDougall, G. 1994. Predictors of metamemory in older adults. *Nurs Res* **43**, 212–18.

McDowd, J. and Birren, J. 1990. Aging and attentional processes. In *Handbook of the Psychology of Aging*, 3rd edn, ed. J. Birren and K. Schaie, pp. 222–33. San Diego: Academic Press.

Meiran, N. and Jelicic, M. 1995. Implicit memory in Alzheimer's disease: a meta-analysis. *Neuropsychology* **9**, 1–13.

Moeller, J., Ishikawa, T., Dhawan, V. et al. 1996. The metabolic topography of normal aging. *J Cereb Blood Flow Metab* **16**, 385–98.

Moscovitch, M. 1982. A neuropsychological approach to memory and perception in normal and pathological aging. In *Aging and Cognitive Processes*, ed. F.I.M. Craik and S. Trehub, pp. 57–88. New York: Plenum Press.

Moscovitch, M. and Winocur, G. 1983. Contextual cues and release from proactive inhibition in young and old people. *Can J Psychol* **37**, 331–44.

Moscovitch, M. and Winocur, G. 1992. The neuropsychology of memory and aging. In *The Handbook of Aging and Cognition*, ed. F. Craik and T. Salthouse, pp. 315–72. Hillsdale, NJ: Lawrence Erlbaum.

Moscovitch, M. and Winocur, G. 1995. Frontal lobes, memory and ageing. *Ann NY Acad Sci* **769**, 119–50.

Neely, A. and Bäckman, L. 1993. Long-term maintenance of gains from memory training in older adults: two 3½-year follow-up studies. *J Gerontol* **48**, P233–7.

Nyberg, L., Nilsson, L.G., Oloffson, U. and Bäckman, L. 1997. Effects of division of attention during encoding and retrieval on age differences in episodic memory. *Exp Aging Res* **23**, 137–43.

Penland, J. 1994. Dietary boron, brain function, and cognitive performance. *Environ Health Perspect* **102** (Suppl.), 65–72.

Perlmutter, M. and Nyquist, L. 1990. Relationships between self-reported physical health and mental health and intelligence performance across adulthood. *J Gerontol Psychol Sci* **45**, P145–55.

Poon, L., Messner, S., Martin, P., Noble, C. and Clayton, G. 1992. Influences of cognitive resources on adaptation and old age. *Int J Aging Hum Dev* **34**, 31–46.

Riley, K. 1994a. Cognitive development. In *Functional Performance in Older Adults*, ed. B. Bondar and M. Wagner, pp. 107–20. Philadelphia: F.A. Davis.

Riley, K. 1994b. Depression. In *Functional Performance in Older Adults*, ed. B. Bonder and M. Wagner, pp. 256–68. Philadelphia: F.A. Davis.

Robertson-Tchabo, E., Hausman, C. and Arenberg, D. 1976. A classical mnemonic for older learners: a trip that works. *Educ Gerontol Int Quart* **1**, 215–26.

Ruth, J. and Coleman, P. 1996. Personality and aging: coping and management of the self in later life. In *Handbook of the Psychology of Aging*, 4th edn, ed. J. Birren and K. Schaie, pp. 308–22. Toronto: Academic Press.

Scheibel, A. 1996. Structural and functional changes in the aging brain. In *Handbook of the Psychology of Aging*, 4th edn, ed. J. Birren and K. Schaie, pp. 105–28. Toronto: Academic Press.

Scogin, F. and Bienias, J. 1988. A three-year follow-up of older adult participants in a memory-skills training program. *Psychol Aging* **3**, 334–7.

Seeman, T., Rodin, J. and Albert, M. 1993. Self-efficacy and cognitive performance in high-functioning older individuals. *J Aging Health* **5**, 455–74.

Shaw, R. 1992. Coping effectiveness in nursing home residents: the role of control. *J Aging Health* **4**, 551–63.

Shimamura, A., Janowsky, J. and Squire, L. 1991. What is the role of frontal lobe damage in memory disorders? In *Frontal Lobe Function and Dysfunction*, ed. H. Levin, M. Eisenberg and A. Benton, pp. 173–95. Toronto: Oxford University Press.

Stigsdotter, A. and Bäckman, L. 1989. Multifactorial memory training with older adults: how to foster maintenance of improved performance. *Gerontology* **35**, 260–7.

Stuss, D., Eskes, G. and Foster, J. 1994. Experimental neuropsychological studies of frontal lobe functions. In *Handbook of Neuropsychology*, Vol. 9. ed. F. Boller and J. Grafman, pp. 149–85. Amsterdam: Elsevier Science.

Stuss, D., Shallice, T., Alexander, M. and Picton, T. 1995. A multidisciplinary approach to anterior attentional functions. *Ann NY Acad Sci* **769**, 191–211.

Uchiyama, C., Mitrushina, M., Satz, P. and Schall, M. 1996. Direct and indirect effects of demographic, medical, and psychological variables on neuropsychological performance in normal geriatric persons: a structural equation model. *J Int Neuropsychol Soc* **2**, 299–305.

Verhaeghen, P., Marcoen, A. and Goossens, L. 1992. Improving memory performance in the aged through mnemonic training: a meta-analytic study. *Psychol Aging* **7**, 242–51.

Verhaeghen, P., Marcoen, A. and Goosens, L. 1993. Facts and fiction about memory ageing: a quantitiative integration of research findings. *J Gerontol Psychol Sci* **48**, P157–71.

Waxman, S. and deGroot, J. 1995. *Correlative Neuroanatomy*, 22nd edn. Norwalk, CT: Appleton & Lange.

Wenk, G. 1989. Nutrition, cognition, and memory. *Top Geriatr Rehab* **5**, 79–87.

West, M. 1993. Regionally specific loss of neurons in the aging human hippocampus. *Neurbiol Aging* **14**, 287–93.

West, R. 1995. Compensatory strategies for age-associated memory impairment. In *Handbook of Memory Disorders*, ed. A. Baddeley, B. Wilson and F. Watts, pp. 482–500. Chichester: John Wiley & Sons.

West, R., Barron, K. and Crook, T. 1992. Everyday memory performance across the life span: effects of age and noncognitive individual differences. *Psychol Aging* **7**, 72–82.

Wilson, B., Baddeley, A. and Evans, J. 1994. Errorless learning in the rehabilitation of memory impaired people. *Neuropsychol Rehab* **4**, 307–26.

Winocur, G., Kinsbourne, M. and Moscovitch, M. 1989. The effect of cuing on release from proactive interference in Korsakoff amnesic patients. *J Exp Psychol Hum Learn Mem* **7**, 56–65.

Winocur, G. and Moscovitch, M. 1983. Paired associate learning in institutionalized and noninstitutionalized old people: an analysis of interference and context effects. *J Gerontol* **38**, 455–64.

Winocur, G. and Moscovitch, M. 1990. A comparison of cognitive function in institutionalized and community dwelling old people of normal intelligence. *Can J Psychol* **44**, 435–44.

Winocur, G., Moscovitch, M. and Freedman, J. 1987a. An investigation of cognitive function in relation to psychosocial variables in institutionalized old people. *Can J Psychol* **41**, 257–69.

Winocur, G., Moscovitch, M. and Stuss, D.T. 1996. Explicit and implicit memory in the elderly: evidence for double dissociation involving medial temporal and frontal lobe functions. *Neuropsychology* **10**, 57–65.

Winocur, G., Moscovitch, M. and Witherspoon, D. 1987b. Contextual cuing and memory performance in brain-damaged amnesics and old people. *Brain Cogn* **6**, 129–31.

Winocur, G. and Weiskrantz, L. 1976. An investigation of paired-associate learning in amnesic patients. *Neuropsychologia* **14**, 97–110.

Wood, L. and Pratt, J. 1987. Pegword mnemonic as an aid to memory in the elderly: a comparison of four age groups. *Educ Gerontol* **13**, 325–39.

Yesavage, J. 1985. Nonpharmacologic treatments for memory losses with normal aging. *Am J Psychiatry* **142**, 600–5.

Yesavage, J. and Rose, T. 1983. Concentration and mnemonic training in elderly subjects with memory complaints: a study of combined therapy and order effect. *Psychiatry Res* **9**, 157–67.

Zarit, S., Gallagher, D. and Kramer, N. 1981. Memory training in the community aged: effects of depression, memory complaint, and memory performance. *Educ Gerontol Int Quart* **6**, 11–27.

Zarit, S., Johannsson, B. and Malmberg, B. 1995. Changes in functional competency in the oldest old: a longitudinal study. *J Aging Health* **7**, 3–23.

Zec, R. 1995. The neuropsychology of aging. *Exp Gerontol* **30**, 432–42.

PART II

Pharmacological approaches

Introduction

Donald T. Stuss

This part, on 'pharmacological approaches', may appear somewhat misplaced in a volume on 'cognitive' rehabilitation. The comparatively small size of the section would also imply a limited amount of applicable knowledge on the topic. Why then has it been situated in a somewhat prominent position early in the book?

The size of the section to some degree reflects the developmental stage of the pharmaceutical approach to cognitive rehabilitation. Also, it indicates our desire to emphasize the more 'cognitive' aspects of this page-limited book, commensurate with our stated objectives. Nevertheless, placement of this section early in the book reflects our belief in the present and future role of neuropharmacological therapy in the treatment of cognitive disorders.

The three chapters exemplify what exists, and what might be expected. The chapter by Arnsten and Smith represents the required scientific approach to pharmacological strategies for neuroprotection and rehabilitation. Using traumatic brain injury as an example, the emphasis is on understanding the mechanisms underlying the cognitive dysfunction after such trauma. In this chapter, Arnsten and Smith convincingly present the case for the appropriate *timing* of pharmacological interventions. Brain trauma results in a secondary injury cascade. Identifying the distinct aspects of the cascade provides the knowledge base to develop therapeutic approaches that target these individual components. While this research is still in the experimental stage, the potential clinical relevance of early treatment to prevent later cognitive dysfunction is exciting.

The second part of this chapter moves into the treatment of cognitive deficits that have already developed after traumatic brain injury. Again, the approach is methodological and thorough. Neuropathological studies direct the researcher to the primary brain regions to be studied, the frontal and temporal lobes (a similar approach was used to understand the cognitive deficits after traumatic brain injury: Stuss et al., 1985). The review of the mechanism of the neuromodulators related to these selective brain regions is the basis for understanding how targeted pharmacological cognitive enhancers might be used to minimize cognitive deficits. At present, this focused research approach has been attempted primarily in nonhuman animals.

The two other chapters in this part of the book represent examples of the clinical applications of known pharmacological interventions. Two groups were selected as examples: traumatic brain injury and Alzheimer's disease. Traumatic brain injury was a natural choice. A large proportion of rehabilitation funds and effort is directed to minimize the devastating effects of traumatic brain injury. John Cassidy, as a practising psychiatrist with a very active neurorehabilitation treatment programme, was asked to describe his current practical approaches. Cassidy places neuropharmacological management in a broader rehabilitative context, which includes a neurological model of treatment, environmental support, behavioural programming, and the use of psychotherapy. This practical lesson cannot be overemphasized. In real life, all needs of the patient must be considered, and an armamentarium of the best established tools used. It is the caregiver's job to understand these needs, and all the factors that might be contributing to the individual's problems. What characterizes this chapter is a practical approach to the neuropharmacological arm of treatment which includes the importance of precise differential diagnosis. Cassidy provides examples to highlight the efficacy of certain drugs, as well as to demonstrate the problems that may result. A case study provides a vibrant example of the specificity of the treatment through the multiple stages of recovery.

The chapter by Leiter and Cummings summarizes pharmacological interventions in Alzheimer's disease. Many may question the relevance of a chapter on Alzheimer's disease in a volume on cognitive rehabilitation. Because this is a progressive disorder, rehabilitation is normally not a considered option. The reasons for including this chapter are several. First, as indicated in the chapter, Alzheimer's disease is becoming an increasingly prevalent cause of cognitive and behavioural disorders. Second, it is an excellent example of the neuropharmacological approach to the amelioration of cognitive and behavioural disorders. Third, as indicated in the introductory chapter, our belief is in rehabilitation of the whole person by whatever means necessary, and that a broad approach is necessary. Alzheimer's disease is one example of the broader approach. The chapter by Leiter and Cummings specifically deals with cognition and behaviour, and acknowledges that behavioural *and* pharmacological interventions are the most effective tools at present. The final reason for including the chapter is our opinion that rehabilitation of some type should be targeted to individuals with progressive disorders and not restricted to those with acute disorders who have a natural recovery course.

The first part of Leiter and Cummings' chapter is a handy primer on the diagnosis and neuropathological changes associated with Alzheimer's disease. The behavioural disturbances such as agitation, delusions and hallucinations, depressions, anxiety, and other problems such as sleep and appetite are described. The organization of the pharmacological management of cognitive deficits reflects the current methods, with an emphasis on general approaches such as cholinergic and neuroprotective treatments. The summary tables, which provide information on usual daily doses for different drugs used to treat Alzheimer's disease, should be extremely useful for the health professional and family caregiver.

The more behaviourally oriented reader might find the Arnsten and Smith chapter a bit daunting, but the information is very relevant to the future of pharmacotherapy in patients with traumatic brain injury. What the scientist will obtain from this chapter is a framework to direct basic science by clinical questions. The chapter by Cassidy is important because it illustrates how a model is helpful to direct treatment, and how pharmacotherapeutic interventions contribute to the overall rehabilitative plan which is directed to specific behaviour. Leiter and Cummings' chapter is an excellent example of what today might be considered 'evidence-based' medicine. Pharmacological interventions directed to specific behavioural disturbances can assist in the entire rehabilitative efforts and therapeutic milieu.

Reference

Stuss, D.T., Ely, P., Hugenholtz, H. et al. 1985. Subtle neuropsychological deficits in patients with good recovery after closed head injury. *Neurosurgery* 17, 37–44.

7

Pharmacological strategies for neuroprotection and rehabilitation

Amy F.T. Arnsten and Douglas H. Smith

Introduction

The ongoing epidemic of traumatic brain injury has only recently been recognized to be a potentially treatable disease process. This new awareness has led to multiple efforts aimed at developing therapeutic strategies to combat both the acute and the chronic pathological sequelae of brain trauma. A primary focus of these studies is the attenuation of posttraumatic cognitive dysfunction, which is the most common and most disabling feature of traumatic brain injury. This chapter summarizes these studies and reviews the proposed mechanisms thought to be responsible for the development and persistence of posttraumatic cognitive dysfunction.

Therapeutic protection at the time of trauma

- Following brain trauma, a cascade of delayed or secondary processes has been shown to potentiate primary mechanical damage.
- The temporal evolution of secondary damage following brain trauma lends itself to manipulation by a variety of therapeutic measures.
- Posttraumatic cognitive dysfunction has been produced in animal models of brain trauma, and has been shown to be attenuated by several therapeutic strategies.
- Selective hippocampal damage appears to be associated with deficits in spatial memory following experimental brain trauma in animals, and may be reduced by therapeutic intervention.

Immediately following traumatic brain injury, a cascade of delayed or secondary processes has been shown to potentiate damage, and to induce injury to regions not directly affected by the initial trauma. These changes may appear within minutes following brain trauma or may evolve over hours or even days and weeks. Through the use of newly developed experimental models of brain trauma, it has been shown that much of the secondary damage may result from an aberrant balance of the brain's endogenous neurochemistry. These neurochemical changes are thought to include dramatic changes in neurotransmitter activity, altered neurotransmitter release, alterations in neurotransmitter reuptake or clearance systems, changes in receptor binding, the synthesis of 'autodestructive' factors and inflammatory mediators, and the alteration of trophic factors. This disregulation of the brain's chemistry may lead to cell swelling, membrane disruption, alterations in regional blood flow, changes in metabolism, and changes in the phenotype of receptor systems (for review see McIntosh et al., 1996a). Recently, traumatic brain injury has also been shown to produce apoptosis of brain cells, possibly initiated through programmed cell death (Rink et al., 1995). Ultimately, these effects may lead to irreparable damage and dysfunction. Fortunately, this temporal evolution of secondary damage lends itself to manipulation or disruption by a variety of therapeutic measures. Moreover, the recent identification of specific properties of secondary injury following trauma has helped in the development of targeted therapy. This chapter reviews some of the presumed mediators of secondary injury and the promising therapeutic measures that may combat the deleterious secondary cascade following brain trauma. Some of the classes of therapies discussed have not yet been evaluated for their effects on posttraumatic cognitive outcome, but are included due to other potentially related efficacious attributes. It is important to note that the majority of studies of acute therapy highlighted here represent data from experimental models of brain trauma in animals. Extensive studies of therapeutic efficacy in the acute setting for human brain trauma patients have only recently been initiated.

Evaluation techniques to determine therapeutic efficacy on cognitive status following experimental brain injury in rodents

Although multiple techniques have been developed to assess cognitive status in rodents, modifications of the Morris water maze paradigm (Morris, 1984) are by far the most commonly utilized for models of brain trauma. Therefore, this discussion is restricted to two generalized paradigms used to determine pharmacological efficacy in rodent models. Water maze paradigms take advantage of the innate behaviour of rodents, which are actually very good swimmers but will vigorously attempt to escape from water. The essential feature of water maze techniques is as follows: rodents are placed into a large circular pool of water, from which they can only escape by climbing onto a hidden platform. The platform is hidden by virtue of being submerged just beneath the surface of water, which is rendered opaque. Thus, the platform offers no local cues to guide escape behaviour. To navigate to the platform, rodents must learn the spatial position of distal visual cues in order to guide them to the escape location. Normal rodents very quickly acclimate to this task and learn to swim directly to the platform site from random starting positions at the circumference of the pool. Two generally distinct water maze paradigms have evolved to assess either spatial memory function or learning ability following experimental brain trauma.

Posttraumatic memory evaluation

Posttraumatic memory function may be evaluated by training the animals prior to brain injury to become highly proficient in their ability to find the platform. Shortly following training, brain trauma is induced or the animals are treated as shams (no injury). From a few days to a few weeks following injury, the animals can be assessed for memory (retention) of the task learned prior to injury. The platform is removed from the maze and the animals are allowed to swim for a short period of time (usually one minute) while a computer tracking system records their swimming patterns. Without the platform in the maze, platform-seeking behaviour is attributed to memory of its previous location. While nonbrain-injured animals will repeatedly swim over or near the platform site, brain-injured animals have been shown to have greatly diminished platform-seeking behaviour, often displaying no apparent retention of the water maze task (Smith et al., 1991, 1992; Fig. 7.1). To express these differences in behaviour, memory scores are derived by determining the number of seconds spent in proximity to the platform site. This technique has been the most extensively utilized to evaluate therapeutic efficacy in models of brain injury.

Posttraumatic learning evaluation

In contrast to the memory/retention paradigms, no training is performed prior to injury. Rather, brain trauma is induced first and the animals are subsequently evaluated for their ability to navigate to the platform at various timepoints following injury. After a series of learning trials in the water maze, the elapsed time necessary to find the hidden platform (escape latency) is usually quite low for noninjured animals. However, brain-injured animals have been shown to have very significantly increased escape latencies, reflecting an impaired ability to learn the location of the hidden platform (Hamm et al., 1992; Pierce et al., 1993; Fig. 7.1).

The obvious need to evaluate cognitive outcome in animal models of brain trauma initiated the development of specialized water maze paradigms early in this decade. Since that time, a multitude of pharmacology studies has been performed using these techniques. However, it is important to note that evaluation of cognitive function in experimental models of brain trauma is only one measure in a battery of outcome tests that

Water Maze Paradigms

Memory/Retention   **Learning/Acquisition**

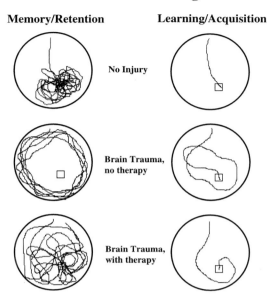

No Injury

Brain Trauma,
no therapy

Brain Trauma,
with therapy

Fig. 7.1 Aerial view of representative water maze swimming patterns seen in a memory/retention paradigm and a learning/acquisition paradigm. Circle, water maze circumference; square, platform location (removed for memory/retention paradigm); continuous line, swimming pattern of rodent. For the memory/retention test, note the improved posttraumatic platform-seeking behaviour, demonstrating preserved memory function in the treated animal compared to the nontreated animal. For the learning/acquisition test, note the decreased posttraumatic escape latency (shorter path length) in the treated animal compared to the nontreated animal, demonstrating enhanced learning ability.

are currently utilized to determine pharmacological efficacy.

Pathophysiological changes and pharmacological intervention following brain trauma

A multitude of mechanisms has been implicated in the pathological posttraumatic sequelae leading to many proposed therapeutic strategies. Therefore, this review focuses on the most currently relevant therapies with the potential for clinical application. Particular empha-

sis is placed on excitatory amino acid (EAA) neurotransmitters owing to their prominence as the most extensively evaluated class of compounds for the treatment of traumatic brain injury.

Excitatory amino acid neurotoxicity

A major component of the secondary neurochemical response to brain trauma is thought to include the acute and marked release of EAA neurotransmitters (e.g. glutamate and aspartate), leading to a pathological overexcitation of EAA subtype receptors (Choi, 1985; Rothman and Olney, 1986; Mayer et al., 1987; Collingridge and Davies, 1989: Collingridge and Lester, 1989). These receptors include the inotropic kainate (KA) and α-amino-3-hydroxy-5-methyl-4-isoxazole propionate (AMPA) receptors, found in both glia and neurons, and the N-methyl-D-aspartate (NMDA) receptor, found only in neurons. Overactivation of the AMPA/KA receptors has been shown to induce a massive influx of NA^+ and efflux of K^+ through receptor-associated monovalent ionophores (Choi, 1985). This ionic shift causes a depolarization sufficient to overcome a voltage-dependent block by Mg^{2+} of the NMDA receptor-associated divalent ionophore. Following ligand activation and removal of the Mg^{2+} block of the NMDA receptor ionophore, a large influx of Ca^{2+} into the neuron may occur (Rothman and Olney, 1986; Mayer and Westbrook, 1987; Collingridge and Davies, 1989; Collingridge and Lester, 1989). It has been proposed that a pathologically sustained increase in intracellular Ca^{2+} may play a central role in the development of secondary cell damage or death by initiating a cascade of deleterious calcium-dependent processes (Young, 1987). The sustained release of glutamate with prolonged postsynaptic excitation has been postulated to lead to (1) early accumulation of intracellular Na^+ (through AMPA and KA receptor gated ionophores), causing acute neuronal swelling; and (2) delayed Ca^{2+} influx (through the NMDA receptor ionophore), initiating a cascade of metabolic disturbances within the neuron (Choi, 1985). More recently, the increase in intracellular free Ca^{2+} following an excitotoxic event has also been linked both to the influx of Ca^{2+} through nonNMDA receptors (KA and AMPA receptors) (Iino, Ozawa and Tsuki, 1990; Hume,

Dingledine and Heinemann, 1991) and to the inositol triphosphate-mediated release of Ca^{2+} from intracellular stores triggered by EAA stimulation of another EAA receptor, the EAA metabotropic receptor (Sugiyama, Ito and Hirono, 1987; Schoepp, Bockaert and Sladeczek, 1990a).

Brain trauma, excitatory amino acids and cognitive dysfunction

In several animal models of brain trauma, and subsequently in patients, in-vivo intracerebral microdialysis techniques have demonstrated an acute and marked increase in extracellular EAAs following injury (Faden et al., 1989; Nilsson et al., 1990; Katayama et al., 1990; Palmer et al., 1993). In concert with these findings, changes in cation homeostasis have been observed following experimental brain injury. Atomic absorption spectrophotometric analysis has demonstrated that total tissue concentrations of Na^+ and Ca^{2+} are increased following brain injury in the rat, while the total tissue concentrations of Ca^{2+}, K^+ and Mg^{2+} decrease (Soares et al., 1992; Fineman et al., 1993; Smith et al., 1993a). In addition, extracellular K^+ concentration has been observed to increase substantially following experimental brain injury (Katayama et al., 1990). Moreover, intracellular free Mg^{2+} concentrations ($[Mg^{2+}]_i$), assessed using ^{31}P magnetic resonance spectroscopy (MRS), have been shown to decrease dramatically following experimental brain trauma (Vink et al., 1988a; Smith et al., 1994).

An important aspect of EAA neurotoxicity following trauma is the general role of EAA receptors in cognition. EAA neurotransmission has been shown to play a major role in normal cognitive processes. Long-term potentiation has been shown to be mediated, in part, by the influx of calcium through NMDA receptors (Bliss and Lomo, 1973; Collingridge and Bliss, 1987; Collingridge and Davies, 1989). Long-term potentiation is considered to be the synaptic analogue of memory (Morris and Baker, 1983) because studies have demonstrated that antagonists acting at the NMDA receptor induce both a blockade of long-term potentiation and a cognitive impairment (Morris et al., 1986; Collingridge and Bliss, 1987; Morris, 1989; Davis, S., Butcher and Morris, 1992).

Through excitotoxic processes, damage and/or dysfunction of the EAA receptor network might therefore impede production of normal long-term potentiation and thus disrupt normal cognitive processes. Indeed, in the clinical setting, the most common and most persistent sequela of brain trauma is cognitive dysfunction, including memory and learning deficits (Levin, 1985).

Recently, a series of studies has linked EAA neurotoxicity with posttraumatic cognitive dysfunction. In addition, these studies may have identified an anatomical substrate responsible for this dysfunction. Several groups have characterized both learning and memory deficits following experimental brain injury in the rat and mouse, using neurobehavioural tests such as the Morris water maze and eight-arm radial maze (Morris, 1984; Lyeth et al., 1990; Smith et al., 1991). It has been demonstrated that the extent of posttraumatic retrograde amnesia correlates with the magnitude of selective hippocampal neuronal cell loss in the hippocampus in the CA3 and dentate hilar subfields of the hippocampus (Smith et al., 1991, 1992; Hicks et al., 1993). It has been well established that the hippocampus plays a major role in spatial learning and memory (Scoville and Milner, 1957; Eichenbaum, Stewart and Morris, 1990) and that selective damage to it will impair memory function. The apparent selective vulnerability of the hippocampus to trauma may be a result of having the highest concentration of various subtypes of EAA receptors in the brain (Monaghan and Cotman, 1986; Nakanishi, 1992). Following experimental brain injury in the rat, decreases in NMDA receptor binding have been observed in the hippocampus (Miller et al., 1990), and long-term potentiation has been found to be suppressed (Miyazaki et al., 1992). In other rat brain-injury studies, consistent posttraumatic loss of neurons has been observed in the ipsilateral CA3 and dentate hilar regions of the hippocampus, which is associated with a deficit in long-term potentiation production and a dysfunction of spatial learning in the Morris water maze (Sutherland, Sutton and Feeney, 1993). These findings have led several investigators to postulate that posttraumatic cognitive deficits may result, in part, from excitotoxic events. EAA neurotoxicity may specifically target the hippocampus, inducing neuronal cell loss, cellular stress, and/or dysfunction, thereby disrupting normal synaptic transmission. Taken together, these observations have served as the basis for the development of several pharmacological compounds aimed at attenuating potential trauma-induced EAA-induced neurotoxicity. Recent studies have demonstrated that EAA receptor antagonists may attenuate posttraumatic spatial memory dysfunction and protect neurons in the hippocampus. These efforts have provided further evidence of a potential mechanistic link between posttraumatic EAA neurotoxicity, cognitive deficits, and hippocampal dysfunction.

Excitatory amino acid modulation following brain trauma

Due to the broad acceptance of the role of EAA neurotoxicity in the deleterious posttraumatic sequelae, many pharmacological compounds affecting EAA neurotransmission systems have been assessed in several experimental models of brain injury. While the majority of outcome parameters used in these studies did not involve cognitive evaluation, it can be argued that any measured attenuation of posttraumatic EAA neurotoxicity may have general implications for cognitive outcome. The following is a compendium of studies utilizing EAA receptor antagonists and effectors, grouped according to outcome parameters, that have demonstrated efficacy in the treatment of traumatic brain injury. Due to the complicated scheme of these experimental studies, the effects of each subclass of EAA receptor modulation are summarized and dosing regimens are excluded (for a detailed review, see Smith and McIntosh, 1996). It is important to note that not all compounds in each class share similar effects.

Competitive NMDA receptor antagonism
Originally, competitive antagonists proved difficult to use due to their poor blood–brain permeability. Nonetheless, 3-(2-carboxypiperizin-4yl)-propyl-1-phosphonic acid (CPP) was shown to improve neurological motor outcome (Faden et al., 1989), while 2-amino-5-phosphovaleric acid (APV) was shown to decrease trauma-induced hypermetabolism (Kawamata et al., 1992). More recently developed competitive NMDA receptor antagonists, including cis-4-(phospho-methyl)-2-piperidine carboxylic acid (CGS19755), appear to have a greater blood–brain barrier permeability (Murphy et al., 1988; Schoepp et al., 1990b). Although CGS19755 showed no beneficial effects on neurological motor outcome (hemiparesis; Smith et al., 1990), in another study administration of this NMDA competitive antagonist was shown to decrease glutamate release (Panter and Faden, 1992). However, a recently completed Phase III clinical trial with CGS19755 did not demonstrate efficacy of this compound in brain-injured patients.

NMDA receptor-associated ionophore blockade
Compounds evaluated thus far include phencyclidine and ketamine, previously identified as dissociative anaesthetics (Kemp, Foster and Wong, 1987), the antitussive compound dextromethorphan, and its derivative dextrorphan (Kemp et al., 1987), dizocilopine (MK801; Wong, Knight and Woodruff, 1988), and a nonpsychotropic cannabinoid HU-211 (7-hydroxy-tetrahydrocannabinol 1,1-dimethylheptyl; Feigenbaum et al., 1989). Phencyclidine was actually the first EAA receptor antagonist to demonstrate efficacy in an experimental brain trauma model by attenuating posttraumatic neurological motor deficits (Hayes et al., 1988). MK801 was also shown to improve neurological motor outcome and reduce cerebral oedema formation (Shapira et al., 1990). More recently, both dextromethorphan and HU-211 have been shown to improve neurological motor function and decrease regional oedema formation (Shohami, Novikov and Mechoulam, 1993). In addition, dextrorphan has been shown to improve motor outcome, maintain intracellular magnesium concentration (Faden et al., 1989), and decrease glutamate release (Panter and Faden, 1992). Ketamine has been shown to improve cognitive outcome (Smith et al., 1993a) and maintain cation homeostasis (Shapira et al., 1993) following experimental brain injury. In considering the clinical utility of this class of compounds, it is important to note that MK801 as well as ketamine and phencyclidine have been shown to produce pathological changes in neurons, including vacuolization of neurons in the cingulate gyrus (Olney, Labruyere and Price, 1989). In addition, these compounds have been shown to induce expression of the stress protein heat

shock protein (Sharp et al., 1991). These observations have sparked a debate concerning the potential therapeutic utility versus the possible inherent neurotoxicity of these compounds.

Modulation of the NMDA receptor by magnesium
Correction of posttraumatic hypomagnesic states has been observed following the exogenous administration of magnesium salts (i.e. $MgCl_2$ and $MgSO_4$; McIntosh et al., 1988c). Magnesium therapy has also been shown to improve cognitive outcome (Smith et al. 1993a), decrease neurological motor dysfunction (McIntosh et al., 1988c, 1989), and decrease regional cerebral oedema formation (Okiyama et al., 1995) following experimental brain injury.

Magnesium therapy is currently being used clinically for pregnancy-related hypertension (eclampsia) at doses far exceeding the 7–10 mg/kg dose suggested for brain trauma therapy. Therefore, salts are attractive compounds for the treatment of brain injury, due to their current clinical use for other pathologies.

NMDA receptor-associated glycine site modulation
The co-agonist of the NMDA receptor, glycine, has been shown to be an absolute requirement for NMDA receptor activation (Johnson and Ascher, 1987; Kleckner and Dingledine, 1988). Currently, one selective antagonist of this site, indole-2-carboxylic acid (I2CA), has demonstrated efficacy following experimental brain trauma (Smith et al., 1993b). However, two broad-spectrum EAA antagonists, kynurenate (KYNA) and 6-cyano-7-nitroquinoxaline-2,3-dine (CNQX), which antagonize both the NMDA receptor-associated glycine site and AMPA/KA receptors, have also been shown to be efficacious in models of brain trauma (Kawamata et al., 1992; Smith et al., 1993a; Hicks, Smith and McIntosh, 1994). In a comparison study, I2CA and KYNA have been shown to improve neurological motor outcome and cognitive outcome, to decrease regional cerebral oedema, and to maintain total tissue cation homeostasis (Smith et al., 1993b). Whereas KYNA proved superior in attenuating increases in total tissue Ca^{2+}, I2CA more significantly attenuated posttraumatic changes in Mg^{2+}, K^+, Na^+ and Zn^+. When administered intracerebrally through a microdialysis cannula, KYNA has

also been shown to reduce the release of K^+ and decrease a hypermetabolic response to experimental trauma (Kawamata et al., 1992). Moreover, intravenous administration of KYNA has been shown to reduce the posttraumatic loss of hippocampal neurons, which appears to be associated with its ability to improve posttraumatic memory dysfunction (Hicks et al., 1994).

NMDA receptor-associated polyamine site modulation
Eliprodil (SL82.0715) has been shown to decrease cortical lesion volume in a model of brain injury even when the initial dose was delayed for up to 18 hours following trauma (Toulmond et al., 1993). This study is particularly suggestive of a prolonged window of opportunity following brain trauma.

AMPA/KA receptor modulation
The two broad-spectrum EAA antagonists KYNA and CNQX act as competitive antagonists at AMPA/KA receptors. The efficacy of KYNA has been described under the NMDA receptor-associated glycine site antagonist grouping. CNQX has been shown to decrease local posttraumatic hypermetabolism when administered via an intracerebral microdialysis cannula (Kawamata et al., 1992). The AMPA/KA receptor may also be modulated in a noncompetitive fashion by the 2,3-benzodiazepine muscle relaxant GYKI 52466 (1-(4-aminophenyl)-4-methyl-7,8-methylenedioxy-5H-2,3-benzodiazepine HC1; Dovevan and Rogawski, 1993). In an initial study in an animal model, GYKI has also been shown to improve cognitive outcome dramatically following experimental brain injury (Hylton et al., 1995).

Excitatory amino acid metabotropic receptor modulation
Excitatory amino acid metabotropic receptors are the most recent class of EAA receptors to be evaluated following experimental brain injury. Prolonged alterations in the function of metabotropic receptors have been shown in the hippocampi of brain-injured animals (Delahunty et al., 1995a, 1995b). It was also found that the metabotropic receptor antagonist alpha-methyl-4-carboxyphenylglycine (MCPG) improved posttraumatic

cognitive outcome and neurological motor outcome when administered intracerebroventricularly prior to experimental brain injury (Gong et al., 1995).

Excitatory amino acid release inhibitors

A recent approach for posttraumatic EAA modulation is the inhibition of EAA release. BW1003C87 (5-[2,3,5-trichlorophenyl]pyrimidine-2,4-diamine ethane sulfonate) and 619C89 (4-amino-2-[4-methyl-1-pipera-zinyl]-5-[2,3,5-trichlorophenyl] pyrimidine mesylate monohydrate), derivatives of lamotrigine, have been shown to inhibit veratrine-stimulated but not K^+-stimulated glutamate release, potentially by reducing ion flux through voltage-gated Na^+ channels (Miller et al., 1986; Meldrum et al., 1992). In separate studies using the same experimental model of brain trauma, 619C89 has been shown to improve cognitive deficits (Voddi et al., 1995), while BW1003C87 has been shown to reduce cerebral oedema formation (Okiyama et al., 1995). A very recent report has shown that another related compound, Riluzole, attenuated both cognitive and neuro-motor dysfunction following experimental brain injury (McIntosh et al., 1996b).

Excitatory amino acid modulation summary

These data of posttraumatic modulation of EAAs support the hypothesis of EAA neurotoxicity. It appears that an acute and marked release of EAA neurotrans-mitters occurs following trauma, targeting selectively vulnerable regions in the brain rich in EAA receptors, including the hippocampus, leading to secondary neuronal cell destruction or damage. The positive effects of EAA modulation on posttraumatic memory function help to confirm the hypothesis of the role of EAAs in the selective delayed damage to cognitive systems. In particular, the posttraumatic effects of KYNA on memory, hippocampal neuronal sparing, maintenance of Ca^{2+} homeostasis in the hippocampus, and attenuation of oedema formation in the hippocam-pus support the concept of a mechanistic link between posttraumatic EAA neurotoxicity, cognitive dysfunction and hippocampal damage.

Despite the apparent failure of CGS19755 in clinical trials, many newer EAA modulating compounds are currently being evaluated for their efficacy in brain-injured patients.

Calcium channel blockers

The potential role of a sustained increase in intracellu-lar free calcium in the pathogenesis of secondary brain injury has led to several investigations of therapeutic modulation of calcium channels. In an experimental model of brain trauma, Hovda and colleagues (1991) observed a regional increase in calcium for at least 48 hours following injury, suggesting that a prolonged window exists for therapeutic intervention. In a similar model of brain trauma, Okiyama et al. (1992, 1994) demonstrated that (S)-emopamil, a phenylalkylamine calcium channel/$5HT_2$ antagonist, reduced regional cerebral oedema formation, dramatically improved neurological motor outcome, and attenuated cognitive dysfunction. A subsequent study revealed that this compound also significantly attenuated a trauma-induced reduction in regional cerebral blood flow (Okiyama et al., 1994). In contrast to these promising experimental studies, a clinical study with the dihydro-peridine calcium channel antagonist nimodipine dem-onstrated no beneficial effects in brain-injured patients (Teasdale, 1991). Moreover, in the same experimental model which demonstrated efficacy of (S)-emopamil, evaluation of posttraumatic treatment with nimodipine showed no benefit (Gentile et al., 1993).

Opiate peptide modulation

Following brain trauma, changes in the concentrations of endogenous opiate peptides have been implicated in the pathophysiological secondary sequelae (Faden, Jacobs and Holaday, 1981; Young et al., 1981; Flamm et al., 1982). It has been suggested that release of these peptides may elicit profound effects on the cardiovascu-lar system, including decreasing regional blood flow and inducing a hypotensive response to injury. In addition, these compounds may interact with the EAA neuro-transmission systems. In experimental models of brain trauma in both the cat and the rat, a nonselective opiate receptor blocker, naloxone, reversed posttraumatic hypotension and increased brain perfusion pressure

(Hayes et al., 1983; Robinson et al., 1987; McIntosh, Fernyak and Faden, 1991). In subsequent studies, Win 44,441–3, an antagonist of the κ-opiate receptor, was shown to improve cardiovascular function, regional cerebral blood flow, and survival following experimental brain injury in the rat (McIntosh et al., 1987). In addition, nalmefene, also a κ-opiate receptor antagonist, maintained the concentration of intracellular magnesium (Vink et al., 1990).

Opiate peptide antagonists, thyrotropin-releasing hormone and its analogues CG-3703 and YM-14673, have been shown to attenuate neurological motor dysfunction following experimental brain injury in rats (Faden, 1989; McIntosh, Vink and Faden, 1988a). CG-3703 has also been shown to improve posttraumatic cardiovascular status, intracellular metabolic status, and survival (McIntosh, Vink and Faden, 1988b; Vink, McIntosh and Faden, 1988b). The actions of these compounds have also been attributed to modulation of serotonergic systems (Salzman, Hirofugi and Knight, 1987).

Despite these promising data, clinical evaluation of opiate antagonists for brain trauma therapy may not be forthcoming due to the lower potential efficacy of naloxone compared to methylprednisolone in a spinal cord injury clinical trial (NASCIS 2; Bracken et al., 1990, 1992).

Catecholamine modulation

Similar to the posttraumatic release in EAAs, it has been proposed that there is a similar response of catecholamines. Early studies of brain-injured patients demonstrated that serum norepinephrine levels were elevated commensurately with the severity of injury (Clifton et al., 1983). More recently, a correlation between the elevation of circulating norepinephrine and Glasgow coma scores has been observed (Hamill et al., 1987). Relatively early work with an experimental model of brain trauma demonstrated that amphetamine accelerated the recovery from neurological motor dysfunction (Feeney, Gonzales and Law, 1981). While it has been suggested that brain trauma may result in a decreased inhibitory neurotransmitter action of norepinephrine, the efficacy of amphetamine may potentially reflect a partial balancing of this derangement.

Cholinergic modulation

An increase in acetylcholine has also been observed in the cerebrospinal fluid following traumatic brain injury in both humans and animals (Ruge, 1945; Bornstein, 1946). In addition, a posttraumatic derangement of cholinergic receptors and an increased regional turnover of acetylcholine have been observed (Saija et al., 1988, 1989). Because of these observations, the anticholinergic scopolamine has been extensively evaluated for therapeutic efficacy in a model of experimental traumatic brain injury. Scopolamine was shown to attenuate various components of transient behavioural suppression and reversed long-term motor deficits following brain trauma (Lyeth et al., 1988a, 1988b). Curiously, scopolamine administered in combination with morphine demonstrated an additive effect in improving neurological motor dysfunction following brain injury (Patel et al., 1992; Lyeth et al., 1992). Additional studies have shown that scopolamine also reverses posttraumatic elevations in regional acetylcholine turnover (Saija et al., 1988, 1989). Whereas the clinical availability of scopolamine may make it an attractive compound for evaluation in human brain trauma victims, the profound psychomimetic effects at the presumed effective dose pose a substantial barrier. Nevertheless, the evaluation of related compounds with fewer psychomimetic effects may eventually be considered for clinical evaluation.

Free radical inhibition

Like all forms of tissue injury, brain trauma is thought to release or initiate the formation of highly reactive free radicals. This increase in free radicals may produce secondary or delayed damage to cellular membranes, primarily through the process of lipid peroxidation (Demopoulos et al., 1980). Polyunsaturated fatty acids, found most prevalently incorporated in lipids forming cellular membranes, are the most vulnerable to free radical attack (Gutteridge and Halliwell, 1990). In addition, this free radical lipid peroxidation has been shown to be accelerated in the presence of free reactive iron (Halliwall, 1992). Endogenous defence mechanisms have been identified, which use antioxidants or free radical scavengers to neutralize free radical-generated lipid peroxidation. Following injury to the central nervous system, the concentration of these endogenous antioxidants has been shown to be severely depleted, suggesting that this endogenous defence mechanism may become overwhelmed, potentially permitting uncontrolled progression of peroxidative damage to cellular membranes (Hall et al., 1989). Moreover, the brain has been suggested to be especially prone to lipid peroxidation following injury because its membrane lipids are especially rich in polyunsaturated side chains and due to the high concentration of intracellular iron, which may be released following tissue damage (Halliwell, 1992). This feature may be compounded by traumatic disruption of the vasculature, thus introducing additional free iron to the tissue through erythrocyte chromatolysis.

Following a recent study, the Second National Acute Spinal Cord Injury Study (NASCIS 2), in which significant beneficial effects of high-dose methylprednisolone were reported (Bracken et al., 1990, 1992), high-dose glucocorticoids have become the standard treatment for spinal cord injury. The primary attribute of methylprednisolone is thought to be its strong antioxidant properties. Nevertheless, there has been debate about the utility of steroid treatment in head injury in the light of the potentially deleterious side-effects of high-dose therapy. Ongoing experimental studies conducted to consider this point have demonstrated that a series of nonglucocorticoid steroid analogues of methylprednisolone, referred to as 21-aminosteroids or lazeroids, were equal if not superior inhibitors of lipid peroxidation in nervous tissue, without glucocorticoid activity (Braughler et al., 1987). U-74006F (Tirilzad or Freedox) has been shown to be efficacious in experimental models of traumatic brain injury. Hall and colleagues (1988) demonstrated improved grip strength following brain trauma in mice treated with U-74006F. It was also found that treatment with U-74006F enhanced survival at one week postinjury. In subsequent studies of experimental brain injury in rats, McIntosh and coworkers (1992) found that animals treated with U-74006F following injury showed significantly less cerebral oedema formation compared to vehicle-treated injured animals, and showed improved regional total

issue cation homeostasis. In addition, in this model, brain-injured animals receiving U-74006F also showed significantly reduced postinjury mortality. Sanada and colleagues (1993) also demonstrated that U-74006F administration improved neurological motor outcome in brain-injured rats.

In addition to U-74006F, another antioxidant, deferoxamine, which acts as an iron chelator, has also been shown to improve neurological outcome following concussive traumatic brain injury in mice (Panter, Braughler and Hall, 1992).

These findings have led to the initiation of randomized Phase III clinical trials of U-74006F in the treatment of traumatic brain injury in multiple medical centres throughout the world. The final report of that study is pending. In addition, a Phase II study of polyethylene glycol (PEG) conjugated to the free radical scavenger super oxide dismutase (SOD), collectively PEG–SOD, has demonstrated a decreased duration of increased intracranial pressure and decreased mortality in severely brain-injured patients treated with PEG–SOD (Muizelaar et al., 1993). However, preliminary results of a very recently completed Phase III trial with this compound failed to demonstrate an efficacious response.

Hypothermia

A recently revisited therapeutic approach for attenuating the secondary cascade of brain trauma is to maintain the tissue in relative stasis by using hypothermia techniques. Hypothermia treatment has been sporadically attempted for brain trauma victims over the past 50 years. However, early studies yielded mixed results, with much debate about appropriate controls and evaluation techniques. Recent experimental evidence suggests hypothermia attenuates EAA release and free radical production, thus potentially attenuating the secondary pathogenic neurochemical cascade. In animal models of brain trauma, hypothermic treatment has also been recently shown to attenuate neurological motor dysfunction (Clifton, et al., 1991; Lyeth, Jiang and Liu, 1993) and improve histopathological damage (Jiang et al., 1992; Taft et al., 1993; Dietrich et al., 1994). Results from preliminary clinical trials may suggest that modern hypothermia techniques are effective in improving the outcome following brain trauma (Clifton et al., 1993; Marion et al., 1993). A standardized hypothermia technique for brain trauma patients is currently being evaluated in a multicentred trial initiated by the National Institutes of Health in the USA.

Neurotrophic factor therapy

An increase in the concentration of endogenous neurotrophic factors in the brain has been observed following various types of injury (Varon, Hagg and Manthorpe, 1991). This response is thought to reflect an adaptive protective mechanism that delivers trophic (growth) factors to injured regions in need of revitalization and maintenance. Administration of neurotrophic factors has been shown to prevent neuronal death in various brain lesion and ischaemia experimental models (Williams et al., 1986; Kromer, 1987; Hagg et al., 1990; Shigeno et al., 1991). Recently, the neurotrophic factors nerve growth factor and basic fibroblast growth factor have been shown to attenuate cognitive deficits following experimental brain injury (Dietrich et al., 1996; Sinson, Voddi and McIntosh, 1996). These effects have even been observed with therapy delayed for one day following brain trauma. Whereas nerve growth factor was not shown to spare hippocampal neurons following injury, basic fibroblast growth factor did appear to be neuroprotective. More recent studies have shown that administration of nerve growth factor reduces apoptotic cell death following experimental brain injury (Sinson et al., 1997).

Protease inhibition

Pathological overactivation of proteases is thought to occur following brain trauma, potentially playing a major role in tissue damage. It has been shown that the cysteine protease calpain has prolonged activation following experimental brain injury, the extent of which correlated with neuronal degeneration and death (Saatman et al., 1995, 1996). The activation of calpain may result from the posttraumatic increases in the intracellular concentration of calcium. Once activated, calpain may degrade many cellular components, including cytoskeletal proteins (Siman, Baudry and

Lynch, 1984). These observations have led to suggestions that calpain inhibitors may be neuroprotective following brain trauma. Recently, the calpain inhibitor AK295 (Z-leu-aminobutyric acid-CONH(CH$_2$)$_3$ morpholine) has been shown to improve memory and neurological motor outcome following experimental brain trauma in the rat (Saatman et al., 1996). This finding offers hope for the treatment of delayed posttraumatic damage, specifically injury to neuronal processes such as in diffuse axonal injury.

Summary of acute protection following brain trauma

The compendium of studies detailed above offers compelling evidence that a secondary injury cascade occurs immediately following brain trauma, and that this cascade may be attenuated by a variety of therapeutic means. Furthermore, the identification of specific components of this cascade has allowed targeted therapy to be developed and utilized in the experimental arena. We wait in anticipation for these therapies to be shown to be efficacious in the clinical setting.

Treatment of established cognitive deficits

- Most cognitive enhancers under development act by modulating cortical processing, and thus require a relatively intact cortex to be effective. Therefore, it is unlikely that substantial improvement will be garnered from pharmacological treatment in patients with extensive cortical degeneration.

Patients with long-standing brain damage due to trauma often exhibit cognitive deficits associated with lesions to the prefrontal cortex and medial temporal lobe structures such as the hippocampus. As described above, medial temporal lobe structures are important for recent memory and the formation of new, long-term memories (Mishkin, 1978, 1982; Zola-Morgan and Squire, 1985), whereas the prefrontal cortex uses working memory to guide behaviour appropriately (Goldman-Rakic, 1987). The cognitive abilities of the prefrontal cortex are particularly evident when memory must be used to overcome interference from irrelevant stimuli or prepotent response tendencies (Malmo, 1942; Bartus and Levere, 1977). Inhibition of prepotent, inappropriate responses is required during reversals of discrimination problems, and lesions to the orbital and ventromedial prefrontal cortex produce robust reversal deficits (Mishkin et al., 1969; Ridley et al., 1993).

In order to develop intelligent pharmacological strategies for treating these persisting cognitive deficits, we must first understand the neurochemical mechanisms which influence the prefrontal cortex and the medial temporal cortex. The following is a brief review of mechanisms currently known to influence these structures. The focus of this review is on studies of nonhuman primates, as it is not clear that lessons learned in rodents extend to the primate cortex. While it can be argued that the general architecture and function of the temporal lobes are relatively conserved between rodents and primates, differences in the frontal lobes between these groups are certainly extensive. In monkeys, prefrontal cortex function is often assessed using spatial working memory tasks such as delayed response and delayed alternation, whereas medial temporal lobe function is often assessed using a recognition memory task, delayed nonmatch-to-sample. The prefrontal cortex and the medial temporal lobe both receive rich innervations of the neuromodulators dopamine, norepinephrine, serotonin (5HT), and acetylcholine. The following discusses how these transmitters influence higher cortical function, and the potential for developing cognitive enhancers for treating memory impairment.

Neurotransmitter modulation of the prefrontal cortex

Dopamine

It has been appreciated for almost 20 years that dopamine is essential to the proper functioning of the prefrontal cortex (Brozoski et al., 1979). Dopamine depletion in the prefrontal cortex impairs spatial working memory in monkeys, marmosets and rats (Brozoski et al., 1979; Simon, 1981; Bubser and Schmidt, 1990; Roberts et al., 1994). Dopamine acts at both the D1 and D2 families of receptors, and the D1 family appears particularly important for dopamine's beneficial effects on prefrontal cortex cognitive function (Sawaguchi and Goldman-Rakic, 1991, 1994). Thus, one might expect that drugs that mimic dopamine at D1 receptors would enhance prefrontal cortex cognitive

function. Systemic administration of D1 agonists have been found to produce small improvements in prefrontal cortex cognitive function in both young and aged monkeys (Arnsten et al., 1994). However, it is important to note that these improvements were dose dependent, and that small increases in dose led to significantly worsened performance. Cognitive performance can also be worsened by increasing doses of stimulants such as methylphenidate (Bartus, 1979).

It is now appreciated that excessive dopamine receptor stimulation is as detrimental to prefrontal cortex cognitive function as insufficient dopamine receptor stimulation (Arnsten and Goldman-Rakic, 1990; Arnsten et al., 1994; Murphy, Roth and Arnsten, 1994; Williams and Goldman-Rakic, 1995; Murphy et al., 1996a, 1996b; Verma and Moghaddam, 1996; Zahrt, Taylor and Arnsten, 1996). Thus, increasing doses of D1 agonist, whether administered systemically (Arnsten et al., 1994) or locally into the prefrontal cortex (Zahrt et al., 1996), produce impaired working memory performance. Dopamine's detrimental actions may be particularly apparent under conditions in which there has been damage to dendrites and spines (see Arnsten, 1997, for discussion). These findings suggest that D1 agonists may not be ideal as cognitive enhancers.

Interestingly, increased dopamine receptor stimulation in the prefrontal cortex occurs naturally in response to stress. Even mild, psychological stressors can increase dopamine turnover in the prefrontal cortex in rodents (reviewed in Deutch and Roth, 1990). This mechanism may have particular relevance to brain-damaged individuals if their injuries render activities of daily living more stressful. The authors' research in monkeys and rats indicates that stress can produce prefrontal cortex cognitive deficits through a hyperdopaminergic mechanism (Arnsten and Goldman-Rakic, 1990; Murphy et al., 1994, 1996a, 1996b). Performance was protected by pretreatment with agents that either prevented the rise in prefrontal cortex dopamine turnover (Murphy et al., 1996b), or blocked dopamine receptors (Arnsten and Goldman-Rakic, 1990; Murphy et al., 1994, 1996a). Interestingly, both D1 and D2 receptor-selective agents were effective in this regard, suggesting that dopamine has detrimental actions at both the D1 and D2 families of receptors. Only very low doses of dopamine receptor antagonists were useful; higher doses often produced side-effects and further impaired cognition (e.g. Murphy, Roth and Arnsten, 1997). These findings suggest that patients with prefrontal cortex cognitive deficits who experience high levels of stress might benefit from very low doses of dopamine receptor blockers such as clozapine.

In summary, the finding that dopamine and dopamine agonists produce an inverted U-shaped dose–response curve may complicate the clinical use of these compounds. Dose titration would be critical if stimulants or D1 agonists were to be tested clinically. Furthermore, dopamine agonists have not been tested in monkeys with prefrontal cortex lesions, and it is likely that they would lose much of their beneficial effect if many of the prefrontal cortex neurons had degenerated. Finally, very low doses of dopamine antagonists might actually be useful in patients who experience a high degree of stress.

Norepinephrine

Although most research has focused on dopamine mechanisms affecting the prefrontal cortex, accumulating evidence indicates that norepinephrine has an equally important influence on prefrontal cortex cognitive functioning (see Arnsten, Steere and Hunt, 1996, for review). Norepinephrine has marked, beneficial effects on prefrontal cortex cognitive function through actions at postsynaptic, alpha-2 receptors in this region. Thus, either systemic administration or local intra-prefrontal cortex infusion of α-2 adrenergic agonists improves spatial working memory performance, whereas systemic or local administration of the α-2 adrenergic antagonist yohimbine impairs performance (Arnsten and Goldman-Rakic, 1985; Arnsten, Cai and Goldman-Rakic, 1988; Li and Mei, 1994b; Arnsten, 1997). In contrast, performance was not impaired by local infusion of the α-1 receptor antagonist prazosin or the β receptor antagonist propranolol, highlighting the important relationship between the prefrontal cortex and α-2 receptor mechanisms (Li and Mei, 1994b). Preliminary electrophysiological data suggest that α-2 agonists improve prefrontal cortex function by enhancing delay-related activity of the region's pyramidal neurons in monkeys performing a delayed response task (Li and Mei 1994a), whereas yohimbine suppresses memory-related activity (Li and Mei, 1994a; T. Sawaguchi, personal communication).

A number of lines of evidence indicate that norepinephrine's beneficial effects at α-2 receptors localized *post*synaptic to norepinephrine terminals. Thus, α-2 agonists become more, rather than less, effective in young monkeys in whom the presynaptic element has been destroyed or depleted with 6-hydroxydopamine (Arnsten and Goldman-Rakic, 1985) or reserpine (Cai et al., 1993). Similarly, α-2 agonists are more effective in aged monkeys with naturally occurring catecholamine loss (Arnsten et al, 1988). These agents are particularly effective under conditions of high interference or distraction when the prefrontal cortex is challenged (Jackson and Buccafusco, 1991; Arnsten and Contant, 1992).

In addition to their cognitive-enhancing properties, α-2 agonists also induce hypotension and sedation, side-effects that limit their clinical use in many patient populations. In order to develop superior pharmacological treatments for prefrontal cortex cognitive deficits, it is important to understand the receptor subtype mechanisms underlying the beneficial effects of α-2 agonists. Alpha-2 receptor subtypes were originally recognized in pharmacological studies (Bylund, 1985; Boyajian and Leslie, 1987). Later, three α-2 receptor subtypes were cloned in the primate: the α-2A, the α-2B and the α-2C receptors whose genes reside on chromosomes 10, 2 and 4, respectively (Kobilka et al., 1987; Regan et al., 1988; Lomasney et al., 1990). Accumulating evidence indicates that the cognitive-enhancing effects of α-2 agonists are consistent with an α-2A pharmacological profile. Low doses of agonists such as guanfacine and UK-14,304 with higher affinity for the α-2A subtype are able to improve delayed response performance without hypotensive and sedative side-effects, while agonists such as clonidine and B-HT920 with high affinity for the α-2B and α-2C receptors improve delayed response performance at higher doses which also induce marked hypotension and sedation (Arnsten et al., 1988; Arnsten and Leslie, 1991). Furthermore, the improvement in delayed response performance can be reversed by yohimbine, which has high affinity for α-2A receptors, but not by prazosin, which has high affinity for α-2B and α-2C receptors in addition to its α-1 blocking properties (Arnsten and Goldman-Rakic, 1985). Interestingly, the α-2A receptor is most prevalent in the prefrontal cortex, and electronmicrographic analysis has demonstrated postsynaptic localization of α-2A immunoreactivity in the monkey prefrontal cortex (Aoki et al., 1994).

Alpha-2 adrenergic agonists have been shown to improve prefrontal cortex cognitive deficits in some patient populations. Clonidine has been shown to improve prefrontal cortex cognitive tasks such as the Trails B, Word Fluency and Stroop tasks in patients with schizophrenia (Fields et al., 1988) or Korsakoff's syndrome (Mair and McEntee, 1986; Moffoot et al., 1994). In support of a prefrontal cortex mechanism, single photon emission computed tomography (SPECT) imaging studies of Korsakoff's patients have shown that clonidine's beneficial effects on word fluency correlated with increased regional cerebral blood flow in the left prefrontal cortex, the cortical region most affiliated with performance of this task (Moffoot et al., 1994). Clonidine's beneficial effects in Korsakoff's patients appear to result from actions at postsynaptic receptors, as the drug was most effective in those patients with greatest norepinephrine loss (McEntee and Mair, 1990).

The symptoms of attention deficit hyperactivity disorder are also thought to involve prefrontal cortex dysfunction (Mattes 1980; Chelune et al., 1986; Gorenstein and Mammato, 1989; Loge, Staton and Beatty, 1989; Benson, 1991; Barkley, Grodzinsky and DuPaul, 1992; Shue and Douglas, 1992), and clonidine and guanfacine have been helpful in this disorder (Hunt, Mindera and Cohen, 1985; Chappell et al., 1995; Horrigan and Barnhill, 1995; Hunt, Arnsten and Asbell, 1995). In particular, guanfacine has produced significant improvement on the continuous performance task, a test of sustained attention and impulse inhibition that relies on the prefrontal cortex (Chappell et al., 1995).

Although the above results suggest that α-2 agonists might be helpful in the treatment of prefrontal cortex cognitive deficits associated with brain trauma, it is important to note that monkey studies demonstrate that α-2 agonists lose their cognitive-enhancing effects when the prefrontal cortex is ablated (Arnsten and

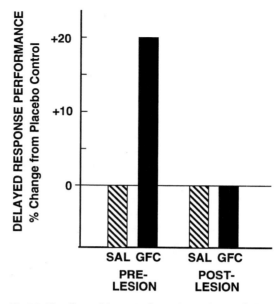

Fig. 7.2 The effects of the α-2A adrenergic agonist guanfacine (0.0011 mg/kg i.m., 2 hours pretreatment) on the delayed response performance of aged monkey number 445 before (left) and after (right) sustaining a bilateral lesion to the dorsolateral prefrontal cortex. The results represent the percentage change from saline (placebo) control performance. GFC, guanfacine; SAL, saline. (Arnsten, unpublished results.)

Goldman-Rakic, 1985; Arnsten and van Dyck, 1997). As can be seen in Fig. 7.2, the α-2 agonist guanfacine improved working memory performance in a normal aged monkey prelesion. However, the drug lost all beneficial effects after the monkey underwent a bilateral prefrontal cortex lesion. These data indicate that an intact cortex is necessary for α-2 agonists to exhibit their cognitive-enhancing actions. Interestingly, the sedative effects of clonidine are retained postlesion (Arnsten and van Dyck, 1997), consistent with a thalamic (Buzsaki et al., 1991) and/or locus ceruleus mechanism (Berridge and Foote, 1991) underlying the sedative actions of these compounds. The loss of cognitive-enhancing properties in monkeys with cortical ablations may have particular relevance to patients with brain damage, as cortical trauma may remove the substrate needed for the beneficial actions of α-2 agonists. This cautious stance is supported by the findings that α-2 agonists have no beneficial effect in patients with Alzheimer's disease (Mohr et al., 1989; Schlegel et al., 1989; Crook et al., 1992), another disorder involving cortical degeneration.

Serotonin

To date, there is little evidence that 5HT alters dorsolateral prefrontal cortex function. Depletion of 5HT from the dorsolateral prefrontal cortex had no effect on spatial working memory performance in monkeys (Brozoski et al., 1979). In rats, depletion of serotonin or serotonin antagonist treatment has often been shown to improve reference memory tasks that depend upon posterior cortical or hippocampal function, but these treatments generally do not alter the performance of working memory tasks (Altman and Normile, 1986, 1988; Normile and Altman, 1988; Altman et al., 1990). In aged monkeys, $5HT_3$ receptor antagonists have no effect on spatial working memory performance, although these agents do improve the performance of a visual discrimination task that depends upon the inferior temporal cortex (Arnsten et al., 1997). These findings are consistent with rodent studies showing improvement on reference memory tasks with serotonin receptor blockade or depletion, and suggest that 5HT may impede posterior cortical function while having little effect on prefrontal cortex function. However, further experiments with more selective 5HT receptor agents will be necessary for a better understanding of how 5HT mechanisms may influence prefrontal cortex function.

Acetylcholine

Although studies of systemically administered cholinergic antagonists would suggest an important role for acetylcholine in the prefrontal cortex, there have been few studies which have addressed this issue explicitly in primates. Bartus' pioneering research demonstrated that systemic administration of the muscarinic antagonist scopolamine could induce working memory deficits in young monkeys (Bartus and Johnson, 1976; Bartus, 1982), and similar learning and memory deficits were observed in humans treated with scopolamine

(e.g. Drachman, 1981). These studies suggest that blocking the cholinergic input from the basal forebrain to the prefrontal cortex results in marked prefrontal cortex dysfunction. This interpretation is generally supported by lesion studies in lower primates, in which lesions to the basal forebrain impair reversal learning abilities associated with the orbital prefrontal cortex (Ridley et al., 1985; Roberts et al., 1992). However, more recent studies in higher primates have shown that lesions of the basal forebrain have surprisingly little effect on learning and memory performance (Aigner et al., 1987; Voytko et al., 1994), although they do increase susceptibility to scopolamine treatment. In their landmark study, Voytko et al. (1994) produced extensive lesions of the medial septum, diagonal band of Broca and nucleus basalis of Meynert in cynomolgous monkeys and observed little effect on the performance of prefrontal cortex tasks such as delayed response or discrimination reversal, even with difficult, long-delay conditions. These results suggest that the marked deficits observed with scopolamine on memory tasks may result from drug actions on other cholinergic systems, e.g. profound effects on thalamic physiology and thus on thalamocortical activation. However, more direct studies will be needed to define the role of cholinergic mechanisms in the prefrontal cortex (for example examining the effects of scopolamine infusion into the prefrontal cortex of monkeys performing a delayed response task), and other cortical areas. It is noteworthy that the basal forebrain lesion produced by Voytko et al. (1994) did impair performance of the Posner task of visuospatial attention. As this task relies on the integrity of the parietal association cortex (Posner et al., 1984), these data suggest that cholinergic mechanisms may be especially important for parietal cortical function.

Neurotransmitter modulation of medial temporal lobe

There has been little or no research on the neurochemical needs of nonprefrontal cortical regions in higher primates, including the medial temporal lobe. Although many studies have examined neurochemical influences on hippocampal and amygdala function in rodents, it is not clear that all these findings extend to primates. For example, numerous studies have shown that cholinergic lesions or antagonists impair, while agonists improve, memory tasks dependent on the hippocampus in rodents (reviewed in Fibiger, 1991). Thus, researchers have assumed that cholinergic influence from the basal forebrain is critical to the proper functioning of the medial temporal lobe. However, Voytko et al. (1994) found that extensive cholinergic lesions depleting cortical and hippocampal acetylcholine in higher primates had no effect on recognition memory tasks such as the delayed nonmatch-to-sample task which are dependent on medial temporal lobe function. These negative effects may be due to postlesion compensatory mechanisms, or cholinergic mechanisms may not be as critical for medial temporal lobe function in primates as they are in rodents. This remains an important area for future research. It should be noted that numerous cholinergic-enhancing drugs have been tested in patients with Alzheimer's disease, and no study has shown truly impressive improvement in memory function. The outcome measures commonly employed in investigational Alzheimer's disease drug trials generally stress the memory functions of the medial temporal lobe (Rosen, Mohs and Davis, 1984). Tacrine has emerged as the first Food and Drug Administration-approved agent for the treatment of Alzheimer's disease, but demonstrates only modest efficacy in large-scale clinical trials (Davis, K.L. et al., 1992; Farlow et al., 1992; Knapp et al., 1994). Similarly, the $5HT_3$ receptor antagonist ondansetron has recently been tested in patients with Alzheimer's disease in multicentre trials in the USA and abroad, and these studies also failed to demonstrate improvement (Glaxo Inc., personal communication). Although it is not clear that negative results in Alzheimer patients would extend to patients with brain trauma, they limit optimism for this approach.

Conclusions

Researchers are currently developing pharmacological treatments for established cognitive impairment. However, as these agents mimic neuromodulators such as norepinephrine, they may require an intact cortical architecture as the substrate for their beneficial actions. Thus, it is less likely that these agents will be effective in patients with extensive cortical damage. A better focus for treating cognitive deficits associated with brain trauma may be administering agents that restrict neurodegenerative processes, both acutely posttrauma and subacutely. These agents may decrease the spread of the lesion and thus limit the development of widespread cognitive deficits.

Despite the recent inability to show efficacy in clinical studies evaluating some of the compounds highlighted in this chapter (i.e. U-74006F, CGS19755 and PEG–SOD), enthusiasm to find a useful therapy has not waned. The apparent 'failure' of the recent clinical trials is not thought to reflect an error in the hypothesis of mechanisms of secondary injury, but rather the choice of specific therapies and the methods of clinical evaluation. Currently, a Phase III clinical trial is underway, evaluating the effect of posttraumatic hypothermia. In addition, a multitude of new agents is currently in the early phases of clinical evaluation (for review, see McIntosh et al., 1996a). These efforts demonstrate a consensus that secondary injury can be controlled but that it may be necessary to develop new-generation compounds and greatly revise clinical outcome measures.

Major difficulties confounding the clinical evaluation of therapeutic efficacy in acute brain trauma include the ability to diagnose accurately the severity and type of injury. Without a specific diagnosis, appropriate application of therapies is not easy to define. Brain trauma actually represents a spectrum of injuries from simple contusion to diffuse axonal injury (for review, see McIntosh et al., 1996a). It is therefore questionable if any one treatment can remedy all forms of traumatic brain damage. For example, in the acute setting, is it reasonable to treat a patient with an EAA receptor antagonist although damage is thought to be confined to the white matter? Clearly, the diagnosis of the type of brain trauma is paramount prior to treatment with standardized regimens. These observations have sparked debate concerning the design of clinical trials pertaining to exclusion criteria. A high percentage of severely brain-injured patients have diffuse axonal injury, which may best respond to nonreceptor-based therapy (e.g. protease inhibitors). In contrast, patients with mild brain trauma are more likely to have a contusion injury, for which receptor-based therapy may be appropriate. However, because brain trauma patients form an incredibly heterogeneous population, a clear-cut diagnosis remains a significant challenge.

Another difficulty of most clinical trials is the almost exclusive inclusion of moderate-to-severe brain-injured patients. It has been questioned whether this is the most ideal group to evaluate due to the extensiveness of injuries and the impracticability of performing extensive functional outcome measures, including cognitive evaluation. Currently under consideration is the inclusion of mild-to-moderate brain-injured patients into clinical trials. This group represents a much greater number of patients, thus enrollment may be improved and the time frame of the clinical trial accelerated. In addition, it is much easier to perform refined evaluation of cognitive status in these patients. The typically uncomplicated injuries in the mild-to-moderate brain trauma patients may also be more amenable to treatment regimens.

Ideally, a cocktail of protective agents, or 'polypharmacy', might be tailored in accordance with the severity and type of trauma, selectively targeting all aspects of the injury. However, at present, we anxiously wait for just one brain trauma therapy to prove efficacious. By attenuating the development of cognitive dysfunction in the acute setting following trauma, it seems most probable that the severity of persistent cognitive deficits would also be greatly reduced. Clearly, the ultimate goal is to develop an arsenal of therapies for brain trauma that can both combat the acute deleterious cascade and elevate cognitive status in patients with established disabilities.

References

Aigner, T.G., Mitchell, S.J., Aggleton, J.P. et al. 1987. Effects of physostigmine and scopolamine on recognition memory in monkeys with ibotinic-acid lesions of the nucleus basalis of Meynert. *Psychopharmacology* 92, 292–300.

Altman, H.J. and Normile, H.J. 1986. Enhancement of the memory of a previously aversive habit following pretest administration of a variety of serotonergic antagonists in mice. *Psychopharmacology* 90, 24–7.

Altman, H.J. and Normile, H.J. 1988. What is the nature of the role of the serotonergic nervous system in learning and memory: prospects for development of and effective treatment strategy for senile dementia. *Neurobiol Aging* 9, 627–38.

Altman, H.J., Normile, H.J., Galloway, M.P., Ramirez, A. and Azmitia, E.C. 1990. Enhanced spatial learning in rats following 5, 7-DHT-induced serotonergic deafferentation of the hippocampus. *Brain Res* 518, 61–6.

Aoki, C., Go, C.-G., Venkatesan, C. and Kurose, H. 1994. Perikaryal and synaptic localization of alpha-2A-adrenergic receptor-like immunoreactivity. *Brain Res* 650, 181–204.

Arnsten, A.F.T. 1997. Catecholamine regulation of the prefrontal cortex. *J Psychopharmacol* 11, 151–62.

Arnsten, A.F.T., Cai, J.X. and Goldman-Rakic, P.S. 1988. The alpha-2 adrenergic agonist guanfacine improves memory in aged monkeys without sedative or hypotensive side effects. *J Neurosci* 8, 4287–98.

Arnsten, A.F.T., Cai, J.X., Murphy, B.L. and Goldman-Rakic, P.S. 1994. Dopamine D1 receptor mechanisms in the cognitive performance of young adult and aged monkeys. *Psychopharmacology* 116, 143–51.

Arnsten, A.F.T. and Contant, T.A. 1992. Alpha-2 adrenergic agonists decrease distractability in aged monkeys performing a delayed response task. *Psychopharmacology* 108, 159–69.

Arnsten, A.F.T. and Goldman-Rakic, P.S. 1985. Alpha-2 adrenergic mechanisms in prefrontal cortex associated with cognitive decline in aged nonhuman primates. *Science* 230, 1273–6.

Arnsten, A.F.T. and Goldman-Rakic, P.S. 1990. Stress impairs prefrontal cortex cognitive function in monkeys: role of dopamine. *Soc Neurosci Abstr* 16, 164.

Arnsten, A.F.T. and Leslie, F.M. 1991. Behavioral and receptor binding analysis of the alpha-2 adrenergic agonist, UK-14304 (5 bromo-6 [2-imidazoline-2-yl amino] quinoxaline): evidence for cognitive enhancement at an alpha-2 adrenoceptor subtype. *Neuropharmacology* 30, 1279–89.

Arnsten, A.F.T., Lin, C.H., van Dyck, C.H. and Stanhope, K.J. 1997. The effects of 5HT-3 receptor antagonists on cognitive performance in aged monkeys. *Neurobiol Aging* 18, 21–8.

Arnsten, A.F.T., Steere, J.C. and Hunt, R.D. 1996. The contribution of α-2 noradrenergic mechanisms to prefrontal cortical cognitive function: potential significance to attention deficit hyperactivity disorder. *Arch Gen Psychiatry* 53, 448–55.

Arnsten, A.F.T. and van Dyck, C.H. 1997. Monoamine and acetylcholine influences on higher cognitive functions in non-human primates: relevance to the treatment of Alzheimer's disease. In *Pharmacological Treatment of Alzheimer's Disease: Molecular and Neurobiological Foundations*, ed. J.D. Brioni and M.W. Decker, pp. 63–86. New York: John Wiley and Sons.

Barkley, R.A., Grodzinsky, G. and DuPaul, G.J. 1992. Frontal lobe functions in attention deficit disorder with and without hyperactivity: a review and research report. *J Abnorm Child Psych* **20**, 163–88.

Bartus, R.T. 1979. Four stimulants of the central nervous system: effects on short-term memory in young vs. aged monkeys. *J Am Geriatr Soc* **27**, 289–97.

Bartus, R.T. 1982. Effects of cholinergic agents on learning and memory in animal models of ageing. In *Aging*, Vol. 19, *Alzheimer's Disease: a Report of Progress in Research*, ed. S. Corkin, J.H. Growden, K.L. Davis, E. Usdin and R.J. Wurtman, pp. 271–80. New York: Raven Press.

Bartus, R.T. and Johnson, H.R. 1976. Short-term memory in the rhesus monkey: disruption from the anti-cholinergic scopolamine. *Pharmacol Biochem Behav* **5**, 39–46.

Bartus, R.T. and Levere, T.E. 1977. Frontal decortication in rhesus monkeys: a test of the interference hypothesis. *Brain Res* **119**, 233–48.

Benson, D.F. 1991. The role of frontal dsyfunction in attention deficit hyperactivity disorder. *J Child Neurol* **6**, S9–S12.

Berridge, C.W. and Foote, S.L. 1991. Effects of locus coeruleus activation on electroencephalographic activity in neocortex and hippocampus. *J Neurosci* **11**, 3135–45.

Bliss, T.V.P. and Lomo, T. 1973. Long-lasting potentiation of synaptic transmission in the dentate area of the anaesthetized rabbit following stimulation of the perforant path. *J Physiol (Lond)* **232**, 331–56.

Bornstein, M. 1946. Presence and action of acetylcholine in experimental brain trauma. *J Neurophysiol* **9**, 349–66.

Boyajian, C.L. and Leslie, F.M. 1987. Pharmacological evidence for alpha-2 adrenoceptor heterogeneity: differential binding properties of [3H]rauwolscine and [3H]idazoxan in rat brain. *J Pharmacol Exp Ther* **241**, 1092–8.

Bracken, M.B., Shepard, M.J., Collins, W.F. et al. 1990. A randomized, controlled trial of methylprednisolone or naloxone in the treatment of acute spinal cord injury. *N Engl J Med* **322**, 1405–11.

Bracken, M.B., Shepard, M.J., Collins, W.F. et al. 1992. Methylprednisolone or naloxone treatment after acute spinal cord injury: 1 year follow-up data. *J Neurosurg* **76**, 23–31.

Braughler, J., Pregenzer, J., Chase, R., Duncan, L., Jacobsen, E. and McCall, J. 1987. Novel 21-aminosteroids as potent inhibitors of iron-dependent lipid peroxidation. *J Biol Chem* **262**, 10434–40.

Brozoski, T., Brown, R.M., Rosvold, H.E. and Goldman, P.S. 1979. Cognitive deficit caused by regional depletion of dopamine in prefrontal cortex of rhesus monkey. *Science* **205**, 929–31.

Bubser, M. and Schmidt, W. 1990. 6-OHDA lesion of the rat prefrontal cortex increases locomotor activity, impairs acquisition of delayed alternation tasks, but does not affect uninterrupted tasks in the radial maze. *Behav Brain Res* **37**, 157–68.

Buzsaki, G., Kennedy, B., Solt, V.B. and Ziegler, M. 1991. Noradrenergic control of thalamic oscillation: the role of alpha-2 receptors. *Eur J Neurol* **3**, 222–9.

Bylund, D.B. 1985. Heterogeneity of alpha-2 adrenergic receptors. *Pharmacol Biochem Behav* **22**, 835–43.

Cai, J.X., Ma, Y., Xu, L. and Hu, X. 1993. Reserpine impairs spatial working memory performance in monkeys: reversal by the alpha-2 adrenergic agonist clonidine. *Brain Res* **614**, 191–6.

Chappell, P.B., Riddle, M.A., Scahill, L. et al. 1995. Guanfacine treatment of comorbid attention deficit hyperactivity disorder and Tourette's syndrome: preliminary clinical experience. *J Am Acad Child Adolesc Psychiatry* **34**, 1140–6.

Chelune, G.J., Ferguson, W., Koon, R. and Dickey, T.O. 1986. Frontal lobe disinhibition in attention deficit disorder. *Child Psychiatry Hum Dev* **16**, 221–34.

Choi, D.W. 1985. Glutamate neurotoxicity in cortical cell culture is calcium dependent. *Neurosci Lett* **58**, 293–7.

Clifton, G.L., Allen, S., Barrodale, P. et al. 1993. A phase II study of moderate hypothermia in severe brain injury. *J Neurotrauma* **10**, 263–71.

Clifton, G.L., Jiang, J.Y., Lyeth, B.G., Jenkins, L.W., Hamm, R.J. and Hayes, R.L. 1991. Marked protection by moderate hypothermia after experimental traumatic brain injury. *J Cereb Blood Flow Metab* **11**, 114–21.

Clifton, G., Robertson, C., Kyper, K., Taylor, A.A., Dhenkne, R.D. and Grossman, R. 1983. Cardiovascular response to severe head injury. *J Neurosurg* **59**, 447–54.

Collingridge, G.L. and Bliss, T.V.P. 1987. NMDA receptors – their role in long-term potentiation. *Trends Neurosci* **10**, 288–93.

Collingridge, G.L. and Davies, S.N. 1989. NMDA receptors and long-term potentiation in the hippocampus. In *The NMDA Receptor*, ed. J.C. Watkins and G.L. Collingridge, pp. 123–35. Oxford: IRL Press.

Collingridge, G.L. and Lester, R.A.J. 1989. Excitatory amino acid receptors in the vertebrate central nervous system. *Pharmacol Rev* **41**, 143–210.

Crook, T., Wilner, E., Rothwell, A., Winterling, D. and McEntee, W. 1992. Noradrenergic intervention in Alzheimer's disease. *Psychopharmacol Bull* **28**, 67–70.

Davis, K.L., Thal, L.J., Gamzu, E.R. et al. 1992. A double-blind, placebo-controlled multicenter study of tacrine for Alzheimer's disease. *N Engl J Med* **327**, 1253–9.

Davis, S., Butcher, S.P. and Morris, R.G.M. 1992. The NMDA receptor antagonist D-2-amino-5-phosphonopentanoate (DAP5) impairs spatial learning and LTP in vivo at intracerebral concentrations comparable to those that block LTP in vitro. *J Neurosci* **12**, 21–34.

Delahunty, T.M., Jiang, J.Y., Black, R.T. and Lyeth, B.G. 1995a. Differential modulation of carbachol and trans-ACPD-stimulated phosphoinositide turnover following traumatic brain injury. *Neurochem Res* **20**, 405–11.

Delahunty, T.M., Jiang, J.Y., Gong, Q.Z., Black, R.T. and Lyeth, B.G. 1995b. Differential consequences of lateral and central fluid percussion brain injury on receptor coupling in rat hippocampus. *J Neurotrauma* **12**, 1045–57.

Demopoulos, H.B., Flamm, E.S., Pietronigro, D.D. and Seligman, M.L. 1980. The free radical pathology and the microcirculation in the major central nervous system disorders. *Acta Phys Scand* Suppl. **492**, 91–119.

Deutch, A.Y. and Roth, R.H. 1990. The determinants of stress-induced activation of the prefrontal cortical dopamine system. *Prog Brain Res* **85**, 367–403.

Dietrich, D.W., Alonso, O., Busto, R. and Finklestein, S.P. 1996. Posttreatment with intravenous basic fibroblast growth factor reduces histopathological damage following fluid-percussion brain injury in rats. *J Neurotrauma* **13**, 309–16.

Dietrich, W.D., Alonso, O., Mordecai, R.B., Globus, Y.T. and Ginsberg, M.D. 1994. Post-traumatic brain hypothermia reduces histopathological damage following concussive brain injury in the rat. *Acta Neuropathol (Berlin)* **87**, 250–8.

Dovevan, S.D. and Rogawski, M.A. 1993. GYKI 52466, a 2,3-benzodiazepine, is a highly selective, noncompetitive antagonist of AMPA/kainate receptor responses. *Neuron* **10**, 51–9.

Drachman, D.A. 1981. The cholinergic system, memory and ageing. In *Aging*, Vol. 17, *Brain Neurotransmitters and Receptors in Aging and Age-related Disorders*, ed. S.J. Enna, T. Samorajski and B. Beer, pp. 255–68. New York: Raven Press.

Eichenbaum, H., Stewart, C., and Morris, R.G.M. 1990. Hippocampal representation in place learning. *J Neurosci* **10**(11), 3531–42.

Faden, A.I. 1989. TRH analog YM-14673 improves outcome following traumatic brain and spinal cord injury in rats: dose–response studies. *Brain Res* **486**, 228–35.

Faden, A.I., Demediuk, P., Panter, S.S. and Vink, R. 1989. The role of excitatory amino acids and NMDA receptors in traumatic brain injury. *Science* **244**, 789–800.

Faden, A.I., Jacobs, T.P. and Holaday, J.W. 1981. Opiate antagonist improves neurologic recovery after spinal injury. *Science* **211**, 493–4.

Farlow, M., Gracon, S.I., Hershey, L.A., Lewis, K.W., Sadowsky, C.H. and Dolan-Ureno, J. 1992. A controlled trial of tacrine in Alzheimer's disease. *JAMA* **268**, 2523–9.

Feeney, D.M., Gonzales, A. and Law, W.A. 1981. Amphetamine restores locomotor function after motor cortex injury in the rat. *Proc West Pharmacol Soc* **24**, 15–17.

Feigenbaum, J.J., Bergmann, F., Richmond, S.A. et al. 1989. Non-psychotropic cannabinoid acts as a functional N-methyl-D-aspartate receptor blocker. *Proc Natl Acad Sci USA* **86**, 9584–7.

Fibiger, H.C. 1991. Cholinergic mechanisms in learning, memory and dementia: a review of recent evidence. *Trends Neurosci* **14**, 220–3.

Fields, R.B., Van Kammen, D.P., Peters, J.L. et al. 1988. Clonidine improves memory function in schizophrenia independently from change in psychosis. *Schiz Res* **1**, 417–23.

Fineman, I., Hovda, D.A., Smith, M., Yoshino, A. and Becker, D.P. 1993. Concussive brain injury is associated with a prolonged accumulation of calcium: a ^{45}Ca autoradiographic study. *Brain Res* **624**, 94–102.

Flamm, E.S., Young, W., Demopoulos, H.B., Decrescito, V. and Tamasula, J.J. 1982. Experimental spinal cord injury: treatment with naloxone. *Neurosurgery* **10**, 227–31.

Gentile, N., Smith, D.H., Burhans, C. and McIntosh, T.K. 1993. Cognitive and neurologic functions and hippocampal neuronal loss after nimodipine in fluid percussion brain injury. *J Neurotrauma* **10**, S193 (Abstract).

Goldman-Rakic, P.W. 1987. Circuitry of the primate prefrontal cortex and the regulation of behavior by representational memory. In *Handbook of Physiology, the Nervous System, Higher Functions of the Brain*, ed. F. Plum, pp. 373–417. Bethesda: American Physiological Society.

Gong, Q.Z., Delahunty, T.M., Hamm, R.J. and Lyeth, B.G. 1995. Metabotropic glutamate antagonist MCPG in the treatment of traumatic brain injury in rats. *Brain Res* **700**(1–2), 299–302.

Gorenstein, E.E. and Mammato, C.A. 1989. Performance of inattentive–overactive children on selected measures of prefrontal-type function. *J Clin Psychol* **45**, 619–32.

Gutteridge, J.M.C. and Halliwell, B. 1990. The measurement and mechanism of lipid peroxidation in biological systems. *Trends Biochem Sci* **15**, 129–35.

Hagg, T., Vahlsing, H.L., Manthorpe, M. and Varon, S. 1990. Nerve growth factor infusion into the denervated adult rat hippocampal formation promotes its cholinergic reinnervation. *J Neurosci* **10**, 3087–92.

Hall, E.D., Yonkers, P.A., Horan, K.L. and Braughler, J.M. 1989. Correlation between attenuation of post-traumatic spinal cord ischemia and preservation of tissue vitamin E by the 21-aminosteroid U74006F. Evidence for an in vivo antioxidant mechanism. *J Neurotrauma* **6**, 169–76.

Hall, E.D., Yonkers, P.A., McCall, J.M. and Braughler, J.M. 1988. Effects of the 21-aminosteroid U74006F on experimental head injury in mice. *J Neurosurg* **68**, 456–61.

Halliwell, B. 1992. Reactive oxygen species and the central nervous system. *J Neurochem* **59**, 1609–23.

Hamill, R.W., Woolf, P.D., McDonald, J., Lee, L.A. and Kelley, M. 1987. Catecholamines predict outcome in traumatic brain injury. *Ann Neurol* **212**, 438–43.

Hamm, R.J., Dixon, C.E., Gbadebu, D.M. et al. 1992. Cognitive deficits following traumatic brain injury by controlled cortical impact. *J Neurotrauma* **9**, 11–20.

Hayes, R.L., Galinet, B.J., Kulkarne, P. and Becker, D.P. 1983. Effects of naloxone on systemic and cerebral responses to experimental concussion brain injury in cats. *J Neurosurg* **58**, 720–8.

Hayes, R.L., Jenkins, L.W., Lyeth, B.G. et al. 1988. Pretreatment with phencyclidine, an N-methyl-D-aspartate antagonist, attenuates long-term behavioral deficits in the rat produced by traumatic brain injury. *J Neurotrauma* **5**, 259–74.

Hicks, R.R., Smith, D.H., Lowenstein, D.H., Saint Marie, R.L. and McIntosh, T.K. 1993. Mild experimental brain injury in the rat induces cognitive deficits associated with regional neuronal loss in the hippocampus. *J Neurotrauma* **10**, 405–14.

Hicks, R.R., Smith, D.H. and McIntosh, T.K. 1994. Kynurenate is neuroprotective following experimental brain injury in the rat. *Brain Res* **655**, 91–6.

Horrigan, J.P. and Barnhill, L.J. 1995. Guanfacine for treatment of attention-deficit-hyperactivity disorder in boys. *J Child Adolesc Psychopharmacol* **5**, 215–23.

Hovda, D.A., Yoshino, A., Fireman, I., Smith, M. and Becker, D.P. 1991. Intracellular calcium accumulates for at least 48 hours following fluid percussion brain injury in the rat. *Proc Am Assoc Neurol Surg* **1**, 452.

Hume, R.I., Dingledine, R. and Heinemann, S. 1991. Identification of a site in glutamate receptor subunits that controls calcium permeability. *Science* **253**, 1028–31.

Hunt, R.D., Arnsten, A.F.T. and Asbell, M.D. 1995. An open trial of guanfacine in the treatment of attention deficit hyperactivity disorder. *J Am Acad Child Adolesc Psychiatry* **34**, 50–4.

Hunt, R.D., Mindera, R.B. and Cohen, D.J. 1985. Clonidine benefits children with attention deficit disorder and hyperactivity: reports of a double-blind placebo-crossover therapeutic trial. *J Am Acad Child Psychiatry* **24**, 617–29.

Hylton, C., Perri, B.R., Voddi, M.D. et al. 1995. Non-NMDA antagonist GYKI 52466 enhances spatial memory after experimental brain injury. *J Neurotrauma* (Abstract) **12**, 124.

Iino, M., Ozawa, S. and Tsuki, K. 1990. Permeation of calcium through excitatory amino acid receptor channels in cultured rat hippocampal neurons. *J Physiol Lond* **424**, 151–65.

Jackson, W.J. and Buccafusco, J.J. 1991. Clonidine enhances delayed matching-to-sample performance by young and aged monkeys. *Pharmacol Biochem Behav* **39**, 79–84.

Jiang, J.Y., Lyeth, B.G., Kapasi, M.Z., Jenkins, L.W. and Povlishock, J.T. 1992. Moderate hypothermia reduces blood–brain barrier disruption following traumatic brain injury in the rat. *Acta Neuropathol* **84**, 495–500.

Johnson, J.W. and Ascher, P. 1987. Glycine potentiates the NMDA response in cultured mouse brain neurons. *Nature* **325**, 529–31.

Katayama, Y., Becker, D.P., Tamura, T. and Hovda, D.A. 1990. Massive increases in extracellular potassium and the indiscriminate release of glutamate following concussive brain injury. *J Neurosurg* **73**, 889–900.

Kawamata, T., Katayama, Y., Hovda, D.A., Yoshino, Y. and Becker, D.P. 1992. Administration of excitatory amino acid antagonists via microdialysis attenuates the increase in glucose utilization seen following concussive brain injury. *J Cereb Blood Flow Metab* **12**, 12–24.

Kemp, J.A., Foster, A.C. and Wong, E.H.F. 1987. Non-competitive antagonists of excitatory amino acid receptors. *Trends Neurosci* **10**, 294–8.

Kleckner, N.W. and Dingledine, R. 1988. Requirement for glycine in activation of NMDA receptors expressed in *Xenopus* oocytes. *Science* **241**, 835–7.

Knapp, M.J., Knopman, D.S., Solomon, P.R., Pendlebury, W.W., Davis, C.S. and Gracon, S.I. 1994. A 30-week randomized controlled trial of high-dose tacrine in patients with Alzheimer's disease. *JAMA* **271**, 895–91.

Kobilka, B.K., Matsui, H., Kobilka, T.S. et al. 1987. Cloning, sequencing, and expression of the gene encoding for the human platelet alpha-2-adrenergic receptor. *Science* **238**, 650–6.

Kromer, L.F. 1987. Nerve growth factor treatment after brain injury prevents neuronal death. *Science* **235**, 214–16.

Levin, H.S. 1985. Outcome after head injury. Part II. Neurobehavioral recovery. In *Status Report on Central Nervous System Trauma Research*, pp. 281–99. Bethesda: National Institute of Neurological and Communicative Disease and Stroke.

Li, B.-M. and Mei, Z.-T. 1994a. Alpha-2 adrenergic modulation of prefrontal neuronal activity related to working memory in monkeys. *Abstracts of the 3rd Congress of Federation of Asian and Oceanian Physiological Societies*, p. 96.

Li, B.-M. and Mei, Z.-T. 1994b. Delayed response deficit induced by local injection of the alpha-2 adrenergic antagonist yohimbine into the dorsolateral prefrontal cortex in young adult monkeys. *Behav Neurol Biol* **62**, 134–9.

Loge, D.V., Staton, R.D. and Beatty, W.W. 1989. Performance of children with ADHD on tests sensitive to frontal lobe dysfunction. *J Am Acad Child Adolesc Psychiatry* **29**, 540–5.

Lomasney, J.W., Lorenz, W., Allen, L.F. et al. 1990. Expansion of the alpha-2-adrenergic family: cloning and characterization of a human alpha-2-adrenergic receptor subtype, the gene for which is located on chromosome 2. *Proc Natl Acad Sci USA* **87**, 5094–8.

Lyeth, B.G., Dixon, C.E., Hamm, R. et al. 1988a. Effects of anticholinergic treatment on transient behavioral suppression physiological responses following concussive brain injury to the rat. *Brain Res* **488**, 88–97.

Lyeth, B.G., Dixon, C.E., Jenkins, L.W. et al. 1988b. Effects of scopolamine treatment on long-term behavioral deficits following concussive brain injury to the rat. *Brain Res* **452**, 39–97.

Lyeth, B.G., Jenkins, L.W., Hamm, R.J. et al. 1990. Prolonged memory impairment in the absence of hippocampal cell death following traumatic brain injury in the rat. *Brain Res* **526**, 249–58.

Lyeth, B.G., Jiang, J.Y. and Liu, S. 1993. Behavioral protection by moderate hypothermia initiated after experimental traumatic brain injury. *J Neurotrauma* **10**, 57–64.

Lyeth, B.G., Ray, M., Hamm, R. et al. 1992. Postinjury scopolamine administration in experimental traumatic brain injury. *Brain Res* **569**, 281–6.

Mair, R.G. and McEntee, W.J. 1986. Cognitive enhancement in Korsakoff's psychosis by clonidine: a comparison with l-dopa and ephedrine. *Psychopharmacology* **88**, 374–80.

Malmo, R.B. 1942. Interference factors in delayed response in monkeys after removal of frontal lobes. *Neurophysiology* **5**, 295–308.

Marion, D.W., Obrist, W.D., Carlier, P.M., Penrod, L.E. and Darby, J.M. 1993. The use of moderate therapeutic hypothermia for patients with severe head injuries: a preliminary report. *J Neurosurg* **79**, 354–62.

Mattes, J.A. 1980. The role of frontal lobe dysfunction in childhood hyperkinesis. *Comp Psychiatry* **21**, 358–69.

Mayer, M. and Westbrook, G. 1987. The physiology of excitatory amino acids in the vertebrate central nervous system. *Prog Neurobiol* **28**, 197–276.

McEntee, W.J. and Mair, R.G. 1990. The Korsakoff syndrome: a neurochemical perspective. *Trends Neurosci* **13**, 340–4.

McIntosh, T.K., Fernyak, S. and Faden, A.I. 1991. The effects of naloxone hydrochloride treatment after experimental traumatic brain injury in the rat. *J Cereb Blood Flow Metab* Suppl. 2, S734.

McIntosh, T.K., Hayes, R.L., DeWitt, D.S., Agura, V. and Faden, A.I. 1987. Endogenous opioids may mediate secondary damage after experimental brain injury. *Am J Physiol* **253**, E565–74.

McIntosh, T.K., Smith, D.H., Meaney, D.F., Gennarelli, T.A. and Graham, D.I. 1996a. Neuropathological sequelae of experimental brain injury: relationship to neurochemistry and biomechanics. *Lab Invest* **74**, 315–42.

McIntosh, T.K., Smith, D.H., Voddi, M., Perri, B.R. and Stutzmann, J.-M. 1996b. Riluzole, a novel neuroprotective agent, attenuates both neurologic motor and cognitive dysfunction following experimental brain injury in the rat. *J Neurotrauma* **13**, 767–80.

McIntosh, T.K., Thomas, M.J., Smith, D.H. and Banbury, M.

1992. The novel 21-aminosteroid U74006F attenuates cerebral edema and improves survival after brain injury in the rat. *J Neurotrauma* **9**, 33–40.

McIntosh, T.K., Vink, R. and Faden, A.I. 1988a. Beneficial effect of the TRH analog CG-3703 on brain bioenergetics and survival following traumatic brain injury in rats. In *Perspectives in Shock Research*, ed. A. Lever, pp. 415–20. New York: R. Liss.

McIntosh, T.K., Vink, R. and Faden, A.I. 1988b. An analogue of thyrotropin-releasing hormone improves outcome after brain injury: 31P-NMR studies. *Am J Physiol* **257**, R785–92.

McIntosh, T.K., Vink, R., Yamakami, I. and Faden, A.I. 1988c. Magnesium deficiency exacerbates and pretreatment improves outcome following traumatic brain injury in rats. 31P Magnetic resonance spectroscopy and behavioral studies. *J Neurotrauma* **5**, 17–31.

McIntosh, T.K., Vink, R., Yamakami, I. and Faden, A.I. 1989. Magnesium protects against neurological deficit after brain injury. *Brain Res* **482**, 252–60.

Meldrum, B.S., Swan, J.H., Leach, M.J. et al. 1992. Reduction of glutamate release and protection against ischemic brain damage by BW1003C87. *Brain Res* **593**, 1–6.

Miller, A.A., Sawyer, D.A., Roth, B. et al. 1986. Lamotrigine. In *New Anticonvulsant Drugs*, ed. B.S. Meldrum and R.J. Porter, pp. 165–77. London: John Libbey.

Miller, L.P., Lyeth, B.G., Jenkins, L.W. et al. 1990. Excitatory amino acid receptor subtype binding following traumatic brain injury. *Brain Res* **526**, 103–7.

Mishkin, M. 1978. Memory in monkeys severely impaired by combined but not by separate removal of amygdala and hippocampus. *Nature* **273**, 297–8.

Mishkin, M. 1982. A memory system in the monkey. *Phil Trans R Soc Lond B* **298**, 85–95.

Mishkin, M., Vest, B., Morris, M. and Rosvold, H.E. 1969. A reexamination of the effects of frontal lesions on object alternation. *Neuropsychology* **7**, 357–63.

Miyazaki, S., Katayama, Y., Lyeth, B.G. et al. 1992. Enduring suppression of hippocampal long-term potentiation following traumatic brain injury in rat. *Brain Res* **585**, 335–9.

Moffoot, A., O'Carroll, R.E., Murray, C., Dougall, N., Ebmeier, K. and Goodwin, G.M. 1994. Clonidine infusion increases uptake of Tc-exametazime in anterior cingulate cortex in Korsakoff's psychosis. *Psychol Med* **24**, 53–61.

Mohr, E., Schlegel, J., Fabbrini, G. et al. 1989. Clonidine treatment of Alzheimer's disease. *Arch Neurol* **46**, 376–8.

Monaghan, D.T. and Cotman, C. 1986. Identification and properties of N-methyl-D-aspartate receptors in rat brain plasma membranes. *Proc Natl Acad Sci USA* **83**, 7532–6.

Morris, R.G.M. 1984. Developments of a water maze procedure for studying spatial learning in the rat. *J Neurosci Methods* **11**, 47–60.

Morris, R.G.M. 1989. Synaptic plasticity and learning: selective impairment of learning rats and blockade of long-term potentiation in vivo by the N-methyl-D-aspartate receptor antagonist AP5. *J Neurosci* 9, 3040–57.

Morris, R.G.M., Anderson, E., Lynch, G.S. and Baudry, M. 1986. Selective impairment of learning and blockade of long-term potentiation by an N-methyl-D-aspartate receptor antagonist. *Nature* 319, 774–6.

Morris, R.G.M. and Baker, M. 1983. Does long-term potentiation/synaptic enhancement have anything to do with learning or memory? In *The Neuropsychology of Memory*, ed. L. Squires and N. Butters, pp. 521–35. New York: Guilford Press.

Muizelaar, J.P., Marmarou, A., Young, H.F. et al. 1993. Improving the outcome of severe head injury with the oxygen radical scavenger polyethylene glycol-conjugated superoxide dismutase: a phase II trial. *J Neurosurg* 78, 375–82.

Murphy, B.L., Arnsten, A.F.T., Goldman-Rakic, P.S. and Roth, R.H. 1996a. Increased dopamine turnover in the prefrontal cortex impairs spatial working memory performance in rats and monkeys. *Proc Natl Acad Sci USA* 93, 1325–9.

Murphy, B.L., Arnsten, A.F.T., Jentsch, J.D. and Roth, R.H. 1996b. Dopamine and spatial working memory in rats and monkeys: pharmacological reversal of stress-induced impairment. *J Neurosci* 16, 7768–75.

Murphy, B.L., Roth, R.H. and Arnsten, A.F.T. 1994. The effects of FG7142 on prefrontal cortical dopamine and spatial working memory in rat and monkey. *Soc Neurosci Abstr* 20, 1018.

Murphy, B.L., Roth, R. and Arnsten, A.F.T. 1997. Clozapine reverses the spatial working memory deficits induced by FG7142 in monkeys. *Neuropsychopharmacology* 16, 433–7.

Murphy, D.E., Hutchinson, A.J., Hurt, S.D., Williams, M. and Sills, M.A. 1988. Characterization of the binding of [³H]-CGS 19755: a novel N-methyl-D-aspartate antagonist with nanomolar affinity in rat brain. *Br J Pharmacol* 95, 932–8.

Nakanishi, S. 1992. Molecular characterization of the family of metabotropic glutamate receptors. In *Excitatory Amino Acids*, ed. R. Simon, pp. 21–2. New York: Time Medical Publishers.

Nilsson, P., Hillered, L., Ponten, U. and Urgerstedt, 1990. Changes in cortical extracellular levels of energy-related metabolites and amino acids following concussive brain injury in rats. *J Cereb Blood Flow Metab* 10, 631–7.

Normile, H.J. and Altman, H.J. 1988. Enhanced passive avoidance retention following posttrain serotonergic receptor antagonist administration in middle-aged and aged rats. *Neurobiol Aging* 9, 377–82.

Okiyama, K., Rosenkrantz, T.S., Smith, D.H., Gennarelli, T.A. and McIntosh, T.K. 1994. (S)-Emopamil attenuates regional cerebral blood flow reduction following experimental brain injury. *J Neurotrauma* 11, 83–95.

Okiyama, K., Smith, D.H., Gennarelli, T.A., Simon, R.P., Leach, M. and McIntosh, T.K. 1995. The sodium channel blocker and glutamate release inhibitor BW1003C87 and magnesium attenuate regional cerebral edema following experimental brain injury in the rat. *J Neurochem* 64(2), 802–9.

Okiyama, K., Smith, D.H., Thomas, M.J. and McIntosh, T.K. 1992. Evaluation of a novel calcium channel blocker, (s)-emopamil, on regional cerebral edema and neurobehavioral function after experimental brain injury. *J Neurosurg* 77, 607–15.

Olney, J.W., Labruyere, J. and Price, M. 1989. Pathological changes induced in cerebrocortical neurons by phencyclidine and related drugs. *Science* 244, 1360–2.

Palmer, A.M., Marion, D.W., Botscheller, M.L., Swedlow, P.E., Styren, S.D. and DeKosky, S.T. 1993. Traumatic brain injury-induced excitotoxicity assessed in a controlled cortical impact model. *J Neurochem* 61, 2015–24.

Panter, S.S., Braughler, J.M. and Hall, E. 1992. Dextran-coupled deferoxamine improves outcome in a murine model of head injury. *J Neurotrauma* 9, 47–53.

Panter, S.S. and Faden, A.I. 1992. Pretreatment with the NMDA antagonists limits release of excitatory amino acids following traumatic brain injury. *Neurosci Lett* 136, 165–8.

Patel, P.M., Drummond, J.C., Mitchell, M.D., Yaksh, T.L. and Cole, D.J. 1992. Eicosanoid production in the caudate nucleus and dorsal hippocampus after forebrain ischemia: a microdialysis study. *J Cereb Blood Flow Metab* 12, 88–95.

Pierce, J.E.S., Smith, D.H., Eison, M.S. and McIntosh, T.K. 1993. The nootropic compound BMY-2150Z improves spatial learning ability in brain injured rats. *Brain Res* 624, 199–208.

Posner, M.I., Walker, J.A., Friedrich, F.J. and Rafal, R.D. 1984. Effects of parietal injury on covert orienting of visual attention. *J Neurosci* 4, 1863–74.

Regan, J.W., Kobilka, T.S., Yang-Feng, T.L., Caron, M.G., Lefkowitz, R.J. and Kobilka, B.K. 1988. Cloning and expression of a human kidney cDNA for an alpha-2 adrenergic receptor subtype. *Proc Natl Acad Sci USA*, 85, 6301–5.

Ridley, R.M., Baker, H.F., Drewett, B. and Johnson, J.A. 1985. Effects of ibotinic acid lesions of the basal forebrain on serial reversal learning in marmosets. *Psychopharmacology* 86, 438–43.

Ridley, R.M., Durnford, L.J., Baker, J.A. and Baker, H.F. 1993. Cognitive inflexibility after archicortical and paleocortical prefrontal lesions in marmosets. *Brain Res* 628, 56–64.

Rink, A., Fung, K.-M., Trojanowski, J.Q., Lee, V.M.-Y., Neugebauer, E. and McIntosh, T.K. 1995. Evidence of apoptotic cell death after experimental traumatic brain injury in the rat. *Am J Pathol* 147, 1575–83.

Roberts, A.C., Robbins, T.W., Everitt, B.J. and Muir, J.L. 1992. A specific form of cognitive rigidity following excitotoxic lesions of the basal forebrain in marmosets. *Neuroscience* 47, 251–64.

Roberts, A.C., Salvia, M.A., Wilkinson, L.S. et al. 1994. 6-Hydroxydopamine lesions of the prefrontal cortex in monkeys enhance performance on an analog of the Wisconsin Card Sort Test: possible interactions with subcortical dopamine. *Neuroscience* **14**, 2531–44.

Robinson, S.E., Lyeth, B.G., Jenkins, L.W. et al. 1987. The effect of naloxone pretreatment on behavioral responses to concussive brain injury in the rat. *Neurosci Abstr* **2**, 1254.

Rosen , W.G., Mohs, R.C. and Davis, K.L. 1984. A new rating scale for Alzheimer's disease. *Am J Psychiatry* **141**, 1356–64.

Rothman, S.M. and Olney, J.W. 1986. Glutamate and the pathophysiology of hypoxic–ischemic brain damage. *Ann Neurol* **19**, 105–11.

Ruge, D. 1945. The use of cholinergic blocking agents in the treatment of craniocerebral injuries. *J Neurosurg* **11**, 77–83.

Saatman, K.E., Bozyczko-Coyne, D., Siman, R., Marcy, V. and Gennarelli, T.A. 1995. Calpain I activation following experimental brain injury. *J Neurotrauma* **12**, 138 (Abstract).

Saatman, K.E., Murai, H., Bartus, R.T., Hayward, N.J., Perri, B.R. and McIntosh, T.K. 1996. The calpain inhibitor AK295 improves outcome following experimental brain injury. *Proc Natl Acad Sci USA* **93**(8), 3428–33.

Saija, A., Hayes, R.L., Lyeth, B.G., Dixon, E., Yamamoto, T. and Robinson, S. 1988. The effect of concussive head injury on central cholinergic neurons. *Brain Res* **452**, 303–11.

Saija, A., Robinson, S.E., Lyeth, B.G. et al. 1989. The effects of scopolamine and traumatic brain injury on central cholinergic neurons. *J Neurotrauma* **5**, 161–70.

Salzman, S.K., Hirofugi, C. and Knight, P.B. 1987. Treatment of experimental spinal trauma with thyrotropin-releasing hormone: central serotonergic and vascular mechanisms factor. *Cent Nerv Sys Trauma* **4**, 181–96.

Sanada, T., Nakamura, T., Nishimura, M.C., Isayama, K. and Pitts, L.H. 1993. Effect of U74006F on neurologic function and brain edema after fluid percussion injury in rats. *J Neurotrauma* **10**(1), 65–71.

Sawaguchi, T. and Goldman-Rakic, P.S. 1991. D1 dopamine receptors in prefrontal cortex: involvement in working memory. *Science* **251**, 947–50.

Sawaguchi, T. and Goldman-Rakic, P.S. 1994. The role of D1-dopamine receptors in working memory: local injections of dopamine antagonists into the prefrontal cortex of rhesus monkeys performing an oculomotor delayed response task. *J Neurophysiol* **71**, 515–28.

Schlegel, J., Mohr, E., Williams, J., Mann, U., Gearing, M. and Chase, T.N. 1989. Guanfacine treatment of Alzheimer's disease. *Clin Neuropharmacol* **12**, 124–8.

Schoepp, D., Bockaert, J. and Sladeczek, F. 1990a. Pharmacological and functional characteristics of metabotropic excitatory amino acid receptors. *Trends Pharmacol Sci* **11**, 508–15.

Schoepp, D.D., Ornstein, P.L., Leander, J.D. et al. 1990b. Pharmacological characterization of LY233053: a structurally novel tetrazole-substituted competitive N-methyl-D-aspartic acid antagonist with a short duration of action. *J Pharmacol Exp Ther* **255**, 1301–8.

Scoville, W.B. and Milner, B. 1957. Loss of memory after bilateral hippocampal lesions. *J Neurol Neurosurg Psychiatry* **20**, 11–21.

Shapira, Y., Lam, A.M., Artu, A.A., Eng, C. and Soltow, L. 1993. Ketamine alters calcium and magnesium in brain tissue following experimental head trauma in rats. *J Cereb Blood Flow Metab* **13**, 962–8.

Shapira,Y., Yadid, G., Cotev, S., Niska, A. and Shohami, E. 1990. Protective effect of MK-801 in experimental brain injury. *J Neurotrauma* **7**, 131–9.

Sharp, F., Jasper, P., Hall, J., Noble, L. and Sagar, S.M. 1991. MK-801 and ketamine induce heat shock protein HSP72 in injured neurons in posterior cingulate and retrosplenial cortex. *Ann Neurol* **30**, 801–9.

Shigeno, T., Mima, T., Takakura, K. et al. 1991. Amelioration of delayed neuronal death in the hippocampus by nerve growth factor. *J Neurosci* **11**, 2914–19.

Shohami, E., Novikov, M. and Mechoulam, R. 1993. A non-psychotropic cannabinoid, HU-211, has cerebroprotective effects after closed head injury in the rat. *J Neurotrauma* **10**, 109–19.

Shue, K.L. and Douglas, V.I. 1992. Attention deficit hyperactivity disorder and the frontal lobe syndrome. *Brain Cogn* **20**, 104–24.

Siman, R., Baudry, M. and Lynch, G. 1984. Brain fodrin: substitute for calpain I, an endogenous calcium-activated protease. *Proc Natl Acad Sci USA* **81**, 3572–6.

Simon, H. 1981. Dopaminergic A10 neurons and the frontal system. *J Physiol* **77**, 81–95.

Sinson, G., Perri, B.R., Trojanowski, J.Q., Flamm, E.S. and McIntosh, T.K. 1997. Neurotrophin infusion improves cognitive deficits and decreases cholinergic neuronal cell loss and apoptotic cell death following experimental traumatic brain injury. *J Neurosurg* **86**(3), 511–18.

Sinson, G., Voddi, M. and McIntosh, T.K. 1996. Combined fetal neural transplantation and nerve growth factor infusion: effects on neurological outcome following fluid-percussion brain injury in the rat. *J Neurosurg* **84**, 655–62.

Smith, D.H., Lenkinski, R.E., Meaney, D.F., Ross, D.T., McIntosh, T.K. and Gennarelli, T.A. 1994. Experimental diffuse axonal injury in miniature swine: metabolic consequences. *J Neurotrauma* **11**(1), 128 (Abstract).

Smith, D.H., Lowenstein, D.H., Hicks, R.R., Perlman, K.G. and

McIntosh, T.K. 1992. Experimental brain injury induces long-term memory dysfunction associated with bilateral hilar neuronal cell loss. *Neurosci Abstr* **18**(1), 170.

Smith, D.H. and McIntosh, T.K. 1996. Traumatic brain injury and excitatory amino acids. In *Neurotrauma*, ed. R. Narayan, J. Willberger and J.T. Povlishock, pp. 1445–58. New York: McGraw-Hill.

Smith, D.H., Okiyama, K., Gennarelli, T.A. and McIntosh, T.K. 1993a. Magnesium and ketamine attenuate cognitive dysfunction following experimental brain injury. *Neurosci Lett* **157**, 211–14.

Smith, D.H., Okiyama, K., Thomas, M.J., Claussen, B. and McIntosh, T.K. 1991. Evaluation of memory dysfunction following experimental brain injury using the Morris Water Maze. *J Neurotrauma* **8**, 259–69.

Smith, D.H., Okiyama, K., Thomas, M.J. and McIntosh, T.K. 1993b. Effects of the excitatory amino acid receptor antagonists kynurenate and indole-2-carboxylic acid on behavioral and neurochemical outcome following experimental brain injury. *J Neurosci* **13**, 5383–92.

Smith, D.H., Thomas, M.J., Soares, H.D. and McIntosh, T.K. 1990. Differential effects of competitive and non-competitive N-methyl-D-aspartate (NMDA) receptor antagonists in experimental brain injury. *FASEB J* **4**(3), 773 (Abstract).

Soares, H.D., Thomas, M., Cloherty, K. and McIntosh, T.K. 1992. Development of prolonged focal cerebral edema and regional cation change following experimental brain injury in the rat. *J Neurochem* **58**, 1845–52.

Sugiyama, H., Ito, I. and Hirono, C. 1987. A new type of glutamate receptor linked to inositol phospholipid metabolism. *Nature Lond* **325**, 531–3.

Sutherland, R.J., Sutton, R.L. and Feeney, D.M. 1993. Traumatic brain injury in the rat produces anterograde but not retrograde amnesia and impairment of hippocampal LTP. *Proceedings of the Second International Neurotrauma Meeting* (Abstract).

Taft, W.C., Yang, K., Dixon, C.E., Clifton, G.L. and Hayes, R.L. 1993. Hypothermia attenuates the loss of hippocampal microtubule-associated protein 2 (MAP2) following traumatic brain injury. *J Cereb Blood Flow Metab* **13**, 796–802.

Teasdale, G. 1991. A randomized trial of nimodipine in severe head injury: HIT 1. *J Neurotrauma* **37**, S545–50.

Toulmond, S., Serrano, A., Benavides, J. and Scatton, B. 1993. Prevention by eliprodil (SL 82.0715) of traumatic brain damage in the rat. Existence of a large (18 h) therapeutic window. *Brain Res* **620**, 32–41.

Varon, S., Hagg, T. and Manthorpe, M. 1991. Nerve growth factor in CNS repair and regeneration. *Adv Exp Biol Med* **296**, 267–76.

Verma, A. and Moghaddam, B. 1996. NMDA receptor antagonists impair prefrontal cortex function as assessed via spatial delayed alternation performance in rats: modulation by dopamine. *J Neurosci* **16**, 373–9.

Vink, R., McIntosh, T.K., Demediuk, P., Weiner, M.W. and Faden, A.I. 1988a. Decline in intracellular free Mg^{2+} is associated with irreversible tissue injury following brain trauma. *J Biol Chem* **263**, 757–61.

Vink, R., McIntosh, T.K. and Faden, A.I. 1988b. Treatment with the thyrotropin releasing hormone analog CG3703 restores magnesium homeostasis following traumatic brain injury in rats. *Brain Res* **460**, 184–8.

Vink, R., McIntosh, T.K., Romhanyi, R. and Faden, A.I. 1990. Opiate antagonist nalmefene improves intracellular free Mg^{2+}, bioenergetic state and neurological outcome following traumatic brain injury in rats. *J Neurosci* **10**, 3524–30.

Voddi, M.D., Perri, B.R., Perlman, K.G., Smith, D.H., Leach, M. and McIntosh, T.K. 1995. The pre-synaptic glutamate release inhibitor BW619C89 attenuates memory dysfunction following experimental brain injury. *J Neurotrauma* **12**(1), 146.

Voytko, M.L., Olton, D.S., Richardson, R.T., Gorman, L.K., Tobin, J.T. and Price, D.L. 1994. Basal forebrain lesions in monkeys disrupt attention but not learning and memory. *J Neurosci* **14**, 167–86.

Williams, G.V. and Goldman-Rakic, P.S. 1995. Blockade of dopamine D1 receptors enhances memory fields of prefrontal neurons in primate cerebral cortex. *Nature* **376**, 572–5.

Williams, L.R., Varon, S., Peterson, G.M. et al. 1986. Continious infusion of nerve growth factor prevents basal forebrain neuronal death after fimbria fornix transection. *Proc Natl Acad Sci USA* **83**, 9231–5.

Wong, E.H.F., Knight, A.R. and Woodruff, G.N. 1988. MK-801 labels a site on the N-methyl-D-aspartate receptor channel complex in rat brain membranes. *J Neurochem* **50**, 274–81.

Young, W. 1987. The post-injury response in trauma and ischemia. Secondary injury or protective mechanisms? *Cent Nerv Sys Trauma* **4**, 27–51.

Young, W., Flamm, E.S., Demopoulos, H.B., Tomasula, J.J. and Decrescito, V. 1981. Naloxone ameliorates post-traumatic ischemia in experimental spinal contusion. *J Neurosurg* **55**, 209–19.

Zahrt, J., Taylor, J.R. and Arnsten, A.F.T. 1996. Supranormal stimulation of dopamine D1 receptors in the prefrontal cortex impairs spatial working memory in rats. *Soc Neurosci Abstr* **22**, 1128.

Zola-Morgan, S. and Squire, L.R. 1985. Medial temporal lesions in monkeys impair memory on a variety of tasks sensitive to human amnesia. *Behav Neurosci* **99**, 22–34.

8

Neuropharmacological contributions to the rehabilitation of patients with traumatic brain injury

John W. Cassidy

Introduction

- Traumatic brain injury patients with behavioural dysfunction require specially adapted rehabilitation programmes.
- Understanding the underlying pathophysiology is crucial to making a meaningful diagnosis and prognosis.

The neuropharmacological management of patients with acquired brain injuries has a celebrated history. Beginning in the late 1960s and roughly extending through the mid-1970s, pharmacologically induced behavioural control was essentially associated with the reintroduction of coma. The backlash from such interventions was inevitable, and from the late 1970s through the early 1990s all psychotropics were summarily banished from the rehabilitation pharmacopoeia. Instead, patients were essentially permitted to express any type of dysregulated behaviour as long as they were trailed by 1:1 or 2:1 staff supervision or exiled to the hinterlands of the 'State Psychiatric Hospital.' Obviously, either approach missed the point: patients must regain behavioural control so they can participate in necessary rehabilitative therapies designed to reduce their level of disability as efficiently as possible. Thus, a more contemporary approach to these patients incorporates elements of both philosophies into a coherent treatment programme. These elements include a neurological rehabilitative model of treatment, environmental prothesis, behavioural programming, and psychotherapeutic techniques in addition to appropriate neuropharmacological management.

The neurological model of rehabilitation, with its focus on accurate diagnosis and understanding of the natural history of the disorder under consideration, has been extremely helpful in evolving the standard of care provided to patients with acquired brain injuries. However, its principal weakness has been the lack of consideration given to the behavioural disorders that commonly accompany these conditions. The extension of this model of rehabilitation to a behaviourally disordered patient population requires a concomitant understanding of neuropsychiatry. While seemingly a daunting leap of faith, such a development is little more than the logical evolution of the constructs already familiar to those working with this model. This augmentation remains predicated upon two important constructs: diagnosis and prognosis. In this context, a meaningful diagnosis must go beyond giving a label to the dysregulated behaviour (e.g. aggression) and include an assessment of how this problem is understood syndromically. From a conceptual perspective, aggression is much like 'fever'; it is a sign to the treating clinician that something is wrong, but it does not inform him or her of what is wrong. Without such information, treatment interventions are at best 'shot gun' and at worst inappropriate.

The assessment

- Secondary complications must be evaluated when a traumatic brain injury patient develops a behavioural disorder.
- Re-evaluation of injury characteristics provides a template for possible outcomes.
- Patient evaluation must also consider premorbid and environmental factors that may be contributing to behaviour dysfunction.

Table 8.1 Medical complications

Pulmonary	*Nutrition*
Acute cardiac failure	Malnutrition
Adult respiratory distress syndrome	Haemothorax
	Hypoventilation/ hyperventilation
Airway obstruction	
	Neurogenic pulmonary oedema
Apnoea	
	Neurogenic ventilation/ perfusion defect
Atelectasis	
	Pre-existing pulmonary disease
Chest wall injuries	
Diaphragm paralysis/rupture	Pneumonia
Embolism	Pneumothorax
	Pulmonary contusion/ oedema
Cardiovascular	
Cardiac dysrhythmias	
Deep venous thrombosis	
Pulmonary embolism	
Disseminated intravascular coagulation	
Fluid–electrolytes	
Hyponatraemia	
Hypernatraemia	
Diabetes insipidus	

Table 8.2 Neurologic complications

Depressed sensorium
  Drug reactions
  Metabolic disorders
  Infection
  Primary brain complications
    Haematoma or hygroma
    Seizures
    Hydrocephalus
    Cerebrospinal fluid leak
    New trauma
    Traumatic aneurysm
Spasticity
Unrecognized spinal cord injury
Pain syndromes

Table 8.3 Psychiatric complications following traumatic brain injury

Amnestic disorder
Anxiety disorder
Delirium
Dementia
Impulse control disorder
Mood disorder
  Depressive
  Bipolar
Personality change
Psychotic disorder
Sleep disorder
Somatoform disorder

Secondary complications

When a patient with a traumatic brain injury develops a comorbid behavioural disorder, the first response of the treatment team must be to look for evolving secondary complications, be they medical, neurological or psychiatric. This task routinely falls to the attending physicians and nursing staff. However, given that other team members spend a great deal of time with these patients, it is incumbent upon each treating clinician to notice and report all deviations from the expected to the appropriate 'case-manager'. Tables 8.1, 8.2 and 8.3 list the important diagnostic considerations in each specialty area.

Secondary medical complications occur more frequently than one might expect. Vigilant nursing and expectant medical care are the appropriate antidotes for many of these difficulties. Although the issue of drug side-effects has been reviewed *ad nauseum*, a full medication review is warranted for any patient whose condition unexpectedly deteriorates. Table 8.4 lists some common medications with the potential to produce delirium. A full discussion of any of these medical conditions is beyond the scope of this chapter, but can be found in a number of standard texts on the subject.

Neurological complications can eventuate into neurosurgical emergencies. The slowly expanding subdural haematoma or the insidious evolution of obstructive hydrocephalus can lead to dysregulation of behaviour and unexpected regression in functioning

Table 8.4 Medications with potential to cause regression in cognitive function

Antibiotic	NSAIIs	Sedative–hypnotic
Acyclovir	Phenylbutazone	Barbiturates
Amphotericin B		Benzodiazepines
Cephalexin	*Antiparkinson*	Glutethimide
Chloroquine	Amantadine	
Isoniazid	Benztropine	*Sympathomimetic*
Metronidazole	Biperiden	Amphetamines
Rifampin	Carbidopa	Disulfiram
	Levodopa	Metrizamide
Anticholinergic		Phenylephrine
Atropine	*Analgesic*	Phenylpropanolamine
Belladonna alkaloids	Opiates	Propylthiouracil
Phenothiazines	Salicylates	Quinacrine
Scopolamine	Synthetic narcotics	Theophylline
Tricyclic antidepressants		
	Cardiac	*Over-the-counter*
Anticonvulsant	β-blockers	Compoz
Phenobarbital	Clonidine	Excedrin PM
Phenytoin	Digitalis	Sleep-Eze
	Disopyramide	Sominex
Antiemetics	Lidocaine	
Promethazine	Mexiletine	*Miscellaneous*
	Quinidine	Aminophylline
Antihistamine	Procainamide	Bromides
Cimetidine		Chlorpropamide
Promethazine	*Drug withdrawal*	Lithium
	Alcohol	
Anti-inflammatory	Barbiturates	
Corticosteroids	Benzodiazepines	

Notes:
Modified from Wise and Brandt (1987, p. 301).

that, if not immediately reversed, can result in death. Seizures are another late neurological complication that can produce deviation from an expected trajectory of recovery. Although perhaps less common than once believed, these disorders are now far more treatable than ever before, given the recent introduction of several new anticonvulsant medications.

Reassessment of the patient's initial injury characteristics must be undertaken when unexpected behavioural disorders present. Most helpful is a review of the initial emergency medical service and emergency department records. Very often, the contribution of focal contusional or diffuse hypoxaemic–ischaemic injury is underestimated. Focal contusional injury is readily seen on neuroimaging studies and produces 'stroke-like' sequelae and recovery trajectory. When focal contusional injury occurs in the frontal or anterior temporal cortices, concomitant behavioural disorders are frequently seen. This type of injury is a harbinger of a nondiffuse axonal injury recovery curve. Rather than following a 12–18-month trajectory to social and vocational re-entry, these patients plateau at four to six months and they are left with substantial executive dysfunction that often produces enduring behavioural disorders. The clinical hallmarks of diffuse hypoxaemic–ischaemic injury are cardiopulmonary or pulmonary arrest, profound hypotension and significantly increased intracranial pressure. These

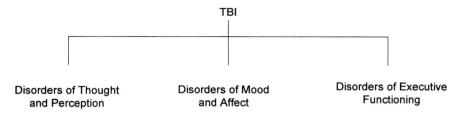

Fig. 8.1 Categories of neuropsychiatric disorders following traumatic brain injury. TBI = traumatic brain injury.

patients plateau early and have far worse outcomes and more behavioural problems than those with diffuse axonal injury alone. Unrelenting amnesia with associated parkinsonian motor abnormalities is commonly seen in patients with this type of injury. These constructs are further elaborated in Chapters 10 and 18.

A number of behavioural disorders can occur early in the course of rehabilitation. These are conceptualized as falling into one of three rubrics (Fig. 8.1). Not surprisingly, most rehabilitative clinicians have been reluctant to use psychiatric diagnostic strategies to conceptualize these problems; however, the extension of the neurological model requires that we do so. Historically, as has been the case with the physical expressions of neurological disability, clinicians have focused on the surface manifestations of the behavioural problems that present in these patient populations. Subjective clinical impressions or rating scales, such as the Katz Adjustment Scale or the Overt Aggression Scale, have been used in these circumstances. Thus, when describing behavioural disorders, the extant rehabilitation literature is replete with considerations of aggression, agitation, disorders of conduct, disorders of will, or disinhibition. However, these characterizations are no more helpful to a treating clinician using the neurological model of rehabilitation than is the broad diagnosis of 'traumatic brain injury'. Although not yet traceable to a distinct neuropathology, a formal diagnostic inquiry can lead to the diagnosis of a well-described neuropsychiatric syndrome that has treatment designed to decrease handicap.

The evaluation of the patient

The evaluation of the patient with acquired brain injury and comorbid behavioural problems begins where thoughtful consultations always do, i.e. with taking a history and performing an examination. Ideally, one should carefully evaluate the premorbid functioning of the patient, the characteristics of the injury, and the current living environment.

Premorbid issues

A structured interview with the family, focusing on previous neuromedical or neuropsychiatric disorders, will begin to elucidate premorbid functioning. In addition, external validators such as education, military and vocational histories should be requested when possible. These adjunctive sources can help balance retrospective falsification that may occur following injury. Previous substance abuse or criminal history must be explicitly sought, for they are rarely spontaneously disclosed. A detailed family history may identify specific familial neuropsychiatric diatheses that may aid both diagnosis and treatment.

The environment

The evaluation of behaviour in relationship to the treatment environment is vital. Issues central to any behavioural analysis should be considered: antecedent behaviours noted by the staff, particular precipitating environmental stimuli, and the consequences already occurring in the treatment environment when the behaviour is seen. Diurnal variation is common and may be related to an underlying neuropsychiatric syndrome, a cyclic reinforcer in the milieu, such as morning activities of daily living, shift changes for the nursing staff, or fatigue.

The clinical examination

The next step in the analysis is the clinical examination, which should incorporate elements of naturalistic behavioural observation, a psychiatric mental status, and an extended neurological examination. Behavioural observation should test hypotheses already gleaned from the history. Whenever possible, direct observation of antecedent environmental factors as well as the problematic behaviour is necessary. In particular, inferences regarding premeditation, volition, confusion and psychosis should be evaluated. Episodic behaviours will require examination of the patient during the expression of the targeted behaviour. At times, manifestations of the syndrome noted in the latter circumstances will not be evident when the patient is in behavioural control.

Following the above, one begins the extended neuro-psychiatric examination, which ideally includes a structured evaluation of cortical functioning. A model that incorporates elements from Strub and Black (1988), Taylor (1981), and Folstein, Folstein and McHugh (1975) fulfills these criteria. Special attention should be directed towards the patient's arousal and attention, orientation, speech, perception, affect and memory. This approach helps refine the focus of possible neuroanatomical abnormalities that may have pharmacological implications (Flor-Henry, 1983). It also establishes a clinical baseline of cognitive functioning which can be easily followed over time to monitor both beneficial and deleterious effects of any prescribed medication.

Next, the clinician should proceed to a comprehensive neurological examination. This examination may allow for further anatomical localization, as well as identifying concomitant conditions that may affect medication selection. As an example, a patient with prominent parkinsonian features secondary to hypoxaemic–ischaemic injury to the basal ganglia would be a poor candidate for high-potency neuroleptics, even if psychosis were evident. This evaluation allows the clinician to assess the language and motor effects seen with certain classes of medication in relationship to a pre-established baseline. Correlation of this information with the results of neuroimaging, electroencephalographic and neuropsychological testing will often suggest underlying pathophysiological processes involved in the expression of the maladaptive behaviour.

During the acute phase of rehabilitation, many of these behavioural difficulties pass with the clearing of posttraumatic amnesia and require little more than temporary environmental modification. However, if behavioural disabilities persist, they are often the problems that prevent full participation in rehabilitation and delay discharge. This is the group of patients that generally become rehabilitative outliers.

Destructive behaviour

Persistent aggression is one such problem. Although we all seem to know conceptually what aggression is, it has been a difficult construct to define operationally. In some settings, agitation is the descriptor of choice, in others, irritability. For the purposes of this chapter, the phrase destructive behaviour will be used to subsume all of the terms listed above. Destructive behaviour is defined as behaviour that results in partial or complete injury to the physical or psychological integrity of a person or object. However, neither destructive behaviour nor aggression is a diagnosis, but rather a sign or a behavioural manifestation that serves to indicate the presence of malfunction or disease. This sign is a component of many neurobehavioural syndromes and therefore always has a differential diagnosis.

Syndromes associated with destructive behaviour

Delirium

- Delirium is commonly associated with destructive behaviour, often as a patient emerges from a coma.
- Pharmacological interventions are directed at containment and tranquillization.
- Prolonged delirium following traumatic brain injury can evolve into other neuropsychiatric syndromes.

Delirium is a syndrome which affects arousal, attention, orientation, perception (e.g. visual and auditory illusions or hallucinations), motoric activity (generally increased), mood and memory. Many patients show diurnal variation in symptoms as well as disturbed sleep cycles. It is one of the more common syndromes associated with destructive behaviour seen early in the course of rehabilitation, often occurring as the patient emerges from coma. The problematic behaviour can range from periods of uncontrollable restlessness (during which wandering and the disconnection of intravenous lines can occur) to florid episodes of uncontrollably destructive behaviour.

Although delirium can be a consequence of the injury itself, other aetiological factors need to be ruled out. Independent of brain injury, delirium represents a potentially life-threatening syndrome, with mortality rates at one year reported by some centres to be as high as 35 per cent (Rabins and Folstein, 1982). A full review of this topic is beyond the scope of this chapter, and interested readers are referred to Strub and Black (1988) and Lipowski (1980) for further details. However, all medications should be carefully reviewed because many, including commonly prescribed agents such as phenytoin and analgesics, have been implicated in inducing this condition.

There are no controlled treatment studies with idiopathic, delirious traumatic brain injury or similar patients (Wise and Brandt, 1987). Rather, there are series or case reports that currently guide the clinical management of these patients (Lipowski, 1980; Wise and Brandt, 1987). Given that this condition is principally biologically mediated, neuropharmacological agents and environmental manipulations become the treatments of choice.

Generally, most pharmacological interventions for delirium are directed at containment and tranquillization. Intravenous haloperidol is considered the drug of choice, administered either as a bolus (Lipowski, 1980) or as a continuous drip (Fernandez et al., 1988). Given its relative specificity for dopamine receptors, it produces little hypotension, has few if any anticholinergic effects, and does not suppress the respiratory drive (Wise and Brandt, 1987). Sos and Cassem (1980) and Tesar, Murray and Cassem (1985) have used this agent extensively in idiopathic, agitated deliriums with good results and little morbidity. Interestingly, when this medication is given intravenously, it produces fewer extrapyramidal side-effects than when administered orally (Menza et al., 1987). Following traumatic brain injury, the lowest possible effective doses should be employed. Thus, 2 mg may be administered every 30 minutes until reasonable control has been achieved or a maximum of 15 mg per 24 hours. Acceptable results have also been obtained when low-dose benzodiazepines are combined with neuroleptics (Adams, 1984). One to two milligrams of lorazepam administered intravenously or intramuscularly may reduce the dose of haloperidol needed to produce the desired clinical outcome. Delirium is usually time limited and begins to end with the clearing of the posttraumatic amnesia. Thus, these interventions need to be carefully reviewed on a daily basis. Once the patient has stabilized, the haloperidol should be gradually reduced over a period of three to five days rather than abruptly discontinued (Wise and Brandt, 1987). Clinical experience suggests that a prolonged delirium following traumatic brain injury can evolve into a number of neuropsychiatric syndromes as the patient's consciousness clears. These syndromes include secondary psychoses, amnestic disorder or dementia.

Management also focuses on environmental prothesis. To that end, it attempts to reduce the handicapping conditions of the patient and provide for the safety of all concerned. This environment must be controlled and quiet. The notion that a stimulating environment helps a damaged central nervous system recover is unfounded. Therefore, all nonessential personnel should be excluded from the treatment milieu. The environment must be as clear of obstacles as possible, overhead paging systems should be eliminated and, when necessary, 1:1 staffing should be provided. Diurnal variation in lighting and activity should be maintained. Focus must be maintained on providing respiratory support, intravenous and enteric access to sustain life. Thus, restraints may become necessary if the patient consistently compromises the integrity of these supports. When such measures are employed, the staff must be prepared to explain the rationale behind their use to the patient's family. The so-called 'Craig bed' cannot provide this level of support to the patient and its use should be avoided under most circumstances. Behavioural and psychosocial strategies are less effective at this point in time.

As delirium clears, a patient can be handicapped by a number of psychiatric disorders best conceptualized (at first, at least) as secondary to the underlying neuro-

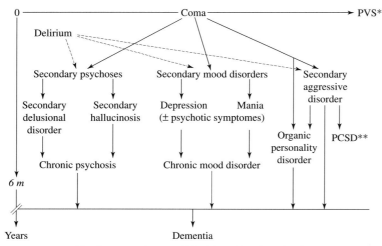

Fig. 8.2 Secondary psychiatric syndromes.

pathology. These difficulties fall into three broad categories: mood disorders, disorders of thought or perception, and disorders principally characterized by frontal systems deficits. They may evolve into a number of more specific diagnoses, as shown in Fig. 8.2.

Secondary psychotic disorders, delusional disorders and hallucinosis

• Perceptual distortion or delusional thinking can complicate recovery; it may be accompanied by destructive behaviour.
• If symptoms continue beyond several days, become commanding in nature, or behaviour cannot be reasonably contained, pharmacological intervention is warranted.
• Available antipsychotic agents offer numerous options; the side-effect profile should influence their choice.

In other patients, initial recovery is complicated primarily by the presence of perceptual distortions or delusional thinking (Shapiro, 1939; Achte, Hillbom and Aalberg, 1969; Davison and Bagley, 1969). Frequently, these sensory and cognitive difficulties are accompanied by destructive behaviour which can be quite unpredictable. These symptoms are transient and will

abate spontaneously with the clearing of consciousness. Under these circumstances, no pharmacological intervention is warranted. In the acute stages of rehabilitation, several circumstances can alter this recommendation. First, the disturbances continue beyond several days. Second, the hallucinations or delusions become 'commanding' in nature, i.e. the individual is 'told to do' certain life-threatening things, like harm himself or others. Third, the accompanying destructive behaviour cannot be contained within the treatment milieu.

There are no controlled studies to guide the pharmacological therapy of the traumatic brain injury patient with a secondary psychotic disorder. However, there are numerous controlled studies of the use of these agents in patients with idiopathic psychotic disorders (Donaldson, Gelenberg and Baldessarini, 1983; Janicak et al., 1993) and some case reports in the traumatic brain injury literature. Selection of an appropriate agent is determined more by the wish to avoid certain side-effects than by drug specificity. The recent introduction of risperidone and olanzapine has simplified this process, as both medications are relatively free of the motor, cardiovascular and anticholinergic side-effects that plagued older antipsychotic agents. The older antipsychotic agents cluster into two categories. The first, low-dose, high-potency agents such as pimozide, haloperidol, thiothixene or fluphenazine lack anticholinergic and autonomic effects. However, they are more likely to cause pseudo-parkinsonian side-effects such as tremor, gait disturbance and akathisia. The second, high-dose, low-potency drugs such as chlorpromazine and thioridazine are less likely to produce motor side-effects but are more sedating and produce both anticholinergic and autonomic side-effects. Both groups are now reserved for the treatment of refractory patients who fail to respond to either risperidone or olanzapine.

Clozapine, another atypical antipsychotic, has an important but limited role to play in those with traumatic brain injury and chronic psychoses. It is the most effective antipsychotic agent currently available in the USA. Like risperidone and olanzapine, clozapine produces few if any extrapyramidal effects and has not been implicated in causing tardive dyskinesia (Anden and Stock, 1973). In fact, it may improve dyskinetic movements in patients who already manifest this disorder. However, it is epileptogenic, profoundly sedating and can produce agranulocytosis. Thus, it should be used cautiously in patients with a high risk of seizures or in those being treated with carbamazepine or other agents likely to suppress bone marrow functioning. Clozapine may be used in conjunction with sodium valproate for patients with seizure disorders for whom no other neuroleptic alternatives exist. In addition, the Food and Drug Administration requires that patient's receiving this medication have weekly blood counts before their seven-day supply of medication can be released from a pharmacy. Hypotension, tachycardia and hyperptyalism also need to be carefully monitored. Michals et al. (1993) reported their experience in using this agent with nine traumatic brain injury patients in 1992. All patients were in the very late phases of postacute rehabilitation. Approximately one-third of these patients had a positive response to this medication. However, two of the nine had its use precluded by the onset of seizures.

Secondary mania

- The treatment of secondary mania is generally effective with lithium, carbamazepine, sodium valproate or a combination thereof.

Disorders primarily involving mood and its accompanying neurovegetative signs may also present early in the course of rehabilitation in association with destructive behaviour. Secondary mood disorder, manic type, is generally seen toward the end of posttraumatic amnesia. If this condition occurs later, a second pathophysiological process, such as the development of a subdural haematoma, seizure disorder, or intracerebral infection, should be sought. These patients will present with pressured speech, flight of ideas (often grandiose in nature), motoric hyperactivity and insomnia. Their sensorium is usually clear, but they may become confused as their condition worsens.

No controlled studies have been done with destructive traumatic brain injury patients with a secondary mania. The neuropsychiatric literature describes controlled studies of the agents discussed below used with patients who suffer from idiopathic mania. Rare case reports have included traumatic brain injury patients.

As seen in the secondary psychotic disorders, if psychosis accompanies these symptoms, a brief trial of a neuroleptic is indicated by clinical experience. However, if psychosis is not present and the difficulties persist beyond seven to ten days, lithium should be considered as its efficacy has been conclusively demonstrated in controlled neuropsychiatric studies (Schou, 1988). Some clinicians have been concerned about the epileptogenic potential of lithium, yet Erwin et al. (1973) actually reported a 36 per cent reduction in the number of seizures seen in 17 lithium-treated, epileptic patients. Close blood monitoring (twice per week) is suggested, especially early after the initiation of treatment until steady-state conditions are reached.

During the past two decades, anticonvulsants have demonstrated efficacy in the treatment of both primary and secondary mania. Ballenger and Post (1980) were the first to study systematically the use of carbamazepine in controlled trials for this indication. Carbamazepine may be used as a single agent or in combination with lithium. Although there have been reports of neurotoxicity when these two agents have been used in combination, they are rare (Shukla et al., 1987). An adequate therapeutic response is often obtained with blood levels in the 8–10 ng/dl range (Folks et al., 1982; Rall and Schleifer, 1985). In uncontrolled trials, McElroy et al. (1987) and McElroy and Pope (1988) have used sodium valproate for these syndromes. This group reported two patients who had secondary mania caused by traumatic brain injury which responded to valproate (Pope et al., 1988). Of particular interest was the fact that neither patient had responded to other more standard treatments before the valproate trial. Freeman et al. (1992), in a controlled study, noted that this agent may be of greater benefit than lithium to individuals with 'mixed mania' often associated with destructive behaviour. Blood levels need to be monitored and should be maintained between 55 and 100 ng/dl, although most investigators have found the higher end of the therapeutic range to be optimal (McElroy et al., 1989).

Secondary depression

- Secondary depression often responds to selective serotonin reuptake inhibitors (SSRIs); the presence of psychosis may require the addition of an antipsychotic.

Depression should always be considered in the differential diagnosis of destructive behaviour. This is especially true if a patient who has been otherwise stable begins to deteriorate behaviourally.

No controlled studies with traumatic brain injury patients who sustained moderate or severe injuries have been reported. The controlled nontraumatic brain injury but neuromedical literature (especially that concerning itself with poststroke depression) is relatively abundant and supports the efficacy of antidepressants in treating such conditions. Varney, Martzke and Roberts (1987) reported an uncontrolled series of 51 traumatic brain injury patients who responded positively to thymoleptic therapy. Similarly, Cassidy reported a series of nine severe traumatic brain injury patients treated with the newer SSRI fluoxetine. In an uncontrolled open trial, more than 60 per cent of these individuals benefitted from treatment, with few side-effects (Cassidy, 1989). Thus, depressed traumatic brain injury patients manifesting destructive behaviour should be tried on an antidepressant. Newer agents such as the SSRIs (fluoxetine, fluvoxamine, paroxetine or sertraline) should be considered the drugs of choice.

However, depression and destructive behaviour associated with psychosis will require treatment with both an antidepressant and an antipsychotic medication. This has been demonstrated in a controlled fashion in the psychiatric literature (Spiker et al., 1985), and clinical experience with traumatic brain injury patients concurs.

Secondary aggressive disorder

- Psychostimulants or dopamine agonists may have an impact on the treatment of secondary aggressive disorder.

Another proposed syndrome seen after the patient has emerged from coma is organic aggressive disorder, described by Silver, Yudofsky and Hales (1987). In this disorder, destructive behaviour is seen, while difficulties with orientation are less pronounced than in delirium. Abnormalities in thought content or perception do not predominate and a change in personality is not a requirement of diagnosis. Quasicontrolled studies exist in the traumatic brain injury literature. Numerous case reports exist in both the nontraumatic brain injury and traumatic brain injury neurobehavioural literature.

Rao, Jellinek and Woolston (1985), in a quasicontrolled study, have treated this group of patients successfully with oral haloperidol with doses in the 2–15 mg per day range. They reported no significant differences in rehabilitative outcome between the treated and control groups. Nevertheless, the period of posttraumatic amnesia was significantly longer in the treated group. However, this difference may be attributable to increased severity of neurological impairment in the treatment group. Theoretical challenges to this study have been partially based on an earlier study by Feeney, Gonzalez and Law (1982) in which it was reported that haloperidol impaired motor recovery following brain injury in animal models, presumably by disrupting dopaminergic transmission. Although the applicability of these findings to humans is unknown at this time, they stimulated the search for other agents with which to treat these patients.

Trials with various antidepressants have been one response to this dilemma. Jackson, Corrigan and Arnett (1985) were the first to report the use of amitriptyline for aggression in 1985. In that report, they discussed a patient who responded to 50 mg of amitriptyline administered orally at bedtime. Their group (Mysiw, Jackson and Corrigan, 1988) did a follow-up study involving 20 patients with secondary aggression. Dosages of this agent ranged up to a maximum of 150 mg per day. However, like the Rao study, only 50 per cent of the treatment group cleared posttraumatic amnesia. Again, the nontreated group was not a true control group since the patients had already had a return of continuous memory and did not exhibit behavioural difficulties significant enough to warrant entry into the treatment group. A few case reports of organically impaired (but not head-injured) patients with aggression have shown a good response to the serotonergically active antidepressant trazodone. The mean dose of trazodone has been 200 mg, but some clinicians have used up to 600 mg per day in divided doses.

A nonbenzodiazepine anxiolytic, buspirone, may also come to play a role in the treatment of these patients. At low doses, it is a direct 5-HT$_{1A}$ agonist (Eison and Temple, 1986). Levine (1988) presented a case report using this agent in a patient with traumatic brain injury and organic aggressive syndrome. Sustained improvement occurred at 10 mg given three times per day. In general, the side-effects of buspirone are few and mainly confined to mild sedation. However, a few scattered reports have been found which suggest buspirone may produce akathisia and tinnitus (Levine, 1988; Patterson, 1988).

Psychostimulants such as dextroamphetamine and methylphenidate have also been tried in case reports of traumatic brain injury patients with secondary aggression (Haas and Cope, 1985). Results have been mixed and occasionally patients would develop what appeared to be tolerance to these medications. Amantadine, a direct and indirect dopamine agonist, has been used with some success in these patients. Chandler, Barnhill and Gualtieri (1988) reported two relatively acute cases who responded satisfactorily to this agent following failure with other medications. Amantadine had a favourable toxicity profile and was not epileptogenic. Other direct-acting dopamine agonists such as bromocriptine, pergolide and low-dose apomorphine may also benefit certain individuals who do not respond to amantadine or the indirect-acting psychostimulants.

Although not well studied in patients with acute secondary aggressive disorder, adrenergically active agents have been considered as second-line drugs by experienced clinicians. The author prefers to use a transdermal clonidine patch (0.2–0.6 mg/day for a week) for these patients, an agent which is discussed in detail below.

Partial complex epilepsy

Late-onset, partial complex epilepsy may also be rarely associated with episodic, nondirected destructive behaviour. Historically, patients with intermittent explosive disorder have been considered a subset of this group, and limbically active anticonvulsants, such as carbamazepine and sodium valproate, are therefore the drugs of choice (Eames, 1989). Accompanying so-called interictal personality disturbances are rarely responsive to anticonvulsants alone. Paranoid delusions may develop, even years after the onset of seizures, which require concomitant management with neuroleptics. This is also true of associated mood disturbances that require treatment with appropriate thymoleptics (Humphries and Dixon, 1988).

Secondary personality disorder

- Beta blockers and α-2 agonists are used to control episodic destructive behaviour or organic personality disorder.
- Lithium is an additional option, even without evidence of primary affective disorder.
- Psychostimulants are useful when destructive patients are inattentive or underaroused.

More chronic destructive disorders occurring with personality change and independently of major mood or perceptual abnormalities may be seen after the sensorium has cleared. They are usually episodic in nature and often related to persistent frontal system deficits or disconnection syndromes. Various labels have been given to the former condition, ranging from frontal aggression to organic personality disorder, explosive type. Rare controlled studies exist in the traumatic brain injury and neuromedical literature, although there are abundant case reports.

Elliott (1987) first reported on the use of propranolol, a beta-adrenergic receptor blocker, in patients with organic difficulties and agitation. All of these patients in this open study improved with doses ranging between 60 and 1600 mg per day. A number of similar studies followed Elliott's report, demonstrating improvement in 86 per cent of more than 200 patients treated with this agent (Yudofsky, Williams and Gorman, 1981; Volavka, 1988). However, Greendyke et al. (1986) reviewed the use of propranolol in a double-blind crossover study, and although they found a statistical reduction in the number of assaults in the treatment group, the absolute number was not markedly decreased. Silver et al. offer guidelines for the use of this agent (Silver et al., 1987).

With the increased use of propranolol, the initial enthusiasm regarding its role in secondary personality disorder has waned. This has occurred for several reasons. First, it takes considerable time to titrate gradually upwards towards the recommended target dose of 640 mg per day. Second, the drug must be withheld due to clinically significant postural hypotension that occurs on a regular basis in this patient population. Third, it can take many weeks after reaching a relatively high dose to know whether the medication will be effective and this amount of time is not generally available for most 'managed care' patients.

Therefore, other alpha and beta blockers have been evaluated. In case reports, nadolol has been reported to be efficacious in doses between 40 and 160 mg per day. The utility of this agent suggests that peripheral as well as central mechanisms may be important in the usefulness of this class of drugs (Polakoff, Sorgi and Ratey, 1986). Greendyke and Kanter (1986) reported their use of pindolol (up to 60 mg per day) in similar patients. This agent appears to have an advantage over propranolol in that it produces less hypotension, apparently due to its intrinsic sympathomimetic activity.

Clonidine, an α-2 agonist, has been shown to benefit some of these patients. It acts primarily on the presynaptic α-2 autoreceptor, effectively inhibiting noradrenergic activity throughout the central nervous system. Side-effects include sedation and postural hypotension. There is a significant 'first-pass' effect on blood pressure, so the initial dose is preferably small and given at bedtime. The amount is then gradually titrated up to approximately 0.6 mg per day (Rudd and Blaschke, 1985). A transdermal preparation of this agent is available providing sustained release of up to 0.3 mg/day over a week.

Lithium carbonate has also been prescribed under these circumstances and is associated with a comparatively large literature in the head-injured population. Lithium has been used in the treatment of syndromes associated with destructive behaviour with or without associated head injury (Morrison et al., 1973; Sheard, 1975). Hale and Donaldson (1982) reported its use in five patients broadly diagnosed as having organic brain syndrome. However, three of the five individuals in this study had major head trauma. Each of the patients demonstrated improvement on lithium treatment, with blood levels between 0.6 and 0.8 mEq/l. None of the patients in this group had evidence of a primary affective disorder. Three of the subjects reported improved cognitive functioning while being treated with this agent; however, this has not been a consistent finding throughout all studies. Haas and Cope (1985) reported a single case of aggression that was unresponsive to benzodiazepines, neuroleptics, propranolol and methylphenidate. Lithium was significantly helpful. The response to lithium occurred within several days. Lithium levels ranged up to 0.8 mEq/l. Williams and Goldstein (1979) reported on its effectiveness in a number of patients with organic brain syndromes including one case associated with cerebrovascular accident. Again, none of the patients had a clearcut mood disorder and agitation was severe in most. Glenn et al. (1989) reported on the use of lithium in ten traumatic brain injury patients described as aggressive or affectively unstable. Six of these patients had a positive response to this intervention, although one 'regressed' after the seventh week of the study. Adverse neurological effects were noted in three of these patients; however, only one was being treated with lithium alone.

Serotonergically active agents that reduce most forms of destructive behaviour have been used in this syndrome as well. Ratey, Komry and Gaffar (1992) reported using buspirone to treat agitation and maladaptive behaviour in two patients with acquired brain injuries.

Low doses in the range of 10–15 mg/day were found effective for these patients. Generally, the response to this agent is rapid. Therefore, Gualtieri and Evans (1988) recommend discontinuing buspirone if it is not effective within several days following its initiation.

Direct and indirect dopamine agonists have also been used in this syndrome. In particular, psychostimulants have been used to treat destructive patients when they are inattentive and underaroused. Dextroamphetamine and methylphenidate have been the primary agents used. Lipper and Tuchman (1987) reported the first case in which dextroamphetamine was tried. The patient was described as agitated and depressed in addition to having memory and cognitive problems. He was apparently unresponsive to amitriptyline or a perphenazine–amitriptyline combination. Dextroamphetamine was successfully employed, with gradually increasing doses up to 15 mg twice a day. The medication was briefly discontinued; however, its reinstitution did not lead to another positive response. Since that report, a number of clinical investigators have reported the effectiveness of methylphenidate and pemoline in similar situations (Evans, Gualtieri and Patterson, 1987; Gualtieri and Evans, 1988).

Mooney and Hass (1993) reported a controlled study in which methylphenidate was used to treat 'anger' in postacute traumatic brain injury patients who sustained severe injuries. A randomized, pretest, posttest, placebo control group, single-blind design was employed to evaluate the effectiveness of this agent. Several interesting findings were reported: short-term treatment with the active agent significantly reduced 'anger' in this patient population. Patients with higher pretreatment anger scores responded better to methylphenidate than those with lower pretreatment anger scores. Further, this drug reduced the level of general psychopathology in the treatment group without producing significant adverse effects. However, attention, as measured by a variety of neuropsychological tests, unexpectedly did not improve with treatment.

Speech et al. (1993) came to the opposite conclusion regarding dysregulated behaviour in a double-blind, placebo-controlled randomized study of methylphenidate using a crossover design. This is particularly problematic because these two studies are among the best in the pharmacological treatment of behavioural disturbances following traumatic brain injury. However, the two study designs are not equivalent in several important ways. First, the length of treatment in the Speech study is significantly shorter, one week compared to six weeks in the Mooney study. Second, the Speech study has more than 50 per cent women, whereas Mooney studied men exclusively. Third, Speech grouped moderate and severe traumatic brain injury patients together; Mooney and Haas (1993) restricted their study to those with severe injuries only. Finally, different outcome measures were used in an attempt to determine the effects of the active compound.

Clinical experience suggests the usefulness of methylphenidate despite the conflicting reports. Furthermore, given its relatively benign side-effect profile and potentially rapid onset, it remains the initial drug of choice for this disorder. However, adrenergically active agents run a close second.

Other cognitive disorders

Although less dramatic in their presentation than disorders presenting with destructive behaviour, cognitive impairments are often the great limiting step in the rehabilitation of patients with traumatic brain injury. Despite a significant descriptive and basic science literature of these disorders, controlled trials of neuropharmacological interventions are few in number and equivocal in results. Interested readers are referred to a 1994 review by Wroblewski and Glenn.

Dementia

In later stages of rehabilitation and community re-entry, other syndromes associated with destructive behaviour begin to emerge. For some patients the global central nervous system dysfunction of delirium will evolve into the more permanent problem of dementia. In others, it appears to be the final common pathway into which many other disorders devolve.

Controlled treatment studies do not exist for this syndrome, nor are there any clearly defined traumatic brain injury case reports. Thus, treatment is guided by non-traumatic brain injury case reports, clinical experience, and the attempt to treat potentially treatable subsyndromes of this condition.

When evaluating these patients, it is quite important to consider the 'pseudodementia' of depression in the differential diagnosis. Many clinicians have suggested at least a six-week trial of an antidepressant in this subgroup of patients because the prognosis for those with frank dementia is so poor. Neuroleptics have been used in this population with varying degrees of success (Salzman, 1987). However, given the chronicity of this condition, newer agents that do not produce tardive dyskinesia are the drugs of choice. Occasionally, benzodiazepines have been successfully used in those who have agitation associated with dementia. For this indication, oxazepam is the most frequently used agent from this class of medications (Deberdt and Bagley, 1978). More recently, buspirone has been used successfully to manage destructive behaviour occurring with dementia (Colenda, 1988). Given its benign side-effect profile, this medication should be considered the drug of choice in this subgroup of patients. Theoretically, other serotonergically active agents should be effective as well. Thus, a trial of fluoxetine, fluvoxamine, sertraline or paroxetine may be warranted if buspirone fails to improve the condition.

Case study

At the time of his work-related injury, W.D. was 21 years old. He was struck by an automobile while riding his bicycle and was immediately rendered unconscious. Emergency Medical Service records indicated that he had an initial Glasgow Coma Score of 3. He was in respiratory distress and intubated at the scene. Upon arrival at the emergency department, his postresuscitation Glasgow Coma Score had risen to 6. His initial brain computerized tomography (CT) scan revealed diffuse petechial haemorrhages and bilateral intraventricular bleeding. A ventriculostomy was placed for two weeks to control increased intracranial pressure. True coma lasted for five days, but he remained mute for over a month. He remained confused throughout his acute hospitalization. Subsequent brain CT scans revealed the following: left orbital frontal and inferior opercular contusions, right thalamic infarcts, bilateral posterior and periventricular encephalomalacia. Two months postinjury he was transferred to an acute rehabilitation hospital. In that setting, the patient remained confused and extremely agitated. He spent the majority of his days restrained in a chair bolted to the floor. When released from restraints, he would unpredictably strike out at staff and on one occasion assaulted a staff member, breaking her jaw. His treating physician tried a number of medications in an attempt to improve his behaviour. These included: pindolol, amantadine and lorazepam. The patient did not benefit from these interventions. A repeat brain CT revealed a 3×3 cm left orbital and frontal polar contusion and moderate diffuse cerebral atrophy.

Six months postinjury, the patient remained confused and agitated, with a Galveston Orientation and Amnesia Test (GOAT) score of 40. During a phase of increased agitation, the amantadine was discontinued and the patient's GOAT score decreased to 17. Subsequent trials on buspirone and carbamazepine were not particularly helpful. Buspirone was discontinued and doxepin was begun, together with low-dose haloperidol. The dosage of pindolol was increased and lithium was added to his medication regimen. On these agents, his aggression persisted and he required eight staff members to complete activities of daily living and ten to restrain him when he became violent. He was subsequently referred to a behavioural rehabilitation programme at five months postadmission.

At the time of admission to the programme, he was confused, with a GOAT in the midthirties, acutely agitated, extremely perseverative and aphasic. Admission medications included: haloperidol 2 mg i.m. t.i.d., lithium carbonate 600 mg p.o. b.i.d., 900 mg p.o. q.h.s. and lorazepam 2 mg i.m. Q4h p.r.n. agitation. The manifestation of his destructive behaviour showed no discernible pattern and was extremely unpredictable. His mental status examination revealed significant suspiciousness in thought content and hypervigilance. General physical examination was essentially unremarkable. Neurological examination revealed profound parkinsonism, bilateral hyperreflexia and frontal release signs on the right. Repeat brain CT revealed a left frontal and right parietal infarcts and a hydrocephalus ex vacuo. An EEG demonstrated left frontal slowing, but no electrographic seizures.

All of the patient's medications were discontinued and he was observed for two weeks free of medication. During this time, it was noted that his disorder of thought content worsened and he exhibited frank paranoia and appeared to be responding to internal stimuli. Although his parkinsonism improved when he stopped taking haloperidol, it did not completely abate. He did not clear posttraumatic amnesia. At the end of 14 days, he was begun on clozapine and restarted on amantadine. His environment was simplified and no staff other than those trained in the management of aggressive behaviour were permitted to interact with him. On 300 mg a day of clozapine and amantadine, he exhibited considerable improvement in his thought disorder and subsequently in his destructive behaviour. At day 14, the restraints were discontinued and he was permitted to ambulate with assistance in the treatment milieu.

Subsequently, it was noted that his destructive behaviour would re-emerge when he became frustrated performing tasks that he felt were 'beneath' his abilities. Therefore, clonidine and labetalol were added to his medications. With the addition of these medications, he began to respond to behavioural cues and was able to perform all activities of daily living with only stand-by assistance. Six months after entry into the programme, he was able to make the transition to a community-based residential facility.

This patient's course emphasizes the effect of focal contusional and diffuse hypoxaemic injury on outcome. These neuropathological substrates produced fixed deficits that were unresponsive to standard remediative therapies. Furthermore, it became clear that the secondary delusional disorder producing abnormalities in his thought content had been unresponsive to haloperidol and that other medications 'generically' prescribed to improve 'phenotypic' agitation were unsuccessful in altering the course of his condition. Using the extension of the neurorehabilitation model, it became clear that both newer antipsychotic agents and medications designed to aid secondary personality disorder were necessary to improve his condition. Implementation of these more specific therapies reduced his level of disability and permitted his transfer to a less restrictive and less costly treatment environment.

Beyond psychopharmacology

- Treatment settings are enhanced by the provision of a quiet, secure and safe environment.
- Behavioural interventions need to be consistent and appropriate to the situation.
- Psychotherapy should provide an active coaching technique focusing on practical problem solving and acceptance of deficits.

As much as any of us might wish for a magic elixir that transforms maladaptive, dysregulated behaviour into appropriate and controlled conduct, such an agent does not yet exist and probably never will. Therefore, other nonpharmacological strategies must be employed to help improve these patients' outcome. These approaches centre on the use of environmental prosthesis, behavioural programming and psychotherapeutic techniques. A full discussion of each is beyond the scope of this chapter, and the interested reader is referred to a number of texts that focus exclusively on these strategies (Wood and Eames, 1989; Eames, Haffey and Cope, 1990) and to other chapters in this volume. However, a few comments are warranted. First, although we all wish to believe that most treatment programmes are comprehensive enough to care for even the worst of traumatic brain injury outliers, the fact of the matter is that they are not; nor should they be. The attempt to be all things to all patient populations produces inescapable mediocrity for the whole. Very few programmes see enough outliers to become expert in their management. Therefore, it becomes incumbent upon general programmes to recognize the need to refer these patients to specialized settings where the major focus of treatment centres on these handicapping conditions.

Second, environmental prosthesis must occur in even the most basic of neurorehabilitation settings. As noted above, such prosthesis centres on creating a quiet, secure and safe treatment milieu, an environment that is the antithesis of most acute rehabilitation hospital settings. However, it can be created if the will to do so exists both clinically and administratively. The constant background din of television sets, overhead paging systems and modern cleaning equipment is not conducive to healing a damaged central nervous system in which inattentiveness and slowed processing speed must be overcome for learning to occur.

Third, inconsistently applied and ill-conceived 'cookbook' behavioural programming is worse than none at all. It rapidly devolves into a draconian punishment system that demoralizes both patients and staff. Therefore, most general programmes are well advised to confine their behavioural interventions to time-out and praise. Disruptive behaviour is best dealt with by brief periods of time-out in a quiet-room. Generally, within five minutes the calmer patient is quietly encouraged to re-enter the treatment milieu and retry the activity or interaction that precipitated his or her dysregulated response. Praise, for even the smallest successes, goes a long way towards providing the only 'positive reinforcement' most of us, including our brain-injured patients, need to continue to persevere at tasks that must be accomplished despite our reluctance to believe that such mastery can be achieved.

Fourth, psychotherapy is not a technique to be practised just because a patient and a clinician can both talk. It is rarely indicated for those with significant cognitive impairment or major psychiatric sequelae. Standard practice must be modified to a more active, coaching technique that focuses on practical day-to-day problem solving and acceptance of those deficits that are unlikely to improve with time. Although improvement of self-awareness is a noble goal of psychotherapy, it is rarely achieved in those with true anosognosia. Finally, an hour's worth of psychotherapy once a week is no substitute for repeated encouragement from a caring staff, genuinely interested in the welfare of its patients.

Conclusions

Behaviourally disordered patients test the mettle of every rehabilitation programme. Many of these patients are best managed at specialized centres. However, a significant minority can be managed by a rehabilitation hospital dedicated to the neurological model of rehabilitation[1] if hospital staff have the will to extend the model to deal with the neuropsychiatric complications of acquired brain injury. Such a programme must be able to provide a prosthetic environment designed to ameliorate handicap and employ appropriate neuropharmacological interventions that treat behavioural complications aggressively, but with informed compassion for the individuals who find themselves disabled by disorders of the mind as well as those emanating only from its organic substrate.

Endnote

1 A detailed review of the neurological model of rehabilitation can be found in Mills, V.M., Cassidy, J.W. and Katz, D.I., eds. 1997. *Neurological Rehabilitation: a Guide to Diagnosis, Prognosis and Treatment*. Malden, MA: Blackwell Science.

References

Achte, K.A., Hillbom, E. and Aalberg, V. 1969. Psychosis following war brain injuries. *Acta Psychiatr Scand* 45, 1–18.

Adams, F. 1984. Neuropsychiatric evaluation and treatment of delirium in the critically ill cancer patient. *Cancer Bull* 36, 156–60.

Anden, N.E. and Stock, G. 1973. Effect of clozapine on the turnover of dopamine in the corpus striatum and in the limbic system. *J Pharm Pharmacol* 25, 346–8.

Ballenger, J.C. and Post, R.M. 1980. Carbamazepine in manic–depressive illness: a new treatment. *Am J Psychiatry* 137, 782–90.

Cassidy, J.W. 1989. Fluoxetine: a new serotonergically-active antidepressant. *J Head Trauma Rehabil* 4, 67–9.

Chandler, M.C., Barnhill, J.L. and Gualtieri, C.T. 1988. Amantadine for the agitated head-injury patient. *Brain Inj* 2, 309–11.

Colenda, C.C. 1988. Buspirone in treatment of agitated dementia patients. *Lancet* 1, 1169.

Davison, K. and Bagley, C.R. 1969. Schizophrenia-like psychosis associated with organic disorders of the central nervous system. *Br J Psychiatry* 4, 113–84.

Deberdt, R. and Bagley, C.R. 1978. Oxazepam in the treatment of anxiety in children and the elderly. *Acta Psychiatr Scand* 274(s), 104–10.

Donaldson, S.R., Gelenberg, A.J. and Baldessarini, R.J. 1983. The pharmacologic treatment of schizophrenia: a progress report. *Schizophr Bull* 504–27.

Eames, P. 1989. Risk–benefit considerations in drug treatment. In *Models of Brain Injury Rehabilitation*, ed. R.L. Wood and P. Eames, pp. 164–82. London: Chapman and Hall.

Eames, P., Haffey, W.J. and Cope, D.N. 1990. Treatment of behavioral disorders. In *Rehabilitation of the Adult and Child with Traumatic Brain Injury*, ed. M. Rosenthal E.R. Griffith, M.R. Bond and J.D. Miller, pp. 410–32. Philadelphia: F.A. Davis.

Eison, A.S. and Temple, D.L. 1986. Buspirone: review of its pharmacology and current perspectives on its mechanism of action. *Am J Med* 80, 1–9.

Elliott, F.A. 1987. Propranolol for control of belligerent behavior following acute brain damage. *Ann Neurol* 1, 489–91.

Erwin, C.W., Gerber, J., Morrison, S.D. and James, J.F. 1973. Lithium carbonate and convulsive disorders. *Arch Gen Psychiatry* 28, 646–8.

Evans, R.W., Gualtieri, C.T. and Patterson, D. 1987. Treatment of chronic closed head injury with psychostimulant drugs: a controlled case study and an appropriate evaluation procedure. *J Nerv Ment Dis* 175, 106–10.

Feeney, D., Gonzalez, A. and Law, W. 1982. Amphetamine, haloperidol, and experience interact to affect rate of recovery after motor cortex injury. *Science* 217, 855–7.

Fernandez, F., Holmes, V., Adams, F. and Kavanaugh, J. 1988. Treatment of severe, refractory agitation with a haloperidol drip. *J Clin Psychiatry* 49, 239–41.

Flor-Henry, P. 1983. *Cerebral Basis of Psychopathology.* Boston: J. Wright.

Folks, D.G., King, L.D., Dowdy, S.B. et al. 1982. Carbamazepine treatment of selected affectively disordered inpatients. *Am J Psychiatry* 139, 115–17.

Folstein, M.F., Folstein, S.E. and McHugh, P.R. 1975. Minimental state. A practical method for grading the cognitive state of patients for the clinician. *J Psychiatr Res* 12, 189–95.

Freeman, T.W., Clothier, J.L., Pazzaglia, P., Lisen, M. and Swann, A.C. 1992. A double-blind study of valproate and lithium in the treatment of acute mania. *Am J Psychiatry* 149, 108–11.

Glenn, M.B., Wroblewski, B., Parziale, J. and Levine, L. 1989. Lithium carbonate for aggressive behavior or affective instability in ten brain-injured patients. *Am J Phys Med Rehabil* 68, 221–6.

Greendyke, R.M. and Kanter, D.R. 1986. Therapeutic effects of pindolol on behavioral disturbances associated with organic brain disease: double-blind study. *J Clin Psychiatry* 47, 423–6.

Greendyke, R.M., Kanter, D.R., Schuster, D.B., Verstreate, S. and Wootton, J. 1986. Propranolol treatment of assaultive patients with organic brain disease: double-blind, crossover placebo controlled study. *J Nerv Ment Dis* 174, 290–4.

Gualtieri, C.T. and Evans, R.W. 1988. Stimulant treatment for the neurobehavioral sequelae of traumatic brain injury. *Brain Inj* 2, 273–90.

Haas, J.F. and Cope, N. 1985. Neuropharmacologic management of behavior sequelae in head injury: a case report. *Arch Phys Med Rehabil* 66, 472–4.

Hale, M.S. and Donaldson, J.O. 1982. Lithium carbonate in the treatment of organic brain syndrome. *J Nerv Ment Dis* 170, 362–5.

Humphries, H.R. and Dixon, P.S. 1988. Hypomania following complex partial seizures. *Br J Psychiatry* 152, 571–2.

Jackson, R.D., Corrigan, J.D. and Arnett, J.A. 1985. Amitriptyline for agitation in head injury. *Arch Phys Med Rehabil* 66, 180–1.

Janicak, P.G., Davis, J.M., Preskorn, S.H. and Ayd, F.J., eds. 1993. *Principles and Practice of Psychopharmacolotherapy.* Baltimore: Williams & Wilkins.

Levine, A.M. 1988. Buspirone and agitation in head injury. *Brain Inj* 2, 165–7.

Lipowski, Z.J. 1980. Delirium updated. *Compr Psychiatry* 21, 190–6.

Lipper, S. and Tuchman, M.M. 1987. Treatment of chronic posttraumatic organic brain syndrome with dextroamphetamine: first reported case. *J Nerv*

McElroy, S.L., Keck, P.E., Pope, H.G. and Hudson, J.I. 1989. Valproate in psychiatric disorders: literature review and clinical guidelines. *J Clin Psychiatry* 50, 23–9.

McElroy, S.L. and Pope, H.G. 1988. *Use of Anticonvulsants in Psychiatry, Recent Advances.* Clifton, NJ: Oxford Health Care.

McElroy, S.L., Pope, H.G. and Keck, P.E. 1987. Sodium valproate: its use in primary psychiatric disorders. *J Clin Psychopharmacol* 7, 16–24.

Menza, M., Murray, G., Holmes, V. and Rafuls, W.A. 1987. Decreased extrapyramidal symptoms with intravenous haloperidol. *J Clin Psychiatry* 48, 278–80.

Michals, M.I., Crismon, M.L., Roberts, S. and Childs, A. 1993. Clozapine response and adverse effects in nine brain-injured patients. *J Clin Psychopharmacol* 13, 198–203.

Mooney, G.F. and Haas, L.J. 1993. Effect of methylphenidate on brain injury-related anger. *Arch Phys Med Rehabil* 74, 153–60.

Morrison, S.D., Erwin, C.W., Gianturco, D.T. and Gerber, C.J. 1973. Effect of lithium on combative behavior in humans. *Dis Nerv Syst* 34, 186–9.

Mysiw, W.J., Jackson, R.D. and Corrigan, J.D. 1988. Amitriptyline for post-traumatic agitation. *Am J Phys Med Rehabil* **67**, 29–33.

Patterson, J.F. 1988. Akathisia associated with buspirone. *J Clin Psychopharmacol* **8**, 296–7.

Polakoff, S.A., Sorgi, P.J. and Ratey, J.J. 1986. The treatment of impulsive and aggressive behavior with nandolol. *J Clin Psychopharmacol* **6**, 125–26.

Pope, H.G., McElroy, S.L., Satlin, A., Hudson, J.I., Keck, P.E. and Kalish, R. 1988. Head injury, bipolar disorder, and response to valproate. *Compr Psychiatry* **29**, 34–8.

Rabins, P.V. and Folstein, M.F. 1982. Delirium and dementia. *Br J Psychiatry* **140**, 149.

Rall, T.W. and Schleifer, L.S. 1985. Drugs effective in the therapy of the epilepsies. In *The Pharmacological Basis of Therapeutics*, 7th edn, ed. A.G. Gilman, L.S. Goodman, T.W. Rall et al. pp. 446–72. New York: Macmillan.

Rao, N., Jellinek, M. and Woolston, D.C. 1985. Agitation in closed head injury: haloperidol effects on rehabilitation outcome. *Arch Phys Med Rehabil* **66**, 30–4.

Ratey, J.J., Komry, V. and Gaffar, K. 1992. Low-dose buspirone to treat agitation and maladaptive behavior in brain-injured patients: two case reports. *J Clin Psychopharmacol* **12**, 363–4.

Riblet, L.A., Taylor, D.P., Eison, M.S. and Stanton, H.C. 1981. Pharmacology and neurochemistry of buspirone. *J Clin Psychiatry* **43**, 11–18.

Rudd, P. and Blaschke, T.F. 1985. Antihypertensive agents and the drug therapy of hypertension. In *The Pharmacological Basis of Therapeutics*, ed. A.G. Gilman, L.S. Goodman, T.W. Rall et al., pp. 784–805. New York: Macmillan.

Salzman, C. 1987. Treatment of agitation in the elderly. In *Psychopharmacology: the Third Generation of Progress*, ed. H.Y. Meltzer. New York: Raven Press.

Schou, M. 1988. Lithium treatment of manic–depressive illness. *JAMA* **259**, 1834–6.

Shapiro, L.B. 1939. Schizophrenia-like psychosis following head injuries. *IMJ* **10**, 150–254.

Sheard, M.H. 1975. Lithium in the treatment of aggression. *J Nerv Ment Dis* **160**, 108–18.

Shukla, S., Cook, B.L., Mukherjee, S., Godwin, C. and Miller, M.G. 1987. Mania following head trauma. *Am J Psychiatry* **144**, 93–6.

Silver, J.M., Yudofsky, S.C. and Hales, R.E. 1987. Neuropsychiatric aspects of traumatic brain injury. In *Textbook of Neuropsychiatry*, ed. R.E. Hales and S.C. Yudofsky, pp. 179–90. Washington, DC: American Psychiatric Press.

Sos, J. and Cassem, N.H. 1980. Managing postoperative agitation. *Drug Therapy* **10**, 103–6.

Speech, T.J., Rao, S.M., Osmon, D.C. and Sperry, L.T. 1993. A double-blind controlled study of methylphenidate treatment in closed head injury. *Brain Inj* **4**, 333–8.

Spiker, D.G., Weiss, J.C., Dealy, R.S. et al. 1985. The pharmacological treatment of delusional depression. *Am J Psychiatry* **142**, 430–6.

Strub, R.L. and Black, F.W. 1988. *Neurobehavioral Disorders: a Clinical Approach*. Philadelphia: F.A. Davis.

Taylor, M.A. 1981. *The Neuropsychiatric Mental Status Examination*. New York: SP Medical and Scientific Books.

Tesar, G.E., Murray, G.B. and Cassem, N.H. 1985. Use of high-dose intravenous haloperidol in the treatment of agitated cardiac patients. *J Clin Psychopharmacol* **5**, 344–7.

Varney, N.R., Martzke, J.S. and Roberts, R.J. 1987. Major depression in patients with closed head injury. *Neuropsychology* **1**, 7–9.

Volavka, J. 1988. Can aggressive behavior in humans be modified by beta blockers? *Postgrad Med*, 163–8.

Williams, K.H. and Goldstein, G. 1979. Cognitive and affective responses to lithium in patients with organic brain syndrome. *Am J Psychiatry* **136**, 800–3.

Wise, M.G. and Brandt, G.T. 1987. Delirium. In *Textbook of Neuropsychiatry*, ed. R.E. Hales and S.C. Yudofsky, pp. 89–106. Washington, DC: American Psychiatric Press.

Wood, R.L. and Eames, P., eds. 1989. *Models of Brain Injury Rehabilitation*. London: Chapman and Hall.

Wroblewski, B.A. and Glenn, M.B. 1994. Pharmacological treatment of arousal and cognitive deficits. *J Head Trauma Rehabil* **9**(3), 19–42.

Yudofsky, S., Williams, D. and Gorman, J. 1981. Propranolol in the treatment of rage and violent behavior in patients with chronic brain syndromes. *Am J Psychiatry* **138**, 218–20.

9

Pharmacological interventions in Alzheimer's disease

Fredda L. Leiter and Jeffrey L. Cummings

Introduction

- The prevalence of Alzheimer's disease is increasing as the population ages. The associated changes in cognition and behaviour present a growing burden on health care.

Alzheimer's disease is an increasingly important cause of disability as the population ages. At the turn of the century, 4 per cent of the USA population was over 65 years old, and today 13 per cent are over age 65. By the year 2030, an estimated 20 per cent of the population will be within this age group (Department of Health and Human Services, 1990; World Health Organization, 1992). The current prevalence of dementia ranges from an estimated 5 to 10 per cent in the 65 or older age group and up to 47 per cent among those aged 85 years old and above (Evans et al., 1989; Bachman et al., 1992).

In the past ten-year period, the cost of caring for demented patients rose from $12 billion to $30 billion per year (Hay and Ernst, 1987). Alzheimer's disease, which accounts for 35–60 per cent of progressive dementias evaluated in hospital and clinic-based settings, accounts for more cases of dementia than any other condition (Cummings and Benson, 1992).

Alterations in cognition and behaviour in Alzheimer's disease interfere with function and require the increasing involvement of family and institutional caretakers as the patient deteriorates. Cognitive deficits include difficulties with recent and remote memory, language, visuospatial and visuoconstructive function, calculation, praxis, abstraction and judgment (Cummings and Benson, 1992). Neuropsychiatric manifestations of Alzheimer's disease include personality changes, delu-

sions, hallucinations, mood alterations, sleep disorders, appetite changes, disturbances in sexual function, and alterations in psychomotor activity (Reisberg et al., 1987; Cummings and Victoroff, 1990; Mega et al., 1996). The neuropsychiatric disturbances of this disease are difficult to manage, cause concern for patient safety, and produce more psychological distress for caretakers than the cognitive deficits. Unfortunately, the prevention or cure of Alzheimer's disease is not likely in the near future. Therefore, behavioural and pharmacological interventions are the most effective approaches at the present time.

This chapter describes the clinical manifestations, criteria for diagnosis, and nature and distribution of pathological changes of Alzheimer's disease. The pharmacological and nonpharmacological treatments of the neuropsychiatric manifestations are discussed, and treatment of the cognitive deficits is presented.

Clinical characteristics

- The clinical course of the disease is divided into three stages, each placing specific demands on treatment and care.

Patients with Alzheimer's disease demonstrate progressive decline in intellect, have variable neuropsychiatric alterations, and eventually exhibit compromised motor ability (Cummings and Benson, 1992). Progress is variable, with survival ranging from 1 to 15 years, and disease duration averaging 8 to 12 years after diagnosis (Masterman, Craig and Cummings, 1995). The clinical course can be divided into three stages (Cummings and Benson, 1992).

Stage 1 spans approximately the first three years of the disease. The initial manifestation of the disease is nearly always memory disturbance. There is difficulty learning new material and some difficulty with recall of remote information. Deficits in visuospatial skills include impairment in copying complex constructions and geographic disorientation. Patients may become lost in familiar surroundings or while driving. There are difficulties with word finding and naming. Spontaneous speech may be empty, with circumlocution. Personality changes include indifference and occasional irritability. There may be sadness or delusions. Neurological examination is normal. Electroencephalogram (EEG) is normal and magnetic resonance imaging (MRI) and computed axial tomography (CT) are normal or reveal only mild atrophy. Positron emission tomography (PET) and single photon emission computed tomography (SPECT) reveal bilateral parietotemporal hypometabolism or hypoperfusion.

During this initial stage of Alzheimer's disease, patients have impairment of intellectual function, but their preserved social skills may lead observers to underestimate their disability. The extent of deterioration may become evident only when an unusual or stressful situation arises.

In *stage 2*, lasting between three and ten years, remote and recent recall become more severely impaired. Construction ability and spatial orientation continue to decline. Ideomotor apraxia occurs. There is fluent aphasia and acalculia. Indifference and irritability continue, and delusions may be present. Restlessness and pacing are common. There is slowing of background rhythm on EEG. CT and MRI may be normal, or may reveal mild atrophy and ventricular enlargement.

During *stage 3*, after between 8 and 12 years of disease duration, intellectual function severely deteriorates. The patient has limb rigidity and flexed posture. Urinary and faecal incontinence occur. Primitive reflexes such as grasp and suck emerge. The EEG demonstrates diffuse slowing of electrocerebral rhythms. CT and MRI reveal ventricular dilatation and sulcal enlargement. PET and SPECT typically demonstrate biparietal and frontal lobe hypometabolism and hypoperfusion. Ultimately, patients die of aspiration pneumonia, urinary tract infection, asphyxiation (from putting objects in their mouth), or infected decubitus ulcers.

Criteria for the diagnosis of Alzheimer's disease

A work group of the National Institute of Neurological and Communicative Disorders and Stroke and the Alzheimer's Disease and Related Disorders Association (NINCDS/ADRDA) established criteria for the diagnosis of Alzheimer's disease (McKhann et al., 1984). These criteria differentiate between definite, probable and possible diagnoses. Patients have definite Alzheimer's disease when they meet clinical criteria for probable Alzheimer's disease and there is histopathological evidence of Alzheimer's disease obtained by biopsy or autopsy. Probable Alzheimer's disease is established by clinical examination and documented by a structured clinical questionnaire and neuropsychological testing. There must be deficits in two or more areas of cognition as well as progressive worsening of memory and other cognitive functions. There is no disturbance of consciousness. Onset is between age 40 and 90, and there is no systemic or other brain disease that could produce a dementia syndrome. Symptoms must be present for at least six months. The diagnosis of possible Alzheimer's disease is made: when the onset, presentation or progression of the dementia syndrome is atypical but no alternate aetiology is found; when there is a systemic or other brain disease present that can produce a dementia, but is not considered to be the cause of the dementia; or when a single intellectual function progressively declines and there is no identifiable cause.

The fourth edition of the Diagnostic and Statistical Manual of Mental Disorders (DSM IV; American Psychiatric Association, 1994) also provides criteria for the diagnosis of Alzheimer's disease. These criteria include the development of multiple cognitive deficits manifested by both memory impairment and one or more of the following: aphasia, ideomotor apraxia, agnosia, disturbed executive function (planning, organizing, sequencing, abstracting). These cognitive deficits cause significant impairment in social or occupational functioning and represent a significant decline from a previous level of functioning. There is gradual onset and continuing cognitive deterioration. The cognitive deficits are not due to other central nervous system conditions or systemic disorders that cause dementia and are not substance induced.

The differential diagnosis of AD includes many treatable causes of cognitive and behavioural changes in the elderly. The elderly often take prescribed and over-the-counter medications that can affect mental status. Dementia may be caused by systemic illnesses such as thyroid disease, B12 deficiency, and by pulmonary, cardiac, renal or hepatic conditions. Neurological disorders that may have a presentation similar to Alzheimer's disease are brain tumour, stroke, hydrocephalus, and infectious processes such as human immunodeficiency virus (HIV) and syphilis. Symptoms of depression such as impaired memory and concentration and psychomotor retardation can mimic the manifestations of Alzheimer's disease, but are reversible with appropriate treatment. Other dementias, such as frontotemporal dementias, Lewy body dementia, vascular dementias and the dementia of Parkinson's disease, may be misdiagnosed as Alzheimer's disease (Miller et al., 1994).

Neuropathological changes

On gross examination, the brains of Alzheimer's disease patients are atrophic, with most pronounced atrophy in the temporoparietal and anterior frontal regions (Cummings and Benson, 1992). On histological examination of the cerebral cortex, neurofibrillary tangles, neuritic plaques, granulovacuolar degeneration, and amyloid angiopathy are evident. Neurofibrillary tangles are abnormal collections of filaments in neuronal cytoplasm that are seen in normal ageing as well as in other syndromes such as elderly Down's syndrome, post-encephalitic parkinsonism, and dementia pugilistica. Neuritic plaques are found outside the neuron, and have a centre of amyloid, surrounded by abnormal dendrites and axons (Schneider and Tariot, 1994). Neuritic plaques can also be seen in other conditions such as elderly Down's syndrome or lead encephalopathy. The location and extent of neuronal changes correlate with the severity and type of intellectual deficits. Medial temporal and temporoparietal junction areas are most severely affected.

In Alzheimer's disease, specific types of neurons are destroyed. The neurons of the association cortices, cholinergic neurons of the nucleus basalis of Meynert, serotonergic cells in the raphe, and adrenergic cells of locus coeruleus are most affected (Masterman et al., 1995). Less consistent and less marked deficiencies in noradrenergic, serotonergic and GABA-aminobutyric acid neurotransmitters are evident.

Pharmacological treatment of Alzheimer's disease

- Two important considerations guide the use of pharmacological treatment: age-associated alterations in pharmacokinetics and pharmacodynamics; and the potential benefits of pharmacological and behavioural interventions.

Pharmacological treatment of Alzheimer's disease targets behavioural symptoms such as agitation, sleep disturbances, aggression, and apathy; mood and thought content disorders such as depression, anxiety, delusions and hallucinations; or cognitive symptoms such as memory, language, visuospatial function and praxis.

Before the initiation of treatment, general guidelines for pharmacotherapy in the elderly should be considered, as pharmacodynamics and pharmacokinetics are altered in this population (Cummings and Benson, 1992). Absorption may be affected by alterations in gastrointestinal motility or blood flow, absorptive surface, and gastric pH. Distribution is affected by decreased lean body mass, total body water, and serum albumin; body fat is increased, and there are changes in protein binding. Metabolism is affected by decreased liver mass and blood flow and decreased oxidative ability. Excretion is reduced due to decreased renal blood flow, glomerular filtration rate, and tubular secretion. These changes may lead to toxicity when a drug that is given in a dose appropriate for a younger patient is administered to an elderly individual.

The following guidelines for the pharmacological treatment of the elderly demented patient help optimize drug management (Cummings and Benson, 1992). If possible, pharmacological treatment should be minimized and nonpharmacological approaches used.

A careful medication history is crucial. Specific target symptoms for treatment should be determined and response to treatment carefully observed. The patient should be given clear, simple written and verbal instructions, and compliance with these instructions must be evaluated throughout the course of treatment. The drug is introduced at one-third to one-half the dose recommended for younger adults, and the dose increased by small amounts. A maintenance dose with minimal side-effects is then given, even if full resolution of the target symptom is not obtained. It is important to be aware of potential drug interactions, and to simplify the drug regimen as much as possible. The use of medication should not be avoided because of advanced age or diagnosis of dementia. If the patient does not respond to lower doses, and does not have side-effects at higher doses, dosages appropriate for younger adults may be used.

Treatment of behavioural disturbances

- Pharmacotherapy has been effective in treating several behavioural disturbances, including: agitation; delusions and hallucinations; depression; anxiety; sleep, appetite and sexual disturbances; and abnormal psychomotor activity.
- Specific medications and dosages employed are outlined in Tables 9.1 to 9.4.

The behavioural symptoms of Alzheimer's disease can be more disruptive than the cognitive symptoms. Treatment of the behavioural symptoms can improve the patient's quality of life, decrease caretaker burden and delay institutionalization (Swanwick, 1995). This section describes the behavioural symptoms of Alzheimer's disease, their possible aetiologies, and their treatment.

Agitation

Agitation is common in both home and institutional settings. Although there has been no consistent definition of agitation in the literature, a commonly used definition describes it as 'inappropriate verbal, vocal, or motor activity that is not explained by needs or confusion per se' (Cohen-Mansfield and Billig, 1986).

Agitation encompasses a number of behaviours, including physical or verbal aggression, restlessness, pacing, screaming or repeated requests (Deutsch and Rovner, 1991). Restraints are used in many settings to prevent harm to patients and caretakers and to enable the provision of care to patients. However, restrained patients often remain agitated, sustain falls, and have complications such as damage to skin, joints and bone, deconditioning, incontinence of urine and faeces, and faecal impaction. The use of restraints may even escalate agitation (Swanwick, 1995).

Nonpharmacological interventions should be considered before drug treatment. Adaptation of the environment to the patient's needs is essential (Winograd and Jarvik, 1986). Excessive visual and auditory stimuli should be eliminated, the patient should be allowed to have familiar items at hand, and a regular schedule should be maintained. The patient should have as much freedom as possible, with appropriate safeguards such as handrails or restriction within a safe perimeter. It is useful to reinforce positive behaviours verbally and to minimize negative behaviours with distractions such as music or other activities (Gerdner and Swanson, 1993). Catastrophic reactions, which are often associated with the early stages of dementia, respond to behavioural interventions. These reactions are acute episodes of agitation and dysphoria, which occur when patients cannot perform routine tasks. Catastrophic reactions are short lived and are precipitated by specific situations (Whitehouse and Geldmacher, 1994).

Treatment is guided by determination of the specific cause of agitation. First, delirium should be excluded. Next, specific causes for pain, such as decubiti, faecal impaction, or discomfort related to arthritis or other medical conditions, should be explored and alleviated. If perceptual disturbances, thought disorders or depression are present, medications can be prescribed accordingly.

There are few studies that specifically address the treatment of agitation in dementia patients, and in many reports it is not separated from other behavioural symptoms. The populations studied are often heterogeneous and include patients with dementia of aetiologies other than Alzheimer's disease, as well as other neurological disorders such as trauma. Patients studied

Table 9.1 Medications for agitation

Class	Agent	Usual daily dose (range), mg
Conventional antipsychotics	Haloperidol (Haldol)	1 (0.5–3)
	Fluphenazine (Prolixin)	1 (1–5)
	Thiothixene (Navane)	2 (1–10)
	Thioridazine (Mellaril)	25 (10–75)
	Risperidone (Risperdal)	1 (0.5–6)
Novel anti- psychotics	Clozapine (Clozaril)	50 (12.5–100)
	Olanzapine (Zyprexa)	10 (5–15)
Non-neuroleptics	Trazodone (Desyrel)	100 (100–400)
	Buspirone (Buspar)	15 (15–30)
	Carbamezapine (Tegretol)	400 (200–1200)
	Divalproex (Depakote)	425 (250–3000)
	Lithium (Eskalith)	900 (300–1200)
	Lorazepam (Ativan)	1 (0.5–6)

may include those with comorbid psychiatric disorders. Studies have used differing items on a variety of behavioural rating scales to quantify agitation (Risse and Barnes, 1986; Schneider, Pollock and Syness, 1990). Agents used to treat agitation in demented patients include antipsychotic agents, trazodone, benzodiazepines, anticonvulsants, propranolol, buspirone and lithium (Risse and Barnes, 1986; Steele, Lucas and Tune, 1986; Schneider et al., 1990; Cummings and Benson, 1992; Table 9.1).

Neuroleptics are consistently and moderately effective in controlling agitation in demented patients. However, no particular neuroleptic is more efficacious than another (Risse and Barnes, 1986; Schneider et al., 1990). The agitated behaviours that respond best to neuroleptics are excitement, hostility, belligerence and emotional lability. Neuroleptics alleviate other causes of agitation such as suspiciousness, hallucinations and insomnia, but are less effective in treating behaviours such as pacing and calling out. Decreased sociability, deficits in self-care, and indifference do not improve, and may be exacerbated due to sedation and lethargy (Risse and Barnes, 1986).

The choice of neuroleptic is determined by the side-effect profile and the patient's behavioural symptoms and medical condition. Low doses can be useful in con-trolling agitation with a lower incidence and severity of side-effects. The complete effect of neuroleptics may not be seen for one to two months after an appropriate dose is obtained (Zubenko et al., 1992). Patients should not be maintained on neuroleptics for unnecessarily long periods of time, as agitation occurs episodically. The patient's drug regimen should be periodically reviewed, and neuroleptics tapered and discontinued if agitation or other behavioural symptoms resolve (Risse and Barnes, 1986). Close monitoring and resumption of medication for symptom recurrence will reassure care-takers, who may be reluctant for medication to be discontinued.

Extrapyramidal symptoms that may occur as side-effects of neuroleptics include dystonia, parkinsonian symptoms and akathisia. Dystonia may manifest acutely as muscle spasm of the head, neck, tongue and eyes; dystonias of the trunk and lower extremities may affect gait. Younger patients are more likely to develop acute dystonias than elderly patients.

Parkinsonian symptoms include rigidity, tremor, shuffling gait and akinesia, e.g. difficulty initiating movement (Marder and Van Putten, 1995). Neuroleptic-induced parkinsonism is more common in elderly individuals and with the use of high-potency neuroleptics. Alzheimer's disease patients can be particularly susceptible to extrapyramidal symptoms (Reisberg et al., 1987). Parkinsonian side-effects may improve with reduction of the dose of neuroleptic or with an antiparkinsonian agent such as amantadine. Anticholinergic antiparkinsonian agents are not recommended in the elderly and are contraindicated in Alzheimer's disease.

Akathisia is an unpleasant subjective sensation of restlessness, which causes patients to pace or move their feet while sitting. Akathisia can cause anxiety or irritability (Marder and van Putten, 1995). It may respond to propranolol (Hyman, Arana and Rosenbaum, 1995; Wright and Cummings, 1996). When initiating and evaluating neuroleptic treatment, it is essential to differentiate between akathisia and increased agitation, and between akinesia and decreased cooperativeness; increasing the medication inappropriately can exacerbate these side-effects.

Tardive dyskinesia occurs in patients treated chronically with neuroleptics. Individuals with tardive dyskinesia manifest abnormal movements, including lip smacking or facial grimacing, as well as writhing movements of the trunk, fingers and toes. Elderly patients, especially elderly women, are more likely to develop tardive dyskinesia than younger patients. In addition, discontinuation of neuroleptics is less likely to resolve this problem in the elderly (Marder and van Putten, 1995).

Sedation is a commonly reported side-effect of neuroleptics. Orthostatic hypotension and anticholinergic effects (dry mouth, blurred vision, urinary retention, constipation) are also seen. Anticholinergic effects may interfere with cognition, but in the low doses used in elderly patients this may be avoided (Reisberg et al., 1987).

High-potency agents such as haloperidol, fluphenazine and thiothixene are associated with a low frequency of sedative, hypotensive and anticholinergic effects, and a high frequency of extrapyramidal symptoms. Low-potency neuroleptics such as thioridazine are more likely to have sedative, hypotensive and anticholinergic effects, and are less likely to cause extrapyramidal symptoms (Hyman et al., 1995). Risperidone, a newer neuroleptic, may cause postural hypotension and sedation, but does not have anticholinergic effects. It can cause extrapyramidal symptoms but is less likely than the low-potency agents to do so. Clozapine is an atypical antipsychotic that has the advantage of producing few extrapyramidal symptoms and little tardive dyskinesia. It is useful in patients who cannot tolerate other antipsychotics due to akathisia or parkinsonian symptoms. Side-effects include agranulocytosis (1 per cent), which requires weekly monitoring of white blood cells, seizures, postural hypotension, sedation and tachycardia. Clozapine has anticholinergic properties and may increase confusion at higher doses. Olanzapine, a recently introduced novel antipsychotic, has an effect profile similar to that of clozapine but does not cause agranulocytosis.

Medications that affect the serotonergic system have been found to be useful in the treatment of agitation of Alzheimer's disease. Trazodone blocks the reuptake of serotonin, and buspirone acts as a partial agonist of serotonin (Raskind, 1995). Uncontrolled studies have demonstrated that trazodone decreases agitation and aggressive behaviours in the absence of depression when neuroleptics have been unsuccessful (Raskind, 1995). The advantage of trazodone is its lack of induction of extrapyramidal symptoms. Side-effects include sedation, postural hypotension and priapism. Buspirone has also been anecdotally reported to diminish agitated behaviours, and it does not cause sedation or interfere with motor performance (Hyman et al., 1995).

Antimanic drugs such as carbamazepine and divalproex have been effective in the treatment of agitation, irritability and aggressive behaviours in bipolar patients (Essa, 1986; Risse and Barnes, 1986; Mazure, Druss and Cellar, 1992; Tariot et al., 1994; Raskind, 1995; Lott, McElroy and Keys, 1995). Lithium has been useful in the treatment of agitated symptoms in patients with neurological disorders and in Alzheimer's disease patients with comorbid psychiatric conditions (Risse and Barnes, 1986), but not in demented patients without comorbid psychiatric illness (Raskind, 1995). In the elderly, lithium may cause increased cognitive deficits and confusion, even at therapeutic levels. Lithium clearance decreases and its half-life may double due to decreased renal function in the elderly.

If agitation is related to anxiety, benzodiazepines may be useful, particularly a shorter-acting agent such as lorazepam, which depends minimally on hepatic metabolism. However, benzodiazepines may cause paradoxical agitation, and they are most useful in patients with rare episodes of agitation; they should not be used when continuous treatment is required. Buspirone is an alternative to benzodiazepines that may produce fewer mental status changes. Inderal may decrease agitation and assaultive behaviour in patients with neurological disease, but it has side-effects of bradycardia, hypotension, decreased cardiac output, and worsening of chronic pulmonary disease. It has also been reported to cause confusion, depression and sleep disturbances (Risse and Barnes, 1986).

Delusions and hallucinations

A delusion is a false, fixed belief that has no basis in reality and is not accepted by the patient's culture. A hallucination is a disturbance in perception that has no basis in external reality (Scheiber, 1988). Psychosis is a syndrome in which the main feature is the presence of prominent delusions or hallucinations (American Psychiatric Association, 1994).

In Alzheimer's disease, hallucinations occur less frequently than delusions (Wragg and Jeste, 1989). Patients may be aware that they are experiencing false perceptions, or may endorse the experience as real. A sudden onset of hallucinations may indicate delirium, and the patient should be evaluated medically (Cummings et al., 1987). The patient should also be assessed for sensory deficits, poor eyesight, or impaired hearing, which may cause hallucinations.

Ten to 73 per cent of Alzheimer's disease patients have delusions at some point during the illness (Wragg et al., 1989). Hallucinations or delusions were reported in one study by caregivers in approximately 50 per cent of patients (Rabins, Mace and Lucas, 1982). Persecutory delusions are the most frequent type of delusion: in a study of Alzheimer's disease patients, 30 per cent were found to have persecutory beliefs (Cummings et al., 1987). Alzheimer's disease patients may have different types of delusions: of theft; that their house is not their home; that they have been abandoned by their family; that a spouse or other family member is an imposter (Capgras syndrome); or that there is an unseen person living in their home (phantom boarder) (Reisberg et al., 1987; Cummings and Victoroff, 1990). There have also been reports of de Clerambault's syndrome (an untrue belief that the individual is involved in a romance, often with a person of higher social stature); 'picture sign' (the belief that individuals on television or in the newspaper are real); or parasitosis (a false belief of infestation) (Wright and Cummings, 1996).

A consistent relationship between the stage of Alzheimer's disease and the frequency of delusions has not been determined. Some studies state that delusions are more likely to occur in patients with more intact cognitive function (Wragg and Jeste, 1989). It has been postulated that cognitive function must be intact to some extent in order to maintain a delusion (Cummings et al., 1987). Several studies have noted that psychotic symptoms in Alzheimer's disease patients correlate with a more rapidly deteriorating course.

The pathophysiology of delusions in Alzheimer's disease has not been determined. Psychotic Alzheimer's disease patients have been found to have more intact noradrenergic systems, which may contribute to the development of psychosis (Zubenko et al., 1991). Cholinergic deficits may also have a role in the occurrence of delusions; delusions commonly occur with anticholinergic toxicity, and delusions in Alzheimer's disease may resolve with the administration of physostigmine (Cummings, Gorman and Shapira, 1993). Dysfunction of the limbic system is associated with delusions, and there is marked cholinergic deficiency in limbic structures (Cummings, 1985). Neuroleptics, which block dopamine function, and physostigmine, which enhances cholinergic function, both alleviate psychosis associated with Alzheimer's disease (Wright and Cummings, 1996).

Neuroimaging studies using computerized tomography have not demonstrated differences between delusional and nondelusional Alzheimer's disease patients. However, differences have been noted in EEG studies of Alzheimer's disease patients (Burns, Jacoby and Levy, 1990a; Lopez et al., 1992). One study demonstrated that delusional Alzheimer's disease patients more frequently have abnormal EEGs and increased delta and theta activity (Lopez et al., 1991).

As noted in the section above on agitation, delusions can contribute to other behavioural disturbances. These behavioural disturbances may result in management difficulties and in institutionalization of the Alzheimer's disease patient. Neuroleptics are effective treatment (see above).

Depression

The prevalence of major depressive episodes among patients with Alzheimer's disease ranges in frequency from 0 to 87 per cent, with most studies reporting that between 40 and 50 per cent of Alzheimer's disease patients have depressive symptoms (Wragg and Jeste, 1989). The variation in frequency may be related to the assessment of patients in different settings, the use of differing methods of reporting symptoms, and differing diagnostic criteria for Alzheimer's disease and for depression. Depressive symptoms are more common (40–50 per cent) than major depressive episodes (10–20 per cent) in Alzheimer's disease (Masterman et al.,

1995). Depressed mood is more frequent in Alzheimer's disease patients than in normal elderly populations (Wragg and Jeste, 1989).

Alzheimer's disease patients rarely meet all the criteria for major depression, and the presentation of depression may vary greatly in the Alzheimer's disease patient, ranging from agitation and psychosis to abulia and lethargy. Depressive symptoms such as sad affect and feelings of hopelessness and helplessness are common in Alzheimer's disease, and may be difficult for patients to express due to deficits in language (Whitehouse and Geldmacher, 1994). The diagnosis of a depressive syndrome is also difficult because neuro-vegetative symptoms of depression such as sleep, energy, appetite and sexual disturbance are behavioural symptoms shared with Alzheimer's disease (Mendez et al., 1990). Depressive symptoms may be related to alterations in dopaminergic, serotonergic and adrenergic neurotransmitter systems. Both the locus ceruleus and the raphe nuclei, which are sources of these neurotransmitters, are involved in Alzheimer's disease (Zubenko and Moossy, 1988; Mendez et al., 1990).

Depression in the Alzheimer's disease patient is treatable, and psychopharmacological interventions can improve the quality of life for both patients and their families. In a study of treatment with imipramine of Alzheimer's disease patients with and without depression, both groups improved from baseline depression scale scores (Reifler et al., 1989). Alzheimer's disease patients treated with 1-deprenyl demonstrated a small decrease in the Brief Psychiatric Rating Scale scores for anxiety/depression, physical tension and agitation, and a trend towards decreased anergia and hostility (Tariot et al., 1987).

The treatment of depression in the elderly includes selective serotonin reuptake inhibitors (SSRIs), tricyclic antidepressants (TCAs), monoamine oxidase inhibitors (MAOIs), and electroconvulsive therapy (ECT) (Table 9.2).

The SSRIs include fluoxetine, paroxetine and sertraline. Their efficacy has been demonstrated to be equivalent to that of the TCAs, and they induce less orthostatic hypotension and cardiotoxicity, and fewer anticholinergic side-effects. Possible side-effects include insomnia, agitation and weight loss (Salzman, Satlin and Burrows,

Table 9.2 Medications for depression

Agent	Usual daily dose (range), mg
Nortriptyline (Pamelor)	50 (50–100)
Desipramine (Norpramin)	50 (50–150)
Trazodone (Desyrel)	100 (100–400)
Fluoxetine (Prozac)	40 (20–80)
Sertraline (Zoloft)	50 (50–200)
Paroxetine (Paxil)	20 (10–50)
Venlafaxine (Effexor)	100 (50–300)
Nefazodone (Serzone)	400 (200–600)
Buspirone (Wellbutrin)	75 (150–300)

1995). Initiation of treatment with small doses and slowly increasing the daily dosage are recommended.

Tricyclic antidepressants have been useful in the improvement of neurovegetative symptoms, mood and function in daily activities in the elderly. Use of secondary amine tricyclics such as nortriptyline and desipramine is preferable to tertiary amine tricyclics, because they produce less severe side-effects (Salzman et al., 1995). Tertiary amine tricyclics have more potent interaction with alpha-adrenergic, histaminergic and muscarinic receptors and are more likely to cause postural hypotension, sedation and anticholinergic effects. Prior to the initiation of a TCA, a physical examination and electrocardiogram should be obtained. Initial doses of 10–25 mg qhs are recommended, with slow titration upwards, to maximize response and minimize side-effects.

Augmentation of antidepressant treatment or a combination of antidepressants may improve depressive symptoms in patients who do not improve after an adequate initial trial. Lithium, L-triiodothyronine, or another antidepressant may maximize response without the delay involved in changing the initial therapy (Hyman et al., 1995).

The dietary restrictions, possibility of drug interactions, and side-effect profile of MAOIs preclude their being the first-choice antidepressant treatment in Alzheimer's disease.

Electroconvulsive therapy is usually employed as a second-line treatment in the elderly if the patient has failed to respond to antidepressant medications or

Table 9.3 Medications for anxiety

Agent	Usual daily dose (range), mg
Lorazepam (Ativan)	1 (0.5–6)
Oxazepam (Serax)	30 (20–60)
Buspirone (Buspar)	30 (15–45)

Table 9.4 Medications for insomnia

Agent	Usual daily dose (range), mg
Trazadone (Desyrel)	100 (100–400)
Temazepam (Restoril)	15 (15–30)
Lorazepam (Ativan)	1 (0.2–4)
Nortriptyline (Pamelor)	25 (20–75)
Thioridazine (Mellaril)	25 (10–75)
Chloral hydrate (Webcon)	500 (500–1000)

cannot tolerate the side-effects of medication. ECT may be indicated as a first-line treatment if there is severe suicidality, malnutrition, or positive prior response to ECT. In the dementia patient, cognition does not deteriorate after ECT, and may even improve with the alleviation of depression. Temporary adverse effects on memory may be minimized by consideration of electrode placement, frequency of treatments and medications used during the course of ECT treatment (Pritchett, Kellner and Coffey, 1994).

Anxiety

Approximately 40 to 60 per cent of Alzheimer's disease patients experience anxiety. Anxiety regarding upcoming events is the most common symptom (Mendez et al., 1990). Benzodiazepines have been used to treat anxiety in the elderly, but they are most appropriately used to treat acute episodes of anxiety that have a specific precipitant (Table 9.3; Dubovsky, 1994). Patients with cognitive or psychomotor impairment do not tolerate these medications well. Elderly patients may experience sedation, ataxia, psychomotor slowing and cognitive impairment. Buspirone, a nonbenzodiazepine anxiolytic, has been used in anxiety disorders in the elderly as it is less likely to impair cognitive function. However, the onset of action is delayed and reports of efficacy in clinical and research experience are inconsistent (Dubovsky, 1994; Salzman et al., 1995).

Sleep, appetite and sexual disturbances

Disturbances of sleep and diurnal rhythm
Elderly individuals have less stage 3, stage 4 and REM sleep and more wakefulness than younger adults. These changes are exaggerated in Alzheimer's disease patients (Winograd and Jarvik, 1986; Deutsch and Rovner, 1991).

A study of 175 Alzheimer's disease patients reported insomnia in 45 per cent (Merriam et al., 1988). Caretakers in a study of 54 patients described night awakening in 37 patients; 59 per cent reported this as a severe problem (Rabins et al., 1982). Sleep disturbances such as frequent awakenings and difficulty falling asleep were reported in 45 per cent of a group of 126 Alzheimer's disease patients (Swearer et al., 1988). Diurnal rhythm disturbances were present in 14 of 57 Alzheimer's disease patients (Reisberg et al., 1987).

Pharmacotherapy may improve sleep disturbances (Table 9.4). Sedating antidepressants are useful in low doses, and intermediate or short-acting benzodiazepines may be used short term. Benzodiazepines must be used cautiously as they may cause confusion, depression, incontinence, decreased balance, increased cognitive impairment and paradoxical agitation. Low-dose chloral hydrate or low doses of sedating neuroleptics may be useful (Winograd and Jarvik, 1986; Wright and Cummings, 1996). The patient should be assessed for adverse medication effects or medical conditions such as sleep apnoea that may interfere with sleep. Adequate sleep hygiene includes reinforcement of a pattern of daytime activity and nocturnal sleep, avoidance of noise, light and extremes of temperature, and of alcohol (nightcaps) and caffeine (Swanwick, 1995).

Disturbances in eating behaviour
Alzheimer's disease patients often have alterations of appetite and eating. Changes in eating behaviours were reported in 60 per cent of 55 patients and were described as problematic by 55 per cent of the caregivers (Rabins et al., 1982). Forty-six per cent of 126 patients had altered eating behaviours (Swearer et al.,

1988), and 74 per cent of Alzheimer's disease patients in one study had either increased or decreased appetite (Merriam et al., 1988).

Disturbances in sexual activity

Most Alzheimer's disease patients demonstrate diminished interest in sexual activity, but some have periods of increased sexual activity. Sexual aggression is unusual in Alzheimer's disease patients; the behaviour may be alleviated in male patients with medroxyprogesterone administered intramuscularly (Cooper, 1987). Kluver-Bucy syndrome, which involves disturbed sexual behaviour as well as hyperorality, hypermetamorphosis, emotional placidity and agnosia, may occur in Alzheimer's disease patients.

Disturbances in psychomotor activity

An abnormal or inappropriate increase in motor or verbal behaviour can interfere with the care of the Alzheimer's disease patient. These behaviours include agitation, motor restlessness, purposeless fingering movements (carphologia), pacing or wandering. Psychomotor disturbances may occur in the absence of other neuropsychiatric disorders in Alzheimer's disease, and may not correlate with the severity of dementia (Cummings and Victoroff, 1990).

Motor restlessness has been observed in 21–60 per cent of Alzheimer's disease patients (Reisberg et al., 1987; Merriam et al., 1988; Teri, Larson and Reifler, 1988); wandering has been observed in 10–61 per cent (Merriam et al., 1988; Teri et al., 1988); and aggression or assaultiveness has been reported in 18–65 per cent (Rabins et al., 1982; Reisberg et al., 1987; Swearer et al., 1988). In addition to Alzheimer's disease, psychomotor disturbances may be caused by delirium, psychosis, mood disorders, systemic conditions, intoxications and sensory alterations. It is important to consider akathisia in patients on neuroleptic medications as a possible cause of psychomotor restlessness (Cummings and Victoroff, 1990).

Wandering is a potentially dangerous behaviour in both inpatient and community-dwelling Alzheimer's disease patients. Several wandering patterns have been described: exit seekers are trying to leave; self-

Table 9.5 Medications studied for amelioration of cognitive deficits or slowing of disease progression

Agent	Mechanism of action
Choline	Acetylcholine precursor
Phosphatidylcholine (lecithin)	Acetylcholine precursor
Bethanacol	Muscarinic receptor agonist
Physostigmine	Acetylcholinesterase inhibitor
Tacrine (Cognex)	Acetylcholinesterase inhibitor
Donepezil (Aricept)	Acetylcholinesterase inhibitor
L-deprenyl (Selegiline)	MAO-B inhibitor
Hydergine	Metabolic enhancer
Piracetam	Nootropic agent
Nerve growth factor	Maintenance of cholinergic systems
Nimodipine	Calcium channel blocker
Indomethacin	Anti-inflammatory agent

stimulators manipulate the door handle, but without the intention of leaving; akathisiacs exhibit restlessness, pacing and fidgeting; modellers follow others, and will leave the building in order to follow another person (Deutsch et al., 1991; Swanwick, 1995). Differing non-pharmacological treatments may be appropriate for each type: the exit seeker should be allowed to follow his or her plan until intervention is needed and, if possible, be allowed to return to the ward without correction or confrontation; the stimulator may be distracted with alternative tasks or with music. Other interventions include placing alarms on the patient or the doors and avoiding restraints (Swanwick, 1995).

Pharmacological management of cognitive deficits

- Three main approaches to treating cognitive impairments focus on cholinergic function, neuroprotective agents, or cerebral metabolism enhancers.
- Potential new treatments are directed towards the pathogenesis of Alzheimer's disease.

Pharmacological interventions can also target the aetiologies of cognitive disturbances in Alzheimer's disease (Table 9.5). Restitutive strategies address derangements of neurotransmitter systems. Neuroprotective agents may reduce oxidative metabolism, block calcium entry into cells, or inhibit the effects of excitatory amino acids. Antiamyloid agents have promise for interrupting the pathophysiological cascade of Alzheimer's disease (Schneider and Tariot, 1994; Salzman et al., 1995).

Cholinergic treatments

The cholinergic hypothesis posits that decreased cholinergic input to the cortex results in or contributes to the cognitive deficits associated with Alzheimer's disease. The hypothesis is supported by the severe cholinergic deficits in limbic and temporoparietal neocortical areas, and the ability of anticholinergic agents to interfere with cognition (Perry et al., 1978; Perry, 1986). In Alzheimer's disease, there is significant loss of cholinergic cell bodies in the nucleus basalis, and reduced activity of cerebral cortical choline acetyltransferase, which is necessary for acetylcholine synthesis (Schneider, 1993). The cholinergic deficit has been correlated with the degree of cognitive impairment in Alzheimer's disease (Perry et al., 1978), and improvement of cholinergic function has been a focus of treatment. The strategies employed include the administration of precursors, stimulation of muscarinic cholinergic receptors, enhancement of acetylcholine release, and inhibition of acetylcholinesterases that catabolize acetylcholine.

Acetylcholine precursors have been used to increase the synthesis of acetylcholine. Choline and phosphatidylcholine (lecithin) have been demonstrated to increase levels of acetylcholine in the brains of rats. In humans, the administration of choline increases choline levels in the blood and cerebrospinal fluid. However, acetylcholine precursors have not improved cognition in patients with Alzheimer's disease (Becker and Giacobini, 1988).

Muscarinic receptor agonists act through direct activation of postsynaptic cholinergic receptors; their use has been limited by side-effects on blood pressure, vision and salivation (Masterman et al., 1995). Intracranial infusion of the muscarinic agonist bethanacol resulted in improvements in behaviour and mood, and some studies showed benefits for cognition (Penn

et al., 1988; Read et al., 1990). Several muscarinic agonists have been developed or are under study.

Acetylcholinesterase inhibitors have been most widely used in the treatment of the cognitive deficits of Alzheimer's disease. Inhibition of acetylcholinesterase decreases the breakdown of acetylcholine and prolongs its action. Physostigmine, tacrine and donepezil are currently available cholinesterase inhibitors. Physostigmine is a reversible, short-acting (half-life of 30 minutes) cholinesterase inhibitor. Long-term trials of oral physostigmine have shown it to be moderately effective in improving memory (Becker and Giacobini, 1988; Stern, Sano and Mayeux, 1988).

Tacrine is a reversible anticholinesterase with a longer duration of action than physostigmine. It was approved by the United States Food and Drug Administration in 1993 for the palliative treatment of Alzheimer's disease. At high doses, it also has effects on sodium and potassium channels, muscarinic receptors, and monoamine metabolism and uptake (Davis and Powchik, 1995). It is quickly absorbed after oral administration and is cleared in the liver by first-pass metabolism (Schneider, 1993). The half-life of tacrine is 1.5 to 4 hours. There is substantial variation among individuals in its absorption, distribution and metabolism. The concentration of tacrine in the brain is ten times the plasma concentration (Schneider, 1993). Velnacrine is a metabolite of tacrine which is less potent in acetylcholinesterase inhibition and has less variability in pharmacokinetics (Schneider, 1993).

Clinical trials of tacrine used differing sample sizes and a variety of assessment scales, dosages and study designs, so that comparisons among studies are difficult (Schneider, 1993). An early trial of tacrine by Summers, Majovsky and Marsh (1986) demonstrated cognitive improvement on psychometric testing in 10 of 17 subjects, and subjective global improvement in 16 out of 17 subjects. A randomized, double-blind, placebo-controlled crossover study of tacrine plus lecithin demonstrated cognitive improvement at high tacrine doses (Eagger, Levy and Sahakian, 1991). Davis et al. (1992) selected patients who had an initial response to tacrine in order to identify those more likely to respond to later therapy with this drug. In a subsequent double-blind phase, these patients received placebo or the tacrine dose that they had responded to in the earlier phase. The patients on tacrine had a smaller decline in cognitive function, mainly in word recognition, during the period of treatment. Farlow et al. (1992) demonstrated that patients treated with tacrine performed significantly better than those on placebo on cognitive tests measuring word recall, naming of objects and fingers, language and word finding. The study was a double-blind, placebo-controlled, parallel-group study of 468 outpatients in 23 centres. In addition, clinician-rated and caregiver-rated scales of clinical global impression of change demonstrated significant dose-related improvement. Knapp et al. (1994) conducted a randomized, double-blind, placebo-controlled, parallel-group study of 663 patients at 33 centres; patients on 160 mg/day demonstrated statistically significant and clinically observed improvements on objective cognitive tests, clinician-rated and caregiver-rated global evaluations, and quality-of-life assessments. Patients on the 160 mg dose demonstrated a larger treatment effect than patients in previous studies at lower doses of tacrine.

Adverse effects of tacrine include nausea and vomiting, diarrhoea, dyspepsia and anorexia, which are dose dependent. Hepatotoxic effects occur in almost half of the patients, but no deaths have been associated with tacrine hepatotoxicity. Alanine aminotransferase (ALT) elevation is not accompanied by increased alkaline phosphatase or bilirubin, and is not dose related (Davis and Powchik, 1995). In clinical trials, 49 per cent of patients had one increased ALT measurement, 25 per cent had three times the normal ALT concentration, and 2 per cent had greater than 20 times normal concentration. Peak incidence of ALT elevation occurs between six and eight weeks of treatment with tacrine and 90 per cent of increased ALT levels occur by the twelfth week of treatment (Davis and Powchik, 1995).

After tacrine therapy has been initiated, ALT levels should be monitored every other week for 24 weeks. After any dose increase, the levels should be monitored every other week for at least six weeks. It is recommended that tacrine be discontinued if serum ALT is more than five times the upper limit of normal. Patients who have had elevations in serum ALT may be rechallenged with tacrine. In a study of 145 patients with ALT increases between three and ten times the upper normal limit, 127 patients were able successfully to resume tacrine. The mechanism of hepatic injury has been shown on biopsy to be direct injury to hepatic cells or immune-mediated injury (Watkins et al., 1994).

In order to be considered for tacrine treatment, the individual should have a diagnosis of Alzheimer's disease, normal baseline liver functions, and a reliable caregiver who will administer the medication and arrange the blood tests. The risk–benefit ratio should be considered in patients with asthma, renal disease, bradycardia, hypotension, sick sinus syndrome, epilepsy, or metabolic disorders. The initial dose is 40 mg/day, divided into four doses. The dose is increased to 80 mg/day after six weeks, to 120 mg/day after 12 weeks, and to 160 mg/day after 18 weeks. The ALT level should be measured before treatment begins and every other week for a minimum of six weeks after the last dose increase. It is monitored every three months when patients are on stable doses (Davis and Powchik, 1995). A predictor of response to tacrine treatment is adequate blood level.

Kaufer, Cummings and Christine (1996) conducted an open-label study to determine the effects of tacrine on behavioural symptoms in Alzheimer's disease patients. Behaviour significantly improved and the most responsive symptoms were anxiety, apathy, hallucinations, abnormal motor behaviours and disinhibition. The results were most apparent in patients with moderate dementia.

Donepezil (Aricept) is a reversible cholinesterase inhibitor recently approved by the Food and Drug Administration for the treatment of mild to moderate Alzheimer's disease. Its chemical structure differs from tacrine in that it does not include an acridine group, which has been associated with hepatotoxicity. Therapy is initiated at 5 mg at bedtime and may be increased to 10 mg after a four-week period, according to clinical judgement. It is given once a day, due to its long half-life of 70 hours (Doraiswamy, 1996). In a 30-week study, donepezil has been demonstrated to improve cognition and global functioning (Rogers et al., 1996).

The most common adverse effects of donepezil are nausea, diarrhoea and vomiting. These effects are usually mild and resolve as treatment continues. It has been reported anecdotally that patients who cannot tolerate the 10 mg dose are able to continue the medication at 5 mg. Monitoring of ALT and AST monitoring is not necessary. Due to its cholinergic effects, donepezil should be used with caution in patients with ulcer disease, on nonsteroidal anti-inflammatory agents, with asthma or bladder outflow difficulties, or on other cholinergic agents. At the present time, there have been no studies comparing the beneficial effects of tacrine and donepezil (Doraiswamy, 1996).

Metrifonate is another cholinesterase inhibitor currently in development. It has been used since 1962 as an antihelminthic. It is initiated with a loading dose and then a maintenance dose is used. Common side-effects are abdominal pain, diarrhoea, flatulence, nausea and leg cramps.

Neuroprotective treatments

The MAO-B inhibitor 1-deprenyl (selegiline) has been proposed as therapy for slowing the progression of the cognitive symptoms of Alzheimer's disease. The putative mechanism of action is inhibition of monoamine oxidase B, reduction in free radical generation, and preservation of neuronal membranes with enhancement of neuronal survival (Goad et al., 1991). Patients with mild Alzheimer's disease who were administered 1-deprenyl in a 15-month double-blind, placebo-controlled trial did not demonstrate slowed progression of the disease (Burke et al., 1993). In an open pilot study of 1-deprenyl in 14 Alzheimer's disease patients, statistically significant improvements in agitation and depression were noted on objective scales and in caregiver scales; recall was improved but verbal fluency decreased (Schneider, Pollock and Zemansky, 1991). In a single-blind study of eight Alzheimer's disease patients, there were clinically significant improvements in orientation, recall, caregiver stress, behaviours such as paranoid and delusional ideation, hallucinations, disturbed activity, anxiety and phobias (Goad et al., 1991). Additional studies of the efficacy of selegiline in Alzheimer's disease are underway, and other antioxidants such as vitamin E are also being investigated.

Enhancers of cerebral metabolism

Hydergine was the only medication approved by the Food and Drug Administration for Alzheimer's disease before tacrine. It is an ergoloid mesylate which was initially thought to be a cerebral vasodilator. The main mechanism of action is now considered to be metabolic enhancement as hydergine can improve neurotransmitter activity and neuronal metabolism. A double-blind, placebo-controlled study of 80 Alzheimer's disease patients for 24 weeks demonstrated no beneficial effects (Thompson et al., 1990). A meta-analysis of all studies concluded that the agent may produce mild beneficial effects (Schneider and Olin, 1994).

Nootropic agents enhance cerebral metabolism without any direct effect on neurotransmitters. Although they are derivatives of GABA, they have no effect on GABA receptors. They may reduce platelet activity and diminish red blood cell adherence to vessel walls, as well as enhance central cholinergic activity (Schneider and Tariot, 1994). Nootropic agents include piracetam, oxiracetam, pramiractam and aniracetam. Clinical investigations have not demonstrated significant effects in dementia (Vernon and Sorkin, 1991).

Research into treatments for cognitive symptoms

Potential new treatments are directed toward the pathogenesis of Alzheimer's disease. There is a relationship between β-amyloid deposition and neuronal death. It has been proposed that alterations in amyloid precursor metabolism promote the production and aggregation of β-amyloid. Neuronal cytoskeletal abnormalities result in synapse loss and neuronal degeneration. Future treatments could target proteinases that produce the β-amyloid protein or the assembly of β-amyloid into neurotoxic configurations (Cordell, 1994).

As noted above, Alzheimer's disease patients have cell degeneration and neuronal loss in the cholinergic system. Data suggest that nerve growth factor is necessary to maintain cholinergic systems, and preliminary animal studies have demonstrated that nerve growth factor administered intracerebrally is effective in decreasing lesion-induced cholinergic deficits and cognitive impairments. Nerve growth factor treatment has been studied in a small number of Alzheimer's disease patients (Lapchak, 1993; Olson, 1993; Hefti, 1994).

Calcium ion-activated cytotoxic mechanisms are

involved in the death of cholinergic cell bodies, and it has been suggested that a calcium-channel blocker such as nimodipine may be useful as palliative therapy in Alzheimer's disease (Branconnier et al., 1992).

Immune mechanisms in the pathogenesis of Alzheimer's disease have been explored. A large number of immune system proteins has been found to be associated with the characteristic Alzheimer's disease lesions. Increased levels of immunoglobulin receptors, complement receptors, major histocompatibility glycoproteins on reactive microglia, and increased number of cytokines have been found. Complement activation has been the most significant finding, but no agents have been found to intervene at this step (McGeer and Rogers, 1992). A double-blind placebo-controlled study of 44 Alzheimer's disease patients treated with indomethacin demonstrated improvement on cognitive testing, while patients receiving placebo showed a decline; however, over 20 per cent of patients on indomethacin had adverse effects, mainly gastrointestinal (Rogers et al., 1993).

Caregivers

Over the course of Alzheimer's disease, caregivers must cope with the patients' deterioration in cognition and changing behavioural symptoms. The burden of care of Alzheimer's disease patients is significant, and the needs of caretakers must be addressed. Cohen and Eisdorfer (1988) have found clinically significant depression in 55 per cent of caregivers of Alzheimer's disease patients. Caregivers also experience anxiety, anger and resentment, and their subjective sense of burden contributes significantly to the decision to place the patient in an institution (Brown, Potter and Foster, 1990). Family members can help alleviate the burden by assisting with caregiving activities: visiting the patient and caregiver, and staying with the patient so that the caregiver can engage in pleasurable activities. This assistance may improve the caregiver's ability to cope with the chronic stress of caring for the Alzheimer's disease patient (Scott, Roberto and Hutton, 1986).

Interventions to lessen caregiver distress include providing information about the illness and about caring for the dementia patient. Useful books include *The 36-Hour Day* (Mace and Rabins, 1991) and *Understanding Alzheimer's Disease* (Aronson, 1988). Information about techniques to improve patient safety and activities of daily living, as well as about respite services such as day care or home care is helpful. Counselling and support groups address issues such as coping with feelings of guilt, loneliness, inadequacy and anger, and with conflicting emotions regarding institutionalization; enabling caregivers to engage in activities for their own enjoyment; coping with conflicting roles and responsibilities; and developing a support system (Magai, Hartung and Cohen, 1995). Information regarding available resources can be obtained from the local chapter of the Alzheimer's Association.

A potential source of distress for the caregiver is an alteration in the sexual relationship. There may be no change in the patient, or decreased or increased libido may occur. The caregiver spouse may not wish to continue sexual activities, or may feel the loss of the sexual relationship. These problems should be explored with caregivers, with suggestions for redirecting undesired sexual attention or encouraging desirable affection (Cummings and Benson, 1992).

Legal assistance is usually necessary at some point during the course of a dementing illness. Counselling regarding financial planning, mental competence and conservatorship, and decisions concerning medical treatment may be needed. Advance planning to appoint a surrogate decision maker for economic and medical issues should occur early in the disease course (Overman and Stoudemire, 1988).

Conclusions

Alzheimer's disease will become an increasingly important medical problem, for as the population ages, the number of individuals in distress and the economic burden on society grow. The nature of the disease, with its diverse symptoms, its long duration and progressive deterioration, necessitates a multiplicity of treatments. In the elderly population it is necessary at the outset to define the differential diagnosis for any symptoms in order to determine if there is a treatable cause, to attempt nonpharmacological treatment in the first instance, and to use guidelines for pharmacological treatment as outlined in this chapter.

Research into the treatment of cognitive symptoms has addressed multiple possible mechanisms for the deficits of Alzheimer's disease. The anticholinesterase inhibitors have become a focus of treatment. Neuroprotective drugs, antiamyloid agents, nootropics, and neurotropic medications are under vigorous investigation. In the future, these agents may possibly be employed very early in the disease in order to ameliorate its devastating effects.

References

American Psychiatric Association 1994. *Diagnostic and Statistical Manual of Mental Disorders*, 4th edn. Washington, DC: American Psychiatric Press.

Aronson, M.K. ed. 1988. *Understanding Alzheimer's Disease.* New York: Charles Scribner's Sons.

Bachman, D.L., Wolf, P.A., Linn, R. et al. 1992. Prevalence of dementia and probable senile dementia of the Alzheimer type in the Framingham Study. *Neurology* **42**, 115–19.

Becker, R.E. and Giacobini, E. 1988. Mechanisms of cholinesterase inhibition in senile dementia of the Alzheimer's type: clinical, pharmacological and therapeutic aspects. *Drug Dev Res* **12**, 163–95.

Branconnier, R.J., Branconnier, M.E., Walsh, T.M. et al. 1992. Blocking the CA^{2+}-activated cytotoxic mechanisms of cholinergic neuronal death: a novel treatment strategy for Alzheimer's disease. *Psychopharmacol Bull* **28**, 175–81.

Brown, L.J., Potter, J.F. and Foster, B.G. 1990. Caregiver burden should be evaluated during geriatric assessment. *J Am Geriatr Soc* **38**, 455–60.

Burke, W.J., Roccaforte, W.H., Wengel, S.P. et al. 1993. L-deprenyl in the treatment of mild dementia of the Alzheimer's type: results of a 15-month trial. *J Am Geriatr Soc* **41**, 1219–25.

Burns, A., Jacoby, R. and Levy, R. 1990a. Psychiatric phenomena in Alzheimer's disease. I: Disorders of thought content. *Br J Psychiatry* **157**, 72–6.

Burns, A., Jacoby, R. and Levy, R. 1990b. Psychiatric phenomena in Alzheimer's disease. II: Disorders of perception. *Br J Psychiatry* **157**, 76–81.

Burns, A., Jacoby, R. and Levy, R. 1990c. Psychiatric phenomena in Alzheimer's disease. III: Disorders of mood. *Br J Psychiatry* **157**, 81–6.

Burns, A., Jacoby, R. and Levy, R. 1990d. Psychiatric phenomena in Alzheimer's disease. IV: Disorders of behaviour. *Br J Psychiatry* **157**, 86–94.

Cohen, D. and Eisdorfer, C. 1988. Depression in family members caring for a relative with Alzheimer's disease. *J Am Geriatr Soc* **36**, 885–9.

Cohen-Mansfield, J. and Billig, N. 1986. Agitated behaviors in the elderly. I. A conceptual review. *J Am Geriatr Soc* **34**, 711–21.

Cooper, A.J. 1987. Medroxyprogesterone acetate (MPA) treatment of sexual acting out in men suffering from dementia. *J Clin Psychiatry* **48**, 368–70.

Cordell, B. 1994. β-Amyloid formation as a potential therapeutic target for Alzheimer's disease. *Annu Rev Pharmacol Toxicol* **34**, 69–89.

Cummings, J.L. 1985. Organic delusion: phenomenology, anatomical correlations, and review. *Br J Psychiatry* **146**, 184–97.

Cummings, J.L. and Benson, D.F. 1992. *Dementia: a Clinical Approach*, 2nd edn. Boston: Butterworth–Heinemann.

Cummings, J.L., Gorman, D.G. and Shapira, J. 1993. Physostigmine ameliorates the delusions of Alzheimer's disease. *Biol Psychiatry* **33**, 536–41.

Cummings, J.L., Miller, B., Hill, M.A. et al. 1987. Neuropsychiatric aspects of multi-infarct dementia and dementia of the Alzheimer's type. *Arch Neurol* **44**, 389–93.

Cummings, J.L. and Victoroff, J.I. 1990. Noncognitive neuropsychiatric syndromes in Alzheimer's disease. *Neuropsychiatry Neuropsychol Behav Neurol* **3**, 140–58.

Davis, K.L. and Powchik, P. 1995. Tacrine. *Lancet* **345**, 625–30.

Davis, K.L., Thal, L.J., Gamzu, E.R. et al. 1992. A double-blind, placebo-controlled multicenter study of tacrine for Alzheimer's disease. *N Engl J Med* **327**, 1253–9.

Department of Health and Human Services 1990. *Healthy People 2000: National Health Promotion and Disease Prevention Objectives*. Washington, DC: Department of Health and Human Services.

Deutsch, L.H., Bylsma, F.W., Rovner, B.W. et al. 1991. Psychosis and physical aggression in probable Alzheimer's disease. *Am J Psychiatry* **148**, 1159–63.

Deutsch, L.H. and Rovner, B.W. 1991. Agitation and other noncognitive abnormalities in Alzheimer's disease. *Psychiatr Clin North Am* **14**, 341–51.

Doraiswamy, P.M. 1996. Current cholinergic therapy for symptoms of Alzheimer's disease. *Prim Psychiatry* November, 56–68.

Dubovsky, S.L. 1994. Geriatric neuropsychopharmacology. In *Textbook of Geriatric Neuropsychiatry*, ed. C.E. Coffey and J.L. Cummings, pp. 595–631. Washington, DC: American Psychiatric Press.

Eagger, S.A., Levy, R. and Sahakian, B.J. 1991. Tacrine in Alzheimer's disease. *Lancet* **337**, 989–92.

Essa, M. 1986. Carbamazepine in dementia. *J Clin Psychopharmacol* **6**, 234–6.

Evans, D.A., Funkenstein, J., Albert, M.S. et al. 1989. Prevalence of Alzheimer's disease in a community population of older persons. *JAMA* **262**, 2551–6.

Farlow, M., Gracon, S.I., Hershey, L.A. et al. 1992. Controlled trial of tacrine in Alzheimer's disease. *JAMA* **268**, 2523–9.

Gerdner, L.A. and Swanson, E.A. 1993. Effects of individualized music on confused and agitated elderly patients. *Arch Psychiatr Nurs* **7**, 284–91.

Goad, D.L., Davis, C.M., Leim, P. et al. 1991. The use of selegiline in Alzheimer's patients with behavior problems. *J Clin Psychiatry* **52**, 342–5.

Hay, J.W. and Ernst, R.L. 1987. The economic costs of Alzheimer's disease. *Am J Public Health* **77**, 1169–75.

Hefti, F. 1994. Development of effective therapy for Alzheimer's disease based on neurotrophic factors. *Neurobiol Aging* **15**, S193–4.

Hyman, S.E., Arana, G.W. and Rosenbaum, J.F. 1995. Antipsychotic drugs. In *Handbook of Psychiatric Drug Therapy*, pp. 5–42. Boston: Little, Brown and Company.

Kaufer, D.I., Cummings, J.L. and Christine, D. 1996. Effect of tacrine on behavioral symptoms in Alzheimer's disease: an open label study. *J Geriatr Psychiatry Neurol* **9**, 1–6.

Knapp, M.J., Knopman, D.S., Solomon, P.R. et al. 1994. A 30-week randomized controlled trial of high-dose tacrine in patients with Alzheimer's disease. *JAMA* **271**, 985–91.

Lapchak, P.A. 1993. Nerve growth factor pharmacology: application to the treatment of cholinergic neurodegeneration in Alzheimer's disease. *Exp Neurol* **124**, 16–20.

Lopez, O.L., Becker, J.T., Brenner, R.P. et al. 1991. Alzheimer's disease with delusions and hallucinations: neuropsychological and electroencephalographic correlates. *Neurology* **41**, 906–12.

Lopez, O.L., Becker, J.T., Rezek, D. et al. 1992. Neuropsychiatric correlates of cerebral white-matter radiolucencies in probable Alzheimer's disease. *Arch Neurol* **49**, 828–34.

Lott, A.D., McElroy, S.L. and Keys, M.A. 1995. Valproate in the treatment of behavioral agitation in elderly patients with dementia. *J Neuropsychiatry Clin Neurosci* **7**, 314–19.

Mace, N.L. and Rabins, P.V. 1991. *The 36-Hour Day: a Family Guide to Caring for Persons with Alzheimer's Disease, Related Dementing Illnesses, and Memory Loss in Later Life.* Baltimore: Johns Hopkins University Press.

Magai, C., Hartung, R. and Cohen, C.I. 1995. Caregiver distress and behavioral symptoms. In *Behavioral Complications in Alzheimer's Disease*, ed. B.A. Lawlor, pp. 223–43. Washington, DC: American Psychiatric Press.

Marder, S.R. and Van Putten, T.V. 1995. Antipsychotic medications. In *Textbook of Psychopharmacology*, ed. A.F. Schatzberg and C.B. Nemeroff, pp. 247–61. Washington, DC: American Psychiatric Press.

Masterman, D.L., Craig, A.H. and Cummings, J.L. 1995. Alzheimer's disease. In *Treatments of Psychiatric Disorders*, ed. G. Gabbard, pp. 479–513. Washington, DC: American Psychiatric Press.

Mazure, C.M., Druss, B.G. and Cellar, S.S. 1992. Valproate treatment of older psychiatric patients with organic mental syndromes and behavioral dyscontrol. *J Am Geriatr Soc* **40**, 914–16.

McKhann, G., Drachman, D., Folstein, M. et al. 1984. Clinical diagnosis of Alzheimer's disease: report of the NINCDS-ARDA Work Group, Department of Health and Human Services Task Force on Alzheimer's Disease. *Neurology.* **34**, 939–44.

McGeer, P.L. and Rogers, J. 1992. Anti-inflammatory agent as a therapeutic approach to Alzheimer's disease. *Neurology* **42**, 447–9.

Mega, M.S., Cummings, J.L., Fiorello, T. et al. 1996. The spectrum of behavioral changes in Alzheimer's disease. *Neurology* **46**, 130–5.

Mendez, M.F., Martin, R.J., Smyth, K.A. et al. 1990. Psychiatric symptoms associated with Alzheimer's disease. *J Neuropsychiatry Clin Neurosci* **2**, 28–33.

Merriam, A.E., Aronson, M.K., Gaston, P. et al. 1988. The psychiatric symptoms of Alzheimer's disease. *J Am Geriatr Soc* **36**, 7–12.

Miller, B.L., Chang, L., Oropilla, G. et al. 1994. Alzheimer's disease and frontal lobe dementias. In *Textbook of Geriatric Neuropsychiatry*, ed. C.E. Coffey and J.L. Cummings, pp. 390–404. Washington, DC: American Psychiatric Press.

Olson, L. 1993. NGF and the treatment of Alzheimer's disease. *Exp Neurol* **124**, 5–15.

Overman, W. Jr and Stoudemire, A. 1988. Guidelines for legal and financial counseling of Alzheimer's disease patients and their families. *Am J Psychiatry* **145**, 177–206.

Penn, R.D., Martin, E.M., Wilson, R.S. et al. 1988. Intraventricular bethanechol infusion for Alzheimer's disease: results of double-blind and escalating-dose trials. *Neurology* **38**, 219–22.

Perry, E.K. 1986. The cholinergic hypothesis – ten years on. *Br Med Bull* **42**, 63–9.

Perry, E., Tomlinson, B., Blessed, G. et al. 1978. Correlation of cholinergic abnormalities with senile plaques and mental test scores in senile dementia. *BMJ* **2**, 1457–9.

Pritchett, J.T., Kellner, C.H. and Coffey, C.E. 1994. Electroconvulsive therapy in geriatric neuropsychiatry. In *Textbook of Geriatric Neuropsychiatry*, ed. C.E. Coffey and J.L. Cummings, pp. 634–59. Washington, DC: American Psychiatric Press.

Rabins, P.V., Mace, N.L. and Lucas, M.J. 1982. The impact of dementia on the family. *JAMA* **248**, 333–5.

Raskind, M.A. 1995. Treatment of Alzheimer's disease and other dementias. In *American Psychiatric Association Textbook of Psychopharmacology*, ed. A.F. Schatzberg and C.B. Nemeroff, pp. 657–67. Washington, DC: American Psychiatric Press.

Read, S.L., Frazee, J., Shapira, J. et al. 1990. Intracerebroventricular bethanechol for Alzheimer's disease: variable dose-related responses. *Arch Neurol* **47**, 1025–30.

Reifler, B.V., Teri, L., Raskind, M. et al. 1989. Double-blind trial of imipramine in Alzheimer's disease patients with and without depression. *Am J Psychiatry* **146**, 45–4.

Reisberg, B., Borenstein, J., Salob, S.P. et al. 1987. Behavioral symptoms in Alzheimer's disease: phenomenology and treatment. *J Clin Psychiatry* **48**, 9–15.

Risse, S.C. and Barnes, R. 1986. Pharmacologic treatment of agitation associated with dementia. *J Am Geriatr Soc* **34**, 368–76.

Rogers, J., Kirby, L.C., Hempelman, S.R. et al. 1993. Clinical trial of indomethacin in Alzheimer's disease. *Neurology* **43**, 1609–11.

Rogers, S.L., Teaneck, N.J., Doody, R. et al. 1996. E2020 produces both clinical global and cognitive test improvement in patients with mild to moderately severe Alzheimer's disease: results of a 30-week phase III trial. *Neurology* **46**, A217.

Salzman, C., Satlin, A. and Burrows, A.B. 1995. Geriatric psychopharmacology. In *Textbook of Psychopharmacology*, ed. A.F. Schatzberg and C.B. Nemeroff, pp. 803–21. Washington, DC: American Psychiatric Press.

Scheiber, S.C. 1988. Psychiatric interview, psychiatric history, and mental status examination. In *Textbook of Psychiatry*, ed. J.A. Talbott, R.E. Hales and S.C. Yudofsky, pp. 163–94. Washington, DC: American Psychiatric Press.

Schneider, L.S. 1993. Clinical pharmacology of aminoacridines in Alzheimer's disease. *Neurology* **43**, S64–S79.

Schneider, L.S. and Olin, J.T. 1994. Overview of clinical trials of hydergine in dementia. *Arch Neurol* **51**, 787–98.

Schneider, L.S., Pollock, V.E. and Syness, S.A. 1990. A metaanalysis of controlled trial of neuroleptic treatment in dementia. *J Am Geriatr Soc* **38**, 553–63.

Schneider, L.S., Pollock, V.E. and Zemansky, M.F. 1991. A pilot study of low-dose 1-deprenyl in Alzheimer's disease. *J Geriatr Psychiatry Neurol* **4**, 143–8.

Schneider, L.S. and Tariot, P.N. 1994. Emerging drugs for Alzheimer's disease. *Med Clin North Am* **78**, 911–34.

Scott, J.P., Roberto, K.A. and Hutton, J.T. 1986. Families of Alzheimer's victims: family support to the caregivers. *J Am Geriatr Soc* **34**, 348–54.

Steel, C., Lucas, M.J. and Tune, L. 1986. Haloperidol versus thioridazine in the treatment of behavioral symptoms in senile dementia of the Alzheimer's type: preliminary findings. *J Clin Psychiatry* **47**, 310–12.

Stern, Y., Sano, M. and Mayeux, R. 1988. Long-term administration of oral physostigmine in Alzheimer's disease. *Neurology* **38**, 1837–41.

Summers, W.K., Majovski, L.V. and Marsh, G.M. 1986. Oral tetrahydroaminoacridine in long-term treatment of senile dementia, Alzheimer type. *N Engl J Med* **20**, 1241–5.

Swanwick, G.R. 1995. Nonpharmacological treatment of behavioral symptoms. In *Behavioral Complications in Alzheimer's Disease*, ed. B.A. Lawlor, pp. 183–207. Washington, DC: American Psychiatric Press.

Swearer, J.M., Drachman, D.A., O'Donnell, B.F. et al. 1988. Troublesome and disruptive behaviors in dementia. *J Am Geriatr Soc* **36**, 784–90.

Tariot, P.N., Cohen, R.M., Sunderland, T. et al. 1987. L-deprenyl in Alzheimer's disease: preliminary evidence for behavioral change with monoamine oxidase B inhibition. *Arch Gen Psychiatry* **44**, 427–33.

Tariot, P.N., Erb, R., Leibovici, A. et al. 1994. Carbamazepine treatment of agitation on nursing home patients with dementia: a preliminary study. *J Am Geriatr Soc* **42**, 1160–6.

Teri, L., Larson, E.G. and Reifler, B.V. 1988. Behavioral disturbance in dementia of the Alzheimer type. *J Am Geriatr Soc* **36**, 1–6.

Thompson, T.L., Filley, C.M., Mitchell, W.D. et al. 1990. Lack of efficacy of hydergine in patients with Alzheimer's disease. *N Engl J Med* **323**, 445–8.

Vernon, M.W. and Sorkin, E.M. 1991. Piracetam: an overview of its pharmacological properties and a review of its therapeutic use in senile cognitive disorders. *Drugs Aging* **1**, 17–35.

Watkins, P.B., Zimmerman, H.J., Knapp, M.J. et al. 1994. Hepatotoxic effects of tacrine administration in patients with Alzheimer's disease. *JAMA* **271**, 992–8.

Whitehouse, P.J. and Geldmacher, D.S. 1994. Pharmacotherapy for Alzheimer's disease. *Clin Geriatr Med* **10**, 339–50.

Winograd, C.H. and Jarvik, L.F. 1986. Physician management of the demented patient. *J Am Geriatr Soc* **34**, 295–308.

World Health Organization 1992. *World Health Statistics: Demographic Trends, Ageing and Noncommunicable Disease.* Geneva: World Health Organization.

Wragg, R.E. and Jeste, D.V. 1989. Overview of depression and psychosis in Alzheimer's disease. *Am J Psychiatry* **146**, 577–87.

Wright, M.T. and Cummings, J.L. 1996. Neuropsychiatric disturbances in Alzheimer's disease and other dementias: recognition and management. *Neurologist* **2**, 207–18.

Zubenko, G.S. and Moossy, J. 1988. Major depression in primary dementia. *Arch Neurol* **45**, 1182–6.

Zubenko, G.S., Moossy, J., Martinez, J. et al. 1991. Neuropathologic and neurochemical correlates of psychosis in primary dementia. *Arch Neurol* **48**, 619–24.

Zubenko, G.S., Rosen, J., Sweet, R.A. et al. 1992. Impact of psychiatric hospitalization on behavioral complications of Alzheimer's disease. *Am J Psychiatry* **149**, 1484–91.

PART III

Clinical and management issues

Introduction

Donald T. Stuss

This section contains chapters which are essential to the success of an overall cognitive rehabilitation approach, apart from the actual neurorehabilitation techniques.

The first two chapters deal with the structure, organization and functioning of rehabilitation programmes. Each provides different lessons to the reader. Both chapters emphasize the importance of all team members having a similar knowledge base and conceptual approach. Mills and Alexander emphasize principles for the administration of a successful cognitive rehabilitation programme. All of the health care professionals involved in the programme for a particular disorder should be aware of the pathophysiology of the disorder and the normal recovery course. That is, rehabilitation must take place in a context of accurate diagnosis, and informed prognosis. Mills and Alexander deliver very important messages: (1) many factors affect successful rehabilitation, and (2) various factors may be relevant at different stages in recovery. This knowledge will influence *what* type of rehabilitation should be given *when*. A case study illustrates these principles. The Mills and Alexander chapter also has practical advice on the continuum of care, programme development and management, and daily operations that will be relevant to the manager of rehabilitation systems.

Christensen and Caetano's description of a rehabilitation day programme for postacute brain-injured patients complements the Mills and Alexander chapter. Their emphasis is more on the conceptual approach to a programme. Their rehabilitation philosophy is holistic, based on Goldstein's ideas that the injured person must be considered as a 'new organism'. The alteration into this new organism is based on the new challenges that the individual must meet, using the altered abilities which are a result of the trauma. Luria's neuropsychological qualitative approach in assessment and treatment provides the methods to ascertain which abilities are available to meet these challenges. What the clinician will appreciate in Christensen and Caetano's chapter is an example of how the programme at the Center for Rehabilitation of Brain Injury is set up.

A major challenge in rehabilitation is the assessment of outcome, because this provides evidence as to what should be rehabilitated as well as to the success of the implemented interventions. The next two chapters address outcome measurement, albeit from very different perspectives. Lincoln uses the World Health Organization framework to indicate what outcomes should be measured: impairment, disability and handicap. Examples of each are provided. The practicality of this chapter is notable, with a review of concepts of validity, reliability, and sensitivity in selecting measurement tools. The real practical advice is the emphasis on practicality itself. The outcome tool is not relevant if its usage is not practical. Interestingly, for a book on 'cognitive' rehabilitation, Lincoln notes that meaningful measures of cognitive disability need to be developed. It is insufficient to note that a patient has a memory loss, for example. The behavioural consequences of the impairment should be operationally and precisely quantified. It is hoped that this challenge will be met by some of the readers of this book.

In Uswatte and Taub's chapter on outcome measurement, we are presented with a model from the domain of physical rehabilitation of how to transfer laboratory findings to the real world. Every rehabilitation clinician has seen this anomaly – a level of recovery of function has been achieved, but somehow this is not adapted to real life. This chapter remarkably illustrates how basic science, in this case animal research on the recovery of motor function, has a significant payoff for human clinical problems. What is reassuring to the clinician is that successful behavioural rehabilitation might be reflected in cortical reorganization, and that together these markers for success might be used to accelerate our knowledge of rehabilitation outcome.

The next two chapters deal with various aspects of mood, motivation, awareness and overt responsiveness. This is such an important but complicated clinical and management issue in cognitive rehabilitation that two somewhat different views on the topic are presented. Feinstein is a practising clinical/research neuropsychiatrist who addresses the effects of mood, affect and motivation on the rehabilitative process. His neuropsychiatric approach uses neuroanatomy as a framework. The effects of the presence and treatment of depression, bipolar affective disorder, pathological laughing and crying, and anxiety are discussed. Special emphasis is given to apathy, which is considered here as an independent disorder of motivation which affects rehabilitation.

Prigatano's chapter starts with an interesting historical context, relating that Lashley and Luria, two prominent neuroscientists, were concerned with the issue of motivational problems in rehabiitation. Prigatano presents a practical approach, emphasizing the importance of the patient becoming actively involved in rehabilitation, with the goal of gaining awareness of deficits and their consequences. Several important factors are addressed: the relationship between aware-

ness and motivation; the relation of denial of illness and awareness; and the maintenance of the appropriate level of motivation for the individual patient. Prigatano's emphasis on the importance of psychotherapy in rehabilitation returns to one of the major themes in this volume – the importance of a multifaceted approach which deals with specific programmes to maximize rehabilitative efforts.

The final chapter in this section, by Proulx, addresses the importance of the family. The chapter is a fitting 'wrap-up' to the section because it continues and expands many of the themes of the earlier chapters. It is an extension of dealing with the whole person in his or her new context. After neurological injury, the patient's family represents both an old and a new context. The rehabilitative efforts can be maximized by understanding the new family dynamics and recruiting the goodwill of the family to assist in treatment.

The complexity of rehabilitative efforts is one lesson of this section. Multiple factors must be considered: management and organizational issues; the conceptual bases of the developed approaches; the importance of and difficulties in measuring outcome; the measurement of real-life outcome; the influence of likely comorbid factors such as changes in mood, lack of insight and awareness of the deficits; and the affective motivation that might be impaired for different reasons. In cognitive rehabilitation, it is inadequate to deal just with a cognitive deficit, even when we can precisely specify it. The rehabilitation of the neurologically impaired patient requires an organized, conceptually solid, team effort, and this team must have knowledge and awareness of the multiple factors that may impede the rehabilitation efforts.

10

Cognitive rehabilitation: leadership and management of the clinical programme

Virginia M. Mills and Michael P. Alexander

Introduction

In an ideal world, the finest neurorehabilitation programmes would integrate the most up-to-date knowledge and research findings about patients' illnesses into the design and operations of their clinical programming. In the real world, most cognitive rehabilitation programmes do not operate by this principle. Cognitive models for cognitive rehabilitation programmes are too often based on assessment and treatment of only the surface manifestations of diseases. The team's approach to treatment is fragmented, and discipline oriented. Many team members have only partial knowledge about the patient's illness and are not familiar with the natural history of the disorder under consideration.

In addition to the incorporation of substantial clinical knowledge, effective clinical programmes should also be consumer oriented in all of their operations, not bound by traditional expectations of treatment disciplines, with managers and leaders who facilitate change and regularly improve the programme's operations. Unfortunately, this commonsense management approach is not regularly practised in neurorehabilitation programmes and many hospital systems.

This chapter offers the authors' view of the critical factors for the develoment and implementation of effective and dynamic neurorehabilitation programmes. The focus is on cognitive rehabilitation, and it is hoped that this outline could serve as a guide to those interested in the administration of these programmes.

In the past few decades, survival rates have dramatically risen for people with catastrophic illness and injury because of advances made in life support and medical management. The number of people with chronic illness and disability is increasing rather than decreasing as we save more lives. Chronic neurological illness produces a large number of people with chronic disability due to cognitive and behavioural impairments. The incidence of traumatic brain injury in the USA is 200/100 000, or about 500 000 new cases per year, establishing it as one of the most serious brain disorders, especially of people under the age of 40 (Kurtzke and Kurland, 1987). Twenty per cent of the 500 000 cases are moderate to severe injuries, leaving these people with many types of impairments but especially impairment in the cognitive domain (Kraus, 1987). Stroke is the third leading cause of death in the USA and the leading cause of rehabilitation hospitalization. Twenty-five per cent of stroke survivors are under the age of 65 and, therefore, stroke is a major cause of lost productivity (Adams and Victor, 1993). People who survive encephalitis or anoxic–hypotensive brain injury make up a much smaller population than those suffering traumatic brain injury or stroke, but often these illnesses result in significant disability with lasting cognitive and behavioural deficits (Hanley, Johnson and Whitley, 1987; Grosswasser, Hohen and Costeff, 1989; Wilson, 1996). The nondegenerative neurological diseases together make up a significant percentage of people in our society who have permanent handicap and disability from their cognitive and behavioural impairments.

Cognitive rehabilitation programmes in the USA were primarily developed for people surviving traumatic brain injury but, over time, other neurological diagnoses (e.g. anoxic–hypoxic brain injury, encephalitis, stroke, postbrain tumour resection) have found their way to these treatment programmes. Cognitive rehabilitation bases its treatment on the presumption that improvement in a cognitive process, skill or functional ability leads to less disability and less handicap. Dr Howard Rusk noted in 1972 that as we add years to peoples' lives, it is our responsibility to add life to their years (Rusk, 1972). Cognitive rehabilitation programmes presume that focused cognitive treatment lessens handicaps caused by cognitive and behavioural impairments.

This chapter reviews some of the principles and assumptions on which to base the administration of a cognitive rehabilitation programme in the areas of: (1) the clinical model, (2) the treatment team, (3) continuum of care, (4) programme development, (5) the leadership and management team, and (6) daily operations. Neurological diseases, as a group, are a leading cause of disability and handicap. Cognitive impairments are frequently the major cause of disability even after excluding patients with dementia of Alzheimer's type.

The clinical model

- If the treatment team does not understand the pathophysiology of symptoms and signs of a given neurological disorder and does not know the natural history of both the disease and the impairments, proper management is impossible, even if the patient happens to improve.

In order to design efficacious treatment models for patients with cognitive problems, it is imperative that clinicians appreciate how the disorder disrupts normal brain function. An understanding of the pathophysiology and natural history of recovery of the common neurological disorders is essential for their appropriate evaluation, proper prognostication and judicious treatment. Despite some similar clinical manifestations, such as not remembering to carry out an activity in the future, neurological illnesses can have diverse patterns of damage to the central nervous system that have vastly different ramifications for rehabilitation. It is beyond the scope of this chapter to review these disorders, and the reader is referred to other chapters in this book and to other texts to learn about the common

neurological diseases suffered by patients undergoing rehabilitation, their pathophysiology, natural history and anticipated outcomes (Mills, Cassidy and Katz, 1997).

It is, however, within the purview of this chapter to review the principles of clinical thinking required for a well-designed neurorehabilitation programme. These principles have been defined in the neurological model of rehabilitation.

The neurological model of rehabilitation

- The pathophysiology of impairments and disabilities determines, in large part, the course of improvement and the probability of a good outcome. Diagnosis in rehabilitation is not just a list of functional impairments. It is, at best, an attempt at accounting for the mechanism, anticipating the prospects and course of recovery, and describing the residual deficits of that recovered patient.

The neurological model of rehabilitation is predicated upon two important constructs: diagnosis and prognosis. In this context, a meaningful diagnosis does not mean simply identification of the brain disease. We take it as a given that rehabilitation efforts are probably misplaced if the underlying disease is unspecified. In the context of rehabilitation, diagnosis must also extend beyond labelling impairments (e.g. poor memory). Rehabilitation diagnosis should specify how the disease disrupted normal brain functioning, how the disruption has produced disability, and the medical and functional prognosis. Thus, it promotes an understanding of a patient's impairments in the context of a particular neuropathological syndrome and integrates the effects of other factors, such as age, premorbid capacity and comorbid conditions, that interact with the central nervous system insult to produce a particular clinical profile in a given individual. This process also permits more meaningful differential diagnosis to distinguish between which problems are directly attributable to the illness or injury and which are not (Mills et al., 1997).

Not all stroke patients are 'left hemi' or 'right hemi'. Not all 'hemis' are the same or accompanied by the same deficits. Even if the 'hemi' parts of patients' disabilities are equivalent, one may be young, the other old; one may be fit, the other deconditioned; one may have neuropathy, the other not; one may have had an initial lacune, the other a fifth or sixth lacune with balance, gait and cognitive problems only emerging as a consequence of the last infarction. Accounting for deficits is the role of diagnosis. Prognosis takes the diagnostic information, viewed within the framework of natural history, and estimates an anticipated recovery profile for the patient. It also describes the trajectory of recovery, identifying the patient's current location on the recovery curve to estimate the improvement and progress yet to be seen. Thus, the observed impairments become understood in the context of a dynamic process, not simply as a static functional independence measure score. It must be apparent, however, that the confidence placed in the delineation of a patient's prognosis is dependent on the accuracy of the initial diagnosis and the time postinjury that the assessment is made. For some types of brain injury, direct diagnosis is difficult and information about the event or disease process causing the insult becomes of paramount importance. If this information is unavailable or is distorted, then diagnostic reliability greatly suffers, accurate prognostication becomes nearly impossible, and rehabilitation goals may be misguided (Mills et al., 1997).

For rehabilitation patients, it is essential to relate prognosis to functional outcome. By that we mean: what is that patient going to be able to do, and when? Will he or she be independent? If so, in what setting and with what kind of support? Conclusive projection of recovery beyond the short term may be limited early in the rehabilitation course. As time passes and patterns of recovery develop, plotting trajectory and prognosis becomes more meaningful and reliable.

This model does not maintain that all recovery is biologically driven. Rather, it accepts that recovery is guided by a complex interaction of biological and other factors including new learning, directed treatment, compensatory strategies, constitutional diatheses and premorbid personality. The relative influence of each of these factors changes with time; the biological factors are most significant early in the course of recovery but wane with time, as psychosocial and learning influences wax in importance. Thus, it becomes clear that early in the course of injury or illness, when biological influences predominate, rehabilitative interventions may have little, if any, direct influence on cognitive recovery. As time progresses and the dominance of biological processes diminishes, directed, restorative treatment can influence the outcome of deficits that are known to be responsive to therapy. Finally, the natural history of the disorder dictates when deficits become relatively fixed, and the practical benefits of therapy directed at remediation plateau. Therapy directed at teaching patients compensatory strategies for impairments is not limited to the natural recovery period and can be of value many years after the illness. Thus, the neurological model of rehabilitation should identify impairments likely to improve spontaneously, regardless of treatment, impairments that can benefit from directed treatment and the optimal timing of those treatments, and impairments that are fixed and, therefore, unresponsive to restorative therapeutic interventions, despite continued deficits (Mills et al., 1997).

Traditional rehabilitation approaches

- The neurological model of rehabilitation proposes fundamental changes to current practice that centre on how the natural history of a disorder or of the disease process dictates treatment.

The neurological model differs in several respects from models of assessment and treatment of the neurological patient that have traditionally been used in clinical rehabilitation. Rehabilitation diagnoses are usually limited to an aetiological diagnostic label plus some clinical consequences, for example 'stroke with right hemiparesis'. Other medical diagnoses may be listed. The assessments distinguish impairments, disabilities and handicaps, but the assessments for impairments and disabilities may be little more than lists of symptoms and signs without attention to how these problems relate to the underlying brain disorder or to where they occur within the recovery process. For instance, when clinicians encounter patients with memory problems, they may perform an evaluation, develop a treatment plan and set goals using clinical experience. Treatment choices are empiric and based on the observable impairments seen in the patient during the consultation (e.g. the patient cannot recall the therapist's name and previous treatments). This approach may be adequate in many situations. It may be insufficient in one of two manners: (1) failure to determine the pathophysiological mechanism of the deficit: impaired attention, arousal, motivation or mood, might masquerade as impaired memory; and (2) failure to consider the natural history of the underlying neurological condition: rapid improvement without treatment might be anticipated (Mills et al., 1997).

In conclusion, the neurological model of rehabilitation proposes fundamental changes to current rehabilitative practice – changes that centre on how the natural history of a disorder or of the disease process dictates treatment.

The team

- The clinical leaders of rehabilitation teams have two major responsibilities: (1) they must ensure that all team members understand the deficit profile within the larger picture of the patient's diagnosis and prognosis; and (2) they must monitor the implementation of the key interventions of the team whatever the discipline-specific goals might be.
- Every member of the team will need training in four areas for the team to function effectively. These areas are: (1) education about the neurological diseases the clinicians will treat; (2) development of treatment plans and goals for patients with complex cognitive problems; (3) development of an appreciation of the treatment possibilities downstream from the clinician's particular epoch of care; and (4) development and use of assessment systems and treatment approaches that are in accord with the fiscal realities of the organization.

Central to rehabilitation tradition is the team approach. Assessment and treatment planning emerge from the combined approach of all the members of the team. Each discipline brings a particular assessment focus and treatment tradition and the overall plan may be more or less shared (interdisciplinary). This approach to assessment presumes that diagnosis is the 'sum of the parts' and that overall treatment will inevi-

tably be appropriate if it is directed towards all discovered impairments. Being cared for by six people who do not understand a disease and its course hardly makes the patient six times as well off as having a single clinician who does not understand the disease. The neurological model presented here takes exception to this assumption.

Not all individual assessments may be essential or appropriate for all disorders or at all times postonset. The larger picture of neurological diagnosis and natural history should guide individual assessments. For instance, patients who are still in a confusional state after traumatic brain injury should not have elaborate neuropsychological evaluations or language assessment batteries. Although data can be gathered and impairments demonstrated, little can be learned in addition to what was already known, i.e. the patient is still in a confusional state. These efforts will have been redundant, and improvident, and irrelevant to the inevitable improvement (Mills et al., 1997).

The clinical leaders of rehabilitation teams have two major responsibilities: (1) they must ensure that all team members understand the deficit profile within the larger picture of the patient's diagnosis and prognosis then, (2) they must monitor the implementation of the key interventions of the team whatever discipline-specific goals they might have.

For example, if a patient has impaired memory and organizational ability, various team members might be required to define the problem (neurologist, speech–language pathologist or neuropsychologist) and identify an effective way for all team members to communicate with the patient. Establishing the underlying mechanism (confusion? amnesia? frontal? aphasia? mixture?) and prognosis would shape the goals of the intervention. If independent use of a time planner becomes a critical goal, every team member must be made familiar with the type of time planner chosen for the patient and the strategies used to train the patient to use the time planner. It would not be the responsibility of one discipline to complete this goal, although one discipline might create the intervention. Pinpointing such critical goals, as opposed to focused, discipline-specific goals, and ensuring that all team members address them require strong leadership.

Every member of the team will need training in four areas for the team to function effectively. First, many clinicians are not extensively educated about the neurological diseases that they will treat and are not knowledgeable about the prognosis of the impairments that those diseases produce. This is particularly true for cognitive impairments. Training programmes in physical therapy, occupational therapy and speech–language pathology often emphasize the assessment of impairments and the development of treatment plans, with little appreciation for the common evolution of these impairments, treated or not. Clinicians will sometimes establish a plan to treat impairments that are fundamentally untreatable or invariably transient even if untreated. Team members need continued training regarding the common diagnostic groups and the treatment approaches that work most effectively for those patients. Experts in the various diagnostic groups should conduct this training. Experience is essential, but it is not an adequate substitute for knowledge about the pathophysiology of impairment and of recovery. Too much education in rehabilitation is within disciplines and not across disciplines, and the teacher is distinguished from the student only by a number of years of experience.

Second, patients with complex cognitive problems will often make many members of a rehabilitation team uncomfortable because of coexisting behavioural problems, concerns that the problems are 'untreatable' or that patients with cognitive problems are at high risk of not being discharged home. Assuming the care of patients with difficult cognitive issues will require all members to shed preconceived notions about the criteria of a 'good candidate' for rehabilitation. Management of these patients may demand the development of new types of services to prepare for safe discharge or home supervision. Family education may be increasingly complex and time consuming. Familiar, predictable physical rehabilitation goals may be largely irrelevant in predicting or preparing a patient for home discharge. In the past, admission committees preferred to recommend rehabilitation for patients who were likely to have a good outcome, determining that other patients with more complex needs were inappropriate for rehabilitation admission. None of the complexities of cognitive

remediation is an adequate excuse for failure to serve these patients if an appropriate treatment team can be assembled. No discipline or admission committee should be empowered to prevent admission to rehabilitation or to accelerate discharge because cognitive impairments and goals make them uncomfortable.

Third, cognitive difficulties often extend far beyond inpatient rehabilitation. All clinicians treating patients with cognitive problems should have an appreciation of the treatment possibilities downstream from their particular epoch of care. All hospital or clinic-based clinicians should appreciate the methods of generalization of new skills learned from the hospital or outpatient setting to the patient's own living environments. This assures a lasting functional outcome. Education of family members and significant others who will be living with the patient is only one essential aspect of this long-term approach.

Fourth, the team's assessment systems and treatment approaches must be in accord with the fiscal realities of the organization. What rehabilitation member ever wanted to provide less for a patient? The best clinical programme in the world will not survive if it is not financially stable. Clinical teams must be given appropriate financial information to allow them to design and implement programmes which will best suit patient needs and allow for the viability of the organization.

Case study

The following case study illustrates the use of the neurological rehabilitation model by a well-functioning team to teach a patient with neurological impairments the use of memory and organizational aids (Gillespie and Kixmiller, 1997).

Traumatic brain injury: patient G.L.

Assessment

G.L. is a 36-year-old, right-handed female and single parent who, before her injury, was working part time as a waitress. She was very active in her community and she had many friends. G.L. was involved in a motor vehicle accident and sustained a severe traumatic brain injury. Her initial Glasgow Coma Scale (GCS) score was 4 to 5 and she had a four-week coma and three and a half-month posttraumatic amnesia. Her head computed tomography (CT) scan also showed a left temporal contusion and scattered petechial haemorrhages. Her initial GCS, long coma and posttraumatic amnesia were clinical symptoms of her severe diffuse axonal injury. In addition, her head CT showed she had a focal injury to part of the brain involved in memory. Given her injury profile, her rehabilitation neurologist anticipated that G.L. would have permanent memory deficits. This prognosis guided the rehabilitation team's goals and treatment plans in both the hospital and outpatient settings during the times G.L. received treatment over a two-year period. Recovery from her focal injury would be anticipated to occur over a six-month period, whereas recovery from her diffuse axonal injury would occur over one to three years.

Following her four-month inpatient rehabilitation programme, G.L. had some insight into her memory impairments and showed good progress in her cognitive functioning. Consistent with this injury profile and history of recovery, neuropsychological testing conducted at one year postinjury indicated that G.L. was completely amnesic for verbal and visual information that had been encoded 30 minutes earlier. Consequently, her prospective memory was very poor. Procedural and skill learning was average and she had good attention and short-term memory. Executive (frontal) processes were generally intact as well. G.L. was frustrated with her memory deficits and showed some reactive depression.

During her second year of recovery, she enrolled in a postacute rehabilitation programme to which she was referred by her neurologist. The results of neuropsychological testing and a functional assessment indicated the severity of her amnesia would be the largest impairment to her independent daily functioning. G.L. was motivated to address memory issues given that she had some insight into her memory deficits. Therefore, compensation for this impairment became the predominant focus of the postacute programme.

The speech evaluation performed in the postacute programme noted that G.L.'s spoken and written language and comprehension were intact for all her functional needs in the community. The functional evaluation, conducted in the patient's home, indicated that while G.L. was familiar with various community resources, she was not using them. She was unable to carry out multistep plans. She could not accurately write down a short message given over the telephone or remember the information on her own when she finished the telephone call. She required moderate verbal cues and assistance to outline a daily schedule and to schedule new appointments. She could not manage her financial affairs, failing to remember which bills she had paid and on several occasionals paying a bill twice. G.L. needed almost constant reminders and prompts to engage in any kind of leisure activity. Prior rehabilitation attempts to institute a note-keeping system to compensate for her memory deficits had been unsuccessful. Notes were scattered all over the house and in her pocketbook. It appeared that her memory aids were actually confusing her more than assisting her. Finally, observations of G.L. in the community indicated that she was unable to recall what she had ordered in a restaurant for lunch or how much money she had to spend. She required a loan to pay the bill.

G.L.'s rehabilitation team consisted of her rehabilitation neurologist, neuropsychologist, speech–language pathologists, therapeutic recreation specialists and case manager. Her neurologist monitored her progress in the programme and provided G.L., her family and the team with details of her overall prognosis. The neuropsychologist helped the team to determine G.L.'s cognitive strengths, which could be used in the training of the memory aid. He also provided G.L. and her family with counselling and education. The speech pathologists and therapeutic recreation specialists worked together to establish measurable treatment goals and provide daily programming to G.L. The case manager ensured her treatment plan was integrated among all team members and communicated to all relevant significant others.

The team decided to train G.L. in the use of an external memory system because she was and would remain incapable of learning and using internally motivated memory strategies.

To institute an external memory system, the team analysed G.L.'s existing cognitive strengths and weaknesses to determine those that might help and hamper the teaching of a memory aid system.

1. While G.L.'s basic undivided attention was intact, she was susceptible to distraction.
2. Initial learning of new information was somewhat slow. G.L. could not recall any information after a delay. Therefore, the team thought she would probably require a great deal of practice, repetition and prompting to learn to use a new memory aid effectively.
3. Whereas G.L. had little executive (frontal) dysfunction, she did exhibit some problem-solving difficulties. There was concern that she might become easily disorganized when attempting to use a memory system in novel situations.
4. There were, however, a number of cognitive strengths to support the attempted use of a memory aid with G.L. Her intellectual capacity was well within the average range, suggesting that she should not have difficulty understanding the purpose and rationale of the aid. Her basic attention was good, suggesting that if the memory aid could be taught in a relatively distraction-free environment, repeatedly and for short intervals, she would probably be able to attend to the teaching and learn to use the aid.

Design and teaching the use of a memory aid
G.L.'s stated goals were to be more independent in all aspects of her life, including driving, cooking, managing her finances and caring for her daughter. The rehabilitation team wanted to teach G.L. to proceduralize the use of a time planner on a daily basis to compensate for her memory deficits. G.L. was already using scraps of paper and several books as a memory system. The team wanted her to use one memory book to reduce disorganization. With assistance, G.L. purchased a new small-sized logbook which could be kept in her purse, in which all of her to-be-remembered information would be recorded and stored. G.L. had previously used a monthly system that was too complex to manage, so she converted to a weekly calendar.

A cued-procedural learning approach was used. The goal was the spontaneous use of the memory log without explicit recall of the treatment plan. Teaching sessions consisted of repetitive practice recording the information in the log, prompted as needed when she could not recall previous learning of the memory system. Because of her limited concentration and slow encoding, the system was introduced in graduated steps across multiple sessions. Because the functional evaluation had previously shown that G.L. had difficulty both recording to-be-remembered information (e.g. taking a message) and understanding later what she had written, a very clear and easily comprehensible note-taking system was devised. G.L. consistently recorded the topic, as well as key words, to assist her in recalling the event (e.g. what, when and where the occurrence occurred). Cues to record messages in this fashion were affixed to each page of her memory log. All areas of the book were labelled as simply as possible to assist with problem-solving and organizational issues. A directory of emergency numbers, most commonly used telephone contacts, and resources was listed in the book as well. Finally, to address difficulties that were noted in the functional evaluation, the team promoted the use of the system with maximal cueing immediately following any occurrence that was to be recorded. They then began to reduce the amount of assistance that was provided. In this way, G.L. was able to learn the system without experiencing too many failures and setbacks.

Generalization and evaluation
At one month, G.L. was using her time planner reliably enough to be able to make and keep track of her appointments independently with only a few mistakes. She continued to require frequent prompts to take her time planner out of her pocketbook to record information. It eventually surfaced that at least a portion of her reluctance to use the time

planner was psychologically motivated in that she did not want to have to rely on this external device to help her remember. She experienced the natural negative social consequences of missing appointments, while still receiving support from the staff. With continued support and encouragement from the staff, her motivation and use of the time planner improved considerably. By the second month of postacute treatment, she was recording important information in her time planner and only required assistance from the staff to check her work for accuracy. There was an unexpected beneficial generalization. Before her injury, G.L. had enjoyed reading novels. She spontaneously discovered that use of the memory book facilitated reading because she could record information such as the general story line or where she had left off reading.

Final outcome and reassessment
At the end of her 20 weeks of treatment in postacute rehabilitation, G.L. was consistently logging her daily activities independently without cues and was using this information to guide her interactions with others. A six-month follow-up showed that she was recording information from the weekends and had become versed in using such information to function more independently.

Continuum of care

- Patients with severe brain injury will receive treatment at several different levels of care during their recovery.
- Reimbursement and fiscal constraints may influence decisions about levels of care.
- Moving patients into the least restrictive and most natural settings for treatment should be a clinical goal as well as a fiscal goal.
- Home, work and school are the most natural settings.
- The management of insurance monies to guarantee adequate postacute care will increasingly become the responsibility of the primary clinical programme.
- A clear diagnosis and functional prognosis will be essential to manage care, determine proper levels

of care, and preserve resources for the duration of care.

Most patients with catastrophic neurological illnesses experience treatment through a continuum of care between the time of their acute illness and their eventual return to daily living in their home or long-term living situation. When patients no longer require critical care services, they are usually transferred from the acute hospital to a rehabilitation centre, subacute nursing programme, chronic hospital, nursing home, assisted living centre or to their own home with some support services. The timing of patient transfer from the acute hospital to a stepdown level of care varies from region to region and in particular between the USA and Canada. Patients in Canada remain in the acute hospital for a longer period than in the USA (Rehabilitation Planning Committee, 1995).

The management of patients along the continuum of care is currently influenced more by financial reimbursement to different levels of care than by best clinical placement for the patient. The length of stay in an acute hospital inpatient setting has decreased dramatically in the USA over the last few years, in part because hospitals are financially rewarded by Medicare for shortening patients' lengths of stay and increasing patient volume. Hospitals developed their own postacute programmes of care or developed preferred referral arrangements for stepdown care placements for their patients to minimize acute hospital lengths of stay. In Canada, reimbursement from Provincial Ministries of Health to chronic hospitals (that mostly serve rehabilitation inpatients) is primarily based upon the prior year's global budget. The global budgets are not affected by an increased volume of inpatients served. Therefore, at the present time there are no financial incentives in the Canadian system to promote increasing the number of inpatients served per year in cognitive inpatient rehabilitation programmes (Rehabilitation Planning Committee, 1995).

At the postacute level of care, the emphasis in the USA is also to move patients as soon as possible into the least intensive care environment that can provide appropriate medical and support services. The practice has spurred the development of sophisticated medical, nursing and rehabilitation services in many non-traditional settings, such as group homes, assisted living centres, outpatient clinics and patients' own homes. Administrative leaders with vision are now developing operations for their rehabilitation services that are as flexible and mobile as possible in order to serve patients in all types of inpatient, residential and home environments.

The rehabilitation treatment of patients with traumatic brain injury was one of the earliest specialties to pioneer change in models of service delivery and treatment setting in the USA. This patient group had persistent cognitive and behavioural impairments that were the major impediments to independent discharge to home, community or work place. Outpatient centres for cognitive rehabilitation have proliferated because they are so much less expensive than inpatient units and because persistent, long-term cognitive deficits are the primary reason for prolonged disability after traumatic brain injury. The treatment setting will increasingly move to the home and community to aid the generalization of skills to the real-life setting. Whatever the setting, there continue to be debates about the clinical efficacy (and cost efficiencies) of remediation of specific cognitive deficits. Most clinicians agree patients receiving appropriate treatment can make significant gains in their functional abilities long after injury (Moore-Sohlberg and Mateer, 1987; Fryer and Haffey, 1987; Ruff et al., 1989; Mills et al. 1992; NIH, 1998). That ecologically meaningful treatments are easily delivered closer to home, work or school seems uncontested.

The cost of rehabilitation for a person with catastrophic illness from the acute rehabilitation stage through long-term management can be enormous. The majority of insurance dollars are spent in the early stages of recovery. It is essential, however, that some of the patients' financial resources are reserved for the postacute stages of recovery to promote the resumption of a productive and meaningful life. Some managed care organizations in the USA have seriously limited treatment following discharge from an inpatient setting and shifted the burden of support to the government or family. Experts are predicting a change in this practice, but in the meantime many young people are not able to receive postacute services following discharge from the acute or rehabilitation hospital (Frank, 1997).

Programme development, leadership and management

- Operating a cognitive rehabilitation programme is complex because the programme must meet the needs of many customers, including patients, family members, payers, government officials and accrediting agencies.
- Administrative and clinical leadership needs to formulate the vision for the future of the programme, including a path to reach that vision.
- Management needs to develop operational systems that serve the clinical efficiency and growth of the programme.
- Clinical leaders have a responsibility to administrative leaders to identify new concepts in clinical care that should become part of the vision and mission of the organization.

Over the last ten years, new and effective models of cognitive rehabilitation have been developed in response to clinical needs. Four factors require attention to develop a successful programme: patient needs, professional expertise, effective management and financial viability.

Who is the customer in cognitive rehabilitation? The patient, of course, is the foremost customer but not the only customer. Planning and operating a rehabilitation programme generate many customers: the patient, family members, the payer for the programme, government officials who regulate health care, and accrediting agencies. Operating a cognitive rehabilitation programme is complex and difficult because it must meet the needs of so many customers. The programme model must be developed and operated with the patient goals as the primary focus while honouring the fiscal, regulatory and social realities.

There are different treatment models available at this time. Some promote direct remediation of underlying neuropsychological deficits, e.g. attention. Some treatment models emphasize compensation strategies for impairments. Others focus on reinforcement of the skills needed for functional community training. Regardless of the treatment model, successful programmes all require expertise in the fundamental impairments of the disorder, and those responsible for clinical leadership must constantly re-evaluate the effectiveness of different treatments.

The successes and failures of cognitive rehabilitation programmes are rooted in their leadership and management. Stephen Covey said leadership is not management and management is not leadership. Leadership is the formulation of a vision for the future, including a plan to reach that vision. Management is the efficient execution of a programme to accomplish the goals of the organization. Covey says leadership often becomes too concerned with managing daily operations and does not focus on the future vision and mission of an organization (Covey, 1989).

Management needs to develop operational systems that serve the clinical efficiency and the growth of the programme. It needs to direct resources to the organization of clinical programmes and to the solution of clinical operating problems. Too often, teams of clinicians are left to solve their own operating problems without being given the authority to make structural changes in operations. Management makes structural decisions, for example concerning the organization of departments that may undermine clinical efficiency.

Consider the common problem of team authority. If clinicians are hired within discipline-specific departments (physician, physical therapy, occupational therapy, speech pathology, neuropsychology, nursing etc.), then evaluations, promotions and salary increases are always tied to that department. Even when assigned to a cognitive programme, the clinician will have no primary responsibility to the programme. The team becomes a committee with specialty groups representing psychiatry, neurology, neuropsychology, speech pathology, occupational therapy, etc. Team members are expected to work together democratically to operate the programme. The performance of such a programme is completely dependent on how well individual professionals can work together to put the programme into operation. If particular professionals leave the programme, the nature of the programme may change dramatically.

In this team structure, no one can be held professionally accountable within the team, and there is no direct resolution for conflicts over different treatment approaches. Although this is not an effective programme structure, it is a common one. Management cannot avoid the responsibility for making decisions about organizational structure that affect care. Some rehabilitation programmes have solved this particular problem by appointing a case manager who is authorized to direct treatment integration. The case manager has the responsibility of ensuring that the team's efforts are well planned, integrated and communicated to all relevant parties such as family members and payers. The case manager is empowered by management and has the authority to hold team members accountable if they do not fulfill their commitment to the team and treatment plan. For example, if a therapist does not perform family teaching before the patient is discharged, this negatively affects the whole team's efforts in preparing the patient and family for discharge. In this matrix organizational structure, the case manager has input into the performance of the individual as a team member and, therefore, team performance becomes relevant to a person's performance evaluation. The input concerning the team member's performance crosses all clinical disciplines, including those of physicians and nurses. In this structure, the case manager needs to have direct communication with administration and not be part of a clinical department such as nursing.

Clinical leaders also have a responsibility to the administrative leadership to identify new concepts in clinical care that should become part of the vision and mission of the organization. It is a realistic vision, revised regularly to meet clinical, social and financial challenges, that ultimately defines the future of any programme. For example, in the past few years the financial viability of rehabilitation hospitals in the USA has often been associated with how well the leadership has been able to create connections with acute care hospitals and offer them a full continuum of postacute care. Those rehabilitation hospitals that did not see this trend and incorporate it into their vision are now experiencing the consequences of a declining census. The acute care hospitals are finding a way to provide the postacute care for their own patients.

Daily operations

- Cognitive rehabilitation programmes need monitoring for their clinical relevance to patients, payers and referral sources.

- Successful programmes need assessment of availability and access of services to the target population.
- Clinical managers must insist on periodic review of clinical efficiency, programme outcomes and monitoring of costs.

Standards for operating cognitive rehabilitation programmes have been available from the Rehabilitation Accreditation Commission in Tucscon, Arizona, for several years (The Rehabilitation Accreditation Commission, 1999). The standards are well developed and can be used as guidelines for those who are starting a programme or revising operations.

In the authors' opinion, a few crucial operating areas should be addressed on a regular basis by management. These areas include programme development, patient access to programmes, patient outcomes and programme costs.

Programme development requires continuous respecification of the present and future needs of the marketplace. An understanding of the marketplace requires managers to have personal interactions with all referral sources and unambiguous surveying of patients. This information should be formally collected and analysed on an ongoing basis to understand the needs of the marketplace. For example, if it were found that a significant number of patients with brain injury referred to cognitive rehabilitation also had drug and alcohol problems, then the programme's clinical leaders would start assessing whether they could develop new programme components to address the drug and alcohol problems of its patients.

Clinical leadership needs to be accountable for reviewing the assessment and treatment planning procedures to ensure they are efficient and incorporate what is known in the research and clinical literature. For example, in the USA, it was only seven years ago that, after admission to an inpatient rehabilitation hospital, the rehabilitation team required two weeks to complete its initial assessment. The assessment procedures were not efficient and were designed for the novice-level practitioner. Now the standard of care in the USA requires the team's assessment to be completed from one to two days after admission for even the most complex rehabilitation patients.

Programmes are analysed using the available information which describes clinical operations and outcomes. The construction and maintenance of meaningful clinical and administrative databases are invaluable to programme development and cost reduction. In the clinical databases, patients must be categorized in meaningful ways in order to evaluate patient outcomes and the effectiveness of care. Administrators can use established clinical tools to construct some of the database information, such as the Functional Independence Measure or the Minimum Data Set (Functional Index Measure). After the bases have been constructed, clinical, administrative and research leadership can use the data to ask questions regarding patient outcomes, discharge disposition, efficiency of care, efficacy of care and other relevant topics. These same databases can also be used for initiates in quality improvement and programme evaluation. Quality improvement, programme evaluation, programme development and research can then all be tied together for the advancement of the programme.

Access systems for referral sources, patients and their families continually need to be made more customer oriented, easily used and quickly responsive to outside inquiries. For example, if families are unwilling to travel more than 30 miles to access services, will the programme consider developing community-based home care or a satellite service?

Clinicians and managers need to define discharge options and other continua of care that patients will interact with as their programme changes. Administrators and clinicians should be very interested in developing follow-up systems to collect information about the preservation of patient outcomes after discharge and the effectiveness of the programme.

Managers must work with clinicians to review the costs of care. Only with collaborate efforts between management and clinicians can new, effective and less costly models of cognitive rehabilitation evolve. The costs of different cognitive rehabilitation programmes vary and relate to salaries and real-estate cost variations across the USA and Canada. Debt service and overhead costs affect the costs of a programme. It is only possible to address costs in a broad way with regards to cognitive rehabilitation. Cost data that are well organized and attributed to a programme (particularly in a multiservice programme) are invaluable to determine if programme costs can be lowered without changing the product. Costs must be attributable to operating systems in a programme as well as to departmental costs, e.g. the cost of intake, assessment, treatment and follow-up versus the cost of each clinical department. If this information is not available, clinicians and administrators use their own judgment to determine what is most valuable to a programme. Their perceptions are not always correct. Administrators cannot make qualitative judgments about different functional systems, services or programmes because they lack the clinical expertise, so they often choose to cut the costs of all services. For example, in a situation in which all services are cut by 5 per cent, transporting patients to the cognitive rehabilitation programme may be adversely affected such that fewer patients access the programme. Does it make sense to cut transportation costs and therefore patient access and revenue? Unfortunately, the authors have commonly witnessed this practice.

In addition, some third-party payers may forbid the use of some less costly labour options; this can prevent reductions in salary costs. Professional disciplines are by their nature protective of their sphere and scope of practice and are reluctant to embrace unlicensed assistant and aid staff into the treatment team. This is still a viable option to help reduce salary costs if patient outcomes can be maintained with the appropriate use of support staff.

The skilful execution of cost reduction with preservation and sometimes improvement in programme operations is a real art. Effective cost reduction requires there to be good operating cost data and a collaborative effort between administrators, clinicians and payer sources to ensure that quality is preserved and the long-term livelihood of the programme is ensured.

Conclusions

This chapter provides a summary of some of the current challenges facing rehabilitation leaders and managers working in the speciality of cognitive rehabilitation. The practice of cognitive rehabilitation will continue to change with the evolution of rehabilitation as a specialty area in health care. This specialty area is likely to receive greater attention in the future, as more people of all ages survive neurological illnesses, with subsequent lasting cognitive impairments. It will only be through the collaborative efforts of clinical and administrative leaders, and researchers, that new and more effective models of care and clinical practices will develop.

References

Adams, R.D. and Victor, M. 1993. Cerebrovascular diseases. In *Principles of Neurology*, 5th edn, ed. R.D. Adams and M. Victor, pp. 669–748. New York: McGraw-Hill.

Covey, S.R. 1989. *The 7 Habits of Highly Effective People*. New York: Simon & Schuster.

Frank, R.G. 1997. Lessons from the great battle: health care reform 1992–1994. *Arch Phys Med Rehabil* **78**, 120–4.

Fryer, J.L. and Haffey, W.J. 1987. Cognitive rehabilitation and community readaptation: outcomes from two program models. *J Head Trauma Rehabil* **2**, 51–63.

Functional Index Measure Buffalo. NY: *Uniform Data System for Medical Rehabilitation*. State University of New York at Buffalo.

Gillespie, A. and Kixmiller, J.S. 1997. Use of the neurologic model in the rehabilitation assessment and treatment of problems with functional memory and daily planning. In *Neurologic Rehabilitation: a Guide to Diagnosis, Prognosis and Treatment Planning*, ed. V.M. Mills, J.W. Cassidy and D.I. Katz, pp. 283–306. Boston: Blackwell Science.

Grosswasser, Z., Hohen, M. and Costeff, H. 1989. Rehabilitation outcome after anoxic brain damage. *Arch Phys Med Rehabil* **70**, 186–8.

Hanley, D.F., Johnson, R.T. and Whitley, R.J. 1987. Yes, brain biopsy should be a prerequisite for herpes simplex encephalitis treatment. *Arch Neurol* **44**, 1289–90.

Kraus, J.F. 1987. Epidemiology of head injury. In *Head Injury*, 2nd edn, ed. P.R. Cooper, pp. 1–25. Baltimore: Williams & Wilkins.

Kurtzke, J.F. and Kurland, L.T. 1987. The epidemiology of neurologic disease. In *Clinical Neurology*, ed. A.B. Baker and R.J. Joynt, pp. 1–143. Philadelphia: Harper & Row.

Mills, V.M., Cassidy, J.W. and Katz, D.I. 1997. *Neurologic Rehabilitation: a Guide to Diagnosis, Prognosis and Treatment Planning*. Boston: Blackwell Science.

Mills, V.M., Nesbeda, T., Katz, D.I. and Alexander, M.P. 1992. Outcomes for traumatically brain-injured patients following post-acute rehabilitation programmes. *Brain Inj* **3**, 219–28.

Moore-Sohlberg, M. and Mateer, C.A. 1987. Effectiveness of an attention-training program. *J Clin Exp Neuropsychol* **9**, 117–30.

NIH 1998. NIH Consensus Development Conference: Rehabilitation of Persons with Traumatic Brain Injury, 1998 Oct 26–28; 160).

Rehabilitation Planning Committee 1995. *Proposal for the Metropolitan Toronto Rehab Network. March 1995.*

Ruff, R.M., Baser, C.A., Johnston, J.W. et al. 1989. Neuropsychological rehabilitation: an experimental study with head-injured patients. *J Head Trauma Rehabil* **4**, 20–36.

Rusk, H.A. 1972. *World to Care For.* New York: Random House.

The Rehabilitation Accreditation Commission 1999. *Standards Manual and Interpretive Guidelines for Medical Rehabilitation,* pp. 170–200. Tucson, AZ: CARF.

Wilson, B.A. 1996. Cognitive functioning of adult survivors of cerebral hypoxia. *Brain Inj* **10**, 863–74.

11

Neuropsychological rehabilitation in the interdisciplinary team: the postacute stage

Anne-Lise Christensen and Carla Caetano

Introduction

The primary purpose of this chapter is to describe a postacute neuropsychological rehabilitation programme, its characteristics, its interacting elements and the growth and change possible after brain injury as a result of such a programme. Psychosocial outcome based on a neuropsychological rather than a medical model of treatment is emphasized. In addition, the importance of a neuropsychological approach to rehabilitation and the role of an interdisciplinary team in creating an effective treatment milieu are addressed. The Center for Rehabilitation of Brain Injury, at Copenhagen University in Denmark, is used as an example of how a day programme functions within these parameters. Emphasis is placed on (a) theoretical premises, (b) selection, (c) evaluation, and (d) treatment procedures to illustrate the manner in which rehabilitation takes place.

A model for neuropsychological rehabilitation

- The wide-ranging and complex needs of patients with acquired brain injury require comprehensive treatment that is neuropsychological rather than medical in orientation.
- Theoretical influences derive from the work of Goldstein, Luria, Ben-Yishay, Diller and Prigatano.
- Determining the timing of interventions is important and treatment methods may vary, being influenced by demographic factors such as: age, the severity of injury, the stage of the recovery process, individual characteristics, and the availability of neuropsycho-

logical evaluations and specialized programmes to plan treatment effectively.

The importance of a holistic, neuropsychologically based approach to the evaluation and treatment of acquired brain injury and the use of an interdisciplinary team in achieving this goal cannot be overemphasized. The literature pertaining to acquired brain injury is replete with observations of the heterogeneity of injury location and individual differences in response to injury. Increased attention has been given not only to the physical and cognitive sequelae of brain injury, but also to disruptions in the emotional, interpersonal and social spheres of functioning which adversely impact patients, often many years postinjury (Thomsen, 1984; Brooks et al., 1986). Thus, factors such as the comprehensiveness, timing and effectiveness of treatment have been considered to be of importance.

There is growing consensus that the broad range and complex needs of patients with acquired brain injury require comprehensive treatment. Earlier approaches to rehabilitation, while commendable, were arguably limited (see Boake, 1991, for a historical overview of the development of cognitive rehabilitation). Changes from a medical treatment approach to what now may be identified as 'neuropsychological' treatment were influenced by Goldstein (1942) and Luria (1966). Goldsten emphasized a psychological rather than purely medical approach to treatment and stressed the importance of distinguishing between symptoms that are a direct result of the brain injury and those symptoms that reflect 'the expression of the struggle of the changed organism to cope with the defect, and to meet the demands of a milieu with which it is no longer equipped to deal' (Goldstein, 1942, p. 69). These symptoms he viewed as consisting of (a) attempts at adaptation which often result in 'catastrophic reactions', i.e. anxiety in failing at a task, and (b) substitute behaviours to avoid dealing with the changes in functioning (and thereby anxiety), termed 'protective mechanisms' (Goldstein, 1952). These latter attributes are defined as withdrawal, perfectionism and unawareness (not due to denial).

Luria (1966) was influential in integrating the neurological methods of his day to create a holistic means of assessing neuropsychological functioning. Furthermore, he stressed using a wide range of neuropsychological tests administered qualitatively to ensure a comprehensive syndrome analysis. He emphasized not only the study of symptoms but also the 'qualification of defects and an analysis of the factors underlying these behavioural defects' (Luria, in Christensen, 1975, p. 7). Thus, the benefits of the Luria approach are in providing a qualitative method in assessment and, by implication, treatment. The assessment approach results in syndrome analysis and the provision of feedback, which, as a treatment form, is elaborated into a psychosocial approach based on the trust and collaboration essential for the functioning of a holistic treatment programme.

These psychosocial and holistic themes led to the subsequent development of day programme treatment approaches, the first established by Ben-Yishay and Diller in the 1970s. For a description of this programme, the reader is referred to Ben-Yishay and Gold (1990); other examples include Prigatano et al. (1986). This type of treatment approach could certainly be described as the 'turning point in this history of cognitive rehabilitation' (Boake, 1991, p. 11), and subsequently led to the inclusion of the interdisciplinary team as an essential element (Diller, 1990).

In addition to the treatment approach selected, the timing of treatment is also important. Whereas acute rehabilitation has been undisputed, the question of recovery time has been debated (Stein, Glasier and Hoffman, 1994). Sbordone, Liter and Pettler-Jennings (1995) note that generally it has been assumed that most recovery following traumatic brain injury takes place within the first six months after injury, and all

recovery occurs within one to two years postinjury. However, their findings indicate that traumatic brain injury patients continue to exhibit significant improvements in their physical, cognitive, emotional and social functioning two years after injury irrespective of the severity of the initial brain injury, and that gradual improvements continue for as much as ten years postinjury. As their data related to patients who received some form of cognitive rehabilitation during this period, their findings suggest that rehabilitation may have aided recovery. If, in fact, the impact of cognitive rehabilitation was negligible, their findings suggest, at the very least, that positive changes in functioning are possible many years after injury. Thomsen (1984, 1992), in 2.5-year 10–15-year and 20-year follow-up studies, similarly notes that improvement is possible many years after injury.

Defining and determining the efficacy of rehabilitation are challenging tasks in that a number of treatment methods exist dependent on such factors as the severity of injury, the stage of the recovery process, and the availability of neuropsychological evaluations to plan treatment effectively. Thus, some treatment approaches focus on self-care or behavioural stability, whereas others may emphasize independent living and improving life quality. In a review of the benefits of rehabilitation for traumatic brain injury, Hall and Cope (1995) conclude that while there is evidence of positive trends in outcome for day treatment programmes (including rehabilitation that takes place at other phases), cost-effectiveness concerns remain and multicentre studies are needed to address some of the methodological difficulties inherent in this area of research. A possible solution may be to focus on cost effectiveness as this pertains to psychosocial outcome subsequent to programme completion and in prolonged follow-up studies.

The Center for Rehabilitation of Brain Injury in Denmark provides one example of how a postacute, holistic, neuropsychologically oriented rehabilitation programme functions. In this context, 'postacute' acquired brain injury patients (of which approximately half are traumatic brain injury patients) are defined as those who, subsequent to injury, have been discharged from hospital and who are deemed medically stable;

'holistic' refers to an interdisciplinary planning and treatment approach; and 'neuropsychological rehabiliation' implies a psychosocial approach to evaluation and treatment, i.e. considering the cognitive, emotional and social impact of the brain injury while also taking into account the physical condition of patients.

The above-mentioned programme type has demonstrated a positive outcome (Christensen et al., 1992; Teasdale and Christensen, 1994) consistent with other postacute rehabilitation programmes of a similar structure (e.g. Prigatano et al., 1984; Ben-Yishay et al., 1987). In addition, a cost–effect study conducted for The Center for Rehabilitation of Brain Injury has indicated the benefits of the programme, i.e. the immediate benefits are less dependence on health and social services and, later, increased use of educational services. At three years, the rehabilitation had paid for itself; thereafter, there continued to be financial benefits for the paying parties (Larsen, Mehlbye and Gørtz, 1991).

A detailed description of The Center for Rehabilitation of Brain Injury may be found in Christensen and Teasdale (1993). Briefly stated, however, the day programme consists of a structured series of individual and group activities in which 15 acquired brain injury patients participate, the purpose of which is to assist return to employment or educational pursuits. The programme runs for an approximately four-month period, from Tuesdays to Fridays, between 9:00 a.m. and 3:00 p.m. Thereafter, an eight-month group-based follow-up is provided. Individual follow-up can continue for a longer period, depending on each individual's need. For those patients who (a) require less emphasis on employment or education and more on life quality, or (b) do not require (or do not have the capacity for) such intensive treatment, a reduced day programme is offered, i.e. fewer hours and activities per week. The patients who participate in this programme are typically older than those entering the full programme. Individual treatment may also be provided for those patients who need limited but intensive treatment.

The following elements of the intensive day programme are discussed as they are crucial to the effective holistic rehabilitation, namely: (a) the theoretical premise on which the rehabilitation is based; (b) the selection of patients to be treated; (c) the evaluation procedures; and (d) the treatment approach.

Theoretical premise

- Postacute, holistic rehabilitation procedures require a sound theoretical base.
- Luria's theory of brain functioning provides a useful foundation for rehabilitation planning.
- A therapeutic milieu that emphasizes trust, collaboration and developing a sense of self-reliance and self-confidence is essential to minimizing the inhibitory forces of self-protection.
- The collaboration of the interdisciplinary team, the primary therapist and the patients themselves is the means by which holistic, neuropsychological rehabilitation can be achieved.

As holistic rehabilitation aims at a comprehensive treatment approach, it is essential that a sound theoretical base exists to guide treatment planning. Thus, an integrated model of brain functioning should be adhered to. At The Center for Rehabilitation of Brain Injury, treatment is primarily based on the brain-functioning principles and evaluation method of Luria (Luria et al., 1969; Luria, 1966, 1973), who emphasized (a) a functional systems approach to brain–behaviour relationships, consistent with his fundamental concepts (e.g. Mesulam, 1985; Stuss and Benson, 1990), and (b) the importance of recognizing individual differences in the sequelae of brain injury.

The above two premises can be applied in both the evaluation and the treatment of patients. The Luria Neuropsychological Investigation, developed by Christensen (1975) and based on Luria's writings, readily avails itself to a qualitative, syndrome analysis of brain functioning and to the planning of primarily cognitive rehabilitation. This is possible because this type of evaluation addresses both the strengths and the deficits of the patient, including cognitive and personality characteristics, in an individualized rather than a normative manner (see Christensen, Malmros and Townes, 1987; and Christensen, Jensen and Risberg, 1990, for comprehensive accounts of this process).

The centre's day programme consists of both individual and group activities, but the key characteristics of

Luria's approach (described in Christensen, Caetano and Rasmussen 1996) have been elaborated as the basis for treatment. Emphasis is on developing the patient's self-confidence and increasing his or her responsibilities both within and outside the programme, which is achieved by (a) creating a trusting, collaborative and problem-solving therapeutic relationship; (b) individualizing treatment goals within programme activities in an ecologically valid manner; and (c) maintaining a dynamic feedback process not only within the therapeutic relationship, but also in the external environment. It is of paramount importance that these characteristics are adhered to by all members of the rehabilitation team (which, at The Center for Rehabilitation of Brain Injury, consists of ten neuropsychologists and clinical psychologists, one speech and language therapist, one voice therapist, one special education teacher and three physical therapists).

Diller (1990) notes that an effective team must involve members who are able to solve problems beyond their particular knowledge base, and that a 'primary therapist', i.e. one member of the team who is responsible for a patient (other team members providing the necessary additional information required for the patient's care), may be particularly appropriate for brain-injured individuals by making greater consistency possible.

At the Center for Rehabilitation of Brain Injury, the role of the primary therapist is emphasized for this reason, but more specifically to address the specific training of each patient. The primary therapist at this centre is always a neuropsychologist or clinical psychologist, who is responsible for two to three patients simultaneously (patients at the Danish centre are referred to as 'students') and whose duties consist of integrating the evaluation and treatment process for the student, as well as maintaining contact with the student's family and other social systems during the treatment phase and in the follow-up period, which can continue for up to two years.

The role of the primary therapist must be understood in the context of a student-centred milieu. The latter refers to the very active manner in which the staff as a whole aim at fostering a spirit of engagement, hope and growth in the students, so that they are actively responsible for their rehabilitation process. This, once again, is in the spirit of creating an individualized treatment approach based on a collaborative relationship and is made possible by the close contact between the students and staff. For example, a joint staff and student/family meeting takes place at programme start and programme completion. The purpose of these occasions is to create and maintain a sense of rapport between the staff, the students and their significant others.

Selection procedures

- Programmes should be tailored for specific patient groups.
- Patients should be referred to postacute rehabilitation as soon as possible after discharge from hospital.

As previously mentioned, acquired brain injury consists of a complex array of loss of functions and potential life experiences. The definition of admission criteria is important if neuropsychological rehabilitation programmes are to be individually tailored so as to (a) manage the complex needs of the brain-injured individual most effectively, and (b) conduct effective outcome research (Wilson, 1993).

The patients referred to the Danish centre are those who meet the following admission criteria. First and foremost, they have to have a verified brain lesion, be medically stable and in need of active intervention to encourage the recovery process. Other inclusion criteria are: (a) aged at least 16 years of age, (b) able to express an understanding of the need to receive treatment, (c) having the possibility of clarifying and improving their cognitive, emotional and psychosocial functioning so as to return to work or pursue an education, and (d) preferably having support from significant others. Patients who have progressive central nervous system diseases, acute psychiatric illness, who are in need of nursing care, or who have significant substance abuse disorders are excluded from the programme. Those patients who require neuropsychological rehabilitation but do not meet the centre's criteria are evaluated, given advisory consultation and referred to resources elsewhere. The rationale for these selection criteria is related to the goal of the programme, i.e. to create a collaborative therapeutic milieu in which a return to a productive lifestyle is encouraged, and to the type of programme offered, i.e. one which emphasizes individual responsibility, social interaction and group-based problem-solving activities. An important part of this is creating a sense of group affiliation among the students, which is encouraged, for example, by assisting and supporting each other with particular tasks.

At The Center for Rehabilitation of Brain Injury, treatment is focused on adults. It takes place at a university where, through a series of educational courses, the emphasis is on a return to a normal lifestyle consistent with the characteristics of the individual, i.e. following through education or career goals and participating in leisure activities and maintaining interpersonal relationships. Although relevant data have not been published, it would appear that this type of programme best suits those patients with (a) a verified brain lesion, in contrast to those patients who suffer from postconcussion and/or whiplash, and (b) the ability to respond to feedback, so as to promote insight into their condition and future aspirations. This latter attribute can be compared to what Ben-Yishay and his colleagues refer to as the patient's malleability, and is important in achieving treatment objectives. In addition, the programme appears best suited to those patients who have had some life experience and who have the possibility of returning to educational or occupational pursuits. Alternatively, the second type of programme is more appropriate for older adults, and emphasizes life-quality concerns.

Ideally, patients should be referred to the centre as soon as possible after discharge from hospital, but due to the medical community's still-limited acceptance of neuropsychological rehabilitation, the reality is that patients typically get referred only after they have lived at home and/or tried returning to their previous work and have encountered significant difficulties, resulting in emotionally damaging sequelae. The negative emotional sequelae that are often developed by both patients and significant others may then reinforce the patient's cognitive difficulties and protective mechanisms, thereby increasing a sense of failure and helplessness.

It was agreed as early as 1987 that treatment should be initiated and maintained as soon as possible after injury (Christensen and Uzzell, 1988). This decision was based on the view that patients are likely to become increasingly discouraged if early intervention is not given, i.e. their attempts at dealing with their difficulties are often inadequate and their significant others are often confused by not knowing how to deal with the disturbances and reactions of the injured person.

Recent research also seems to be consistent with the view of early intervention as being preferable (e.g. Stein, Glasier and Hoffman, 1994). Thus, whereas patients were previously referred to the centre, on average, two years postinjury (although the range has been as broad as six months to eight years postinjury), in the past two years an increasing number of patients has been referred sooner, i.e. six to eight months after injury.

Evaluation procedures

- The evaluation of brain-injured patients should be comprehensive, i.e. including cognitive, emotional and psychosocial factors as well as taking into consideration physical functioning.
- Neuropsychological assessment should consist of quantitative and qualitative approaches.
- Assessment should be dynamic, i.e. there should be a continuous evaluation of the patient's responses to the treatment plan, and modifications made accordingly.
- Evaluations should be conducted by members of the interdisciplinary team, and this information should be integrated by the primary therapist to form a meaningful, individualized rehabilitation plan.

In an interdisciplinary team approach, evaluations are conducted by each professional but data must be integrated into a meaningful rehabilitation plan throughout the process. This is the procedure followed at The Center for Rehabilitation of Brain Injury and it takes place in a number of stages, summarized in Table 11.1.

Initially, the patients are reviewed by a selection committee consisting of a consulting neurologist, neurosurgeon, physiatrist, the centre's director, a member of the rehabilitation team and an administrative secretary. Medical records are reviewed and a preliminary selection is made. Potential participants are then evaluated

Table 11.1 Assessment periods, and type

| Phase | Type of assessment | | | | |
	Neuropsychological	Communication	Physical	Family/significant others	Other
Selection	LNI[1] Ravens[2]			Interview	Medical review Review of health, social services, referral source
Pre-program	GPI-R[3] EBIQ[4]	Interview	Interview	Interview	If relevant, interview with employer or other sources involved with patient
	WAIS-R[5] (selected subtests) WMS-R[6] (selected subtests) Trails, A, B[7] d2[8] PASAT[9] (modified) MAC[10] Supplementary tests as indicated	Voice Measure of breathing, intonation, articulation Language BDAE[11] (selected subtests) Supplementary tests as needed	Astrand Bicycle Test[12] Modified Harvard Step Test[13] Modified Coopers Running Test[14] Test of fine motor control[15]	GPI-R EBIQ	
During programme	Behaviour observation Mid-programme evaluation of progress in defined goals		Observation, feedback and modification of training goals and activities	Observation and feedback	Feedback of progress, as necessary
Post-programme	Same as preprogramme (includes parallel version of Ravens)				
Follow-up	As needed				

Notes:

 1 Luria's Neuropsychological Investigation (Christensen, 1975).
 2 Ravens Advanced Progressive Matrices (12 item) (Raven 1965).
 3 General Patient Inventory, Revised (The Center for Rehabilitation of Brain Injury).
 4 European Brain Injury Questionnaire (Teasdale et al., 1997).
 5 Wechsler Adult Intelligence Scale, Revised (Wechsler 1981).
 6 Wechsler Memory Scale, Revised (Wechsler, 1987).
 7 Trails A & B (Lezak, 1995).
 8 d2 (Brickenkamp, 1981).
 9 Paced Auditory Serial Addition Test (unpaced) (Gronwall, 1977, unpaced norms by Gade and Mortensen, 1984).
10 Memory Assessment Clinic Battery (Larrabee and Crook, 1991).
11 Boston Diagnostic Aphasia Examination (Goodglass and Kaplan, 1983).
12 Ästrand Bicycle Test (Ästrand and Rodahl, 1970).
13 Harvard Step Test (Asmussen and Hohwü-Christensen, 1980).
14 Coopers Running Test (Cooper, 1968).
15 Test of fine motor control (Mulder, 1997).

Table 11.2 Day programme activities

Individual activities		Group activities	
Type	Hours per week	Type	Hours per week
		Morning meeting	4
Cognitive training	1	Cognitive training	3
Psychotherapy	1–2	Psychotherapy	1.5
Family therapy	Varies as needed	Project groups	1.5
Voice training	0–1, as needed	Lecture series	2
Speech and language therapy	0–3, as needed	Communication skills, study techniques, etc.	2
Physical therapy	1 to as many as needed	Physical therapy	2
Special education	1 to as many as needed	Significant others	2 times per month
Follow-up	As needed	Follow-up	1 × month, 8 months

using the Luria Neuropsychological Investigation and significant others are interviewed. Thereafter, patients are selected for the day programme (Table 11.2).

Once selected for treatment in the day programme, students are evaluated on: (a) further neuropsychological tests by the neuropsychologists, (b) speech, language and voice by the respective therapists, and (c) their physical fitness and motor complaints by the physical therapists.

Of note is that an attempt is made to use the tests in an ecologically valid manner, i.e. test data are also interpreted and administered qualitatively. Thus, even with those tests that are used in a standardized, normative manner, the clinical significance of the task approach is always considered, e.g. the patient's specific cognitive style, compensation patterns, etc. This information and a determination of premorbid functioning and hobbies/interests in comparison to present functioning are regarded as crucial to the effective use of test performance in rehabilitation planning.

Reports of all the test findings are seen by the primary therapist, who then integrates the data into a comprehensive written report that is made available to the student, the referral source and the primary physician. During the middle of the programme and at programme completion, similar evaluations are made by the team and the information is again made available to the above-mentioned parties. This information is used subsequent to programme completion to aid in follow-up and planning of suitable procedures, as, for example, in planning for return to work; the centre is currently collaborating in the development of a work reintegration project.

Direct observations are part of the evaluation process as a means of providing feedback. Prior to programme commencement, an introductory programme of a few days' duration is provided, during which staff and students have the opportunity to meet and get to know one another, and group activities with themes such as life quality and sequelae after brain injury are presented. This process of direct observation and feedback continues throughout the programme as the students participate in individual and group activities with staff members present. Emphasis is placed on encouraging the students to be active participants in this process.

Finally, neuropsychological follow-up assessments are conducted one year and three years after programme completion.

Treatment approach

- Individual rehabilitation takes place within the structure of the day programme.
- Interventions are closely linked to the level of insight the patient has.
- Programme activities should be ecologically valid.
- A therapeutic milieu that emphasizes the possibility

for general development and the reacquisition of specific skills is essential for effective treatment.

Once the initial evaluation procedures are completed, the combined data for each student are discussed in treatment planning meetings, in order to allocate appropriate individual programme activities. Certain activities are prerequisites, whereas others (e.g. speech and language, voice therapy, special education) are selected depending on the student's needs.

At the start of the programme, the staff present a description of the programme, the students introduce themselves and their significant others, and an informal evening meeting follows, during which the therapists, the students and their families socialize together. In this relaxed, social atmosphere, questions may be addressed, rapport established and staff members have the opportunity to observe students within their support systems. At programme completion, there is a meeting conducted in a similar manner and, as part of an evening meeting, the students give feedback on their experiences (an activity inspired by a similar process in the Ben-Yishay programme, i.e. a concluding party at which the students present self-evaluations and plans for the immediate future). In addition, at the mid-programme point, both staff and students participate in a luncheon followed by musical entertainment. Furthermore, in terms of daily functioning, students have lunch together in an eating area within the centre, as do the staff (in close proximity but separate from the students), and staff and students share a common work space, e.g. offices, computers etc., which further encourages a sense of community and interaction.

It is of vital importance that treatment in all the various activities is consistent with the student's level of insight. Deficits in awareness are manifold (Prigatano and Schachter, 1991) and important to the treatment process (Ben-Yishay and Diller, 1993). As much of the treatment at the centre is based on providing feedback, it is important that Goldstein's (1952) 'protective mechanisms' (as previously described) be weighted carefully. Thus, the timing of the intervention is crucial and related to the patient's level of insight. A caring, trusting relationship is, therefore, essential.

Of importance is the individual psychotherapy with the primary therapist (a neuropsychologist or clinical psychologist), who is responsible for integrating information obtained from the student, significant others, and staff members. The individual sessions are used to consolidate the therapeutic relationship, address questions and concerns pertaining to all aspects of brain injury and recovery, and to ensure that the rehabilitation plan has continued relevance and is being followed through. Thus, the primary therapist ensures the smooth flow of the individual rehabilitation process.

Furthermore, there is adherence to Luria's (1963) principle of students with more acute injuries having their deficits retrained while those with longer standing difficulties are trained to make use of specific strategies. Changes in functioning are understood to be occurring as a result of intersystemic or intrasystemic functional reorganization, as described by Luria et al. (1969).

Cognitive training is consistent with Luria's approach. It is essential that the therapist interprets the specific deficits and strengths in terms of a functional systems understanding of brain processes. Thus, deficits are not to be considered in isolation, but as combining to influence functioning in many areas and on many different levels, and the students' response to their condition is also taken into consideration. Cognitive training, therefore, must be individually adapted, and the principles followed through in the group training activities. Initial training tasks are based on the materials developed by Wilson (1987), Sohlberg and Mateer (1989) and Shallice and Burgess (1991) and on various inductive and deductive reasoning tasks. However, as soon as it is possible, training tasks are individually created for each patient. For example, a student may initially participate in paper and pencil attention-training tasks, then progress to identifying and learning compensatory memory strategies and/or developing study-skill techniques. As the programme progresses, greater emphasis is placed on using these strategies to meet the requirements of other programme activities such as the morning meeting or in other contexts outside the programme.

Often, individual therapy within the primary therapist sessions is used to evaluate activities with the student and to explore their ramifications in relation to future goals. Individual therapy also provides the opportunity for training of specific tasks in the here and now; for example, a previously highly skilled guitar teacher who wished to return to teaching after her injury was asked to teach a therapist to play the guitar and feedback was provided on her teaching skills; in another case, a patient who wished to submit job applications was asked to learn to write applications, which were evaluated in individual therapy sessions.

Group activities are run by various staff members, including psychologists, speech and language therapists and/or the special education teacher. Typically, two staff members are present in every group to supervise students. Some group activities, such as the morning meeting, lecture series and the joint student–staff meeting, include all students whereas others require a smaller number of participants to function effectively. These latter activities include the project groups, psychotherapy groups, and cognitive training groups (Table 11.3). Group allocation of the individual student is determined by similarities/differences in premorbid functioning, current cognitive capacity, current language functioning, interpersonal style and personal interests and needs. Group activities aim to be meaningful to the students, and topics/activities are selected so as to be relevant to their lives. For example, the lecture series covers topics related to brain injury, quality-of-life issues, the experiences of previous students, and topics of general interest such as art, music and current events. Group psychotherapy covers topics related to the social and emotional consequences of brain injury. Project groups involve such activities as creating a newsletter, making videos, planning group activities, creating a poster, presenting the centre's activities for an 'open house' day, etc.

Physical training is conducted within the holistic, neuropsychological framework of the programme, i.e. physical deficits and subsequent physical activities are not considered in isolation but are integrated to incorporate the premorbid functioning of the students, their current cognitive difficulties and present interests. Thus, physical *training* rather than physical *treatment* is emphasized, and sport and recreational activities are encouraged. The goals of physical training are to compensate for motor deficits, improve the general level of fitness, and support leisure activities that may be continued after programme completion.

As the evaluation and treatment process is not a static process, and it is the effective functioning of the interdisciplinary team that is essential for maintaining a dynamic, individually oriented treatment approach, weekly conferences are held during the programme period to discuss the student and programme status, and feedback is available daily because of the contact the staff have with each other during and in between programme activities. Furthermore, openness between the team and students is essential to facilitate the development of creative ideas necessary for effective treatment.

Whereas Diller (1990) has correctly pointed out that such a teamwork approach requires flexibility and acceptance of role diffusion, and that this may be regarded as a demanding task, it can be argued, nonetheless, that if the members of the professional team agree on their common goal – namely, to maximize the potential of the brain-injured individual – then professional differences can be regarded as an asset rather than a liability in achieving this common goal.

Although the centre's programme has been influenced by the programmes of Ben-Yishay (Ben-Yishay and Gold, 1990) and Prigatano (Prigatano et al., 1986), certain differences do exist. Whereas all three programmes stress a psychosocial approach with an integrated treatment objective and contact with significant others, differences exist in the form of therapeutic milieu and the use of group-based activities. For example, in contrast to the Ben-Yishay and Gold description, at the Center for Rehabilitation of Brain Injury less use is made of contractual agreement and videotaping as means of changing behaviour and providing feedback. At the Danish centre, emphasis is on developing a collaborative relationship and tailoring activities within the programme to promote general development and reacquisition of specific skills, rather than on using the structure of the programme to make the patients accept treatment. Furthermore, whereas Ben-Yishay and Gold (1990) have a daily session termed 'orientation', the Danish centre has a daily 'morning meeting'. The latter differs from the former by including activities other than orientation and goal setting: namely, encouraging each student to take personal responsibility for a variety of tasks, e.g. chairing the meeting, writing up the minutes and presenting them

Table 11.3 Overview of group activities

Group type	Morning meeting	Cognitive training	Project group	Psychotherapy	Cognitive physical training	Friday lecture	Joint meeting
Characteristics							
Frequency	4 times a week	3 times a week	Once a week	Once a week	Once a week	Once a week	Once a week
Duration	60 minutes	45 minutes	90–120 minutes	90 minutes	120 minutes	90 minutes	30 minutes
Participants	All students 2 staff members	6–7 students 2–3 staff members	6–7 students 2–3 staff members	6–7 students 2 staff members	4 students 2 staff members	All students	All students All staff members
Objectives	General orientation Mobilization of energy Awareness of surroundings Social interaction	Awareness of cognitive difficulties Awareness of strengths and weaknesses Working in group context Identification of alternative strategies	Cooperative interaction Group problem solving	Context for peer discussion Psychosocial awareness Minimize social isolation Personal identity	Improve general fitness level Provide an understanding of the relationship between cognitive dysfunction and difficulties with physical activities Psychosocial interaction	Provide information on topics related to brain injury and general interest	Evaluation Feedback
Task/subject examples	Chairperson of the meeting Leader of the physical exercises Supplier of news/facts	Attention/concentration Speed of processing Memory Problem solving	Plan social events Make video Create newsletter	Sexuality New–old self Future	Fitness exercises Squash Dance activities	Neurosurgery Nutrition The brain	Discussion of problems which arose during the week

Notes:
After Verstraeten (1996).

to the group, providing news items for discussion, leading a brief exercise programme, giving and receiving feedback on these tasks, etc.

Prigatano et al.'s (1986) programme is similar to that of the Danish centre in their emphasis on timing interventions according to the level of awareness the patients develop and in their description of cognitive retraining and cognitive group therapy. However, at the Danish centre the relationship between the primary therapist and the student is stressed by devoting weekly contact specifically to this purpose (as appears to be the case in the Ben-Yishay and Gold description). Thus, whereas these three rehabilitation day programmes share the same objectives and similar treatment approaches, the manner in which they combine and emphasize certain interventions over others may differ. This, the authors believe, is due in part to the cultural differences in Scandinavian and North American education traditions, the former stressing a phenomenological approach and the latter a normative tradition.

Conclusions

Due to the complex and radical nature of acquired brain injury, a holistic, neuropsychologically oriented postacute rehabilitation programme is presented as a means of effectively addressing these issues. The programme in use at The Center for Rehabilitation of Brain Injury is an example of such an approach. Essential to this rehabilitation approach is a model of brain–behaviour functioning for evaluation and rehabilitation planning. In order effectively to individualize the rehabilitation plan within a structured rehabilitation programme, the evaluation process is crucial: not only must the current cognitive, emotional, social and physical status of the patient be identified, but premorbid functioning and future aspirations also need to be considered. Furthermore, the broader psychosocial systems, namely that of significant others, and work/education environments must be taken into account. The evaluation process is not a static one, but rather requires constant monitoring to ensure a consistently appropriate treatment plan, with emphasis on encouraging patients to be aware of their level of skill acquisition.

Treatment can only be effective if rehabilitation goals

are individualized within the various programme activities, which should consist of a combination of individual and group tasks. The individual activities allow for highly specific interventions to be made, while the group activities provide the opportunity for social interaction and support. In order for treatment goals to be achieved, the staff need to work as an interdisciplinary team in which one therapist is the primary therapist. Other staff members must assist the primary therapist in maintaining the effective management of the brain-injured patient's needs. Active collaboration by the patients is essential. The essence of goal setting is to help patients to reintergrate all those elements of self and their responses to the external world that have been brought into disequilibrium by the brain injury. This is done by encouraging an active focus on life goals to overcome the inhibitory and defensive aspects of the difficulties caused by the brain injury.

Whereas a theoretical basis for rehabilitation application is crucial, it is the combination of the various programme elements into a stimulating and ecologically valid therapeutic milieu that is important. The milieu is one which closely resembles 'real life' in terms of task demands and social interactions, while providing a safe environment wherein the self-confidence of the brain-injured individual can be restored. A day programme is often the bridge between the dependency of inpatient hospital care and the demands for self-reliance from the external environment. The combined approach of providing a day programme followed by a period of support during the subsequent phase of returning to occupational or educational pursuits ensures that the patient will not be overextended prematurely, thus reducing the possibility of the development of a negative emotional spiral concerning self-worth and functional ability.

Because of the heterogenous nature of brain injury, the basic questions of what type of rehabilitation should be given to which type of patient at what point in time have not been answered. However, the different programmes offered are intended to serve the needs of different populations, such that the characteristics of one particular programme will be effective for specific constellations of brain injury sequelae. It has been argued that research methodology is required to address these issues in a more stringent manner. (See High, Boake and Lehmkuhl (1995) for an analysis of the difficulties inherent in current studies and recommendations for minimizing these concerns.)

The individual differences inherent in the human brain combined with the vastly different premorbid characteristics of individuals make a single approach highly unlikely to be successful, and it is obvious that a general 'recipe' cannot be provided for the treatment of brain injury. Nonetheless, a general humanistic view – based on findings from other areas such as education and health services which stress growth, stimulation and positive expectations of the person in need of support – can be advocated as providing the guidelines for effective treatment.

References

Asmussen, E. and Hohwü-Christensen, E. 1980. *Idreatsteori – Fysiologi og Kinesiology (Sports Theory – Physiology and Kinesiology)*. Copenhagen: Akademisk Forlag.

Ästrand, I. and Rodahl, K. 1970. Aerobic work capacity in men and women with special reference to age. *Acta Physiol Scand* **49** (Suppl.), 169.

Ben-Yishay, Y. and Diller, L. 1993. Cognitive remediation in traumatic brain injury: update and issues. *Arch Phys Med Rehabil* **74**, 204–13.

Ben-Yishay, Y. and Gold, J. 1990. Therapeutic milieu approach to neuropsychological rehabilitation. In *Neurobehavioural Sequelae of Traumatic Brain Injury*, ed. R.L. Wood, pp. 194–218. New York: Taylor & Francis.

Ben-Yishay, Y., Silver, S.M., Piasetsky, E. and Rattok, J. 1987. Relationship between employability and vocational outcome after intensive holistic cognitive rehabilitation. *J Head Trauma Rehabil* **2**, 35–48.

Boake, C. 1991. History of cognitive rehabilitation following head injury. In *Cognitive Rehabilitation for Persons with Traumatic Brain Injury: a Functional Approach*, ed. J.S.Kreutzer and P.H. Wehman, pp. 3–12. Baltimore: Paul H. Brookes.

Brickenkamp, R. 1981. *Test d2: Aufmerksamkeits-Belastungs-Test: Handanweisung*, 7th edn (*Test d2: Concentration-Endurance Test: Manual*, 7th edn). Göttingen: Verlag für Psychologie.

Brooks, N., Campsie, L., Symington, C., Beattie, A. and McKinlay, W. 1986. The five year outcome of severe blunt head injury: a relative's view. *J. Neurol Neurosurg Psychiatry* **49**, 764–70.

Christensen, A.L. 1975. *Luria's Neuropsychological Investigation. Manual and Test Materials*, 1st edn. New York: Spectrum.

Christensen, A.L., Caetano, C. and Rasmussen, G. 1996. Psychosocial outcome after an intensive neuropsychologically oriented day program: contributing program variables. In *Recovery after Traumatic Brain Injury*, ed. B.P. Uzzell and H.H. Stonnington, pp. 235–46. Mahwah, NJ: Lawrence Erlbaum.

Christensen, A.L., Jensen, L.R. and Risberg, J. 1990. Luria's neuropsychological and neurolinguistic theory. *J Neurolinguistics* **4**, 137–54.

Christensen, A.L., Malmros, R. and Townes, B.D. 1987. Rehabilitation planned in accordance with the Luria neuropsychological investigation: a case history of a patient with left sided aneurysm. *Neuropsychology* **1**, 45–8.

Christensen, A.L., Pinner, E.M., Møller-Pedersen, P., Teasdale, T.W. and Trexler, L.E. 1992. Psychosocial outcome following individualized neuropsychological rehabilitation of brain damage. *Acta Neurol Scand* **85**, 32–8.

Christensen, A.L. and Teasdale, T.W. 1993. A comprehensive and intensive program for cognitive and psychosocial rehabilitation. In *Developments in the Assessment and Rehabilitation of Brain-damaged Patients*, ed. F.J. Stachowiak et al., pp. 465–7. Tubingen: Gunter Narr Verlag.

Christensen, A.L. and Uzzell, B.P. eds. 1988. *Neuropsychological Rehabilitation*. Boston: Kluwer Academic Publishers.

Cooper, K.H. 1968. *Aerobics*. New York: Evans.

Diller, L. 1990. Fostering the interdisciplinary team, fostering research in a society in transition (Congress Presidential Address). *Arch Phys Med Rehabil* **71**, 275–8.

Gade, A. and Mortensen, E.L. 1984. The influence of age, education and intelligence on neuropsychological test performance. Presented at the Third Nordic Conference in Behavioural Toxicology, December, 1994. Aarhus, Denmark.

Goldstein, K. 1942. *Aftereffects of Brain Injuries in War: their Evaluation and Treatment*. London: Heinemann.

Goldstein, K. 1952. Effects of brain damage on personality. *Psychiatry* **15**, 245–60.

Goodglass, H. and Kaplan, E. 1983. *The Assessment of Aphasia and Related Disorders*, 2nd edn. Philadelphia: Lea & Febiger.

Gronwall, D.M.A. 1977. Paced Auditory Serial-Addition Task: a measure of recovery from concussion. *Percept Mot Skills* **44**, 367–73.

Hall, K.M. and Cope, D.N. 1995. The benefits of rehabilitation in traumatic brain injury: a literature review. *J Head Trauma Rehabil* **10**(1), 1–13.

High, W.M., Boake, C. and Lehmkuhl, L.D. 1995. Critical analysis of studies evaluating the effectiveness of rehabilitation after traumatic brain injury. *J Head Trauma Rehabil* **10**(1), 13–26.

Larrabee, G.J. and Crook, T.H. 1991. Computerized memory testing in clinical trials. In *Handbook of Clinical Trials: the*

Neurobehavioural Approach, ed. E.Mohr and P. Brouwers, pp. 293–306. Amsterdam: Swets & Zeitlinger.

Larsen, A., Mehlbye, J. and Gørtz, M. 1991. *Kan Genoptræning Betale sig? En Analyse of de Sociale og Økonomiske Aspekter ved Genoptræning af Hjerneskadede* (Does Rehabilitation Pay? An Analysis of the Social and Economic Aspects of Brain Injury Rehabilitation). Copenhagen: AKF Forlaget.

Lezak, M.D. 1995. *Neuropsychological Assessment*, 3rd edn. Oxford: Oxford University Press.

Luria, A.R. 1963, *Restoration of Function after Brain Injury*, tr. Basil Haigh. London: Pergamon Press. (Original work published 1948.)

Luria, A.R. 1966. *Higher Cortical Functions in Man*. London: Tavistock.

Luria, A.R. 1973. *The Working Brain: an Introduction to Neuropsychology*. Harmondsworth, Middlesex: Penguin.

Luria, A.R., Naydin, V.L., Tsvetskova, L.S. and Vinarskaya, E.N.1969. Restoration of higher cortical function following local brain damage. In *Handbook of Clinical Neurology*, ed. P.J. Vinken and G.W. Bruyn, Vol. 3: *Disorders of Higher Nervous Activity*, pp. 368–433. Amsterdam: North-Holland.

Mesulam, M.M. 1985. *Principles of Behavioral Neurology*. Philadelphia: F.A. Davis.

Mulder, T. 1997. Current topics in motor control: implications for rehabilitation. In *Neurological Rehabilitation*, ed. R.J. Greenwood, M.P. Barnes, T.M. MacMillan and C.D. Ward, Edinburgh: Churchill Livingstone.

Prigatano, G.P., Fordyce, D.J., Zeiner, H.K., Roueche, J.R., Pepping, M. and Wood, B.C. 1984. Neuropsychological rehabilitation after closed head injury in young adults. *J Neurol Neurosurg Psychiatry* 47, 505–13.

Prigatano, G.P., Fordyce, D.J., Zeiner, H.K., Roueche, J.R., Pepping, M. and Wood, B.C. 1986. *Neuropsychological Rehabilitation after Brain Injury*. Baltimore: Johns Hopkins University Press.

Prigatano, G.P. and Schacter, D.L. 1991. *Awareness of Deficit after Brain Injury: Clinical and Theoretical Issues*. New York: Oxford University Press.

Raven, J.C. 1965. *Advanced Progressive Matrices Sets I & II*. London: H.K. Lewis.

Sbordone, R.J., Liter, J.C. and Pettler-Jennings, P. 1995. Recovery of function following severe traumatic brain injury: a retrospective 10-year follow-up. *Brain Inj* 9, 285–99.

Shallice, T. and Burgess, P.W. 1991. Deficits in strategy application following frontal lobe damage in man. *Brain* 114, 727–41.

Sohlberg, M.M. and Mateer, C.A. 1989. *Introduction to Cognitive Rehabilitation: Theory and Practice*. New York: Guilford Press.

Stein, D.G., Glasier, M.M. and Hoffman, S.W. 1994. Pharmacological treatments for brain-injury repair: progress and prognosis. In *Brain Injury and Neuropsychological Rehabilitation: International Perspectives*, ed. A.L. Christensen and B.P. Uzzell, pp. 17–40. Hillsdale, NJ: Lawrence Erlbaum.

Stuss, D.T. and Benson, D.F. 1990. The frontal lobes and language. In *Contemporary Neuropsychology and the Legacy of Luria*, ed. E. Goldberg, pp. 29–49. Hillsdale, NJ: Lawrence Erlbaum.

Teasdale, T.W. and Christensen, A.L. 1994. Psychosocial outcome in Denmark. In *Brain Injury and Neuropsychological Rehabilitation: International Perspectives*, ed. A.L. Christensen and B.P. Uzzell, pp. 35–244. Hillsdale, NJ: Lawrence Erlbaum.

Teasdale, T.W., Christensen, A.-L., Willmes, K. et al. 1997. Subjective experience in brain injured patients and their close relatives: a European Brain Injury Questionnaire study. *Brain Injury* 11(8), 543–63.

Thomsen, I.V. 1984. Late outcome of very severe blunt head trauma: a 10–15 year second follow-up. *J Neurol Neurosurg Psychiatry* 47, 260–8.

Thomsen, I.V. 1992. Late psychosocial outcome in severe traumatic brain injury. Preliminary results of a third follow-up study after 20 years. *Scand J Rehabil Med* 26 (Suppl.), 142–52.

Verstraeten, S. 1996. *Disconnection Syndrome: a Case Report*. Unpublished manuscript.

Wechsler, D. 1981. *Wechsler Adult Intelligence Scale – Revised Manual*. New York: The Psychological Corporation.

Wechsler, D. 1987. *Wechsler Memory Scale – Revised Manual*. San Antonio, TX: The Psychological Corporation.

Wilson, B. 1987. *The Rehabilitation of Memory*. New York: Guilford Press.

Wilson, B.A. 1993. How do we know that rehabilitation works? [Editorial]. *Neuropsychol Rehabil* 3, 1–4.

12

Outcome measurement in cognitive neurorehabilitation

Nadina Lincoln

Introduction

The aim of the chapter is to consider the criteria for selecting outcome measures for evaluating the effects of cognitive neurorehabilitation. The International Classification of Impairments, Disabilities and Handicaps (World Health Organization, 1980) is used as a framework for deciding what to measure. The properties of the ideal outcome measure are discussed. Examples of outcome measures commonly used in clinical studies are provided and their strengths and limitations considered. Finally, areas in which there is scope for further development of outcome measures are presented.

Outcome

- Outcomes may be assessed at the levels of impairment, disability or handicap.
- Disability measures are the most important outcomes for cognitive rehabilitation.
- Quality of life is best assessed as component domains rather than a single measure.

Rehabilitation may be considered in terms of process, structure and outcome. Process consists of the activities which are designed to improve the functioning of the individual. This includes the treatment techniques used by members of the multidisciplinary team, designed to foster recovery or adaptation. Structure refers to the facilities provided to enable the treatments to be administered, such as the environment, staff and equipment. Outcome refers to the result of the rehabilitation endeavour. It is the endpoint of rehabilitation

against which its effectiveness is judged. In cognitive rehabilitation, the aim is to help the patient to function to the maximum level of ability possible within the constraints of deficits resulting from brain damage. In addition, that individual should be as contented and satisfied with his or her condition as is possible, and so should the relatives. The assessment of outcome is the means by which we determine whether rehabilitation has achieved these aims.

Measurement of outcome

The International Classification of Impairments, Disabilities and Handicap (World Health Organization, 1980) provides a useful framework for the selection of appropriate outcome measures. The definitions are as follows.

Impairment: the loss or abnormality of psychological, physiological or anatomical structure or function. It includes cognitive deficits such as disorders of memory, attention, apraxia and aphasia.

Disability: the restriction or lack of ability to perform an activity within the range considered normal for a human being. It is the behavioural consequences of an impairment, such as the loss of ability to walk, dress, earn a living and participate in social activities. It also includes the effects of cognitive impairments on daily life, such as difficulties in telling the time and losing items around the home.

Handicap: the disadvantage, resulting from an impairment or disability, that prevents the fulfillment of a role that is normal (depending on age, sex, social and cultural factors) for that individual. It represents the social, cultural, economic and environmental effects of impairments and disabilities. It will include the disruption to interpersonal relationships that may occur following a head injury.

Usually, an impairment such as visual inattention will give rise to a disability, such as the inability to dress independently, which in turn will give rise to a handicap, namely loss of personal independence. However, some disabilities may not lead to handicap, for example an inability to read may have no effect on the lifestyle of a person who has no desire to read for pleasure and is happy to rely on others for essential reading activities such as dealing with domestic bills. An effective rehabilitation programme would reduce the impairments and the disabilities which are consequent upon those impairments. In many instances, it is not possible to ameliorate the impairment, but nevertheless significant gains may be made by attempting directly to reduce the disability. Although it would be desirable to reduce handicap, this can rarely be achieved directly and it is often not within the remit of the rehabilitation team. Provided the disability has been reduced, the assumption is that it will have a beneficial effect on handicap. Even so, it is clearly important to know whether an intervention has an effect on handicap and therefore it is appropriate to consider measures of handicap as outcome measures for cognitive rehabilitation.

Quality of life is another elusive outcome which relates to handicap in that the less the handicap, the greater the quality of life. Most assessments of quality of life incorporate several domains, which include both disabilities and handicaps. It is beyond the scope of assessment procedures adequately to assess all the domains which contribute to quality of life and produce a satisfactory single quality-of-life measure. For this reason it does not seem practical at present even to attempt to assess quality of life in general, but rather only the specific domains, even though improving the quality of life of those who receive rehabilitation must be the ultimate goal of rehabilitation.

Selection of measures

- Measures of motor, sensory, visual and cognitive impairment provide standardized descriptions of patients.

- Motor impairment measures include measures of tone, strength, control and range of movement.
- The sensory impairment measures used in clinical practice are often unreliable.

In order to choose an outcome measure, it is important to know that the measure meets the requirements of a measurement tool. These requirements are as follows.

Validity: any measure must measure what it purports to measure. For example, measures of activities of daily living should include those activities that most people would consider to be essential for personal independence in daily life. Measures should relate to other measures of the same underlying ability and include all the relevant aspects of the attributes they measure. Hypotheses generated based on the measure should be upheld. For example, one would predict that head-injured people will do less well on a measure of memory than normal subjects, and if this is supported it indicates that the measure has construct validity.

Reliability: any outcome measure should provide the same information if used by different assessors (interrater reliability) or by the same assessor on different occasions (intrarater reliability). If the assessment is to be used to monitor change, it needs to have minimal practice effects and to show no variation simply as a result of repeating the assessment (test–retest reliability).

Sensitivity: outcome measures in rehabilitation may be reliable and valid but unless they are sensitive to change, i.e. able to detect change in ability when change has occurred, and responsive to differences between rehabilitation programmes, they will not evaluate rehabilitation outcome.

Practicality: the selection of outcome measures is dominated by practical constraints. An outcome measure must be short enough to be used in a clinical or research setting, easy to administer and acceptable to patients. Those measures which are tiring, detailed, intrusive or repetitive will not be tolerated. It must also be easy to communicate the findings to others.

Many studies evaluating the effects of cognitive rehabilitation have used single-case experimental designs. Measures are repeated frequently and therefore need to be short, less disruptive to the patient and with minimal practice effects. When using a randomized controlled trial to evaluate an intervention, it is necessary to use measures which have been used in other studies. It is difficult to conduct a trial of cognitive rehabilitation with sufficient patients to be sure that a small difference in outcome has not been missed, yet from a patient's perspective even a small gain in function may be worthwhile. A common strategy to resolve this is to conduct a meta-analysis of several trials, which is facilitated by the use of a common outcome measure. Therefore, the ideal outcome measures need to be valid, reliable, sensitive and practical.

Measures of impairment

Cognitive rehabilitation is designed to improve cognitive abilities. Most cognitive impairments can be assessed by a wide range of measures but few have been designed as measures of outcome. Some cognitive assessments are intended as screening devices, to identify cognitive impairments which require further evaluation. Others are diagnostic tools, to differentiate cognitive impairments from each other. Assessments for screening or diagnostic purposes may not be suitable measures of outcome. Measures of cognitive impairment are mentioned in later chapters and therefore are not reviewed in detail here. However, impairments other than cognitive deficits may affect a patient's response to a cognitive rehabilitation programme, and it is therefore appropriate to assess these. They will not be used as outcome assessments as few cognitive rehabilitation techniques would be expected to decrease, for example, motor impairments. However, the treatment of visual inattention could be predicted to reduce sensory inattention or visual field deficits. For this reason, such assessments are considered. The impairments to be assessed are motor function, sensory function and visual abilities.

Motor function may be subdivided into muscle tone, muscle strength, movement control and range of movement. The main measure of muscle tone is the modified Ashworth Scale (Bohannon and Smith, 1987) for grading spasticity. It is a six-point ordinal scale which measures velocity-dependent resistance to passive movement and, by the addition of a grade, ranks where the resistance appears in the range of movement. It has

good interrater reliability (Sloan et al., 1992) but test–retest reliability seems not to have been established. Muscle strength is generally assessed using the Medical Research Council grades, which are an ordinal scale of power used for both the lower and upper limbs. The grades are widely used in clinical practice but lack sensitivity. A refinement of this scale is the Motricity Index (Demeurisse, Demol and Robaye, 1980), which is useful for a wide range of patients with upper motor neuron weakness. There are also more specific measures of muscle strength which have the advantage of greater sensitivity to change. Grip strength provides a single index of upper limb impairment which covers a wide range of ability. Sunderland et al. (1989) compared grip strength to alternative measures of arm function and found grip strength to be the most sensitive. Dynamometry has been used (Wiles and Karni, 1983; Bohannon and Andrews, 1987) and is reasonably reliable, though lengthy to administer. Impairment measures of control include the pursuit rotor, a measure of hand–eye co-ordination, used for research purposes but rarely in clinical practice. The pursuit rotor is easy and quick to administer but only appropriate for those with mild levels of impairment. Balance is a complex aspect of motor control. Various versions of balance performance monitor are available which record weight distribution laterally and anterior–posteriorly and include indices of sway. These can be used to assess outcomes of treatment (Sackley and Lincoln, 1997) as well as providing a global measure of postural control.

Summed indices encompass several impairments within one index to examine motor function as a composite scale. There have been several motor impairment scales developed for stroke patients, e.g. Rivermead Motor Assessment (Lincoln and Leadbitter, 1979), Motor Club Assessment (Ashburn, 1982), Motor Assessment Scale (Carr et al., 1985), but there are few equivalent measures for those with head injury, though the Rivermead Motor Assessment was originally developed with this group. Motor impairments are assessed in batteries designed for patients with Parkinson's disease, such as Lieberman's Index (Lieberman, 1974) and the Webster Rating Scale (Webster, 1968). However, there is limited information on the reliability of these scales or their sensitivity to change with rehabilitation. The Kurtzke Multiple Sclerosis Rating Scale (Kurtzke,

1965) assesses aspects of motor function in the Functional Systems Scale but lacks sensitivity to intervention. The Expanded Disability Status Scale (Kurtzke, 1983), despite its name, is a measure of impairments in multiple sclerosis based on the number of functional systems which are affected.

Sensory impairment is assessed as part of a clinical examination but there are few standardized scales. Some studies have demonstrated that assessment of sensory impairment is unreliable (Tomasello et al., 1982, Lincoln, Crow and Jackson, 1991), though Lincoln, Jackson and Adams (1998) found that the Nottingham Sensory Assessment can be reliable when administered exactly according to the instructions. Tactile inattention, proprioception and stereognosis are relevant aspects of sensation which may affect the outcome of cognitive rehabilitation. It is important that they are assessed using standardized measures, but there are no tests to be recommended.

Visual impairment will affect patients' ability to perform cognitive assessments and participate in cognitive rehabilitation. Therefore, it needs to be documented, but conventional acuity measurement techniques require language skills, and visual field assessment using standard perimetry may be confounded by the presence of inattention (Walker et al., 1991).

Cognitive impairments are assessed by a wide range of psychological tests. Assessments are available to determine the severity of deficits in language, perception, memory, reasoning, attention, movement disorders and other cognitive functions. These are well described in textbooks of neuropsychology (Spreen and Strauss, 1991; Crawford, Parker and McKinlay, 1992; Lezak, 1995). In order for a cognitive assessment to be used as an outcome measure, it must be sensitive to changes over time but have minimal practice effects. For example, although recognition memory tests are sensitive to differences between individuals, they are not appropriate for evaluating change unless there are parallel versions available. It is for this reason that a memory battery such as the Adult Memory and Information Processing Battery (Coughlan and Hollows, 1985) is more appropriate for measuring the effects of intervention than, for example, the Wechsler Memory Scale – Revised (Wechsler, 1987). Many cognitive tests, while reliable over time, will show sufficient improvement simply as a result of practice to make them insensitive to differences between interventions.

Disability

- Disabilities which need to be measured include motor, functional, emotional and cognitive disabilities.
- The most important outcomes for cognitive rehabilitation are cognitive disabilities, yet the measurement of these is poorly developed.
- Independence in activities of daily living and mood measures provide proxy measures for the outcome of cognitive rehabilitation.
- The Barthel Index, Extended Activities of Daily Living, Frenchay Activities Index and Functional Independence Measure are the most suitable measures of activities of daily living.
- Mood should be assessed on questionnaires designed to detect change.

The main aim of cognitive rehabilitation is the reduction of disability, which includes motor, functional, cognitive, emotional and social disabilities.

Physical disability

Most assessments of motor function are based on impairment, but functional motor skills are important to the patient. Walking is probably the most important outcome of successful rehabilitation. The timed 10 m walk test is a quick, sensitive measure, but may not be practical when patients are assessed at home. Categorical scales of walking ability, such as the Functional Ambulation Category (Holden et al., 1984) and Hauser Ambulation Index (Hauser et al., 1983), are less sensitive. The Rivermead Mobility Index (Collen et al., 1991) is a comprehensive assessment of motor disability which includes sitting, transfers and stairs in addition to walking. It has been used as an outcome measure in rehabilitation studies on stroke (Wade et al., 1992) and has been demonstrated to be sensitive in people with multiple sclerosis (Vaney et al., 1996). Sections on motor disability are included in composite disability scales. For example, the Extended Activities of Daily Living Scale (Nouri and Lincoln, 1987) and the Short Form 36 (Stewart and Ware, 1992) include advanced mobility such as walking outside and climbing several flights of stairs. Many of the composite scales also assess impairment and disability in arm function. The Action Research Arm Test (Lyle, 1981) and Frenchay Arm Test (Heller et al., 1987) have both been used as outcome measures in trials of rehabilitation (Crow et al., 1989; Sunderland et al., 1992).

Functional abilities

The ability to perform functional activities in everyday life may be assessed by scales of activities of daily living. These scales deal with basic personal self-care skills and instrumental activities of daily living. The choice of scale is governed by practical considerations. Some scales assess capabilities, i.e. what the patient can do, for example the Northwick Park (Benjamin, 1976) and Rivermead (Whiting and Lincoln, 1980) activities of daily living scales, and others assess performance, i.e. what the patient does do, for example the Barthel Index (Mahoney and Barthel, 1965) and Functional Independence Measure (Granger, Hamilton and Sherwin, 1986). The reason for asking what a patient does do is that this is more likely to be reliable and in most cases a more accurate reflection of the level of disability. The method of administration influences the content of the scales. Items on continence have to be observed and are not included in scales designed to be administered. Most activities of daily living scales consist of a variety of items which are summed to provide an overall score. Concerns have been expressed about treating such summed indices as ordinal scales, but some have been demonstrated by the use of Guttman scaling to be hierarchical, e.g. Rivermead and Barthel, and others have been shown to be acceptable using a Rasch model, e.g. Barthel and Functional Independence Measure.

The Barthel Index (Mahoney and Barthel, 1965) is a widely used measure of personal activities of daily living which has almost become the gold standard for stroke rehabilitation studies. It is sensitive to differences between rehabilitation interventions (Indredavik et al.,

1991), reliable when administered verbally or by post, and is particularly appropriate in the early stages of rehabilitation or for those with severe disabilities. It is not sensitive to change in community-based patients or those with mild motor impairments. It is most commonly used for stroke and elderly patients but has also been demonstrated to be reliable and valid with other neurological patients. The original index was scored on a 0–100-scale, but this implies a spurious degree of accuracy and the revised 20-point version (Collin et al., 1988) is becoming the standard. Wade (1992) recommends that this is the best activities of daily living measure available. However, there are other measures which differ slightly in format and content. The Katz Index (Katz et al., 1963) is a long-established, reliable index covering items similar to those of the Barthel Index, but instead of giving an overall score provides a descriptive category based on the number of activities in which a person is independent. While this is reasonable, it does not facilitate communication or statistical analysis of results. The Rivermead Scale (Whiting and Lincoln, 1980; Lincoln and Edmans, 1990) covers similar items to the Barthel Index in its self-care scale but also has sections on domestic activities. The Northwick Park Index (Benjamin, 1976) also includes a wider range of activities than the Barthel Index, but has an awkward scale ranging from 17 to 51 which does not lead to easy communication of results. The main limitation of the Barthel Index is its ceiling effect: patients scoring 20 may have significant disabilities in activities of daily living. Therefore, rehabilitation studies may include a measure of instrumental activities of daily living in addition to the Barthel Index.

Two widely used measures of instrumental activities of daily living are the Extended Activities of Daily Living (Nouri and Lincoln, 1987) and the Frenchay Activities Index (Holbrook and Skilbeck, 1983). Each of these includes domestic activities such as preparing meals and washing up, mobility outside the home, leisure and social activities. The former is scored according to whether the item is done independently or with help, and the latter according to the frequency of the item within the previous three or six months. Both scales have been found to be sensitive to differences between rehabilitation interventions (Forster and Young, 1996;

Fuller, Dawson and Wiles, 1996). The Extended Activities of Daily Living Scale is suitable for multi-centre studies as it has been validated as a postal assessment. The original scoring has been modified to make the scale more sensitive (Juby, Berman and Lincoln, 1996). The Frenchay Activities Index is not suitable for use in the early stages of rehabilitation, as the previous three months will include activities prior to the onset of the disability. Cognitive rehabilitation programmes are probably more likely to have an effect on instrumental activities of daily living rather than on personal self-care skills. Therefore, these scales are likely to be more appropriate measures for assessing the generalization of cognitive retraining to daily life skills.

There are some specific aspects of activities of daily living performance that are particularly dependent on cognitive abilities. For example, there is a close relationship between independent dressing skills and perceptual abilities in stroke patients. The Nottingham Dressing Assessment (Walker and Lincoln, 1990) was devised to provide a detailed measure of dressing skills and has been shown to be sensitive to a dressing intervention (Walker, Drummond and Lincoln, 1996). Another specific activity likely to be influenced by cognitive rehabilitation is the ability to participate in leisure activities. There are scales designed to assess leisure participation (Jongbloed and Morgan, 1991; Drummond and Walker, 1994) which have been used in randomized controlled trials of leisure rehabilitation (Jongbloed and Morgan, 1991; Drummond and Walker, 1996).

Most of the above scales have been developed on stroke patients and used in trials of rehabilitation after stroke. Although some have been used with other groups of patients, there is not as much information on the sensitivity of the scales to rehabilitation interventions. The main measure of personal activities of daily living used with a wide range of diagnostic groups is the Functional Independence Measure (Granger et al., 1986). This covers personal self-care and motor activities and has cognitive items on comprehension, expression, social interaction, problem solving and memory. It is particularly appropriate for assessing those with head injury and multiple sclerosis as it includes the cognitive and social aspects. Interrater reliability has been found to be high for items assessing physical disability but low on communication and social cognition sections (Brosseau and Wolfson, 1994; Kidd et al., 1995; Pollak, Rheuault and Stoecker, 1996). Because the effect of a cognitive rehabilitation programme is most relevant to these items, further development of the scale to improve its reliability is clearly needed. Rasch analysis has indicated that the motor and cognitive items form two distinct scales, though this has been questioned by Dickson and Kohler (1996), who identified six factors from a factor analysis of the Functional Independence Measure. It seems that the motor section of the Functional Independence Measure is an acceptable scale of personal independence in the activities of daily living. It is more sensitive to minor changes in the amount of assistance needed than the Barthel Index, but at the expense of some loss of reliability. It may be difficult to use in trials of rehabilitation if it is to be used by an assessor who is not familiar with the patient, but it is a useful measure of progress when administered by those involved in a patient's treatment. The cognitive items form a separate scale, which has not been validated independently of the motor items. The cognitive scale needs independent validation against measures of cognitive function and administration requires prolonged observation of the patient, which means the scale would be difficult to administer in the context of a randomized controlled trial by an independent assessor.

The Functional Assessment Measure, which was developed to assess the specific problems of brain-injured patients (Hall et al., 1993), contains additional items which give greater emphasis to the cognitive, communicative and psychosocial function. McPherson et al. (1996) evaluated the interrater reliability of the Functional Independence Measure and Functional Assessment Measure and found high agreement between the raters, but greatest discrepancies occurred on cognitive, communication and behavioural items. The assessment also took approximately an hour to administer, which is longer than alternative indices. For the Functional Assessment Measure to be used to evaluate the outcome of treatment, particularly cognitive rehabilitation, further work is needed to check the repeat reliability, validity and sensitivity to the effects of different interventions.

The Rivermead Head Injury Follow-Up Questionnaire (Crawford, Wenden and Wade, 1996) has been developed as an outcome measure for patients with mild to moderate head injury. It is a short, simple measure which can be administered by post and at interview. It was found to have good interrater reliability, to be sensitive to changes over time and to detect differences in outcome in a randomized controlled trial (Wade et al., 1997). However, further validation and reliability checks are required and its value with people with severe head injuries needs to be assessed.

Measures of disability for people with multiple sclerosis seem to be few. The Kurtzke scales, although called disability scales, are actually measures of impairment. The Functional Independence Measure (Brosseau and Wolfson, 1994) and Assessment of Motor and Process Skills (Doble et al., 1994) have been used, but there are few data on which to base a decision about the most appropriate measure for this group. The Assessment of Motor and Process Skills requires patients to perform tasks and so takes longer, but it covers instrumental activities of daily living, which may be more important to assess than personal activities of daily living, when the effects of cognitive rehabilitation are being evaluated.

Some measures of activities of daily living are available for those with Parkinson's disease and other movement disorders (Wade, 1992), for example the North-western University Disability Scales (Canter, De la Torre and Mier, 1961), the Self Assessment Parkinson's Disease Disability Scale (Brown et al., 1989) and the Unified Parkinson's Disease Rating Scale (Lang and Fahn, 1989). These mix impairments and disabilities, include items which would not come within the conventional definition of activities of daily living, and there are few reliability studies.

In addition to the condition-specific activities of daily living measures, there are general rehabilitation outcome measures, which are predominantly measures of disability. The Sickness Impact Profile (Bergner et al., 1981), the British version of which is the Functional Limitations Profile (Charlton, Patrick and Peach, 1983), assesses the impact of sickness on daily activities and behaviour. It provides subscales in 12 areas, including ambulation, body care and household management. It is lengthy, though it has been suggested that the subscales could be used on their own (Bowling, 1991).

Mood

Although mood disorders might be considered either as an impairment, i.e. a direct consequence of some underlying pathology, or as a disability, the consequence of impairments, in the context of cognitive rehabilitation they are probably best considered as emotional disabilities. Various mood assessment scales have been developed but relatively few have been validated for patients with neurological disorders. Mood may be assessed by interview or questionnaire, the latter having the advantage of greater standardization and less experience needed to administer the assessment. Those which have a large proportion of items affected by physical disability are likely to be insensitive to mood changes in neurological patients. Many of the mood questionnaires were developed as screening devices to detect significant levels of depression or anxiety. To evaluate the outcome of cognitive neuro-rehabilitation, measures also have to be sensitive to change and therefore not all screening questionnaires will be suitable for this purpose.

The Hospital Anxiety and Depression Scale (Zigmund and Snaith, 1983) is a short, easy measure which provides separate scores for both anxiety and depression. Although it was designed for hospitalized medically ill patients, several items reflect physical disability rather than mood. It is probably more suitable as a screening measure than for assessing outcome. The Wakefield Depression Inventory (Snaith et al., 1971) is also principally a screening measure but is more sensitive than the Hospital Anxiety and Depression Scale to the effects of intervention (Lincoln et al., 1997). The Self-Rating Depression Scale (Zung, 1965) serves a similar purpose but includes items which are not appropriate for the elderly or those with physical disabilities. In contrast, other scales, such as the Beck Depression Inventory (Beck et al., 1961) and Center for Epidemiologic Studies Depression Scale (Radloff, 1977), were designed as measures of the severity of depressive symptoms. They are likely to be more sensitive to the effects of intervention than measures designed for screening purposes.

Cognitive rehabilitation would be expected to decrease the likelihood that someone is depressed. If cognitive impairment is recognized and explained and patients are given strategies to cope with their cognitive problems, they will probably suffer from less depression. Patients may also become less anxious or suffer less general distress. Anxiety measures, apart from the Hospital Anxiety and Depression Scale, have rarely been used as outcome measures for studies of rehabilitation. The most widely used measure of general psychological distress is the General Health Questionnaire (Goldberg and Williams, 1988). The GHQ28 has been found to be sensitive to the effects of rehabilitation (Juby et al., 1996) but may cause problems if administered as a postal assessment because of items about suicide causing distress. There are fewer of these in the GHQ30, but this version does not have subscale scores for different components of psychological distress, which can be useful. The GHQ12 is shorter and has few distressing items, but its sensitivity to the effects of intervention in neurological patients has not been established.

One problem in assessing mood in neurological patients is that many have communication difficulties. There have been attempts to develop scales so that these patients may be assessed. The Delighted–Terrible Faces Scale (Andrews and Withey, 1976) consists of pictorial representations of faces varying in expression from very happy through neutral to very miserable. It has been found to be acceptable in studies of the elderly (Bowling and Browne, 1991) and stroke patients (Anderson, 1992) but the distribution of scores in both studies was skewed. The Stroke Aphasic Depression Questionnaire (Sutcliffe and Lincoln, 1998) was developed to assess mood in aphasic patients. Items that could be observed by relatives or nursing staff were taken from mood questionnaires and rephrased in terms of observable behaviours. The scale was validated in comparison with the Hospital Anxiety and Depression Scale and the Wakefield Depression Inventory and was found to be valid when used by carers but not by nursing staff. The Neuropsychiatric Inventory (Cummings et al., 1994) was developed to assess mood disorders in dementia. Ten domains of psychopathology, such as delusions, dysphoria and anxiety, are rated on the basis of an interview with a carer. The scale has good validity and reliability, but its sensitivity to change in response to treatment has not been established.

Cognitive disability

Cognitive disability is the most important outcome for cognitive rehabilitation. The most common strategy has been to develop a questionnaire that includes items on the behavioural manifestations of a particular cognitive impairment. These items may be completed by patients or relatives, or both, to determine the subjective effects of cognitive impairment on daily life. These effects are important indicators of the outcome of cognitive neurorehabilitation but there are few scales available and not all possible cognitive deficits are included.

Subjective memory impairment has been investigated using the Everyday Memory Questionnaire (Sunderland, Harris and Baddeley, 1983) in studies of stroke (Tinson and Lincoln, 1987), head injury (Sunderland et al., 1984) and multiple sclerosis patients (Taylor, 1990). The questionnaire has been used both for patients to assess their own problems and for relatives to assess the difficulties of the patients. It has validity in that it correlates reasonably well with tests of memory ability, and its reliability is acceptable, though not good. The Cognitive Failures Questionnaire (Broadbent et al., 1982) is similar, with versions both for patients and for others. It is less specific to memory and includes the behavioural consequences of other cognitive deficits. The Subjective Memory Assessment Questionnaire (Davis et al., 1995) is shorter and has been validated for stroke patients. The Memory Failures Questionnaire (Gilewski, Zelinski and Schaie, 1990) contains more items which form four subscales, including one on the use of mnemonics. There is conflicting evidence on the extent to which it correlates with prospective memory (Zelinski, Gilewski and Anthony-Bergstone, 1990; Kinsella et al., 1996), but further development is required.

The behavioural manifestations of visual neglect have also been assessed by questionnaire. Towle and Lincoln (1991) developed the Problems in Everyday Living Questionnaire as a subjective measure of visual neglect. The patient has to report how often problems such as bumping into door frames and making errors when dialling the telephone have occurred. The Catherine Bergego Scale (Azouvi et al., 1996) contains ten items which the patient has to rate according to their severity. It has been found to have good interrater reliability. Validation was by correlation with conventional tests of neglect and with the Barthel Index as a measure of personal independence. Test–retest reliability and sensitivity to change need to be checked. Neither scale has been demonstrated to be sensitive to differences between interventions. An alternative approach has been to ask patients to carry out practical tasks and to observe their performance. Zoccolotti, Antonucci and Judica (1991) describe a scale which differentiates tasks involving the exploration of external space, dealing cards and serving tea from those which relate to one's own body, using a comb or razor. The scales were found to have high interrater reliability and internal consistency and concurrent validity in relation to conventional impairment measures of hemi-inattention.

Ponsford and Kinsella (1991) developed a rating scale of attentional behaviour which showed modest but statistically significant correlations with neuropsychological measures of attention. There was good internal consistency and intrarater reliability but agreement between raters working in different contexts was less satisfactory. The scale was used to monitor the effects of treatment. Scores showed change over time but the results from the rating scales did not correspond to the neuropsychological measures of attention. Discrepancies seemed to occur as a result of emotional factors and expectations of the therapists. This highlights the difficulty of validating such scales, and Ponsford and Kinsella suggested that more concrete descriptions of scale items might reduce this subjectivity. A rating scale for problem-solving behaviours was developed by von Cramon et al. (1991) to evaluate the behavioural effects of treatment. Aspects of problem-solving behaviour were rated according to the frequency of their occurrence. The scale was found to be reliable and sensitive to improvements.

The effects of language problems on everyday life have been investigated in more detail. The Com-municative Activities of Daily Living (Holland, 1980) presents language tasks through role play. This is more sensitive to communication strengths than traditional testing but it is still a test and not a naturalistic observation. The Functional Communication Profile (Sarno, 1969) and Edinburgh Functional Communication Profile (Skinner et al., 1984) provide ratings of practical language behaviour but are very subjective. The Profile of Functional Impairment in Communication (Lindscott, Knight and Godfrey, 1996) contains a detailed analysis of communication skills but requires an experienced assessor.

Assessments of cognitive function which are designed to reflect the cognitive skills needed in everyday life, such as the Rivermead Behavioral Memory Test (Wilson et al., 1985), Behavioral Inattention Test (Wilson, Cockburn and Halligan, 1987), Behavioral Assessment of the Dysexecutive Syndrome (Wilson et al., 1996) and Test of Everyday Attention (Robertson et al., 1994), may be considered to measure disability rather than impairment. They include items which are likely to be predictive of everyday performance rather than assessing everyday performance itself. Although they have the advantage of ecological validity, unlike many assessments of cognitive impairment, they are probably not true disability measures.

Social and occupational disability

Behavioural and psychosocial problems are common consequences of traumatic brain injury and need to be assessed, particularly in the later stages of rehabilitation. Assessment procedures have been criticized for their lack of rigorous evaluation (Hall, 1992). The Neurobehavioral Rating Scale (Levin et al, 1987) is based on behaviour, symptoms and skills measured in a structured clinical setting. The Neurobehavioral Functioning Inventory can be used with informants to record their perceptions of everyday problems (Kreutzer et al., 1996). Neither scale has well-established reliability or validity and neither has been shown to be a sensitive indicator of rehabilitation outcome. However, the scales would seem to be worth developing further as they tap the disabilities which are likely to be associated with cognitive impairment.

Handicap

- There are few measures of handicap.
- The best developed handicap measures are the London Handicap Scale and Short Form 36.
- Global measures which include impairment, disability and handicap are unlikely to be sensitive to the effects of cognitive rehabilitation.

Although it is unlikely that cognitive rehabilitation will have a direct effect on handicap, it may be useful to assess handicap as an effect of an overall rehabilitation package. Many measures overlap with disability scales or indicators of quality of life. Disability relates an individual's circumstances to a normal reference group, whereas handicap relates to the disadvantage for the individual. Handicap is therefore more subjective and inherently more difficult to measure, particularly in people with cognitive impairments. The World Health Organization (1980) developed scales to assess each of the six survival roles, orientation, physical independence, mobility, occupation of time, social integration and economic self-sufficiency. The scales include many components better measured by other scales, and their reliability and validity have not been well documented. These scales were used as the basis for the development of a simpler and more attractive measure of handicap. The London Handicap Scale (Harwood et al., 1994), which generates a profile of handicaps in the same six dimensions and an overall severity score. The validity, reliability and responsiveness were demonstrated in various patient groups. The London Handicap Scale seems to be more acceptable than alternative handicap measures such as the Environmental Status Scale (Mellerup et al., 1981), which has been recommended for people with multiple sclerosis but has been found by others to have limited validity (Stewart, Kidd and Thompson, 1995).

Health-related quality of life is a concept which overlaps with handicap. Generic measures of quality of life, therefore, may be used as indicators of handicap. The Short Form 36 (Stewart and Ware, 1992) is a short questionnaire, derived from the Rand Health Batteries, measuring: physical functioning, social functioning, role limitations due to physical problems, role limitations due to emotional problems, mental health, energy/vitality, pain and general health perception. It has good construct validity (Ware et al., 1993), though there are doubts about its applicability with the elderly (Hill and Harries, 1994). There are also floor effects in physically disabled groups (Freeman et al., 1996). By adding items, Vickrey et al. (1995) created the Multiple Sclerosis Quality of Life 54 Instrument, which was shown to have high internal consistency, test–retest reliability and construct validity, but its responsiveness to change over time has not been evaluated.

There have been attempts to provide simple global measures of outcome which encompass impairment, disability and handicap, such as the Disability Rating Scale (Rappaport et al., 1982). These have the advantages that they can be applied to a wide range of patients and are easy to use. However, as outcome measures, they are relatively insensitive and therefore only useful in large-scale randomized controlled trials. They are unlikely to contribute much to our evaluation of cognitive rehabilitation.

Future developments

- The psychometric properties of most measures need further evaluation.
- Disability measures are needed for the evaluation of outcome in single case experimental design studies.
- Researchers conducting randomized control trials should attempt to reach consensus on a few standard disability measures in order to facilitate meta-analyses.

For each of the measures mentioned, further work is needed to establish the validity and reliability of the scale. In particular, the validity is often only established with one diagnostic group. Disability and handicap measures should be applicable across a wide range of diagnostic groups. Validation studies should be carried out in several groups of patients to confirm the validity of the underlying construct and indicate any condition-specific features of the scale. The reliability needs to be checked in a variety of situations (inpatient, outpatient, hospital, community), conditions and over a variety of time intervals. For most scales this task has hardly yet begun. The issue of sensitivity to the effects of intervention will not be established until there are far more efficacy studies. Most single case experimental design studies use measures of impairment to assess the effect of intervention. However, it is the effect on daily life that is of most concern to patients and their families. Therefore, disability measures need to be developed for use in this context. Few of the measures described above are sensitive to the small changes in ability that need to be detected and many are too long to be administered with the frequency that is necessary in single case experimental design studies. The alternative approach to treatment evaluation is the randomized controlled trial. Several of the measures described above have been found to be sensitive to differences between rehabilitation procedures in randomized controlled trials. However, there have been very few such trials of cognitive rehabilitation. One reason may be that it is hard to recruit sufficient patients within a single centre; we have yet to reach the stage of multi-centre trials of cognitive rehabilitation. However, this requires consensus about which outcome measure to use. Even if we do not achieve the multicentre trial ideal, consistency of outcome measures is important for the purpose of meta-analysis. The main way forward, therefore, seems to be to agree on a group of outcome measures suitable for trials of cognitive neurorehabilitation. These measures need to be developed and refined in terms of their psychometric properties. If this is achieved in the context of research, it will also then be possible to use the measures for the audit of clinical services and the evaluation of the progress of an individual patient in a rehabilitation setting.

Conclusions

Standardized measures are available for evaluating the outcome of cognitive neurorehabilitation. These include measures at the levels of impairment, disability and handicap. At each level, the measures chosen should be reliable, valid, sensitive to the effects of intervention and consistent with those used by other researchers. There is a particular need for the development of measures of cognitive disability.

References

Anderson, R. 1992. *The Aftermath of Stroke: the Experience of Patients and their Families*. Cambridge: Cambridge University Press.

Andrews, F.M. and Withey, S.B. 1976. *Social Indicators of Well Being: Americans' Perceptions of Life Quality*. New York: Plenum Press.

Ashburn, A. 1982. Assessment of motor function in stroke patients. *Physiotherapy* **68**, 109–13.

Azouvi, P., Marchal, F., Samuel, C. et al. 1996. Functional consequences and awareness of unilateral neglect: study of an evaluation scale. *Neuropsychol Rehabil* **6**, 133–50.

Beck, A.T., Ward, C.H., Mendelson, M., Mock, J. and Erbaugh, J. 1961. An inventory for measuring depression. *Arch Gen Psychiatry* **4**, 561–71.

Benjamin, J. 1976. The Northwick Park ADL Index. *Br J Occup Therapy* **39**, 301–6.

Bergner, M., Bobbitt, R.A., Carter, W.B. and Gibson, B.S. 1981. The Sickness Impact Profile: development and final revision of a health status measure. *Med Care* **19**, 787–805.

Bohannon, R.W. and Andrews, A.W. 1987. Inter-rater reliability of hand-held dynamometry. *Phys Therapy* **67**, 931–3.

Bohannon, R.W. and Smith, M.B. 1987. Inter-rater reliability of the modified Ashworth Scale of muscle spasticity. *Phys Therapy* **67**, 206–7.

Bowling, A. 1991. *Measuring Health: a Review of Quality of Life Measurement Scales*. Buckingham: Open University Press.

Bowling, A. and Browne, P. 1991. Social networks, health and emotional well being amongst the oldest old in London. *J Gerontol* **46**, S20–S32.

Broadbent, D.E., Cooper, P.F., Fitzgerald, P. and Parkes, K.R. 1982. The Cognitive Failures Questionnaire (CFQ) and its correlates. *Br J Clin Psychol* **21**, 1–16.

Brosseau, L. and Wolfson, C. 1994. The inter-rater reliability and construct validity of the Functional Independence Measure for multiple sclerosis subjects. *Clin Rehabil* **8**, 107–15.

Brown, R.G., MacCarthey, B., Jahanshahi, M. and Marsden, C.D. 1989. Accuracy of self-reported disability in patients with parkinsonism. *Arch Neurol* **46**, 955–9.

Canter, G.J., De la Torre, R. and Mier, M. 1961. A method for evaluating disability in patients with Parkinson's disease. *J Nerv Ment Dis* **133**, 143–7.

Carr, J.H., Shepherd, R.B., Nordholm, L. and Lynne, D. 1985. Investigation of a new motor assessment scale for stroke patients. *Phys Therapy* **65**, 175–80.

Charlton, J.R.H., Patrick, D.L. and Peach, H. 1983. Use of multivariate measures of disability in health surveys. *J Epidemiol Comm Health* **37**, 296–304.

Collen, F.M., Wade,D.T., Robb, G.F. and Bradshaw, C.M. 1991. The Rivermead Mobility Index: a further development of the Rivermead Motor Assesment. *Int Disabil Studies* **13**, 50–4.

Collin, C., Wade, D.T., Davis, S. and Horne, V. 1988. The Barthel Index: a reliability study. *Int Disabil Studies* **10**, 61–3.

Coughlan, A.K. and Hollows, S.E. 1985. *The Adult Memory and Information Processing Battery.* Leeds: AK Coughlan, St James University Hospital.

Crawford, J.R., Parker, D.M. and McKinlay, W.W. 1992. *A Handbook of Neuropsychological Assessment.* Hove, UK: Lawrence Erlbaum.

Crawford, S., Wenden, F.J. and Wade, D.T. 1996. The Rivermead Head Injury Follow-up Questionnaire: a study of a new rating scale and other measures to evaluate outcome after head injury. *J Neurol Neurosurg Psychiatry* **60**, 510–14.

Crow, J.L., Lincoln, N.B., Nouri, F.M. and De Weerdt, W. 1989. The effectiveness of EMG biofeedback in the treatment of arm function after stroke. *Int Disabil Studies* **11**, 155–60.

Cummings, J.L., Mega, Gray, K., Rosenberg-Thompson, S., Carusi, D.A. and Gornbein, J. 1994. The Neuropsychiatric Inventory: comprehensive assessment of psychopathology in dementia. *Neurology* **44**, 2308–14.

Davis, A.M., Cockburn, J.M., Wade, D.T. and Smith, P.T. 1995. A subjective memory assessment questionnaire for use with elderly people after stroke. *Clin Rehabil* **9**, 238–44.

Demeurisse, G., Demol, O. and Robaye, E. 1980. Motor evaluation in vascular hemiplegia. *Eur Neurol* **19**, 382–9.

Dickson, H.G. and Kohler, F. 1996. The multi-dimensionality of the FIM motor items precludes an interval scaling using Rasch analysis. *Scand J Rehabil Med* **26**, 159–62.

Doble, S.E., Fisk, J.D., Fisher, A.G., Ritvo, P.G. and Murray, T.J. 1994. Functional competence of community dwelling persons with multiple sclerosis using the assessment of motor and process skills. *Arch Phys Med Rehabil* **75**, 843–51.

Drummond, A.E.R. and Walker, M.F. 1996. A randomized controlled trial of leisure rehabilitation after stroke. *Clin Rehabil* **9**, 283–90.

Forster, A. and Young, J. 1996. Specialist nurse support for patients with stroke in the community: a randomized trial. *BMJ* **312**, 1642–6.

Freeman, J.A., Langdon, D.W. and Thompson, A.J. (1996). Health related quality of life in people with multiple sclerosis undergoing in-patient rehabilitation. *J Neurol Rehabil* **10**, 185–94.

Fuller, K.J., Dawson, K. and Wiles, C.M. 1996. Physiotherapy in chronic multiple sclerosis: a controlled trial. *Clin Rehabil* **10**, 195–204.

Gilewski, M.J., Zelinski, E.M. and Schaie, K.W. 1990. The Memory Functioning Questionnaire for assessment of memory complaints in adulthood and old age. *Psychol Aging* **5**, 482–90.

Goldberg, D. and Williams, P. 1988. *A User's Guide to the General Health Questionnaire.* Windsor: NFER-Nelson.

Granger, C.V., Hamilton, B.B. and Sherwin, F.S. 1986. *Guide for Use of the Uniform Data Set for Medical Rehabilitation.* Buffalo, NY: Department of Rehabilitation Medicine, Buffalo General Hospital.

Hall, K.M. 1992. Overview of functional assessment scales in brain injury rehabilitation. *Neurorehabilitation* **2**, 98–113.

Hall, K.M., Hamilton, B.B., Gordon, W.A. and Zasler, N.D. 1993. Characteristics and comparisons of functional assessment indices: Disability Rating Scale, Functional Independence Measure and Functional Assessment Measure. *J Head Trauma Rehabil* **8**, 60–71.

Harwood, R.H., Rogers, A., Dickinson, E. and Ebrahim, S. 1994. Measuring handicap: the London Handicap Scale, a new outcome measure for chronic disease. *Qual Health Care* **3**, 11–16.

Hauser, S.L., Dawson, D.M., Lehrich, J.R. et al. 1983. Intensive immunosuppression in multiple sclerosis: a randomized three-arm study of high dose intravenous cyclophosphamide, plasma exchange and ACTH. *N Engl J Med* **308**, 173–80.

Heller, A., Wade, D.T., Wood, V.A., Sunderland, A., Langton-Hewer, R. and Ward, E. 1987. Arm function after stroke: measurement and recovery over the first three months. *J Neurol Neurosurg Psychiatry* **50**, 714–19.

Hill, S. and Harries, U. 1994. Assessing the outcome of health care for the older person in community settings: should we use the SF36? Outcomes briefing Issue 4. Leeds: UK Clearing House on Health Outcomes, Nuffield Institute for Health.

Holbrook, M. and Skilbeck, C.E. 1983. An activities index for stroke patients. *Age Aging* **12**, 166–70.

Holden, M.K., Gill, K.M., Magliozzi, M.R., Nathan, J. and Piehl-Baker, L. 1984. Clinical gait assessment in the neurologically impaired: reliability and meangingfulness. *Phys Therapy* **64**, 35–40.

Holland, A.L. 1980. *Communicative Activities of Daily Living: a Test of Functional Communication for Aphasic Adults.* Austin, TX: Pro-Ed.

Indredavik, B., Bakke, F., Solberg, R., Riseth, R., Haaheim, L.L. and Holme, J. 1991. Benefit of a stroke unit: a randomized controlled trial. *Stroke* **22**, 1026–31.

Jongbloed, L. and Morgan, D. 1991. An investigation of involvement in leisure activities after stroke. *Am J Occup Therapy* **45**, 420–7.

Juby, L.C., Berman, P. and Lincoln, N.B. 1996. The effect of a stroke rehabilitation unit on functional and psychological outcome: a randomized controlled trial. *Cereb Dis* **6**, 106–10.

Katz, M.M., Ford, A.B., Moscowitz, R.W., Jackson, B.A. and Jaffe, M.W. 1963. Studies of illness in the aged. The index of ADL: a standardized measure of biological and psychosocial function. *JAMA* **185**, 914–19.

Kidd, D., Stewart, G., Baldry, J. et al. 1995. The functional independence measure: a comparative validity and reliability study. *Disabil Rehabil* **17**, 10–14.

Kinsella, G., Murtagh, D., Landry, A. et al. 1996. Everyday memory following traumatic brain injury. *Brain Inj* **10**, 499–507.

Kreutzer, J.S., Marwitz, J.H., Seel, R. and Srio, C.D. 1996. Validation of a neurobehavioral functioning inventory for adults with traumatic brain injury. *Arch Phys Med Rehabil* **77**, 116–24.

Kurtzke, J.F. 1965. Further notes on disability evaluation in multiple sclerosis with scale modifications. *Neurology* **15**, 654–61.

Kurtzke, J.F. 1983. Rating neurologic impairment in multiple sclerosis: an expanded disability status scale (EDSS). *Neurology* **33**, 1444–52.

Lang, A.E.T. and Fahn, S. 1989. Assessment of Parkinson's disease. In *Quantification of Neurological Deficit*, ed. T.L. Munsat, pp. 285–309. Stoneham, MA: Butterworths.

Levin, H.S., High, W.M., Goethe, K.E. et al. 1987. The Neurobehavioral Rating Scale: assessment of the behavioral sequelae of head injury by the clinician. *J Neurol Neurosurg Psychiatry* **50**, 183–93.

Lezak, M.D. 1995. *Neuropsychological Assessment*. New York: Oxford University Press.

Lieberman, A.N. 1974. Parkinson's disease: a clinical review. *Am J Med Sci* **267**, 66–80.

Lincoln, N.B., Crow, J.L. and Jackson, J.M. 1991. The unreliability of sensory assessment. *Clin Rehabil* **5**, 273–82.

Lincoln, N.B. and Edmans, J.A. 1990. A revalidation of the Rivermead ADL scale for elderly patients with stroke. *Age Aging* **19**, 9–24.

Lincoln, N.B., Flannaghan, T., Sutcliffe, L. and Rother, L. 1997. Evaluation of cognitive behavioural therapy for depression after stroke: a pilot study. *Clin Rehabil* **11**, 114–22.

Lincoln, N.B., Jackson, J.M. and Adams, S.A. 1998. Reliability and revision of the Nottingham Sensory Assessment for Stroke Patients. *Physiotherapy* **84**, 358–65.

Lincoln, N.B. and Leadbitter, D. 1979. Assessment of motor function in stroke patients. *Physiotherapy* **65**, 48–51.

Lindscott, R.J., Knight, R.G. and Godfrey, H.P.D. 1996. The profile of functional impairment in communication: a measure of communication impairment for clinical use. *Brain Inj* **6**, 397–412.

Lyle, R.C. 1981. A performance test for the assessment of upper limb function in physical rehabilitation treatment and research. *Int J Rehabil Res* **4**, 483–92.

Mahoney, F.I. and Barthel, D.W. 1965. Functional evaluation: Barthel Index. *Maryland State Med J* **14**, 61–5.

McPherson, K.M., Pentland, B., Cudmore, S.F. and Prescott, R.J. 1996. An inter-rater reliability study of the Functional Assessment Measure (FIM + FAM). *Disabil Rehabil* **18**, 341–7.

Mellerup, E., Fog, T., Raun, N. et al. 1981. The Socio-economic Scale. *Acta Psychiatr Scand* **64** (Suppl. 87), 130–8.

Nouri, F.M. and Lincoln, N.B. 1987. An extended ADL scale for use with stroke patients. *Clin Rehabil* **1**, 301–5.

Pollak, N., Rheuault, W. and Stoecker, J.L. 1996. Reliability and validity of the FIM for persons aged 80 years and above from a multi-level continuing care retirement community. *Arch Phys Med Rehabil* **77**, 1056–61.

Ponsford, J. and Kinsella, G. 1991. The use of a rating scale of attentional behavior. *Neuropsychol Rehabil* **1**, 241–58.

Radloff, L.S. 1977. The CES-D scale: a self report depression scale for research in the general population. *Appl Psychol Meas* **1**, 385–401.

Rappaport, M., Hall, K.M., Hopkins, K., Belleza, T. and Cope, D.N. 1982. Disability rating scale for severe head trauma: coma to community. *Arch Phys Med Rehabil* **63**, 118–23.

Robertson, I.H., Ward, T., Ridgway, V. and Nimmo-Smith, I. 1994. *The Test of Everyday Attention*. Bury St Edmunds: Thames Valley Test Company.

Sackley, C.M. and Lincoln, N.B. 1997. Single blind randomized controlled trial of visual feedback after stroke: effects on stance symmetry and function. *Clin Rehabil* **19**, 536–46.

Sarno, M.T. 1969. *The Functional Communication Profile Manual of Directions*. New York: Institute of Rehabilitation Medicine, New York University Medical Center.

Skinner, C., Wirz, S., Thompson, I. and Davidson, J. 1984. *The Edinburgh Functional Communication Profile*. Oxford: Winslow Press.

Sloan, R.L., Sinclair, E., Thompson, J., Taylor, S. and Pentland, B. 1992. Inter-rater reliability of the Modified Ashworth Scale for spasticity in hemiplegic patients. *Int J Rehabil Res* **15**, 158–61.

Snaith, R.P., Ahmed, S.M., Mehta, S. and Hamilton, M. 1971. Assessment of the severity of primary depressive illness: the Wakefield Self Assessment Depression Inventory. *Psychol Med* **1**, 143–9.

Spreen, O. and Strauss, E. 1991. *A Compendium of Neuropsychological Tests*. New York: Oxford University Press.

Stewart, A.L. and Ware, J.E., eds. 1992. *Measuring Functioning and Well-Being: the Medical Outcomes Study Approach*. Durham, NC: Duke University Press.

Stewart, G., Kidd, D. and Thompson, A.J. 1995. The assessment of handicap: an evaluation of the Environmental Status Scale. *Disabil Rehabil* **17**, 312–16.

Sunderland, A., Harris, J.E. and Baddeley, A.D. 1983. Do laboratory tests predict everyday memory? A neuropsychological study. *J Verb Learn Verb Behav* **22**, 341–57.

Sunderland, A., Harris, J.E. and Gleave, J. 1984. Memory failures in everyday life following severe head injury. *J Clin Neuropsychol* **6**, 127–42.

Sunderland, A., Tinson, D.J., Bradley, E.L., Fletcher, D., Langton-Hewer, R.L. and Wade, D.T. 1992. Enhanced physical therapy improves recovery of arm function after stroke: a randomized controlled trial. *J Neurol Neurosurg Psychiatry* **55**, 530–5.

Sunderland, A., Tinson, D., Bradley, L. and Langton-Hewer, R.L. 1989. Arm function after stroke: an evaluation of grip strength as a measure of recovery and a prognostic indicator. *J Neurol Neurosurg Psychiatry* **52**, 1267–72.

Sutcliffe, L.M. and Lincoln, N.B. 1998. The assessment of depression in aphasic stroke patients: the development of the Stroke Aphasic Depression Questionnaire. *Clin Rehabil* **12**, 451–8.

Taylor, R. 1990. Relationships between cognitive test performance and everyday cognitive difficulties in multiple sclerosis. *Br J Clin Psychol* **29**, 251–3.

Tinson, D.J. and Lincoln, N.B. 1987. Subjective memory impairment after stroke. *Int Disabil Studies* **9**, 6–9.

Tomasello, F., Mariani, F., Fieschi, C. et al. 1982. Assessment of interobserver differences in the Italian multi-center study on reversible cerebral ischaemia. *Stroke* **13**, 32–4.

Towle, D. and Lincoln, N.B. 1991. Development of a questionnaire for detecting everyday problems in stroke patients with unilateral visual neglect. *Clin Rehabil* **5**, 135–40.

Vaney, C., Blaurock, H., Gattlen, B. and Meisels, C. 1996. Assessing mobility in multiple sclerosis using the Rivermead Mobility Index and gait speed. *Clin Rehabil* **10**, 216–26.

Vickrey, B.G., Hays, R.D., Harooni, R., Myers, L.W. and Ellison, G.W. 1995. A health related quality of life measure for multiple sclerosis. *Qual Life Res* **4**, 187–206.

von Cramon, D.Y., von Matthes, von Cramon, G. and Mai, N. 1991. Problem solving deficits in brain-injured patients: a therapeutic approach. *Neuropsychol Rehabil* **1**, 45–64.

Wade, D.T. 1992. *Measurement in Neurological Rehabilitation.* Oxford: Oxford University Press.

Wade, D.T., Collen, F.M., Robb, G.F. and Warlow, C.P. 1992. Physiotherapy intervention late after stroke and mobility. *BMJ* **304**, 609–13.

Wade, D.T., Crawford, S., Wenden, F., King, N.S. and Moss, N.E.G.

1997. Does routine follow-up after head injury help? A randomized control trial. *J. Neurol Neurosurg Psychiatry* **62**, 478–84.

Walker, M.F., Drummond, A.E.R. and Lincoln, N.B. 1996. Evaluation of dressing practice for stroke patients after discharge from hospital. *Clin Rehabil* **10**, 23–31.

Walker, M.F. and Lincoln, N.B. 1990. Reacquisition of dressing skills after stroke. *Int Disabil Studies* **12**, 41–3.

Walker, R., Findlay, J.M., Young, A.W. and Welch, J. 1991. Disentangling neglect and hemianopia. *Neuropsychologia* **29**, 1019–27.

Ware, J.E., Snow, K.K., Kosinski, M. and Gandek, B. 1993. *SF-36 Health Survey Manual and Interpretation Guide.* Boston: The Health Institute, New England Medical Center.

Webster, D.D. 1968. Critical analysis of the disability in Parkinson's disease. *Mod Treat* **5**, 257–82.

Wechsler, D. 1987. *Wechsler Memory Scale Revised.* New York: Psychological Corporation.

Whiting, S.E. and Lincoln, N.B. 1980. An activities of daily living assessment for stroke patients. *Br J Occup Therapy* **February**, 44–6.

Wiles, C.M. and Karni, Y. 1983. The measurement of strength in patients with peripheral neuromuscular disorders. *J Neurol Neurosurg Psychiatry* **46**, 1006–13.

Wilson, B.A., Alderman, N., Burgess, P., Emslie, H. and Evans, J.J. 1996. *Behavioral Assessment of the Dysexecutive Syndrome.* Bury St Edmunds: Thames Valley Test Company.

Wilson, B.A., Cockburn, J. and Baddeley, A. 1985. *The Rivermead Behavioral Memory Test.* Bury St Edmunds: Thames Valley Test Company.

Wilson, B.A., Cockburn, J. and Halligan, P.W. 1987. *Behavioral Inattention Test.* Bury St Edmunds: Thames Valley Test Company.

World Health Organization 1980. *International Classification of Impairments, Disabilities and Handicaps.* Geneva: WHO.

Zelinski, E.M., Gilewski, M.J. and Anthony-Bergstrone, C.R. 1990. Memory functioning questionnaire: concurrent validity with memory performance and self-reported memory failures. *Psychol Aging* **5**, 388–99.

Zigmund, A.S. and Snaith, R.P. 1983. The Hospital Anxiety and Depression Scale. *Acta Psychiatr Scand* **67**, 361–70.

Zoccolotti, P., Antonucci, G. and Judica, A. 1991. A functional evaluation of hemi-neglect by means of a semi-structured scale: personal extrapersonal differentiation. *Neuropsychol Rehabil* **1**, 33–44.

Zung, W.W.K. 1965. A self-rating depression scale. *Arch Gen Psychiatry* **12**, 63–70.

13

Constraint-induced movement therapy: new approaches to outcome measurement in rehabilitation

Gitendra Uswatte and Edward Taub

Introduction

- The development of effective cognitive neurore-habilitation treatments demands instruments that measure functional changes in cognition in the real world.
- The development of instruments to measure the real-world outcomes of a new physical rehabilitation technique, constraint–induced movement therapy, may provide some guidelines for developing new measures in cognitive neurorehabilitation.

The development of new cognitive neurorehabilitation techniques that effectively transfer results obtained in the clinic to the real-life setting will require innovations in measuring techniques. The assessment of treatment effect and compliance is best accomplished through direct, continuous and objective measurement of the target of intervention in the appropriate environment. Although current neuropsychological instruments measure various cognitive abilities (Lezak, 1995), there are no instruments with these desirable qualities that measure cognitive function in the real-life setting.

Constraint-induced movement therapy (e.g. Taub, 1980; Taub et al., 1993) is a new treatment for chronic upper extremity hemiparesis that successfully transfers improvement in the quality and amount of upper extremity use from the clinic to the real-life setting. Physical rehabilitation outcome evaluation instruments, however, do not provide a direct measure of motor function in the real world. Traditional instruments in physical rehabilitation focus on measuring strength, flexibility and coordination in the clinic or laboratory situation (Smith and Clark, 1995). More recent instruments measure functional ability in the home indirectly by clinical observation of activities of daily living performed in the laboratory or clinic (Holbrook and Skilbeck, 1983; Baxter-Petralia et al., 1990; Cress et al., 1996), but the relationship between performance on these instruments and performance in the real-life situation has not been rigorously tested (Keith, 1995). The experimental work conducted by this laboratory and the observations of others (Andrews and Stewart, 1979) suggest that laboratory motor tests indicate a rehabilitation patient's maximum motor ability, but that patients do not necessarily make full use of that ability in the real-life setting. Consequently, it was decided that the constraint–induced movement therapy research project should develop new instruments that measure upper-extremity function directly in the home.

The authors believe that the solutions devised for measuring motor activity outside the clinic hold some lessons for the further development of measurement technology in the field of cognitive neurorehabilitation. This chapter reviews the development of constraint–induced movement therapy, provides a model explaining its operation in terms of learning followed by use-dependent cortical reorganization, presents the measurement instruments used to evaluate the intervention, and discusses the applications of measurement in cognitive neurorehabilitation.

Constraint-induced movement therapy

- Monkeys with a unilateral forelimb deafferentation learn not to use their impaired limb during the initial postoperative period when spinal shock renders the animals incapable of moving their affected limb extensively.

- This phenomenon has been termed learned nonuse.
- The monkeys continue the learned nonuse of their impaired limb after the spinal shock has passed off and they are physically capable of purposive movement.
- Restricting movement of the unaffected limb and/or training of the affected limb over a number of days can overcome this learned nonuse. Both techniques induce massed practice in the use of the affected limb for several consecutive days and, thereby, convert a functionless limb into a limb that is used extensively.
- The same techniques produce substantial increases in affected arm use when applied to people with a stroke-related chronic upper extremity paresis.

Most of the patients worked with to date have been relatively high functioning; however, recent work with lower functioning patients suggests that up to 50 per cent of the stroke population with a unilateral chronic motor deficit may be amenable to substantial improvement through application of constraint-induced movement therapy techniques.

Research with monkeys

Constraint-induced movement therapy, which consists of a family of techniques, is derived from basic research with primates. When a single forelimb is deafferented in a monkey, the animal does not make use of it in the life situation (Mott and Sherrington, 1895; Lassek, 1953). However, by restricting movement of the intact limb for several days, the monkey can be induced to use the deafferented extremity permanently. Training of deafferented limb use also proved to be an effective technique. Initially, conditioned response techniques were employed to train limb use (Knapp, Taub and Berman, 1958, 1963; and Taub and Berman, 1963; Taub, Bacon and Berman, 1965; Taub, Ellman and Berman, 1966; Taub, 1977; Taub et al., 1978). Subsequently, it was found that shaping techniques, which involve increasing behavioural requirements in very small steps (Skinner, 1938, 1968; Morgan, 1974; Panyan, 1980), are considerably more effective (Taub, 1976, 1977).

Several converging lines of evidence suggest that nonuse of a single deafferented limb is a learning phenomenon involving conditioned suppression of movement (Taub, 1977, 1980). The restraint and shaping techniques appear to be effective because they overcome learned nonuse.

Substantial neurological injury usually leads to a shock-like phenomenon, whether at the level of the spinal cord (spinal shock) or brain (diaschisis or cortical shock). Deafferentation initially results in a reduction within the spinal cord in the background level of excitation that keeps neurons ready to respond. This effect is most marked in the deafferented segments of the spinal cord, where the depressed condition of the motor neurons greatly elevates the threshold for excitation necessary to produce movement. With time, recovery processes raise the background level of excitability of motor neurons so that movements, *at least potentially*, can be expressed. In monkeys, the period of spinal shock lasts from two to six months following forelimb deafferentation (Taub, 1977).

The inability of the monkeys to use the deafferented limb due to spinal shock leads to conditioned suppression of use of that limb. Animals with one deafferented limb try to use that extremity in the immediate postoperative situation, but they cannot. Attempts to use the deafferented limb often lead to painful and otherwise aversive consequences such as falls and loss of food. These failures in use constitute punishments that suppress arm use (Kimble, 1961). Meanwhile, the monkeys cope quite well in the laboratory environment on three limbs and are therefore positively reinforced for this pattern of behaviour, which as a result is strengthened. This response set persists, and consequently the monkeys never learn that, several months after the operation, the limb has become capable of movement. The development of learned nonuse is shown in Fig. 13.1.

The restraint of the intact limb several months after unilateral deafferentation serves to overcome this conditioned suppression of movement or 'learned nonuse'. Restriction of the intact limb forces animals to use the deafferented limb or forego feeding, locomotion and other important daily activities with any degree of efficiency. This change in motivation overcomes the learned nonuse of the deafferented limb and

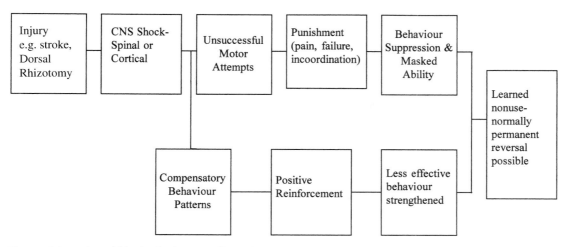

Fig. 13.1 Schematic model for the development of learned nonuse. (From 'Constraint-induced movement therapy for motor recovery after stroke' by David M. Morris, Jean E. Crago, Stephanie C. DeLuca, Rama D. Pidikiti and Edward Taub, 1994, *NeuroRehabilitation*, **9**, p. 31. Copyright 1994 by Elsevier Science Ireland Ltd. Reprinted with permission of the author.)

consequently the animal uses it. The counterconditioning of learned nonuse is shown in Fig. 13.2.

An experiment was carried out to test the learned nonuse formulation directly (Taub, 1977, 1980). Movement of a unilaterally deafferented forelimb was prevented with a restraining device in several animals so that they could not attempt to use that extremity for a period of three months following surgery. The reasoning was that in preventing an animal from trying to use the deafferented limb during the period before the spinal shock had passed off, one should thereby prevent the animal from learning that the limb could not be used during that interval. In conformity with this prediction, the animals were able to use their deafferented extremity in the free situation after the restraint was removed. Suggestive evidence in support of the learned nonuse formulation was also obtained during the course of deafferentation experiments carried out on the day of birth (Taub et al., 1973) and prenatally (Taub et al., 1975; Taub, 1980).

Research with humans

In 1980, it was proposed that learned nonuse might develop in some humans after stroke (Taub, 1980). It

was suggested that this phenomenon could develop in some humans by mechanisms similar to those that operate after deafferentation in monkeys, with the exception that the initial period of motor incapacitation would be due to cortical rather than spinal shock. It was suggested, therefore, that the same techniques that overcome learned nonuse in monkeys following unilateral deafferentation might also constitute a treatment to increase the amount of limb use in humans after stroke.

Constraint-induced movement therapy techniques were first successfully applied to humans with an upper extremity hemiparesis by Steven Wolf (Ostendorf and Wolf, 1981; Wolf et al., 1989) in conformity with the unaffected limb constraint portion of Taub's protocol (1980), but not including the affected limb training component. The 1989 study included stroke and traumatic brain injury patients who were more than one year postinjury and who possessed a minimum of 10 degrees extension at the metacarpophalangeal and interphalangeal joints and 20 degrees extension at the wrist of the affected arm (minimum motor criterion). The patients were asked to wear a sling on the unaffected arm all day for two weeks, except during a half-hour exercise period and sleeping hours. The

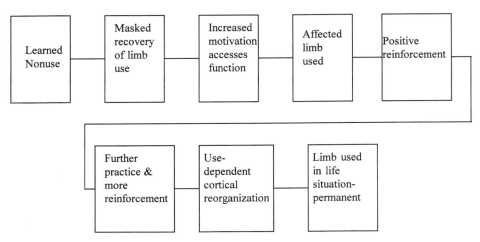

Fig. 13.2 Schematic model of mechanism for overcoming learned nonuse. From 'Constraint-induced movement therapy for motor recovery after stroke' by David M. Morris, Jean E. Crago, Stephanie C. DeLuca, Rama D. Pidikiti and Edward Taub, 1994, *NeuroRehabilitation*, **9**, p. 31. Copyright 1994 by Elsevier Science Ireland Ltd. Reprinted with permission of the author.)

patients demonstrated significant improvements in speed or force of movement, depending on the task, on 19 out of 21 tasks on the Wolf Motor Function Test (Wolf et al., 1989; Taub et al., 1993), a laboratory test involving simple upper extremity movements.

Taub et al. (1993) undertook further work on the application of constraint-induced movement therapy to stroke patients with a chronic upper extremity hemiparesis. This study employed an attention-placebo control group, combined training of the paretic arm with restraint of the contralateral upper extremity, and emphasized transfer of therapeutic gains in the laboratory to the life situation. Four treatment subjects had their unaffected arms restrained in a sling for 14 days and on ten of those days received seven hours of supervised practice using their affected arms. Five control subjects were told they had much greater movement in their affected limbs than they expressed, were led through a series of passive movement exercises in the treatment centre, and were given passive movement exercises to perform at home. All were at least one year poststroke (mean 4 years) and had passed the minimum motor criterion before admission to the study. Treatment efficacy was evaluated using the Wolf

Motor Function Test, the Arm Motor Ability Test (McCulloch et al., 1988; Kopp et al., 1997), and the Motor Activity Log (Taub et al., 1993), which tracks arm use in 14 activities of daily living through a semi-structured interview. The treatment group demonstrated a significant increase in motor ability as measured by the Wolf Motor Function and Arm Motor Ability tests over the treatment period, whereas the control subjects showed no change or a decline in arm motor ability. On the Motor Activity Log, the treatment group showed a large increase in real-world arm use over the two-week period and demonstrated a further small increase in use when tested two years after treatment; the control subjects exhibited no change or a decline in arm use over the same period.

Other experiments (Taub and Crago, 1995; Taub et al., 1995) suggested that there is a family of techniques that can overcome learned nonuse. The interventions that proved effective included placement of a sling on the less-affected arm and shaping of the paretic arm, placement of a half-glove on the less-affected arm as a reminder not to use it, and shaping of the paretic arm, shaping of the paretic arm only, and intensive physical therapy of the paretic arm for five hours a day for ten consecutive weekdays. The therapeutic elements shared by these different techniques appear to be focusing of attention on the paretic arm and massing of practice of the paretic arm. These two effects are induced in most of the techniques by constraining movement of the less-affected arm (Taub and Wolf, 1997).

Initial motor ability of patients

The patients treated to date have almost all had relatively high initial levels of motor ability. This selection has occurred largely because of the minimum motor criterion for entry into treatment. It is estimated that approximately 20–25 per cent of the chronic stroke population meet this motor criterion (Wolf and Binder-Macleod, 1983). However, recent work with lower functioning patients is proving to very promising, suggesting that constraint-induced movement therapy may be applicable to up to 50 per cent of the stroke population with a chronic unilateral motor deficit. The minimum motor criterion for inclusion of lower functioning patients into therapy is 10 degrees extension at the wrist and enough active extension of the fingers to release a tennis ball placed in the hand by the experimenter. Five patients whose initial motor ability fell below the minimum criteria for the higher functioning group and above the minimum criteria for the lower functioning group have been given constraint-induced movement therapy to date. All five lower functioning patients exhibited substantial improvement. The change on the outcome measures was slightly lower than that of the higher functioning patients, while the final level was somewhat lower than that of the higher functioning patients since the lower functioning patients started from a lower initial level of motor ability. One patient with probable Alzheimer's disease was not compliant in wearing the restraint device once out of the laboratory. His treatment gain was more modest than that of the other subjects, but his therapy was also much reduced compared to theirs and was not consistent with the laboratory's protocol. The data suggest that the motor capacity of chronic patients is modifiable in a larger percentage of the population than research originally indicated.

Neurophysiological mechanisms involved in constraint-induced movement therapy

- Cortical reorganization is associated with the effect of constraint-induced movement therapy.
- A neurophysiological prognosticator of the recovery of upper extremity function after stroke may exist.

Recent magnetic source imaging studies with humans, carried out by a group of investigators including one of the coauthors (E.T.), and an intracortical microstimulation study with monkeys suggest that cortical reorganization may be associated with the therapeutic effect of constraint-induced movement therapy. The human imaging studies followed the seminal work of Merzenich and coworkers with monkeys (e.g. Merzenich et al., 1984) and showed that the cortical somatosensory representation of the digits of the left hand was larger in string players than in nonmusician controls (Elbert et al., 1995). Moreover, the representation of the fingers of blind Braille readers, who use several fingers jointly to read, was found to be enlarged (Sterr et al., 1998). These results, in conjunction with research on cortical reorganization in adult phantom limb patients (Flor et al., 1995), suggest that the size of the cortical representation of a body part in adult humans depends on the amount of use of that part. The intracortical microstimulation study demonstrated that, in adult squirrel monkeys which were surgically given an ischaemic infarct in the cortical area controlling the movements of a hand, training of the affected limb results in cortical reorganization of the area surrounding the infarct (Nudo et al., 1996). These findings suggest the possibility that the increase in affected arm use produced by constraint-induced movement therapy results in a use-dependent increase in the cortical representation of the affected arm.

The hypothesis that constraint-induced movement therapy produces a large, use-dependent cortical reorganization in humans with stroke-related hemiparesis of an upper extremity was recently confirmed in two studies. One study used focal transcranial magnetic stimulation (TMS) to map the areas of the brain that control arm movement in six patients with a chronic upper extremity hemiparesis (mean chronicity = six years) before and after constraint-induced movement therapy (Liepert et al., 1998). The investigators found the therapy produced a significant increase in the patients' amount of arm use in the home over the two-week treatment period. Over the same period, they found that the cortical region from which EMG responses of a hand muscle can be elicited by TMS was more than doubled. Kopp et al. (1999) carried out a current source density analysis of the steady-state electroencephalographic motor potential of constraint-induced movement therapy patients. They found that three months after treatment the motor cortex ipsilateral to the affected arm, which normally controls movements of the contralateral arm, had been recruited to generate movements of the affected arm. This effect was not in evidence immediately after treatment and was presumably due to the sustained increase in affected arm use over the three-month follow-up period produced by constraint-induced movement therapy. To the best of the authors' knowledge, these two studies are the first to demonstrate an alteration in brain structure or function associated with *therapy-induced* rehabilitation of movement after central nervous system damage in humans.

Preliminary MRI data collected by Chatterjee et al. suggest that there may be an association between the locus of the infarct and the ability to pass the minimum motor criterion. If the initial findings are confirmed, then the MRIs obtained in the acute phase could serve as a prognosticator of amenability to constraint-induced movement therapy in the chronic phase or, alternatively, suggest preventive treatment in the acute phase itself.

Measurement of constraint-induced movement therapy efficacy and compliance

- Constraint-induced movement therapy outcome is measured in two domains: motor ability in the laboratory and extremity use in the home (i.e. function in the real world).
- Motor ability is assessed in the laboratory using two standard motor tests and two motor tests developed by the authors' laboratory. The standard tests are active and passive range of motion and the Fugl-

Meyer Poststroke Motor Recovery Test. The new tests are the Wolf Motor Function Test and Arm Motor Ability Test.
- Function in the real world is assessed using four measures: Motor Activity Log, Daily Home Treatment Diary, Actual Amount of Use Test, and accelerometry.
- Accelerometry can provide a direct, continuous and objective measure of arm use in the real world.
- Laboratory motor tests indicate the maximum motor ability of patients, whereas real-world measures indicate how much the arm is being used in the home. Direct measures of real-world arm use are necessary because motor ability and the amount of arm use in the home are not strongly related.

Laboratory upper extremity motor ability measures range of motion

Passive and active range of motion measurements are taken with respect to 26 joint motions of the upper extremity. The two primary measures are: (1) the number of joint motions which show a clinically significant change (>5 degrees) from pretreatment to posttreatment; and (2) the average change in range of motion across those joint motions that are outside of normal limits prior to treatment. The range of motion data that have been collected to date have been dominated by a ceiling effect. Patients treated, on average, displayed 84 per cent of normal active range of motion before treatment and 89 per cent of normal active range of motion after treatment. The minimum motor criterion and other exclusion criteria appear to have screened out patients with more restricted range of motion.

Fugl-Meyer Poststroke Motor Recovery Test

The upper extremity portion of this test is a standard laboratory test with an established reliability and validity (Fugl-Meyer et al., 1975; Duncan, Propst and Nelson, 1983; Berglund and Fugl-Meyer, 1986) that measures the coordination, flexibility and sensory capability of the patient's affected arm. Patients are asked to perform simple arm movements and to respond to tactile stimuli; in addition, the examiner passively moves the patient's upper extremity at each of the joints. The synergy of the movements, the response to tactile stimuli, the range of motion, and the occurrence of pain are rated on three-point scales. The ratings for the individual items are summed to produce a subtest score for the upper extremity. The items include abducting the shoulder, grasping a piece of paper between thumb and forefinger, and detecting a light touch to the palmar surface of the hand. The test data in the authors' laboratory also appear to have been dominated by a ceiling effect. The mean score pretreatment was 101 out of a possible 126 points; the mean score posttreatment was 113.

Wolf Motor Function Test

This laboratory motor test, developed specifically to evaluate the effects of constraint-induced movement therapy (Wolf et al., 1989; Taub et al., 1993), measures the ability of patients to perform 19 simple limb movements and tasks with the affected arm. The items include activities such as lifting the affected arm from the test table surface to a box, extending the elbow past a line 40 cm from the initial position, turning over playing cards, and picking up a pencil. Test performance is timed and videotaped and later rated independently by three clinicians blinded to the pretreatment or posttreatment status of the patient. As originally developed, performance time was the primary measure (Wolf et al., 1989). Subsequently, rating scales for quality of movement and functional ability were added (Taub et al., 1993). Currently, only the Functional Ability Scale is used, because the two rating scales appear to measure identical constructs ($r_{QOM,FA} = 0.98$). Patients, on average, demonstrated significant reductions in median performance time, from 6.0 seconds before treatment to 3.2 seconds after treatment, and significant increases in mean functional ability, from 3.5 to 4.0 rating points. The attention-placebo controls did not show significant changes. The reliability and validity of the Wolf Motor Function Test are currently being evaluated by the authors' laboratory.

Arm Motor Ability Test

This laboratory motor test, also developed specifically to evaluate the effects of constraint-induced movement

therapy (McCulloch et al., 1988; Taub et al., 1993, Kopp et al., 1997), measures the ability of patients to perform 13 activities of daily living with their affected arm. Each of the 13 tasks is a complete activity of daily living commonly carried out in the real-life setting, such as putting on a sweater, dialling a telephone number, and unscrewing a jar cap. Test performance is timed and videotaped and later rated on the Functional Ability Scale by three independent clinicians blinded to the treatment status of the patient. For timing and rating, 12 of the tasks are broken down into two to three simpler components. This breakdown into component segments allows for the type of quanitification possible with simpler actions without interfering with the normal flow of movement characteristic of everyday activity. In the 1993 Taub et al. study, patients in the treatment group demonstrated significant decreases in median performance time, from 4.4 seconds to 3.4 seconds, and significant increases in functional ability, from 3.4 to 3.8 rating points. Attention-placebo controls did not show significant changes.

In a study with 33 subacute stroke patients, the Arm Motor Ability Test demonstrated high interrater reliability, internal consistency and construct validity, and good concurrent validity (Kopp et al., 1997). The patients were administered the test and the Motricity Index – Arm Test (Demeurisse, Demol and Robaye, 1980), which assesses motor impairment by rating movement at three upper extremity joints. Half of these patients were given the Arm Motor Ability Test again one week later and the other half two weeks later. The interrater reliabilities (Spearman correlation coefficient) between two observers on the initial test day for functional ability and performance time were 0.98 and 0.99, respectively. The internal consistencies (Chronbach's alpha) on this day for functional ability and performance time were 0.99 and 0.94, respectively. The concurrent validities (Spearman correlation coefficient) between the Arm Motor Ability Test and the Motricity Index – Arm for functional ability and performance time were 0.61 and 0.45, respectively; these values were limited by the relatively low internal consistency of the latter (Kopp et al., 1997). Construct validity was demonstrated by the ability of the Arm Motor Ability Test to detect improvements in motor ability due to spontaneous recovery as measured by the Functional Ability Scale and performance time over the one-week and two-week retest intervals and by its ability to discriminate between the initial improvement at one week and the larger improvement at two weeks as measured by the Functional Ability Scale.

Real-world upper extremity function measures

Motor Activity Log

This semistructured interview measures how much and how well patients use their affected arm for activities of daily living in the home over a specified period. The Motor Activity Log is administered independently to the patient and a significant other or informant. The patient or caregiver is asked to rate how much and how well the patient has used the affected arm for 14 activities of daily living tasks in the past day, week or year. Patients and caregivers use a six-point Amount of Use Scale to rate how much they are using their affected arm and a six-point Quality of Movement Scale to rate how well they are using it. The tasks include such activities as brushing teeth, buttoning a shirt or blouse, and eating with a fork or spoon.

The constraint-induced movement therapy patients treated in the authors' laboratory improved from a mean of 1.2 (1 = very little use) a year before treatment to 3.2 (3 = moderate use, 4 = almost normal amount of use) four weeks after treatment on the Amount of Use Scale and improved from 1.1 (1 = very poor quality of movement) to 3.4 (3 = moderate quality of movement, 4 = almost normal quality of movement) on the Quality of Movement Scale. The caregiver reports indicated similar improvements: 1.1 to 3.1 on the Amount of Use Scale and 0.8 to 3.0 on the Quality of Movement Scale. The interrater reliability within patient and caregiver pairs on both scales was very high, mean InterClass Correlation Type 3,1 (Shrout and Fleiss, 1979) = 0.90. Attention-placebo controls did not show significant changes; mean Quality of Movement Scores remained constant at 1.6 rating points.

The Motor Activity Log has drawbacks that are typically associated with self-report instruments. Patients' ratings may be influenced by experimenter bias or demand characteristics or patients simply may not be able to recall accurately how they used their affected extremity. However, there is no other instrument available for assessing the actual amount of use of affected extremities in the real-life setting. Although there are several global measures of functional independence (Functional Independence Measure: Keith et al., 1987; Barthel Index: Mahoney and Barthel, 1965), these are 'burden of care' assessments that determine to what extent patients can carry out activities of daily living independently, regardless of the function of their affected arm.

Daily home treatment diary

This diary provides an estimate of how well the patient has complied with the main intervention in the home environment. During treatment, patients are instructed to wear a sling or half-glove on the unaffected arm for more than 90 per cent of the time when they are at home and awake. Patients record when the constraint device is on and what activities are engaged in during the day. If patients do not fill out the diary, because of forgetfulness, difficulty writing with the affected hand, or functional illiteracy, the experimenter helps them fill it out upon arrival in the laboratory the next day. If there has been substantial noncompliance with wearing the constraint device, the experimenter attempts to determine the reasons and then problem solves with the patient to help increase compliance. The experimenter calculates the patient's percentage compliance with the constraint protocol on the basis of the diary account. Patients, on average, reported a 74 per cent compliance rate at home.

The daily home treatment diary is subject to the same problems as the Motor Activity Log: experimenter bias, demand characteristics, and inaccurate recall. These biases are especially salient if the experimenter must help the subject to complete the diary.

Actual Amount of Use Test

This observational test measures how much patients spontaneously use their affected arm to perform a set of tasks in the laboratory. It is administered on first entrance into the laboratory before pretreatment testing and again just prior to posttreatment testing. Patients are videotaped as they are unobtrusively led through a standardized scenario of 20 tasks that they might encounter in the clinic on a regular basis (e.g. remove coat, place project card in wallet, fill out form). The patients are not prompted as to what arm to use to accomplish the tasks or informed that they are being tested. Nor are patients told that they are being videotaped during test administration; they have given informed consent to be videotaped when they enter the constraint-induced movement therapy project. Independent clinicians use the videotape to rate the patient's behaviour on the amount of arm use. The patients' performance on the Actual Amount of Use Test is believed to be more closely related to how much they actually use their affected arms in their daily lives than their performance on tests of motor ability in which they are asked to perform tasks specifically with their affected arm.

Although the Actual Amount of Use Test is not subject to the problems associated with self-report measures, the relationship between performance on this in-laboratory test and actual use of the limb in the home has yet to be evaluated experimentally. Preliminary results indicate a large increase in the percentage of activities carried out spontaneously by the affected arm with treatment. Five patients in the sling constraint and shaping group who have been administered the Actual Amount of Use Test so far performed 34 per cent of the tasks attempted with the affected arm before treatment and 64 per cent after treatment. This increase is congruent with the increase in the amount of use reported on the Motor Activity Log.

Accelerometers

Accelerometers can provide a more objective, direct and detailed measure of how much patients use their affected arm in the home situation and how well they comply with the home treatment protocol than interview or in-laboratory observational measures. Accelerometers have been used by fitness researchers, with moderate success, to measure overall physical activity levels in children and adults outside the labora-

tory. These investigators have established that laboratory manipulations of physical activity produce reliable changes in accelerometer recordings (Wong et al., 1981; Nichols, Patterson and Early, 1992; Bouten et al., 1994; Melanson and Freedson, 1995), and have validated accelerometer recordings in the home against self-reports or caregiver reports of physical activity (Patterson et al., 1993; Miller, Freedson and Kline, 1994; Janz, Witt and Mahoney, 1995) and other objective measures of activity, such as heart rate telemetry (Janz, 1994; Makikawa et al., 1994). In physical rehabilitation, accelerometers have been used with initial success to measure overall physical activity in the laboratory (Kochersberger et al., 1996; Veltnic et al., 1996) and the home (Kochersberger et al., 1996), the use of a prosthetic device by transtibial amputees in the home (Stam, Eijskoot and Bussmann, 1995), and the use of the arm to propel a wheelchair in the laboratory (Tajima et al., 1994).

The accelerometers employed in the authors' laboratory are Computer Science Application Inc. Model 7164 Activity Monitor Accelerometers. They are plastic units about the size and weight of a large wristwatch that are based on piezoelectric crystal technology. When the piezoelectric crystal in the accelerometers is subject to acceleration, it deforms and produces a charge. This charge is digitized at a 10 Hz sampling rate and summed over a user-specified epoch. The reported sum is called an activity count; 128 counts represent an acceleration of 2.13 g at 0.75 Hz over a 0.1 second epoch. The Activity Monitors are differentially sensitive to different frequencies of movement; they are relatively insensitive to movements at frequencies below 0.1 Hz and above 3.6 Hz (Computer Science Applications Inc., 1996). This range closely matches the frequency of healthy human arm movement (Foster, McPartland and Kupfer, 1978).

It is proposed that patients should wear Activity Monitors on each arm and the hip during 95 per cent of their waking hours for one week, starting seven days prior to treatment, the two-week treatment period, one week starting 21 days after treatment, and one week starting two years after treatment. The acceleration recordings from these devices will indicate how much the patient is moving the affected arm, the unaffected arm, and the whole body. Activity counts from the affected arm unit will be compared before and after treatment to evaluate the change in arm use due to treatment. Activity counts from the unaffected arm unit during treatment will be used to monitor compliance with the constraint protocol, and activity counts from the hip unit before and after treatment will be used to assess the impact of the intervention on general physical activity. The ratio of affected to unaffected arm activity counts will be compared before and after treatment to evaluate whether there is an increase in the use of the affected arm relative to the unaffected arm. In addition, the data will be examined in five-minute increments to provide a detailed account of the patient's arm movements.

A series of experiments is currently being conducted to provide reliability and validity data for using accelerometers to measure arm use. Experiment 1 examined the relationship between acceleration recordings and simple, standardized arm movements performed by college students in the laboratory. The results suggested that the Activity Monitors provide highly reliable measures of simple arm movement, with high sensitivity to movement parallel to the x and y axes of the units, low sensivity to movement parallel to the z axis, and higher sensitivity to changes in movement speed than distance (Uswatte et al., 1997a). Experiment 2 examined the relationship between acceleration recordings and three parameters of arm movement (speed, excursion, duration) involved in three activities of daily living (vacuuming, shelving, sponging) performed by college students in the laboratory (Uswatte et al., 1997b). The results suggested that the Activity Monitors provide highly reliable measures of activities of daily living-like arm movement, with high sensitivity to the duration of the task and the speed of the arm movement, but low sensitivity to the excursion of the movement. Experiment 3 will evaluate the relationship among accelerometer recordings taken from the arm and observer counts of arm movements and judgements of the duration of task-related arm movement involved in activities of daily living tasks engaged in by constraint-induced movement therapy patients and age-matched controls in the laboratory. Experiment 4 will study the relationship among accelerometer recordings, patient and caregiver diaries of arm use, and observer counts of arm movement in constraint-induced movement therapy patients over five weeks in the home. A high positive correlation between the accelerometer recordings and observation measures and the recordings and diary measures in Experiments 3 and 4 will suggest that the accelerometers are valid measures of arm use in the laboratory and real world, respectively.

The first two experiments and other pilot work suggest that there are some limitations to using accelerometers to measure arm use in the home. First, when measuring arm movement, accelerometers respond more strongly to certain kinds of movement than to others. The sample of movement obtained by accelerometers, however, is likely to be an adequate index of the amount of arm use because activities of daily living tasks generally involve movement components in each of the three spatial axes (Redmond and Hegge, 1985). Second, not all movements of the upper extremity are related to use of the limb (e.g. swinging the arm during ambulation). Third, variation in physical dimensions, pace and coordination across subjects may be so large that the accelerometer measure may be useful only on a within-subjects basis. This may limit the generality of the data obtained in absolute terms, but would not invalidate the use of the accelerometers for obtaining information on the relative change in the amount of extremity movement for individual subjects before and after treatment. Fourth, the variability in the type of tasks performed on different days may limit the accuracy of the accelerometer measure for evaluating upper extremity use in the home by constraint-induced movement therapy patients on a day-to-day basis. However, this variability is likely to be less of a problem when measurements are cumulated over a longer period of time, such as a week. Finally, sudden or shaky upper extremity movements tend to inflate accelerometer recordings in a manner that is not consistent with the actual amount of use of the extremity. Data-smoothing techniques used in psychophysiological research may be of value in substantially reducing this problem. Although these limitations must be given serious consideration, it is not anticipated that they will cause serious problems for measuring upper extremity function in the real world.

Relationship between motor ability and real-world function measures

Laboratory motor tests and real-world outcome measures provide complementary information about patient motor status. On laboratory motor tests, clinicians observe the best a patient is able to achieve when explicitly asked to carry out a movement or task in the laboratory; the results indicate a patient's maximum motor ability. However, this performance does not indicate whether the patient is actually using the extremity for the tested purpose in the life situation. In a study of 29 stroke patients who were consecutive admissions to a rehabilitation facility (Andrews and Stewart, 1979), primary caregivers reported that in 25–45 per cent of cases activities of daily living were performed less well in the home situation than in the laboratory. This observation has been confirmed by every clinician the authors have contacted. Among the patients treated in the authors' laboratory, there were no significant correlations between performance on the pretreatment motor ability tests and the baseline measure of arm use. These observations and the authors' results suggest that the transfer from the laboratory to the home needs to be tested directly.

Indeed, the gap between performance on laboratory tests and the actual amount of extremity use in the home is an index of learned nonuse. Constraint-induced movement therapy operates in this window. It provides a bridge between the laboratory or clinic and the life setting so that the therapeutic gains made in the clinic transfer maximally and contribute to the functional independence of the patient in the real world.

Among the patients treated in the authors' laboratory, there has been a moderately strong, positive relationship between the initial level of arm motor ability and the improvement in arm use produced by therapy: $0.48 < rs < 0.57$, $ps < 0.01$; patients with a high initial level of motor ability have shown larger gains in arm use than patients with a low initial motor ability level. Given that there was no significant relationship between the initial level of arm use and arm ability, this result is congruent with the hypothesis that constraint-induced movement therapy operates in the gap between arm motor ability and arm use: patients with high motor ability have more

room to improve. The relationship between changes in arm motor ability and changes in arm use with treatment is not yet clear.

Cognitive and affective measures

In addition to the use of measures of motor performance, a measure of expectancy and self-efficacy, and a measure of depression, the Zung Depression Inventory (Zung and Durham, 1965), patients in the authors' laboratory are also examined pretreatment and posttreatment using five neuropsychological tests – (1) Mini-Mental State Exam (Bleecker et al., 1988), (2) Cancel-H Test (Gordon et al., 1984), (3) Line Cancellation Task (Albert, 1973), (4) Sentence Repetition Test (Benton and Hamscher, 1983), and (5) Token Test (Benton and Hamscher, 1983). No significant changes between pretreatment and posttreatment performance have been detected on these measures.

Conclusions

- There are no instruments in cognitive psychology or neuropsychology that measure cognitive function directly in the real-life setting.
- New measurement instruments in cognitive neurorehabilitation are needed that provide direct, continuous and objective measures of real-world cognitive activity.

There are no instruments in cognitive psychology or neuropsychology that measure cognitive function directly in the home situation. Traditionally, neuropsychological instruments have been used to diagnose cognitive disorders (Hart and Hayden, 1986). Therefore, cognitive function in the home has not been examined carefully. However, substantial research has been done on the relationship between performance on neuropsychological instruments and activities of daily living function. Investigators have examined the validity of neuropsychological instruments for assessing and predicting functional ability by studying the relationship between performance on neuropsychological tests and laboratory performance tests of activities of daily living and instrumental activities of daily living function (Goldstein, et al., 1992; Richardson, Nadler and Malloy,

1995; Baum et al., 1996), and by studying the relationship between neuropsychological test performance and retrospective questionnaires of home (Searight et al., 1989; McCue, Rogers and Goldstein, 1990; Tuokko and Crockett, 1991) and social functioning (Dunn et al., 1990; Millis, Rosenthal and Lourie, 1994; Kaitaro, Koskinen and Kaipio, 1995). These approaches may be flawed for the same reason that it is wrong to assume that motor ability or function in the clinic reflects motor function in the home. As with motor ability in the clinic and motor function at home, there may be a disparity between cognitive ability in the clinic and cognitive practice at home, as well as between activities of daily living function in the clinic and activities of daily living behaviour at home.

The authors suggest that the approach their laboratory has taken to measure arm use in the real world can serve as a model for measurement procedures in cognitive rehabilitation. Interventions that aim to improve cognitive skills so that people with brain injuries can function better in their daily lives require instruments that measure cognitive activity in the life situation. These instruments might include measures such as the Motor Activity Log, which quantifies retrospective reports from the patient or caregiver, and the Actual Amount of Use Test, which unobtrusively samples the spontaneous behaviour of the patient. Accelerometry, in particular, might serve as a good model because it provides a direct measure of activity in the life setting and avoids the problems of obtaining self-reports from people with brain damage. An instrument parallel to the accelerometer in cognitive neurorehabilitation might be a portable electroencephalographic (EEG) device. This device could provide information on power in different parts of the EEG spectrum while a patient is engaged in different types of activities throughout the day. The activities could be recorded by a caregiver or could be tasks that are carried out with a personal computer whose clock is coordinated with that of the EEG device.

Researchers in cognitive neurorehabilitation may want to adopt the assessment of motor function as a model for the assessment of real-world cognitive function because of the complexity of cognitive activity relative to motor activity. The mechanisms underlying cognitive activity are less well defined and less well understood than those underlying motor activity. In addition, cognitive activity is less easily measured than motor activity because a given observable behaviour is an unreliable index of the cognitive processes with which it may be associated. The approach adopted in the authors' laboratory for the relatively simple task of measuring motor activity may be a useful guide to some ways in which the assessment of cognitive activity in the real world can be carried out.

Acknowledgements

This research was supported by Grant #HD34273–01 from the National Institutes of Health, Grant #94–172 from the Retirement Research Foundation, and a grant from the Center for Ageing, University of Alabama at Birmingham, to Edward Taub; and Grant #B93–629AP from the Rehabilitation Research and Development Service, US Department of Veterans Affairs, to Rama D. Pidikiti and Edward Taub.

The authors would like to thank the following collaborators: Jean E. Crago, Rama D. Pidikiti, Stephanie C. DeLuca, David Morris, Wolfgang Miltner, Bruno Kopp, Seth Spraggins, Scott Moran, Harrison Walker, Jesse Calhoun, Vinayak Sharma, Maneesh Varma, Curtis Beatty, Sharon Shaw, Anjan Chatterjee, Edwin W. Cook, David Edwards, Louis D. Burgio, Thomas A. Novack, Donna M. Bearden, Thomas E. Groomes, William D. Fleming, Cecil S. Nepomuceno, and Neal E. Miller.

References

Albert, M.L. 1973. A simple test of visual neglect. *Neurology* **23**, 658–64.

Andrews, K. and Stewart, J. 1979. Stroke recovery: he can but does he? *Rheumatol Rehabil* **18**, 43–8.

Baum, C., Edwards, E., Yonan, C. and Storandt, M. 1996. The relation of neuropsychological test performance to performance of functional tasks in dementia of the Alzheimer type. *Arch Clin Neuropsychol* **11**, 69–75.

Baxter-Petralia, P., Bruening, L.A., Blackmore, S.M. and McEntee, P.M. 1990. Physical capacity evaluation. In *Rehabilitation of the Hand*, ed. J.M. Hunter, pp. 93–108. St Louis: CV Mosby.

Benton, A.L. and Hamscher, K. 1983. *Multilingual Aphasia Examination*. Iowa City: AJL Associates Inc.

Berglund, K. and Fugl-Meyer, A.R. 1986. Upper extremity function in hemiplegia. A cross-validation study of two assessment methods. *Scand J Rehabil Med* 18, 155–7.

Bleecker, M., Bolla-Wilson, K., Kawas, C. and Agnew, J. 1988. Age-specific norms for the Mini-Mental State Exam. *Neurology* 38, 1565–8.

Bouten, C.V., Westerterp, K.R., Verduin, M. and Janssen, J.D. 1994. Assessment of energy expenditure for physical activity using a triaxial accelerometer. *Med Sci Sports Exerc* 26, 1516–23.

Computer Science Applications Inc. 1996. *Activity Monitor Model 7164* [Manual]. Shalimar, FL: CSA Inc.

Cress, M.E., Buchner, D.M., Questad, K.A., Esselman, P.C., deLateur, B.J. and Schwartz, R.S. 1996. Continuous-scale physical functional performance in healthy older adults: a validation study. *Arch Phys Med Rehabil* 77, 1243–50.

Demeurisse, G., Demol, O. and Robaye, E. 1980. Motor evaluation in vascular hemiplegia. *Eur Neurol* 19, 382–9.

Duncan, P.W., Propst, M. and Nelson, S.G. 1983. Reliability of the Fugl-Meyer assessment of sensorimotor recovery following cerebrovascular accident. *Phys Ther* 63, 1606–10.

Dunn, E.J., Searight, H.R., Grisso, T., Margolis, R.B. and Gibbons, J.L. 1990. The relation of the Halstead–Reitan neuropsychological battery to functional daily living living skills in geriatric patients. *Arch Clin Neuropsychol* 5, 103–17.

Elbert, T., Pantev, C., Wienbruch, C., Rockstroh, B. and Taub, E. 1995. Increased use of the left hand in string players associated with increased cortical representation of the fingers. *Science* 270, 305–7.

Flor, H., Elbert, S., Knecht, C. et al. 1995. Phantom limb pain as a perceptual correlate of massive cortical reorganization in upper limb amputees. *Nature* 375, 482–4.

Foster, F.G., McPartland, R.J. and Kupfer, D.J. 1978. Motion sensing devices in medicine, part I: a report on reliability and validity. *J Inter-Am Med* 3, 4–8.

Fugl-Meyer, A.R., Jaasko, L, Leyman, I., Olson, S. and Steglind, S. 1975. The post-stroke hemiplegic patient: a method for evaluation of physical performance. *Scand J Rehabil Med* 7, 13–31.

Goldstein, G., McCue, M., Rogers, J. and Nussbaum, P.D. 1992. Diagnostic differences in memory test based predictions of functional capacity in the elderly. *Neuropsychol Rehabil* 2, 307–17.

Gordon, W.A., Ruckdeschel-Hibbard, M., Egelko. S. et al. 1984. *Evaluation of the Deficits Associated with Right Brain Damage: Normative Data on the Institute of Rehabilitation Medicine Test Battery*. New York: Institute of Rehabilitation Medicine, New York University Medical Center.

Hart, T. and Hayden, M.E. 1986. The ecological validity of neuro-psychological assessment and remediation. In *Clinical Neuropsychology of Intervention*, ed. B.P. Uzell and Y. Gross, pp. 21–50. Boston: Martinus Nijhoff.

Holbrook, M. and Skilbeck, C.E. 1983. An activities index for use with stroke patients. *Age Aging* 12, 166–70.

Janz, K.F. 1994. Validation of the CSA accelerometer for assessing children's physical activity. *Med Sci Sports Exerc* 26, 369–75.

Janz, K.F., Witt, J. and Mahoney, L.T. 1995. The stability of children's physical activity as measured by accelerometry and self-report. *Med Sci Sports Exerc* 27, 1326–32.

Kaitaro, T., Koskinen, S. and Kaipio, M.L. 1995. Neuropsychological problems in everyday life: a 5-year follow-up study of young severely closed-head-injured patients. *Brain Inj* 9, 713–27.

Keith, R.A. 1995. Conceptual basis of outcome measures. *Am J Phys Med Rehabil* 74, 73–80.

Keith, R.A., Granger, C.V., Hamilton, B.B. and Sherwin, F.S. 1987. The functional independence measure: a new tool for rehabilitation. In *Advances in Clinical Rehabilitation*, Vol. 1, ed. M.G. Eisenberg and R.C. Grzesiak, pp. 6–18. New York: Springer-Verlag.

Kimble, G.S. 1961. *Hilgard and Marquis' Conditioning and Learning*, 2nd edn. New York: Appleton-Century-Crofts.

Knapp, H.D., Taub, E. and Berman, A.J. 1958. Effect of deafferentation on a conditioned avoidance response. *Science* 128, 842–3.

Knapp, H.D., Taub, E. and Berman, A.J. 1963. Movements in monkeys with deafferented forelimbs. *Exp Neurol* 7, 305–15.

Kochersberger, G., McConnell, E., Kuchibhatla, M.N. and Pieper, C. 1996. The reliability, validity, and stability of a measure of physical activity in the elderly. *Arch Phys Med Rehabil* 77, 793–5.

Kopp, B., Kunkel, A., Flor, H. et al. 1997. The Arm Motor Ability Test (AMAT): reliability, validity, and sensitivity to change of an instrument for assessing ADL disability. *Arch Phys Med Rehabil* 78, 615–20.

Kopp, B., Kunkel, A., Muehlnickel, W., Villringer, K., Taub, E. and Flor, H. 1999. Plasticity in the motor system related to therapy-induced improvement of movement after stroke. *Neuroreport* 10, 807–10.

Lassek, A.M. 1953. Inactivation of voluntary motor function following rhizotomy. *J Neuropathol Exp Neurol* 2, 83–7.

Lezak, M.D. 1995. *Neuropsychological Assessment*, 3rd edn. New York: Oxford Press.

Liepert, J., Bauder, H., Sommer, M. et al. 1998. Motor cortex plasticity during constraint-induced movement therapy in chronic stroke patients. *Neurosci Lett* 250, 5–8.

Mahoney, R.I. and Barthel, D.W. 1965. Functional evaluation: the Barthel index. *Mid-state Med J* **14**, 61–5.

Makikawa, M., Imai, K., Shindoi, T., Tanooka, K., Iizumi, H. and Mitani, H. 1994. Microprocessor-based memory device for ambulatory heart rate and physical activity recording. *Methods Info Med* **33**, 94–6.

McCulloch, K., Cook, E.W. III, Fleming, W.C., Novack, T.A., Nepomuceno, C.S. and Taub, E. 1988. A reliable test of upper extremity ADL function [Abstract]. *Arch Phys Med Rehabil* **69**, 755.

McCue, M., Rogers, J.C. and Goldstein, G. 1990. Relationships between neuropsychological and functional assessment in elderly neuropsychiatric patients. *Rehabil Psychol* **35**, 91–9.

Melanson, E.L. and Freedson, P.S. 1995. Validity of the Computer Science Applications, Inc. (CSA) activity monitor. *Med Sci Sports Exerc* **27**, 934–40.

Merzenich, M.M., Nelson, R.J., Stryker, M.P., Cynader, M.S., Shoppmann, A. and Zook, J.M. 1984. Somatosensory cortical map changes following digit amputation in adult monkeys. *J Comp Neurol* **224**, 591–605.

Miller, D.J., Freedson, P.S. and Kline G.M. 1994. Comparison of activity levels using the Caltrac accelerometer and five questionnaires. *Med Sci Sports Exerc* **26**, 376–82.

Millis, S.R., Rosenthal, M. and Lourie, I.F. 1994. Predicting community integration after traumatic brain injury with neuropsychological measures. *Int J Neurosci* **79**, 165–7.

Morgan, W.G. 1974. The shaping game: a teaching technique. *Behav Ther* **5**, 271–2.

Mott, P.W. and Sherrington, C.S. 1895. Experiments upon the influence of sensory nerves upon the movement and nutrition of limbs. *Proc R Soc Lond* **57**, 481–8.

Nichols, J.F., Patterson, P. and Early, T. 1992. A validation of a physical activity monitor for young and older adults. *Can J Sport Sci* **17**, 299–303.

Nudo, R.J., Wise, B.M., SiFuentes, F. and Milliken, G.W. 1996. Neural substrates for the effects of rehabilitative training on motor recovery following ischemic infarct. *Science* **272**, 1791–4.

Ostendorf, C.G. and Wolf, S.L. 1981. Effect of forced use of the upper extremity of a hemiplegic patient on changes in function. *Phys Ther* **61**, 1022–8.

Panyan, M.V. 1980. *How to Use Shaping*. Lawrence, KS: H & H Enterprises.

Patterson, S.M., Krantz, L.C., Montgomery, L.C., Deuster, P.A., Hedges, S.M. and Nebel, L.E. 1993. Automated physical activity monitoring: validation and comparison with physiological and self-report measures. *Psychophysiology* **30**, 296–305.

Redmond, D.P. and Hegge, F.W. 1985. Observations on the design and specification of a wrist-worn human activity monitoring system. *Behav Res Meth* **17**, 659–69.

Richardson, E.D., Nadler, J.D. and Malloy, P.F. 1995. Neuropsychologic prediction of performance measures of daily living skills in geriatric patients. *Neuropsychology* **9**, 565–72.

Searight, H.R., Dunn, E.J., Grisso, T., Margolis, R.B. and Gibbons, J.L. 1989. The relation of the Halstead–Reitan Neuropsychological Battery to ratings of everyday functioning in a geriatric sample. *Neuropsychology* **3**, 135–45.

Shrout, P.E. and Fleiss, J.L. 1979. Intraclass correlations: uses in assessing rater reliability. *Psychol Bull* **86**, 420–8.

Skinner, B.F. 1938. *The Behavior of Organisms*. New York: Appleton-Century-Crofts.

Skinner, B.F. 1968. *The Technology of Teaching*. New York: Appleton-Century-Crofts.

Smith, D.S. and Clark, M.S. 1995. Competence and performance in activities of daily living in patients following rehabilitation from stroke. *Disabil Rehabil* **17**, 15–23.

Stam, H.J., Eijskoot, F. and Bussmann, J.B. 1995. A device for long-term ambulatory monitoring in trans-tibial amputees. *Prosthet Orthot Int* **19**, 53–5.

Sterr, A., Mueller, M.M., Elbert, T., Rockstroh, B., Pantev, C. and Taub, E. 1998. Changed perceptions in Braille readers. *Nature* **391**, 134–5.

Tajima, F., Ogata, H., Lee, K.H., Ookawa, H. and Piciulo, C.M. 1994. Use of an accelerometer in evaluating arm movement during wheelchair propulsion. *Sangyo Ika Daigaku Zasshi* **16**, 219–26.

Taub, E. 1976. Motor behavior following deafferentation in the developing and motorically mature monkey. In *Neural Control of Locomotion*, ed. R. Herman, S. Grillner, H.J. Ralston, P.S.G. Stein and D. Stuart, pp. 675–705. New York: Plenum Press.

Taub, E. 1977. Movement in nonhuman primates deprived of somatosensory feedback. *Exerc Sports Sci Rev* **4**, 335–74.

Taub, E. 1980. Somatosensory deafferentation research with monkeys: implications for rehabilitation medicine. In *Behavioral Psychology in Rehabilitation Medicine: Clinical Applications*, ed. L.P. Ince, pp. 371–401. New York: Williams & Wilkins.

Taub, E., Bacon, R. and Berman, A.J. 1965. The acquisition of a trace-conditioned response after deafferentation of the responding limb. *J Comp Physiol Psychol* **58**, 275–9.

Taub, E. and Berman, A.J. 1963. Avoidance conditioning in the absence of relevant proprioceptive and exteroceptive feedback. *J Comp Physiol Psychol* **56**, 1012–16.

Taub, E. and Crago, J.E. 1995. Overcoming learned nonuse: a

new behavioral approach to physical medicine. In *Biobehavioral Self-Regulation: Eastern and Western Perspectives*, ed. T. Kikuchi, H. Sakuma, I. Saito and K. Tsuboi, pp. 2–9. Tokyo: Springer-Verlag.

Taub, E., Ellman, S.J. and Berman, A.J. 1966. Deafferentation in monkeys: effect on conditioned grasp response. *Science* **151**, 593–4.

Taub, E., Miller, N.E., Novack, T.A. et al. 1993. Technique to improve chronic motor deficit after stroke. *Arch Phys Med Rehabil* **74**, 347–54.

Taub, E., Perrella, P.N., Miller, N.E. and Barro, G. 1973. Behavioral development following forelimb deafferentation on day of birth of monkeys with and without binding. *Science* **181**, 959–60.

Taub, E., Perrella, P.N., Miller, N.E. and Barro, G. 1975. Diminution of early environmental control through perinatal and prenatal somatosensory deafferentation. *Biol Psychiatry* **10**, 609–26.

Taub, E., Pidikiti, R., Deluca, S. and Crago, J. 1995. Effects of motor restriction of an unimpaired upper extremity and training on improving functional tasks and altering brain/behaviors. In *Imaging and Neurologic Rehabilitation*, ed. J. Toole and D.C. Good, pp. 133–54. New York: Demos Publications.

Taub, E., Williams, M., Barro, G. and Steiner, S.S. 1978. Comparison of the performance of deafferented and intact monkeys on continuous and fixed ratio schedules of reinforcement. *Exp Neurol* **58**, 1–13.

Tuokko, H.A. and Crockett, D.J. 1991. Assessment of everyday functioning in normal and malignant memory disordered elderly. In *The Neuropsychology of Everyday Life: Issues in Development and Rehabilitation*, ed. D.E. Tupper and K.D. Cicceroni, pp. 135–82. Boston: Kluwer Academic Publishers.

Uswatte, G., Spraggins, S., Walker, H., Calhoun, J. and Taub, E. 1997. Validity and reliability of accelerometry as an objective measure of upper extremity use at home. Abstract. *Arch Phys Med Rehabil* **78**, 904.

Veltnic, P.H., Bussman, H.B., de Vries, W., Martens, W.L. and Van Lummel, R.C. 1996. Detection of static and dynamic activities using uniaxial accelerometers. *IEEE Trans Rehabil Eng* **4**, 375–85.

Wolf, S.L. and Binder-Macleod, S.A. 1983. Electromyographic biofeedback applications to the hemiplegic patient: changes in upper extremity neuromuscular and functional status. *Phys Ther* **63**, 1393–403.

Wolf, S.L., Lecraw, D.E., Barton, L.A. and Jann, B.B. 1989. Forced use of hemiplegic upper extremities to reverse the effect of learned nonuse among chronic stroke and head-injured patients. *Exp Neurol* **104**, 125–32.

Wong, T.C., Webster, J.G., Montoye, H.J. and Washburn, R. 1981. Portable accelerometer device for measuring human energy expenditure. *IEEE Trans Biomed Eng BME* **28**, 467–71.

Zung, W.W.K. and Durham, N.C. 1965. A self-rating depression scale. *Arch Gen Psychiatry* **12**, 63–70.

14

Mood and motivation in rehabilitation

Anthony Feinstein

Introduction

Patients with an acquired brain injury may present with abnormalities of mood, affect and motivation. Given the disabling nature of these disturbances, accurate clinical assessment is a prerequisite in planning a comprehensive rehabilitation strategy. It is important to realize at the outset that abnormalities in each domain may occur independently of one another, although a more common clinical picture is one in which all domains are affected to varying degrees. The importance in making this clinical distinction cannot be over-emphasized for distinct abnormalities in mood, affect and motivation, as each demands a specific treatment. The clinician who fails to tease out these various features of the mental state thus runs the risk of missing potentially treatable conditions that will adversely impinge on the entire rehabilitation process.

To understand better how such presentations arise in a clinical setting, reference is made to the neural circuitry underpinning these abnormalities. While there is sound empirical evidence elucidating the neural pathways controlling mood and motivation, the pathogenesis of disturbances in affect, i.e. the display of emotion as distinct from subjective feeling, is less clearly understood. Therefore, only brief reference is made to pathogenesis within a clinical perspective in the section of the chapter dealing with pseudobulbar affect, also termed pathological laughing and crying.

The aim of this chapter is to acquaint the reader with a summary of the relevant neuroanatomy of mood and motivation, followed by a description of the clinical features, differential diagnosis and treatment of disorders of mood (depression and mania), affect (pathological laughing and crying), anxiety and motivation. The emphasis is clinical and the approach a practical one for the therapeutic benefits of timely and correct intervention are considerable.

Frontal subcortical circuits and behaviour

- Five, discrete frontal–subcortical neural circuits associated with specific behavioural difficulties have been identified. Three of these relate to disorders of mood and motivation and are mediated via dysregulation of neurotransmitters such as dopamine and serotonin:

dorsolateral prefrontal circuit subserving executive cognitive tasks and mood (depression);

an orbitofrontal circuit linked to mania, obsessive–compulsive disorder and personality change of the disinhibited and labile subtype.

an anterior cingulate pathway associated with motivation.

Five discrete frontal subcortical circuits (Alexander, DeLong and Strick, 1986; Alexander and Crutcher, 1990) have been delineated. All begin in the frontal lobes and project first to the striatum, then to the globus pallidus and substantia nigra, before synapsing in the thalamus, from where the circuit loops back to the frontal lobes. Of the five circuits, three originate in separate prefrontal cortical areas, namely the dorsolateral prefrontal cortex, the lateral orbital cortex, and the anterior cingulate cortex. The remaining two circuits begin in the supplementary motor area and frontal eye fields.

These three main pathways have subsidiary pathways at various stages throughout their course and send and receive connections to and from related limbic structures. As the circuits progress from cortex to subcortex, the neurons funnel into increasingly smaller areas, while maintaining their parallel and distinct anatomical integrity. This 'squeezing' of the circuits helps explain how lesions situated at various points along the pathway give rise to differing clinical presentations.

Behavioural change

Each prefrontal circuit is associated with a specific behavioural syndrome (Cummings, 1993). Lesions localized to the dorsolateral prefrontal cortex produce depression and/or cognitive difficulties characterized by problems with executive functions such as planning, organizing, sequencing and abstracting. A lesion in the lateral orbitofrontal area may produce mania or obsessive–compulsive behaviour. It may also give rise to changes in personality, typically of the labile, disinhibited and aggressive type. Patients may appear irritable and display a lack of social tact. They differ from individuals with dorsolateral prefrontal pathology by performing normally on tests that challenge executive functioning. Anterior cingulate pathology typically produces abnormalities of motivation, and individuals may present as profoundly apathetic or abulic.

Lesions affecting the striatal structures may produce clinical states similar to those described above, depending on the extent to which the pathological process remains localized. This becomes increasingly less likely as the circuit projects posteroinferiorly, so that lesions affecting the globus pallidus or thalamus do not produce a discrete syndrome, but rather a mixture of signs and symptoms. Thus, the clinical picture may be a combination of disinhibition and irritability (orbitofrontal syndrome), reduced motivation and interest (medial frontal–anterior cingulate syndrome) and neuropsychological deficits (dorsolateral prefrontal syndrome).

Mechanisms of behavioural change

Interruptions to these circuits probably translate into behavioural abnormalities via a dysregulation of neurotransmitters such as glutamate, dopamine and serotonin, amongst others. The relationship between dopamine and the anterior cingulate pathway is evidence of this. Apathy results from dysfunction of this circuit (Adair et al., 1996) and may be successfully treated with dopaminergic drugs (Ross and Stewart, 1981). An analogous situation pertains to the neurotransmitter serotinin and the orbitofrontal and dorsolateral prefrontal circuits. Dysfunction of these circuits may produce behavioural change such as depression and obsessive–compulsive disorder that respond favourably to drugs that selectively enhance serotonin availability.

Having briefly outlined some basic neuroanatomy, the remainder of the chapter is devoted to a discussion of the pathogenesis and clinical features of depression, mania, pathological laughing and crying, and impaired motivation.

Depressive disorders

- Clinically significant depression is frequently found in a rehabilitation setting.
- It is associated with cerebral blood flow abnormalities affecting orbitofrontal and dorsolateral prefrontal cortex.
- There is also a link with adverse psychosocial stressors.
- Concomitant physical and cognitive abnormalities may obscure the diagnosis.
- Attention to a patient's thought content and interviewing an informant help in establishing the diagnosis.
- Pharmacotherapy is often effective in treating depression, although patients may prove sensitive to adverse side-effects. Therefore, selective serotonin reuptake inhibitors (SSRIs) are probably the drugs of choice.

Frequency and pathogenesis

There is an accumulating body of evidence suggesting that clinically significant depression, akin to major depression, may be an integral part of many disabling conditions. The most robust data come from the neurological literature, in which lifetime prevalence figures approaching 50 per cent for Parkinson's disease (Starkstein and Robinson, 1989) and multiple sclerosis (Sadovnick et al., 1996) have been noted, well in excess of the 17 per cent figure reported in general population comorbidity surveys (Kessler et al., 1994). Similarly, elevated prevalence rates have been noted with stroke (Robinson and Price, 1982), Huntington's disease (Folstein et al., 1983), traumatic brain injury (Robinson and Jorge, 1994) and Alzheimer's disease (Loreck and Folstein, 1993).

The clinician often faces a dilemma in deciding whether depression is aetiologically related to the physical disorder that has prompted the need for rehabilitation or the chance occurrence of an additional illness or an understandable, psychological reaction to physical disability. While on an individual basis it is never possible to be entirely certain on this score, the absence of the usual female preponderance of patients strongly suggests these mood changes are directly attributable to the neurological process (Clayton and Lewis, 1981). The advent of sophisticated neuroimaging has also more recently provided a means to assess the potential association between depression and cerebral pathology. In stroke patients, an association between left (dominant) anterior placed lesions and more serious depressive illness has been reported (Robinson et al., 1983) and replicated (Eastwood et al., 1989). However, with regard to right-sided lesions, the relationship between lesion site and severity of depression would appear to be more complex and time dependent, i.e. more posterior right-sided lesions associated with early-onset depression, with a delayed onset more closely linked to right anterior-placed lesions (Robinson et al., 1984). Subcortical pathology, in particular stroke affecting the left basal ganglia, has also been associated with depression, severity of the mood change once again being related to more anterior-placed lesions (Starkstein, Robinson and Price, 1987).

The importance of frontal system pathology in the pathogenesis of depression has also been noted in other neuropsychiatric disorders. Depressed as opposed to nondepressed Parkinson's disease patients have significantly lower metabolic activity in the head of the caudate nucleus and orbitofrontal cortex (Mayberg et al., 1990). Similarly, orbitofrontal and inferior prefrontal cortex hypometabolism differentiated depressed from nondepressed Huntington's disease patients (Mayberg et al., 1992). Positron emission tomography findings from both these disorders overlap with neuroimaging data from patients who are depressed but without concomitant neurological disease (Baxter et al., 1989; Bench et al., 1992). Although there is no direct evidence from any of these studies confirming neuronal loss, hypometabolism in brain areas rich in biogenic amine pathways implicates abnormalities in dopamine and catecholamine transmission in patients who become depressed. This is further supported by Parkinson's disease patients endorsing more depressive symptomatology when in the 'off' state (more bradykinetic) than when motor function improves ('on' state) (Friedenberg and Cummings, 1989).

Impressive as these results are, there are disorders in which the link between brain involvement and depression is more equivocal. The best example is multiple sclerosis, for which the lifetime prevalence rate for depression is three times that expected in the general population. Despite the frequency with which clinically significant mood change occurs, the results from neuroimaging studies have been disappointing. Although magnetic resonance imaging is sensitive in detecting and localizing lesions, the number of studies failing to report an association between brain abnormalities and depression (Huber et al., 1987; Ron and Logsdail, 1989) outnumber those that do report such an association (Honer et al., 1987). Rather, the most significant correlates of mood in some magnetic resonance imaging studies have not been cerebral but levels of social stress and support (Feinstein et al., 1992a, Feinstein, Youl and Ron, 1992b). The studies come as timely reminders that despite significant advances in neuroimaging and the mapping in vivo of neural pathways subserving mood, the pathogenesis of depression cannot be divorced from the patient's social context.

The assessment of depression

History

It is important to take a thorough psychiatric history from all patients at their initial assessment. Particularly within a rehabilitation setting, patients may prove poor historians, for a variety of reasons ranging from cognitive impairment to impaired insight, and therefore an informant who knows the patient well (regular contact over many years) should also be interviewed. Depression may be missed in aphasic patients, being obscured by difficulties they have in expressing their distress. However, it is a frequent concomitant and may manifest as grief or catastrophic reactions, major depression and suicide (Benson and Ardila, 1993). The presence of a family history of mental illness and the nature of that illness should be ascertained for there is some evidence that mood change, irrespective of an acquired brain insult, remains consistent within families (Schiffer et al., 1988). In addition, the presence of a premorbid psychiatric history may throw light on the subsequent development of mood change. A detailed social history is mandatory to document relevant stressors (financial, residential, occupational, relationship) and supports that are present. The number of drugs implicated in causing a depressive illness is legion and medication lists should therefore be thoroughly checked (Cummings, 1985).

At a symptom level, it is often difficult to decide what is attributable to depression or the associated physical disorder. This problem frequently occurs with fatigue, which is virtually ubiquitous within a rehabilitation population. Vegetative features such as poor sleep, loss of appetite and sexual interest, considered the hallmarks of depression in a psychiatric population, may also prove misleading. Patients with acquired brain injuries often display abnormalities in these areas independent of mood variation. While it remains essential to document all these changes plus subjective complaints of low mood, specific attention should be addressed to complaints (or observations) which may carry greater weight, such as irritability, feelings of hopelessness, frustration, loss of interest in activities that formerly gave enjoyment and that could still be pursued, social withdrawal and thoughts of suicide or self-harm, the last-mentioned of which should never be overlooked. Epidemiological data point to suicide as a significant cause of morbidity in multiple sclerosis, spinal cord injuries and certain subsets of epileptic patients (Stenager and Stenager, 1992). Finally, the duration of symptoms should be noted, wherever possible corroborating this with an informant. Transient lability in mood may be part of adjusting to disability or a new environment. However, the persistence of a low, nondistractible mood is a more serious development.

Mental state examination

The mental state assessment in depressed patients presents similar difficulties, e.g. how to differentiate the bradykinesia and masked facies of Parkinson's disease from the psychomotor retardation and blunted affect of depression. Conversely, low mood may be incorrectly attributed to patients with disorders of prosody associated with nondominant cerebral pathology (George et al., 1996). Although speech, language and thought form may prove misleading, thought content characterized by cognitive distortions and somatic preoccupations is often the crucial factor that establishes the diagnosis. Often, the diagnosis may only be reached after combining information from history, mental state assessment and the observations of family informants and allied health workers.

Pseudodementia

Depression masquerading as dementia is a problem frequently encountered in rehabilitation settings. One reason is the common occurrence of depression in people with well-established dementia (Caine, 1981). In addition, affective change may herald the onset of cognitive change that will only become more apparent with time. Clinical clues suggestive of depression include a family history of affective disorder and a preserved ability to learn new information. Neuropsychological testing may further help in diagnostic clarification. A three-way comparison of memory testing in brain-damaged, depressed and healthy controls has demonstrated clear performance differences in the brain-damaged groups and has also shown that depression is unlikely significantly to compromise performance (Coughlan and Hollows, 1984). However, these are group findings and caution has been advocated in using neuropsychological testing as an infallible method of detecting pseudodementia (Caine, 1981).

The difficulty of accurate diagnosis is illustrated by the results of a longitudinal study in which a third of cases were found to have been erroneously first diagnosed as demented (Ron et al., 1979).

Adjuncts to diagnosis

The diagnosis of a depressive syndrome is essentially a clinical one. In cases of uncertainty, little help can be obtained from adjunctive methods such as the dexamethasone suppression test, for which the rate of false-positive results as demonstrated in Parkinson's disease is unacceptably high (Frochtengarten et al., 1987). Similarly, rating scales are not a substitute for clinical acumen. They are, however, useful as a research tool and for allowing the patient subjectively to record changes in mood over time. The results need to be interpreted with caution, as many of the better known and most widely used scales are ill-suited to a rehabilitation setting because they contain an unacceptably high number of somatic-based questions, endorsement of which may give rise to false-positive results.

Treatment

There is a paucity of controlled clinical trials for depression within a rehabilitation setting and much of the evidence to date has been anecdotal. However, some general principles do apply. When prescribing antidepressant medication, the physician should be alert to possible drug interactions and patient susceptibility to side-effects because of compromised cerebral dysfunction. There is a case for using an SSRI as a first-choice antidepressant because of the lower incidence of troubling side-effects of these drugs, although they are not without their own problems, i.e. insomnia, sexual dysfunction and apathy. It is prudent to start at lower doses than one would in cases of uncomplicated depression (i.e. 10 mg of an SSRI such as fluoxetine or paroxetine), but should patients tolerate the medication well, there is no reason not to use comparable doses (>20 mg) if clinically indicated. An advantage to some tricyclic antidepressant drugs is the presence of a clear therapeutic window, and careful monitoring of plasma levels may allow the physician to gauge the most effective dose. Electroconvulsive therapy should be considered in

patients who have not responded well to pharmacotherapy. There are no absolute contraindications to the procedure, although patients with raised intracranial pressure or at risk for an intercerebral bleed demand caution and particularly close monitoring. In patients for whom the diagnosis of depression versus dementia is unclear, aggressive treatment for depression may provide the answer.

While supportive psychotherapy for patients and families is advocated, care should be taken in following a purely cognitive approach given the possibility of comorbid intellectual deficits.

Bipolar affective disorder

- Bipolar affective disorder may occur as a sequel to an acquired brain injury and symptoms may be difficult to distinguish from those of a personality change of the disinhibited subtype.
- Manic mood may respond well to mood stabilizers, with benzodiazepine and neuroleptic medication added for sedation and psychotic features respectively.

Secondary mania may follow an acquired brain injury with a frequency that exceeds chance expectation (Schiffer, Wineman and Weitkamp, 1986). A constellation of physical overactivity, elevated (or irritable) mood and grandiose (or persecutory) beliefs should alert the physician to the diagnosis. There may be difficulty in distinguishing mania from a brain disorder causing a personality change of the disinhibited, labile or aggressive subtype (see above). However, while the latter may show disinhibition and grandiose thinking, the presence of the triad of symptoms mentioned above makes the diagnosis of an affective disorder more likely. Similarly, a positive premorbid and family history of affective disorder helps differentiate the two.

With regard to treatment, mood-stabilizing drugs (lithium, carbamazepine and sodium valproate) with a benzodiazepine for sedation are the drugs of choice. Should psychotic symptoms be present, neuroleptic medication will be required. Newer compounds such as risperidone would appear to offer significant benefits given their more favourable side-effect profile. Clozapine would be the neuroleptic of choice in patients with psychosis and coexisting movement disorders. As with depression in the context of an acquired brain injury, the likelihood of adverse side-effects is increased. This may require keeping serum levels of mood-stablizing drugs at the lower end of the therapeutic range, which in practical terms may mean a daily dose of lithium of 600 mg as opposed to the 900–1200 mg used more often in a general psychiatry practice. There is, however, a considerable individual variation in the ability of patients with an acquired brain injury to tolerate side-effects, and therefore generalization becomes hazardous. Rather, the clinician should monitor each case according to its individual merits.

Pathological laughing and crying

- Pathological laughing and crying is a less common, but nevertheless disabling, complication of cerebral damage that responds well to small doses of amitriptyline or levodopa.

This condition has been regarded as synonymous with pseudobulbar affect, in which abnormalities of affect do not correspond to subjective alterations in mood (Poeck, 1969). However, more recent evidence has challenged this assumption (Ross and Stewart, 1987), suggesting at least a degree of overlap between outward displays of emotional dyscontrol and subjective feelings of emotional distress. Although the condition may prove disabling, it is amenable to effective treatment, either with small doses of amitriptyline (Schiffer, Herndon and Rudick, 1985) or, failing that, levodopa (Wolf, Santana and Thorpy, 1979). The precise pathogenesis is unclear, although evidence suggests it is associated with destruction of the serotonergic raphe nuclei in the brain stem or their ascending projections to the cerebral hemispheres (Andersen et al., 1994).

Anxiety disorders

- Whereas individual symptoms of anxiety are common, the prevalence of anxiety disorders in a rehabilitation sample has yet to be reliably established.
- In some disorders, most notably stroke, the occurrence appears to be a frequent one.

The category 'anxiety disorders' is a broad rubric encompassing disorders such as generalized anxiety disorder, obsessive–compulsive disorder and panic dis-order. Anxiety disorders in patients with physical illness, unlike their depressive counterparts, have received virtually no attention. Much of this disinterest has been attributed to the high frequency with which symptoms of anxiety occur in this setting (Popkin and Tucker, 1994). A distinction should therefore be made between isolated symptoms of anxiety, which are extremely common, and a specific syndrome of anxiety, termed 'anxiety disorders due to a general medical condition' by the *Diagnostic and Statistical Manual*, fourth edition (American Psychiatric Association, 1994). Although the prevalence of the latter within a rehabilitation setting has not been accurately ascertained, a review of anxiety syndromes associated with neurological disorders found that it occurred most commonly in patients with cerebral vascular disease, but was also part of the presentation of Huntington's disease, closed head injury, multiple sclerosis, encephalitis and central nervous system tumours, to mention a few of the more common disorders (Hall, 1980). Factors that suggest a causal relationship between the neurological and anxiety disorders are onset after the age of 35 years and an absence of family and personal histories of psychiatric illness. There are no published reports of cerebral correlates for the disorder.

A long list of medications may give rise to anxiety disorders, including steroids, caffeine, bronchodilators, insulin, oestrogens, antihistamines, digitalis and L-dopa.

Disorders of motivation

- Poor motivation (termed apathy) frequently complicates recovery during rehabilitation.
- Apathy may be a primary phenomenon or occur secondary to other disorders such as depression and dementia.
- Reversible causes (biological, psychosocial) should be corrected before resorting to pharmacotherapy as treatment.
- Dopamine-augmenting agents may prove an effective treatment in cases of primary apathy or a useful adjunct in secondary cases.

This discussion, while acknowledging a large and important literature from experimental psychology devoted to motivation, is confined to relevant clinical aspects. The important contributions of Robert Marin (1990; 1991; Marin et al., 1994) in bringing clarity to a loosely defined clinical concept are acknowledged, and this chapter follows Marin's approach in using the term apathy to denote impaired motivation.

Apathy may exist as a *primary*, independent syndrome, unencumbered by abnormalities of mood, fluctuations in level of consciousness or multiple intellectual deficits. As discussed in the section on frontal–subcortical circuits, an example of such a primary state is frontal lobe injury, particularly damage to the anterior cingulate, where impaired motivation is not accompanied by subjective emotional distress. More commonly, however, apathy may be one symptom comprising part of a larger syndrome, and in such cases the disorder of motivation should be regarded as a *secondary* phenomenon. Examples of these syndromes include delirium, dementia, depression and schizophrenia (Marin, 1991).

Before deciding whether apathy is primary or secondary in origin, the following points should be considered (Marin, 1991). Impaired motivation may be: (a) a reflection or exaggeration of premorbid personality traits; (b) part of a numbing of responsiveness and withdrawal induced by overwhelming stress; or (c) a response to altered physiological functioning such as loss of any of the primary senses, motor function and coordination. It may also stem from institutional living (Wing and Brown, 1970).

Apathy and depression

Differentiating apathy as a primary disorder from apathy as part of a depressive syndrome is important for they are not synonymous. The assessment of depressed patients is based on complaints such as social withdrawal, inability to enjoy activities that formerly gave them pleasure, and loss of interest and inactivity with respect to activities of daily living. These changes are unwanted and accompanied by subjective feelings of low mood and a thought content characterized by depressive cognitions such as poor self-esteem and an expectation of future failure. Attempts at social engagement are actively avoided. In more extreme cases, thought and actions may turn to suicide. This contrasts

with a primary apathetic syndrome in which patients may bear a superficial behavioural similarity to the above picture, but do not subjectively experience dysphoria and regard their altered state with emotional indifference (Marin et al., 1994).

Apathy and medical illness

Many neurological disorders are associated with apathy. They share a number of factors that, acting individually or in combination, produce a reduction in motivation (Marin, 1990). These factors include cognitive dysfunction hindering the capacity to focus and direct behaviour, an altered perception of the individual's abilities, and direct involvement of brain regions that control drive, i.e. frontal lobes. Thus, apathy may be found in dementia, basal ganglia disease, Korsakoff's syndrome, and disorders giving rise to indifference or neglect (e.g. right hemisphere stroke).

Medical conditions such as hyperthyroidism and hypoparathyroidism may also produce apathetic-like states, as may drugs ranging from neuroleptics and SSRIs to marijuana.

Mention should be made of two related neurological states that represent extreme forms of apathy. Abulia refers to an impairment of will and an inability to initiate behaviour. In its most extreme form, patients display akinetic mutism, in which they present as awake but unresponsive to sensory stimuli except for visual following. There is an absence of noticeable motor findings such as rigidity and dystonia and patients are unable to speak. An interruption in dopaminergic transmission to a corticolimbic structure such as the anterior cingulate is thought to induce the syndrome (Ross and Stewart, 1981; Devinsky, Morrell and Brent, 1995).

Assessment and treatment of apathy

The assessment of a patient's motivation follows on from the points mentioned above. Thus, history taking should include talking to an informant to ascertain the patient's premorbid personality profile and degree of motivation. The informant may also clarify the degree to which motivation is related to environment. A thorough physical and mental state assessment should elucidate whether the loss of motivation is primary or a symptom of another condition. Although this distinction appears simple in theory, detecting the various contributory factors frequently presents a considerable clinical challenge. Cognitive, perceptual and sensorimotor impairments should be carefully noted and a complete list of all medications obtained.

A first step to treatment is the removal of reversible psychosocial, medical and pharmacological causes of apathy. When apathy is traced to environmental factors, social interventions are called for, whereas psychotherapy is indicated for patients who feel overwhelmed by their disability and the adjustment to their lives this entails. The correction of sensorimotor impairments such as impaired visual acuity should be attended to and appropriate medical treatment (e.g. thyroid supplementation for hypothyroidism) should be initiated. Should apathy be secondary to an existing disorder such as depression, treatment targeted at the latter may successfully alleviate apathy as well. In some cases, however, SSRIs may themselves be implicated in causing poor motivation (Hoehn-Saric, Lipsey and McLeod, 1990).

The observation that a functional deficiency of dopamine can give rise to apathy suggests possible avenues of pharmacological intervention. Thus, treatment with psychostimulants (methylphenidate, dextroamphetamine and magnesium pemoline), direct dopamine agonists (bromocryptine, pergolide) or indirect dopamine agonists (amantadine) may prove helpful (Marin et al., 1995). Dosages should be adjusted according to individual response and tolerance of side-effects. There are reports of patients with profound abulia (Barret, 1991) and akinetic mutism (Ross and Stewart, 1981) responding dramatically to these agents.

Finally, time spent explaining to family members may prevent patients being blamed or criticised for their apparent disinterest and unresponsiveness to well-meaning efforts at their rehabilitation.

Conclusions

Alterations of affect, mood and motivation are frequently found in patients requiring rehabilitation. This chapter highlights certain neural networks associated with these behavioural disturbances and provides a framework for clinical assessment that incorporates biological and psychosocial factors. Treatment targeted at specific disorders may prove singularly effective and should therefore be energetically pursued, while remaining cognisant of the patient's enhanced sensitivity to drug side-effects and interactions. Improvement in mood and motivation may facilitate other aspects of rehabilitation and contribute significantly to enhancing quality of life.

References

Adair, J.C., Williamson, D.J.G., Schwartz, R.L. and Heilman, K.M. 1996. Ventral tegmental area injury and frontal lobe disorder. *Neurology* **46**, 842–3.

Alexander, G.E. and Crutcher, M.D. 1990. Functional architecture of basal ganglia circuits: neural substrates of parallel processing. *Trends Neurosci* **13**, 266–71.

Alexander, G.E., DeLong, M.R. and Strick, P.L. 1986. Parallel organization of functionally segregated circuits linking basal ganglia and cortex. *Ann Rev Neurosci* **9**, 357–81.

American Psychiatric Association 1994. *Diagnostic and Statistical Manual*, 4th edn. Washington, DC: American Psychiatric Association.

Andersen, G., Ingeman-Nielsen, M., Vestergaard, K. and Riis, J.O. 1994. Pathoanatomic correlations between poststroke pathologic crying and damage to brain areas involved in serotonergic neurotransmission. *Stroke* **25**, 1050–2.

Barret, K. 1991. Treating organic abulia with bromocriptine and lisuride: four case studies. *J Neurol Neurosurg Psychiatry* **56**, 718–21.

Baxter, L.R., Schwartz, J.M., Phelps, M.E. et al. 1989. Reduction of prefrontal cortex metabolism common to three types of depression. *Arch Gen Psychiatry* **46**, 243–50.

Bench, C.J., Friston, K.J., Brown, R.G., Scott, L.C., Frackowiak, S.J. and Dolan, R.J. 1992. The anatomy of melancholia – focal abnormalities of cerebral blood flow in major depression. *Psychol Med* **22**, 607–15.

Benson, D.F. and Ardila, A. 1993. Depression in aphasia. In *Depression in Neurologic Disease*, ed. S.E. Starkstein and R.G. Robinson, pp. 152–64. Baltimore: Johns Hopkins University Press.

Caine, E.D. 1981. Pseudodementia: current concepts and future directions. *Arch Gen Psychiatry* **38**, 1359–64.

Clayton, P.J. and Lewis, C.E. 1981. The significance of secondary depression. *J Affect Dis* **3**, 25–35.

Coughlan, A.K. and Hollows, S.E. 1984. Use of memory tests in differentiating organic disorder from depression. *Br J Psychiatry* **145**, 164–7.

Cummings, J.L. 1985. *Clinical Neuropsychiatry*. Orlando: Grune & Stratton.

Cummings, J.L. 1993. Frontal–subcortical circuits and human behaviour. *Arch Neurol* **50**, 873–80.

Devinsky, O., Morrell, M.J. and Brent, A.V. 1995. Contributions of the anterior cingulate cortex to behaviour. *Brain* **118**, 279–306.

Eastwood, M.R., Rifat, S.L., Nobbs, H. and Ruderman, J. 1989. Mood disorder following CVA. *Br J Psychiatry* **154**, 195–200.

Feinstein, A., Kartsounis, L., Miller, D., Youl, B. and Ron, M.A. 1992a. Clinically isolated lesions of the type seen in multiple sclerosis: a cognitive, psychiatric and MRI study. *J Neurol Neurosurg Psychiatry* **55**, 869–76.

Feinstein, A., Youl, B. and Ron, M.A. 1992b. Psychometric, psychiatric and MRI abnormalities in acute optic neuritis. *Brain* **115**, 1403–15.

Folstein, S.E., Abbott, M.H., Chase, G.A., Jensen, B.A. and Folstein, M.F. 1983. The association of affective disorder with Huntington's disease in a case series and in families. *Psychol Med* **13**, 537–42.

Friedenberg, D.L. and Cummings, J.L. 1989. Parkinson's disease, depression and the on–off phenomenon. *Psychosomatics* **30**, 94–9.

Frochtengarten, M.L., Villares, J.C.B., Maluf, E. and Carlini, E.A. 1987. Depressive symptoms and the dexamethasone suppression test in Parkinson patients. *Biol Psychiatry* **22**, 386–9.

George, M.S., Parekh, P.I., Rosinsky, N. et al. 1996. Understanding emotional prosody activates right hemisphere regions. *Arch Neurol* **53**, 665–70.

Hall, R.C.W. 1980. Anxiety. In *Psychiatric Presentations of Medical Illness*, ed. R.C.W. Hall, pp. 13–32. New York: Spectrum Publications.

Hoehn-Saric, R., Lipsey, J.R. and McLeod, D.R. 1990. Apathy and indifference in patients on fluvoxamine and fluoxetine. *J Clin Psychopharmacol* **10**, 343–5.

Honer, W.G., Hurwtiz, T., Li, D.K.B., Palmer, M. and Paty, D.W. 1987. Temporal lobe involvement in multiple sclerosis patients with psychiatric disorders. *Arch Neurol* **44**, 187–90.

Huber, S.J., Paulsen, G.W., Shuttleworth, E.C. et al. 1987. Magnetic resonance imaging correlates of dementia in multiple sclerosis. *Arch Gen Neurol* **44**, 732–6.

Kessler, R.C., McGonagle, K.A. Zhao, S. et al. 1994. Lifetime and 12-month prevalence of DSM-111-R psychiatric disorders in the United States. *Arch Gen Psychiatry* **51**, 8–19.

Loreck, D.J. and Folstein, M.F. 1993. Depression in Alzheimer's disease. In *Depression and Neurologic Disease*, ed. S.E. Starkstein and G. Robinson, pp. 50–62. Baltimore: Johns Hopkins University Press.

Marin, R.S. 1990. Differential diagnosis and classification of apathy. *Am J Psychiatry* **147**, 22–30.

Marin, R.S. 1991. Apathy: a neuropsychiatric syndrome. *J Neuropsychiatry Clin Neurosci* **3**, 243–54.

Marin, R.S., Firinciogullari, S. and Biedrzycki, R.C. 1994. Group differences in the relationship between apathy and depression. *J Nerv Ment Dis* **183**, 235–9.

Marin, R.S., Fogel, B.S., Hawkins, J., Duffy, J. and Krupp, B. 1995. Apathy: a treatable syndrome. *J Neuropsychiatry Clin Neurosci* **7**, 23–30.

Mayberg, H.S., Starkstein, S.E., Sadzot, B. et al. 1990. Selective hypometabolism in the inferior frontal lobe in depressed patients with Parkinson's disease. *Ann Neurol* **28**, 57–64.

Mayberg, H.S., Starkstein, S.E., Peyser, C.E. et al. 1992. Paralimbic frontal hypometabolism in depression associated with Huntington's disease. *Neurology* **42**, 1791–7.

Poeck, K. 1969. Pathophysiology of emotional disorders associated with brain damage. In *Handbook of Clinical Neurology*, Vol. 3, ed. P.J. Vinken and G.W. Bruyn, pp. 343–67. Amsterdam: North Holland Publishing Company.

Popkin, M.K. and Tucker, G.J. 1994. Mental disorders due to a general medical condition. Mood, anxiety, psychotic, catatonic and personality disorders. In *DSM-1V Sourcebook*, Vol. 1, ed. T.A. Widiger, A.J. Frances, A.J. Pincus, M.B. First, R. Ross and W. Davis, pp. 243–76. Washington, DC: American Psychiatric Association.

Robinson, R.G. and Jorge, R. 1994. Mood disorders. In *Neuropsychiatry of Traumatic Brain Injury*, ed. J.M. Silver, S.C. Yudofsky and R.E. Hales, pp. 251–84. Washington, DC: American Psychiatric Press.

Robinson, R.G., Kubos, K.L., Starr, L.B., Rao, K. and Price, T.R. 1983. Mood changes in stroke patients: relationship to lesion location. *Comp Psychiatry* **24**, 555–56.

Robinson, R.G. and Price, T.R. 1982. Post stroke depressive disorders: a follow-up study of 103 patients. *Stroke* **13**, 635–41.

Robinson, R.G., Starr, L.B., Lipsey, J.R., Rao, K. and Price, T.R. 1984. A two year longitudinal study of post stroke mood disorder: dynamic changes in associated variables over the first six months of follow-up. *Stroke* **15**, 510–16.

Ron, M.A. and Logsdail, S.J. 1989. Psychiatric morbidity in multiple sclerosis: a clinical and MRI study. *Psychol Med* **19**, 887–95.

Ron, M.A., Toone, B.K., Garralda, M.E. and Lishman, W.A. 1979. Diagnostic accuracy of presenile dementia. *Br J Psychiatry* **134**, 161–8.

Ross, E.D. and Stewart, R.M. 1981. Akinetic mutism from hypothalamic damage: successful treatment with dopamine agonists. *Neurology* **31**, 1435–9.

Ross, E.D. and Stewart, R.S. 1987. Pathological display of affect in patients with depression and right frontal brain damage. *J Nerv Ment Dis* **175**, 165–72.

Sadovnick, A.D., Remick, R.A., Allen, J. et al. 1996. Depression and multiple sclerosis. *Neurology* **46**, 628–32.

Schiffer, R.B., Herndon, R.M. and Rudick, R.A. 1985. Treatment of pathological laughing and weeping with amitriptyline. *N Engl J Med* **312**, 1480–2.

Schiffer, R.B., Weitkamp, L.R., Wineman, N.M. and Guttormsen, S. 1988. Multiple sclerosis and affective disorder: family history, sex, and HLA-DR antigens. *Arch Neurol* **45**, 1345–8.

Schiffer, R.B., Wineman, N.M. and Weitkamp, L.R. 1986. Association between bipolar affective disorder and multiple sclerosis. *Am J Psychiatry* **143**, 94–5.

Starkstein, S.E. and Robinson, R.G. 1989. Depression and Parkinson's disease. In *Aging and Clinical Practice: Depression and Co-Existing Disease*, ed. R.G. Robinson and P.V. Rabins, pp. 213–48. New York: Igaku-Shoi.

Starkstein, S.E., Robinson, R.G. and Price, T.R. 1987. Comparison of cortical and subcortical lesions in the production of post-stroke mood disorders. *Brain* **110**, 1045–59.

Stenager, E.N. and Stenager, E. 1992. Suicide and patients with neurologic disease. *Arch Neurol* **49**, 1296–303.

Wing, J.K. and Brown, G.W. 1970. *Institutionalism and Schizophrenia*. Cambridge: Cambridge University Press.

Wolf, J.K., Santana, H.B. and Thorpy, M. 1979. Treatment of emotional incontinence with levodopa. *Neurology* **29**, 1435–6.

15

Motivation and awareness in cognitive neurorehabilitation

George P. Prigatano

Introduction

Clinical attempts at neuropsychological rehabilitation have long emphasized the role of personality factors in influencing the symptom picture and the process of adaptation to the effects of brain damage (Goldstein, 1942; Luria, 1963; Prigatano et al., 1986). Personality can be defined as recurring patterns of emotional and motivational responses that develop over the lifetime of the individual. These patterns are highly influenced by cognitive processes as well as by environmental factors. They also reflect the basic 'drive' states of the organism that serve the purpose of survival (Prigatano et al., 1986).

A recurring question in the rehabilitation of brain dysfunctional patients, however, is whether the patient's *motivation* influences not only the process of adaptation but also the actual recovery process (Prigatano, 1988a). A lack of motivation is often identified as a major cause of a patient's failure to benefit from neurorehabilitation (Macciocchi and Eaton, 1995). Emotional and motivational disturbances are also frequently cited as major barriers to successful neuropsychological rehabilitation (Prigatano et al, 1986). Such disturbances are a frequent source of 'burden' on family members (Livingston and Brooks, 1988) and rehabilitation therapists (Gans, 1983; Prigatano et al., 1986). Surprisingly, however, the literature on how to deal with 'motivational problems' in neurorehabilitation is sparse. For example, from 1987 to 1996 no article in the *Journal of Head Trauma Rehabilitation* included the term motivation in its title.

When neuropsychological outcomes and their determinants are studied in patients with traumatic brain injuries, seldom, if ever, is there a direct reference to how motivation influences outcome (Dikmen and Machamer, 1995). Perhaps part of the problem lies in the failure to have a precise definition of motivation and our limited ability to measure it. Articles that emphasize the role of behavioural techniques for increasing or decreasing the frequency of behaviours deemed important to the rehabilitation process do exist in the literature (Jacobs et al., 1996). Yet, although these strategies undoubtedly influence behaviour, they do not necessarily deal with the underlying problem of 'poor motivation'.

This chapter, therefore, reapproaches the problem of impaired motivation on the basis of both clinical and experimental findings, but limited information is available. It also relates this topic to the associated problem of impaired self-awareness after brain injury.

A brief historical perspective

- A passive attitude can develop after brain injury.
- Engaging the patient in rehabilitation helps overcome the passive attitude.
- Psychotherapeutic intervention may be helpful to this process.

Shepherd Ivory Franz (1924) argued that 'The phenomena of recovery are just as important to note as the primary phenomena of defect' (p. 350). He further attempted to argue that 'relearning' after aphasia is indeed possible and may occur several months or years after the brain insult. He was struck by the individual patterns of relearning and, like others, emphasized that the process was often slow.

Later, Karl Lashley (1938, p. 751) noted the following about Shepherd Ivory Franz when considering the question of motivation in 'reeducation' after brain damage.

With the patient of Dr Franz, who had failed to learn the alphabet after 900 repetitions, I tried betting 100 cigarettes that he could not learn it in a week. After 10 trials he was letter perfect and remembered it until the debt was paid. Especially with older patients it is often only under pressure of this sort that rapid progress is made.

Lashley (1938) continued to say that some patients and experimental animals seem to 'develop functional disorders superimposed upon the organic. They are likely to have a *passive* (italics added) attitude and to make little effort to utilize the capacities which they retain' (p. 751). He noted that apparent recovery may really reflect getting over this 'passive attitude'. Finally, Lashley (1938) noted that when the disturbance of motivation seemed to be a direct result of a brain lesion, 'In no experiment have we evidence for any improvement in the general level of motivation' (p. 752).

Luria (1963), in his classic text *Restoration of Function After Brain Injury*, left no doubt as to where he stood on the importance of motivation for recovery. He also related the problem of motivation to the problem of impaired self-awareness (Luria, 1963, p. 232):

As a rule, in the overwhelming majority of cases, reorganization of the functional systems takes place in the process of active and conscious activity, directed towards the compensation of the defect. The patient must be *aware* (italics added) of the disturbance lying at the basis of this defective function; in accordance with his recognized defect, the patient selects adequate methods of reorganizing the disturbed function . . . This active process of restoration of a function naturally demands great will power from the patient, and diligent, steadfast work. It is quite obvious, therefore, that the preservation of a steadfast and intensive motivation, stabilizing the patient's inclination to work on the compensation of his defect, is an essential condition of the successful restoration of the disturbed function.

In describing his own rehabilitation after a stroke, Brodal (1973) emphasized the tremendous effort it took to attempt to move a paretic limb. He also emphasized the usefulness of passive range of motion in rehabilita-

PHILOSOPHICAL PATIENCE IN THE FACE OF SUFFERING

SOCIAL RE-INTEGRATION

CONTROL

MASTERY

AWARENESS

ENGAGEMENT

Fig. 15.1 Global components of neuropsychologically oriented rehabilitation. (Adapted from Ben-Yishay, Y. and Prigatano, G.P., 1990. With permission of F.A. Davis.)

tion because it helped him to re-experience what a normal movement of his arm was like. This observation further connects the fact that the conscious representation of a deficit may not reappear automatically; it may require specific training irrespective of the functional system(s) that is involved.

More recent attempts at neuropsychological rehabilitation of higher cerebral dysfunction have further argued for the importance of overcoming the 'passive' attitude of brain dysfunctional patients and for helping them become motivated to engage in rehabilitation activities (Ben-Yishay and Prigatano, 1990). The process of engaging patients in neuropsychological rehabilitation can be demanding, but it is geared specifically towards overcoming the passive attitude of many brain dysfunctional patients.

Once patients are actively engaged in rehabilitation, they are provided with a variety of training exercises in which they can progressively begin to experience or become aware of their specific deficits and the psychosocial consequences of those impairments. This process helps individuals regain a sense of control and mastery in their lives (Fig. 15.1). While cognitive rehabilitation is an important component of this venture, Prigatano and Ben-Yishay (1999) have attempted to demonstrate that psychotherapeutic interventions also may be very helpful in this process. When approaching the problem of motivation in cognitive neurorehabilitation, one must immediately recognize that both cognitive and personality factors are involved in this process. In many instances cognitive neurorehabilitation is only effectively accomplished when the patients' motivation to participate in the rehabilitation experiences has been fostered, developed and reinforced.

The process of fostering motivation in cognitive neurorehabilitation

- Enter the patients' phenomenological field and engage them in tasks that have relevance for their lives. This may help overcome their resistance to cognitive neurorehabilitation.

When attempting cognitive rehabilitation with brain dysfunctional patients, therapists must begin with the patients' phenomenological experience (Prigatano, 1995a). That is, actual cognitive retraining activities need to begin with some activity that (1) holds the patients' interest, and (2) allows patients to begin to observe their own performance on various tasks. In the context of this work, the therapist as well as the patients may need to perform the task, so that the patients can observe how their performance actually compares to a relatively normal performance. This permits the first comparison of what abnormal versus normal behaviour may be on a given task.

It is important that the tasks presented have a certain 'face validity' for patients. That is, patients must feel that these tasks have something to do with their problem(s). If the tasks are simply reminiscent of school work or do not seem to be directly related to the patients' frustrations, the therapist is less likely to be successful in engaging the patients in the task. Incorporating various cognitive tasks in the context of a day treatment programme has proven most successful in getting patients to engage progressively in rehabilitation activities and to become progressively aware of their strengths and limitations (Prigatano et al., 1986).

In the context of this work, patients have inevitable emotional and motivational reactions to rehabilitation interventions. It is the therapist's responsibility to help manage these reactions and not to convey a punitive message when patients resist rehabilitation activities. It is obvious but often forgotten that therapists are paid for their capacity to engage patients in rehabilitation activities that have the potential of helping patients adapt to their deficits as well as facilitating the underlying recovery process. This task can be difficult and demanding because patients are often irritable, passive, hypoaroused, and/or generally disinterested in certain activities. The converse can also be true. At times, patients may be 'too' motivated. Such individuals may become agitated or anxious if they fail to perform adequately on certain tasks. It is the management of these disturbances that is so crucial to the actual process of cognitive neurorehabilitation. In this regard, it is worthwhile to recognize that motivation in and of itself does not result in improved cognitive functioning. Motivation, however, may be a necessary but insufficient condition for cognitive recovery in some patients.

Motivation: theoretical and research observations

- There may be an inverted U relationship between arousal and performance.
- Incentives influence performance but not necessarily underlying function.

Motivation refers to the complex feeling states that parallel hierarchical goal-seeking behaviour (Simon, 1967). As such, it can be described as the arousal component of behaviour that influences attention (Simon, 1994) and thereby helps in the selection of a plan of action. This arousal component has long been known to relate to performance. Summarizing a literature concerning the relationship between arousal and performance, Thompson (1975) presented the hypothetical relationship depicted in Fig. 15.2. This figure is based on the earlier observations of Hebb (1949), Malmo (1959), and Duffy (1962), as Thompson (1975) acknowledges. Thompson (1975, p. 426) states the following:

The diagram of Figure 10.4 [Fig. 15.2] taken from Hebb, shows the hypothetical relation between state of arousal and degree of successful or integrated behavior. A simple experiment illustrates this inverted U function. A person is asked to perform a simple task like mental arithmetic while squeezing a spring-handle device that measures strength of squeeze. If the subject squeezes very weakly there is little effect on mental arithmetic performance. If he squeezes moderately, his performance on

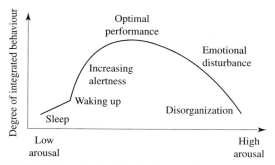

Fig. 15.2 The hypothetical relation between the degree of 'integrated behaviour' – the effective level of function or performance – and the level of arousal. Note the inverted U shape. (Based on Hebb, D.O. 1949. With permission of John Wiley & Sons.

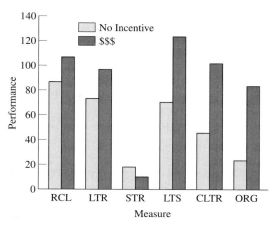

Fig. 15.3 Performance on Buschke Selective Reminding Task with and without monetary incentive. (From Parenté, R. 1994. With permission of *Neurorehabilitation*.)

the task improves. However, if he squeezes very hard, his performance on mental arithmetic deteriorates. In an experiment of this sort, level of arousal is inferred from strength of squeeze.

This phenomenon is clearly seen in neuropsychological rehabilitation. If individuals are hypoaroused or not very motivated, their performance is often substandard or subnormal. If patients can be energized or activated, their performance often improves on a variety of cognitive tasks. An optimal level of arousal, however, seems to be necessary. If their arousal level is too high, patients often do worse on the performance of various cognitive tasks that are utilized in neuropsychological rehabilitation. Thus, motivation is a double-edged sword. Too little or too much can be detrimental to patients and to the rehabilitative process.

The question of how to achieve the optimal level of arousal, attention and feeling states that parallel goal-seeking behaviour is often an issue that the clinician must confront. In this regard, it becomes important for patients to have a realistic view of what they can and cannot do and to choose goals that are appropriate given their cognitive capacities.

In a study with monkeys, Schwartz (1969) showed that the level of reinforcement did not influence motor recovery after experimentally induced cerebral lesions. Under certain conditions, however, the arousal level of the animals was clearly increased. The arousal level per se, however, did not result in improved motor function-

ing. Knowing which behaviours can be influenced by increasing arousal and which behaviours cannot becomes a crucial issue in neurorehabilitation.

In this regard, Parenté (1994) has documented that traumatic brain-injury patients may perform better on learning and memory tests given the right incentives. Using a $100 incentive, he showed that traumatic brain injury patients would perform better on such demanding tasks as the Select Verbal Reminding Test (Fig. 15.3) than if no incentive was given.

Improvement on this verbal and learning memory test, however, does not necessarily mean that the overall capacity to learn and remember has been affected substantially. Rather, it suggests that under certain conditions the incentive to perform a specific task may well result in improved performance on that task only. This finding is comparable with several studies of both brain dysfunctional and nonbrain dysfunctional individuals. It highlights a point made by several theorists that reinforcement and appropriate incentives clearly influence behaviour (Dollard and Miller, 1950). These findings are certainly compatible with what Lashley (1938) observed when discussing Franz's patient who did not learn the alphabet until an appropriate incentive was used.

Parenté (1994) has remarked that perhaps some of

the deficits of traumatic brain injury patients really reflect continuing motivational disturbances. If the right incentive can be established, then the motivational disturbances may be overcome, at least momentarily. An overriding issue, however, continues to be whether motivation per se can be altered without a continuous or daily incentive system.

Finally, experimental animal literature shows similar findings. Levere, Davis and Gonder (1979) demonstrated, for example, that rats would relearn a visual discrimination task after extensive brain lesions provided that the reinforcement was similar to the reinforcement conditions in which they learned the task preoperatively. The appropriate reinforcement can obviously influence some, but not all, behaviour.

Self-awareness: theoretical and research observations

- Disturbances in self-awareness after brain injury are common but poorly understood.
- Different strategies are emerging to deal with these disturbances.

Many traumatic brain injury patients have poor conscious representation of their functional disabilities. They often overestimate their behavioural competencies compared to what their relatives report (Prigatano, Altman and O'Brien, 1990). Although 'denial' has been used in the earlier literature to describe these and other patients (Weinstein and Kahn, 1955), the term may be inaccurate in certain instances. Denial implies a defensive reaction against some painful conflicts with reality. Soon after a severe traumatic brain injury, many patients experience no personal conflict or painful reality. They simply do not perceive the extent of their cognitive impairments or their associated disabilities. Their manner frequently appears 'indifferent' (Prigatano and Klonoff, 1998).

In cognitive neurorehabilitation, it therefore may prove helpful to distinguish between impaired self-awareness and denial of disability (Prigatano and Weinstein, 1996; Prigatano, 1997; Prigatano and Klonoff, 1998). Impaired self-awareness literally means an individual lacks a subjective or phenomenological experience of impaired functioning. In denial of disabil-

ity there is a partial conscious representation of altered function, but confusion about how to deal with or describe the situation remains. In both cases, patients may choose inappropriate goals.

Impairments in the capacity of brain-dysfunctional patients to experience subjectively and to report altered cerebral functioning have been noted since antiquity (Bisiach and Geminiani, 1991). Yet, it remains quite difficult to define human consciousness precisely (Prigatano and Schacter, 1991) and to describe the various forms of altered self-awareness associated with different brain lesions (Prigatano, 1991). Lesions in the frontal region of the brain may specifically alter self-awareness regarding socially inappropriate behaviours as well as creating difficulties in planning and organization. Acute lesions of the inferior parietal lobe may be associated with the phenomenon of anosognosia for hemiplegia. Lesions in the left temporal lobe can alter language function, and patients may be unaware of their language deficits. Bilateral occipital lesions can result in the well-known phenomenon of cortical blindness without individuals recognizing their visual loss.

As partial awareness reappears with time and/or rehabilitation, brain dysfunctional patients may be unable to describe exactly how their functioning has changed. They may, however, have partial awareness of their impairments and associated disabilities. In this latter case, they may often rely on premorbid methods of coping to deal with their limitations. At times, this could be described as the mechanism of denial. This latter group of patients often insists on returning to a previous level of work without appropriate preparation. If given negative feedback, they can be resistant. They may insist that they can perform a variety of daily activities which they are unable to do.

Therapists must be cautious, however, that they do not automatically assume that the level of neuropsychological impairment that patients demonstrate translates directly into the same level of neuropsychological disability, as Wilson (1997) has noted. Patients who have impaired self-awareness might be approached differently from patients who deny their disability.

Different strategies for working with these patients are beginning to emerge (Prigatano, 1997). In the case of impaired self-awareness after brain injury, patients experience no distress, as noted above, but they are perplexed. These individuals often respond positively to structure and guidance that help reduce their perplexity or confusion. As they establish a working relationship with a clinician, who they sense will guide them, they are able to engage in various tasks. Some patients even slowly recognize their limitations.

In the case of denial of disability, patients tend to experience more frustration in addition to confusion. Such patients also lack a clear understanding of what is wrong, but they do sense that something is wrong. If rehabilitation can reduce the patients' daily frustrations (instead of focusing only on confusion), patients often become more cooperative and insightful. This progress is often achieved via such supported activities as a protected work trial, psychotherapy, family intervention and education. Eventually, these patients may be able to choose appropriate goals as they participate in cognitive and neuropsychologically oriented rehabilitation. Allowing them to experience their limitations, albeit in a protected manner, may actually help establish a therapeutic alliance. This type of alliance clearly relates to productivity after neuropsychological rehabilitation (Prigatano et al., 1994).

Clinical examples

- Different patterns of behavioural disturbance have been described in patients who vary in their level of motivation and self-awareness.

Impaired self-awareness as well as denial of disability can interact in complicated ways over time in a given patient (Prigatano and Klonoff, 1998). Patients can also vary in terms of their level of motivation. Different patterns of behavioural disturbances have been described in patients who vary in their level of both motivation and awareness (Prigatano, 1995b). For the purposes of this chapter, two case examples are provided to highlight the important role of motivation and awareness in cognitive neurorehabilitation.

The first case is that of a 50-year-old man who fell from a ladder while at work. Computed tomography revealed bilateral contusions of the frontal lobes. The patient was highly motivated to participate in neuro-

psychologically oriented rehabilitation even though his self-awareness was extremely poor. The patient demonstrated predictable problems of hyperverbality, disinhibition, and poor insight into his limitations. When his behavioural problems were pointed out, he would glibly recognize the difficulties but continue to engage in disruptive behaviours. He was, however, highly motivated to participate in his rehabilitation.

Despite his lack of awareness, this patient was strongly motivated to return to a productive lifestyle. He also had great trust in his physicians, neurorehabilitation therapists, and his wife. His wife clearly emphasized to him the importance of accepting a job that was much less demanding than his previous position. She reinforced the importance of attending a day treatment rehabilitation programme. Finally, she also greatly encouraged him to follow the direction of his therapists despite his behavioural and cognitive limitations.

The patient so trusted his wife that he followed her advice even though he had poor insight into his disability. Eventually, through a considerable amount of structure and cueing, he was able to curb his hyperverbality and inappropriate comments. He returned to a productive lifestyle, albeit in a much less demanding capacity. Although this patient exemplifies a good example of a good psychosocial outcome with poor awareness, he only achieved this success because of his excellent relationships with his wife and therapists.

Typically, poor awareness spells a disastrous psychosocial outcome after neuropsychological rehabilitation, as demonstrated by a 39-year-old man who suffered a severe traumatic brain injury at the age of 21. He was initially evaluated three years after his brain injury. At that time, neuropsychological testing revealed definite evidence of memory impairment as well as disturbances in abstract reasoning.

Whereas the patient was motivated to participate in a neuropsychological rehabilitation programme, he repeatedly minimized his cognitive deficits and emphasized his somatic problems. He would state, for example: 'If I didn't have these headaches, I could do this cognitive task'. It was gently and progressively pointed out to him that the opposite was true. If he could do the cognitive tasks, perhaps he would not develop a headache.

Table 15.1 Motivation in cognitive neurorehabilitation

Issue	Reference
Motivation appears to be a necessary but insufficient condition for good psychosocial adaption to the effects of brain injury	Prigatano (1995a); Prigatano et al. (1986); Prigatano (1988a)
Motivation may improve level of performance on specific tasks without necessarily improving underlying 'capacity' or 'skill'	Lashley (1938); Parenté (1994)
Motivation provides the necessary 'arousal', 'attention' and 'effort' for new learning	Simon (1994); Pribram and McGuinness (1975)
Motivation sustains the patient when engagement in the rehabilitation process is difficult because of various stressors and disappointments	Prigatano (1995a); Prigatano et al. (1986)
Motivation may (in some instances) actually affect recovery processes and the achievement of rehabilitation goals, but the data are sparse	Prigatano and Wong (1997); Schwartz (1969)
'Too much' motivation without adequate awareness can lead to psychosocial deterioration	Prigatano (1995a); Prigatano (1997)

This patient established a fair therapeutic alliance (Prigatano et al., 1994) and eventually returned to employment, albeit at a level below his premorbid status. Unfortunately, however, neither he nor his family ever fully appreciated the extent of his disabilities. With time, he returned to an inappropriate level of work that was incompatible with his abilities. He became more socially isolated and developed suspicious ideation. With time, his thought pattern became clearly delusional and he began to have hallucinatory experiences. The connection between persistent anosognosia and delusions has been described elsewhere (Prigatano, 1988b). In this case, the patient literally had no insight into the extent of his difficulties and yet he experienced repeated failures. The only explanation was that others, rather than himself, were the cause of his limitations. This thought process eventually led to a psychotic breakdown.

Although this patient is a rather dramatic example of how failure to reverse the problem of impaired self-awareness can lead to a disastrous psychosocial outcome after neuropsychological rehabilitation, the case does highlight an important clinical principle. If the underlying impairment of self-awareness is not adequately understood and managed, patients frequently do not develop a good therapeutic working alliance with therapists. The typical result is a failure to

maintain work. This situation is also predictive of a deteriorating psychosocial outcome with time.

Reflecting these observations, Tables 15.1 and 15.2 summarize the key points discussed regarding motivation and awareness in cognitive neurorehabilitation.

The role of psychotherapy in dealing with motivational and awareness problems after brain injury

• A good working or therapeutic alliance with the patient can help overcome the 'passive attitude' encountered in some patients.

An important component to neuropsychological rehabilitation has been psychotherapy with brain dysfunctional patients and, at times, with family members (Prigatano et al., 1986; Prigatano, 1997). Recently, Prigatano and Ben-Yishay (1999) have provided further examples of how psychotherapeutic intervention can help patients.

Ben-Yishay described a case example that demonstrated how a series of well-orchestrated interventions with the patient and family can help the patient cope with feelings of discouragement and a belief that an overriding problem cannot, in fact, be controlled. The reader is referred to that detailed case example because it highlights an important principle that has recently

Table 15.2 Awareness in cognitive neurorehabilitation

Issue	Reference
Disturbances of higher cerebral functioning are often associated with some disturbance in the conscious experience and perception of the self	Prigatano and Schacter (1991); Prigatano and Weinstein (1996); Prigatano (1997)
Impaired self-awareness can lead to a passive (nonengaging) approach to cognitive rehabilitation and, at times, to clear resistance to such activities. Consequently, patients appear 'less motivated' and may not receive adequate rehabilitation	Prigatano et al. (1986); Prigatano (1988a)
Facilitating recovery of impaired self-awareness via a variety of cognitive and interpersonal tasks may aid the process and outcome of neuropsychological rehabilitation, but the data are sparse	Prigatano et al. (1986)
It may be helpful to distinguish impaired self-awareness from denial of disability after brain damage. The distinction may lead to different treatment strategies	Prigatano and Weinstein (1996); Prigatano (1997)

been demonstrated empirically. If patients have a good working or therapeutic alliance with the rehabilitation staff, there is a greater likelihood that they can again become productive after a significant brain injury (Prigatano et al., 1994). Within the context of a therapeutic relationship, patients are often willing to try something that they previously would have been unwilling to try. By establishing a therapeutic relationship, one often overcomes the 'passive attitude' and enables patients to see that performing a series of practical behavioural activities may well improve their adjustment as well as their functional capacities.

While there is nothing 'magical' about psychotherapy, the psychotherapeutic experience can help patients more effectively engage in various aspects of rehabilitation that can help them cope with their disabilities in a more practical manner. An underlying question, however, which continues to be unanswered, is whether motivation per se actually facilitates the recovery process. To date, there is no clear evidence that helps answer this question.

Mechanisms of recovery, motivation and impaired self-awareness

- Speed of finger tapping relates to severity of traumatic brain injury and may recover less than grip strength.

- Speed of finger tapping is often bilaterally slow in traumatic brain injury patients with poor self-awareness.
- The brain mechanism responsible for this 'simple' finger movement may relate to disturbances in motivation and self-awareness.

In his book *Brain and Intelligence. A Quantitative Study of the Frontal Lobes*, Ward Halstead (1947) suggested a four-factor theory of biological intelligence. One of the factors was the 'power', or so-called *P* factor, which partially reflects the 'emotional–conative aspect of all mental activity'. Halstead noted that motor functions were often affected positively or negatively when this *P* factor was affected. Incidental recall on the Tactual Performance Test, speed of finger oscillation (or tapping), and performance on the Flicker Fusion Test significantly loaded on this factor.

Recent studies have shown that speed of finger oscillation relates to the severity of the initial traumatic brain injury (Dikmen et al., 1995) and may not recover as well as grip strength after even mild to moderate head injuries (Haaland et al., 1994). Furthermore, traumatic brain injury patients who show poor self-awareness have slow finger-tapping speeds (Prigatano and Altman, 1990). A recent study has replicated this observation in a cross-cultural investigation with Japanese traumatic brain injury patients who showed poor self-awareness (Prigatano, Ogano and Amakusa, 1997a).

Progressive evidence suggests that the underlying brain mechanisms responsible for 'simple' finger movement actually involve multiple and bilateral brain regions. Work by Frackowiak and colleagues (Weiller et al., 1993), for example, has shown that patients who have recovered from a monoparesis (i.e. who are able to move their fingers to the beat of a metronome comparable to controls) show individual patterns of bilateral cerebral activation. These patterns often involve frontal and parietal regions. Roland (1993) reports similar activation patterns in normal subjects when carrying out a complex finger movement task.

The frontal lobes have long been implicated in motivated behaviour as well as in disturbances of self-awareness (Stuss, 1991). Pribram and McGuinness (1975) suggested that the frontal lobes contribute to the phenomenon of 'intention' whereas the parietal lobes play a key role in 'attention'. Both processes are strongly implicated in the phenomena of motivation and self-awareness.

Patients have to be motivated to tap their fingers at as fast a rate as possible. The author has begun to videotape qualitative differences between patients (Prigatano and Hoffman, 1997). Not uncommonly, 'highly motivated' patients who exhibit poor self-awareness will tap as quickly as they can, often moving the whole hand in an effort to move the key as fast as possible. These individuals often cannot inhibit adjacent finger movements and are exhausted by the task. In such cases, the overmotivation results in less effective movements of the fingers and seems to be correlated with patients' poor insight into their cognitive impairments.

Undoubtedly, with time, other neural cognitive markers will emerge to help us better understand disturbances in motivation and how they are related to disturbances in self-awareness. At this point, however, it can be clinically reported that these dimensions are related, yet seem to be independent. Indications of improvement in both dimensions often relate to the achievement of rehabilitation goals. For example, Prigatano and Wong (1999) have found that improvements in basic cognitive and emotional functioning (as measured by the total score of the Barrow Neurological Institute Screen for Higher Cerebral Functions) were related to the achievement of inpatient rehabilitation goals within four to six weeks after various brain lesions. A subgroup of these patients, who had unilateral stroke, showed achievement of goals paralleled by an increase of speed of finger tapping in the 'unaffected' hand (Prigatano and Wong, 1997). That is, speed of finger tapping in the hand ipsilateral to the lesion was related to goal attainment. Speed of finger tapping in the hand contralateral to the lesion was not. This latter finding suggests that 'undamaged' regions of the brain may be functionally disrupted after brain injury. Specific rehabilitation activities may be needed to 'de-inhibit' these temporarily disturbed functional regions for maximum outcome. Luria (1963) first suggested this concept, which continues to hold promise for the field of neurorehabilitation.

Measuring motivation in studies on cognitive neurorehabilitation

If future research is going to assess adequately how motivational factors influence the processes and outcome of cognitive neurorehabilitation, appropriate measures must be developed. Clinically, several behavioural characteristics often seem to reflect the patient's motivation level (Table 15.3). These behaviours can be measured and might be considered in future studies on cognitive neurorehabilitation.

Conclusions

Whereas patient motivation is often considered a key variable for successful neurorehabilitation (Macciocchi and Eaton, 1995), the empirical data are sparse. Impaired cognitive (and motivational) functioning does seem to relate to the accomplishment of rehabilitation goals (Prigatano and Wong, 1999). It is still unclear whether motivation affects underlying cognitive processes in some generalized and permanent manner.

Efforts at neuropsychological rehabilitation suggest that patients who are motivated to engage in a rehabilitation programme often achieve better psychosocial outcomes (Prigatano et al., 1986). The establishment of a good working alliance between the rehabilitation staff and the patient as well as between the rehabilitation

Table 15.3 Behavioural characteristics implicated in motivation

Time spent on cognitive retraining activities

Number of self-initiated 'practice' activities when learning to compensate for an impairment

Arousal level (perhaps measured by galvanic skin response) when performing various cognitive training tasks

Number of verbal resistance responses to cognitive neurorehabilitation activities (e.g. count number of times the patient makes such comments as 'I don't want to do this'; 'When can I stop this task?)

Number of times patient is 'on time' for appointments

Number of times the patient is willing to make a sacrifice to receive cognitive neurorehabilitation (e.g. willingness of the patient to pay for some portion of the cost of treatment)

Ratings of progressive and improved therapeutic alliance with time and/or training (see Prigatano et al. (1994) for details for how such a rating system is established)

staff and the patient's family appears especially important in achieving a good psychosocial outcome, particularly when return to work is a major rehabilitation goal (Prigatano et al., 1994).

Sometimes patients' self-awareness is poor but their motivation and working alliance with the rehabilitation staff are strong. In such cases, and under very structured circumstances, their psychosocial outcomes may be positive. A more common scenario, however, is that poor self-awareness often results in repeated failures for patients. With repeated failures, patients' psychosocial functioning often declines and sometimes their psychiatric status declines as well.

Clinically, it may be useful to distinguish disorders of impaired self-awareness from denial of disability in cognitive neurorehabilitation. These two interacting disturbances present with different clinical manifestations. In the former, patients are often confused and perplexed. By providing structure and guidance, these individuals can often overcome their passive attitude and engage in rehabilitation in a more productive manner. These individuals can often be guided to make choices that have fewer negative psychosocial con-

sequences. In the case of denial of disability, patients are partially aware of their deficits, but they are frustrated by their limitations. Helping them reduce their frustrations may be the most effective way of establishing a therapeutic alliance and thereby of helping them to manage their residual cognitive and emotional deficits.

Certainly, motivation and awareness seem to be interacting but possibly independent variables. They also may play an extremely important role in recovery phenomena, although researchers have not fully explored this possibility. A number of studies have recently been embarked upon that show that speed of finger tapping not only relates to impaired self-awareness but also to the actual ability to achieve rehabilitation goals after a unilateral cerebrovascular accident (Prigatano and Wong, 1997). Positron emission tomography studies as well as functional magnetic resonance imaging studies suggest that the ability to move the finger rapidly may actually be associated with bilateral cerebral activation involving regions far removed from the sensory motor strip (Weiller et al., 1993). It may be that this 'simple' motor function is, in fact, not so simple and correlates with multiple brain areas of activation. When the brain is damaged, a slow speed of finger tapping may actually reflect a greater diffuseness of dysfunction than has been previously recognized. By exploring the cognitive motor markers of impaired self-awareness and the associated problem with motivation, we will better understand the mechanisms underlying these complicated phenomena. In so doing, we will be able to establish the field of cognitive neurorehabilitation on a firm scientific basis, one that relates it to mechanisms of recovery as well as to mechanisms of deficits.

References

Ben-Yishay, Y. and Prigatano, G.P. 1990. Cognitive remediation. In *Rehabilitation of the Adult and Child with Traumatic Brain Injury*, ed. M. Rosenthal, E.R. Griffith, M.R. Bond et al., pp. 393–409. Philadelphia: F.A. Davis.

Bisiach, E. and Geminiani, G. 1991. Anosognosia related to hemiplegia and hemianopia. In *Awareness of Deficit After Brain Injury*, ed. G.P. Prigatano and D.L. Schacter, pp. 17–39. New York: Oxford University Press.

Brodal, A. 1973. Self-observations and neuro-anatomical considerations after a stroke. *Brain* **96**, 675–94.

Dikmen, S. and Machamer, J.E. 1995. Neurobehavioral outcomes and their determinants. *J Head Trauma Rehabil* **10**, 74–86.

Dikmen, S.S., Machamer, J.E., Winn, H.R. and Temkin, N.R. 1995. Neuropsychological outcome at 1 year post head injury. *Neuropsychology* **9**, 80–90.

Dollard, J. and Miller, N.E. 1950. *Personality and Psychotherapy*. New York: McGraw-Hill.

Duffy, E. 1962. *Activation and Behavior*. New York: John Wiley & Sons.

Franz, S.I. 1924. Studies in re-education. The aphasias. *Comp Psychol* **4**, 349–429.

Gans, J.S. 1983. Hate in the rehabilitation setting. *Arch Phys Med Rehabil* **64**, 176–9.

Goldstein, K. 1942. *Aftereffects of Brain Injury in War*. New York: Grune and Stratton.

Haaland, K.Y., Temkin, N., Randahl, G. and Dikmen, S. 1994. Recovery of simple motor skills after head injury. *J Clin Exp Neuropsychol* **16**, 448–56.

Halstead, W.C. 1947. *Brain and Intelligence. A Quantitative Study of the Frontal Lobes*. Chicago: University of Chicago Press.

Hebb, D.O. 1949. *The Organization of Behavior*. New York: John Wiley & Sons.

Jacobs, H.E., Hart, T., Mory, K.D., Griffin, C., Martin, B.A. and Probst, J. 1996. Single-subject evaluation designs in rehabilitation: case studies on inpatient units. *J Head Trauma Rehabil* **11**, 86–94.

Lashley, K.S. 1938. Factors limiting recovery after central nervous lesions. *J Nerv Ment Dis* **88**, 833–55.

Levere, T.E., Davis, N. and Gonder, L. 1979. Recovery of function after brain damage. Toward understanding the deficit. *Physiol Psychol* **7**, 317–26.

Livingston, M.G. and Brooks, D.N. 1988. The burden on families of the brain injured: a review. *J Head Trauma Rehabil* **3**, 6–15.

Luria, A.R. 1963. *Restoration of Function After Brain Trauma*. London: Pergamon Press.

Macciocchi, S.N. and Eaton, B. 1995. Decision and attribution bias in neurorehabilitation. *Arch Phys Med Rehabil* **76**, 521–4.

Malmo, R.B. 1959. Activation: a neuropsychological dimension. *Psychol Rev* **66**, 367–86.

Parenté, R. 1994. Effect of monetary incentives on performance after traumatic brain injury. *Neurorehabilitation* **4**, 198–203.

Pribram, K.H. and McGuinness, D. 1975. Arousal, activation, and effort in the control of attention. *Psychol Rev* **82**, 116–49.

Prigatano, G.P. 1988a. Emotion and motivation in recovery and adaptation after brain damage. In *Brain Injury and Recovery.*

Theoretical and Controversial Issues, ed. S. Finger, T.E. Levere, C.R. Almli and D.G. Stein, pp. 335–50. New York: Plenum Press.

Prigatano, G.P. 1988b. Anosognosia, delusions, and altered self-awareness after brain injury: a historical perspective. *BNI Quarterly* **4**, 40–8.

Prigatano, G.P. 1991. Disturbances of self-awareness of deficit after traumatic brain injury. In *Awareness of Deficit After Brain Injury: Theoretical and Clinical Issues*, ed. G.P. Prigatano and D.L. Schacter, pp. 111–26. New York: Oxford University Press.

Prigatano, G.P. 1995a. 1994 Sheldon Berrol, MD, Senior Lectureship: the problem of lost normality after brain injury. *J Head Trauma Rehabil* **10**, 87–95.

Prigatano, G.P. 1995b. Personality and social aspects of memory rehabilitation. In *Handbook of Memory Disorders*, ed. B. Baddeley, B. Wilson and F. Watts, pp. 603–14. Chichester: John Wiley & Sons.

Prigatano, G.P. 1997. The problem of awareness in neuropsychological rehabilitation. In *Neuropsychological Rehabilitation*, ed. J. Leon-Carrion, pp. 301–11. Orlando, FL: G.R. Press.

Prigatano, G.P. and Altman, I.M. 1990. Impaired awareness of behavioral limitations after traumatic brain injury. *Arch Phys Med Rehabil* **71**, 1058–64.

Prigatano, G.P., Altman, I.M. and O'Brien, K.P. 1990. Behavioral limitations that traumatic-brain-injured patients tend to underestimate. *Clin Neuropsychol* **4**, 163–76.

Prigatano, G.P. and Ben-Yishay, Y. 1999. Psychotherapy and psychotherapeutic interventions in brain injury rehabilitation. In *Rehabilitation of the Adult and Child with Traumatic Brain Injury*, ed. M. Rosenthal, pp. 271–83. Philadelphia: F.A. Davis.

Prigatano, G.P., Fordyce, D.J., Zeiner, H.K., Roueche, J.R., Pepping, M. and Wood, B.C. 1986. *Neuropsychological Rehabilitation After Brain Injury: Theoretical and Clinical Issues*. Baltimore: Johns Hopkins University Press.

Prigatano, G.P. and Hoffman, B. 1997. Finger tapping and brain dysfunction: a qualitative and quantitative study. *BNI Quarterly* **13**(4), 14–18.

Prigatano, G.P. and Klonoff, P.S. 1998. A clinician's rating scale for evaluating impaired self-awareness and denial of disability following brain injury. *Clin Neuropsychol* **12**, 56–7.

Prigatano, G.P., Klonoff, P.S., O'Brien, K.P. et al. 1994. Productivity after neuropsychologically oriented milieu rehabilitation. *J Head Trauma Rehabil* **9**, 91–102.

Prigatano, G.P., Ogano, M. and Amakusa, B. 1997a. A cross-cultural study on impaired self-awareness in Japanese patients with brain dysfunction. *Neuropsychiatry Neuropsychol Behav Neurol* **10**, 135–43.

Prigatano, G.P. and Schacter, D.L. 1991. *Awareness of Deficit After Brain Injury: Clinical and Theoretical Issues*. New York: Oxford University Press.

Prigatano, G.P. and Weinstein, E.A. 1996. Edwin A. Weinstein's contributions to neuropsychological rehabilitation. *Neuropsychol Rehabil* **6**, 305–26.

Prigatano, G.P. and Wong, J.L. 1997. Speed of finger tapping and goal attainment following unilateral CVA. *Arch Phys Med Rehabil* **78**, 847–52.

Prigatano, G.P. and Wong, J.L., 1999. Cognitive and affective improvement in brain dysfunctional patients who achieve inpatient rehabilitation goals. *Arch Phys Med Rehabil* **80**, 77–84.

Prigatano, G.P., Wong, J.L., Williams, C. and Plenge, K.L. 1997b. Prescribed versus actual length of stay and inpatient neurorehabilitation outcome for brain dysfunctional patients. *Arch Phys Med Rehabil* **78**, 621–9.

Roland, P.E. 1993. *Brain Activation*. New York: Wiley-Liss.

Schwartz, A.S. 1969. Recovery from motor deficit under different motivational conditions. *Physiol Behav* **4**, 57–60.

Simon, H.A. 1967. Motivational and emotional controls of cognition. *Psychol Rev* **76**, 29–39.

Simon, H.A. 1994. The bottleneck of attention: connecting thought with motivation. In *Integrative Views of Motivation, Cognition, and Emotion*, ed. W.D. Spaulding, pp. 1–21. Lincoln, NB: University of Nebraska Press.

Stuss, D.T. 1991. Disturbance of self-awareness after frontal system damage. In *Awareness of Deficit After Brain Injury. Clinical and Theoretical Issues*, ed. G.P. Prigatano and D.L. Schacter, pp. 63–83. New York: Oxford University Press.

Thompson, R.F. 1975. *Introduction to Physiological Psychology*. New York: Harper & Row.

Weiller, C., Ramsay, S.C., Wise, R.J.S., Friston, K.J. and Frackowiak, R.S.J. 1993. Individual patterns of functional reorganization in the human cerebral cortex after capsular infarction. *Ann Neurol* **33**, 181–9.

Weinstein, E.A. and Kahn, R.L. 1955. *Denial of Illness. Symbolic and Physiological Aspects*. Springfield, IL: Charles C. Thomas.

Wilson, B. 1997. Cognitive rehabilitation: how it is and how it might be. *J Int Neuropsychol Soc* **3**, 487–96.

16

Family education and family partnership in cognitive rehabilitation

Guy-B. Proulx

Introduction

A major focus of cognitive rehabilitation is on the acquisition of compensatory strategies that minimize the effects of disability and maximize autonomy in individuals with either stable or progressive neurobehavioural disorders. Rehabilitation has a long history of focusing only on patients and their cognitive impairments. Yet, practical challenges of independent living and social integration of people with brain dysfunction depend as much on the context in which the impairment is expressed as they do on the site of the lesion and the severity of the cognitive impairment. Although cognitive decrements and biomedical issues are an essential starting point, a more interactive approach involving patients' impairments, their environment and the essential role of the family needs much more attention if we are to develop a cogent model of cognitive rehabilitation. Everyone agrees that social integration and functional independence are core objectives of rehabilitation, but generally not enough is done to develop an effective partnership between the rehabilitation professionals and the family. Families must be engaged as soon as possible in the therapeutic process to decrease the burden of cognitive disorders. Lack of early input from the family leads to dysfunctional dynamics that, in turn, compound clinical issues to a frustrating and confusing level for the professionals involved.

This chapter addresses the central role of the family in the rehabilitation process and how efficient family interventions can prevent catastrophic psychosocial complications. Families are an important resource to promote change and help modify habits and roles to deal more appropriately with cognitive impairments.

The central role of the family in rehabilitation

- Financial constraints in the health care system are shifting services from hospital care to 'home care'. At the beginning, this meant increased stress for single 'caregivers'. There is a recent shift, however, to include the family as a whole in order to reduce the burden on single care providers.
- Families provide the information about how patients function in their everyday setting, helping to set the stage for what professionals should look for in their assessments and intervention plans.
- Active participation of the family is necessary to plan for, train and evaluate generalization of rehabilitation gains to the home environment.
- The patient's adaptation to the family is essential to promote optimal outcome.
- Direct family involvement in planning and the delivery of services may be more cost efficient.
- Early identification of dysfunctional families and appropriate referral for counselling are crucial.

Cognitive disorders can cause more harm to patients and their families than they should. In the field of cognitive rehabilitation, increased efforts are being placed on preventing secondary psychosocial complications to brain injury or reducing excessive disability. Active family partnership is essential if the psychosocial costs of cognitive disorders are to be reduced, and the importance of family support has been demonstrated in different patient populations. In a series of dementia studies, Brodaty and his colleagues (Brodaty and Gresham, 1989; Brodaty and Petes, 1991; Brodaty et al., 1993) found that a comprehensive training programme for family caregivers was associated with a lower rate of admission to institutions. They also found that the family training programme was associated with a reduced patient mortality rate. An unexpected finding was that greater family psychological morbidity was associated with shorter survival of patients with dementia, in other words, what occurred in the family had a direct effect on the patients with dementia, even at the level of survival. The link between the quality of family support and clinical outcome has also been established in both head trauma and stroke patients (Lehmann, et al., 1975; Gilchrist and Wilkinson, 1979; Evans et al., 1985; Wagner and Zacchigna, 1988). Married stroke patients, for example, have better outcomes (Henley et al., 1985) and tend to outlive single stroke patients (Abu-Zeid et al., 1978). There is little doubt about the crucial role the family plays in the rehabilitation process.

Lack of family involvement in rehabilitation may be partly a consequence of the way rehabilitation services traditionally have been funded. Until recently, funding went mostly to hospital-based services and, in some cases, to time-limited transitional programmes. Novak, Bergquist and Bennett (1992) believe that this system prevents there being a clear definition of the specific role of families in rehabilitation programmes. Accordingly, because involvement was even discouraged in many cases, families would fall into familiar roles and habits which were not always appropriate for dealing with the consequences of cognitive impairments. Novak et al. stress the need for new definitions for the roles of family members, and highlight education and training as the essential factors that promote the recovery process. Lezak (1978, 1988) has shown the importance of providing families with better information about how to interact with people who have cognitive impairments in order to readjust their demands and expectations realistically. Kay and Cavallo (1994) reinforce this opinion and state that much of what professionals perceive as dysfunctional in families is the result of their being uninformed, underinvolved, and not having basic needs met, all of which may be preventable with appropriate interventions.

Education of the family

Clear information and education regarding the impact of cognitive impairments on everyday behaviour, better coping skills on the part of both patients and families, as well as assistance in finding appropriate community support services all reduce barriers to effective rehabilitation. In a three-year follow-up study of 125 families dealing with cognitive disorders in the elderly, Smyth, Urman and Nathanson (1990) found that families wanted more information about:
the nature of brain dysfunction
how to cope with memory (cognitive) impairments
how to deal with challenging behaviours
how other families cope
how to cope with their own stress
available community support services.

The focus on education is important because rehabilitation, essentially, is teaching people with a disability to recalibrate their family life with the ultimate goal of generalizing cognitive rehabilitation gains to the home setting. The role education plays is even more important to the field of cognitive rehabilitation because understanding how 'learning' takes place and how learning abilities become impaired following brain injury is crucial to any treatment programme (Wilson, 1986). Common sense also tells us that to be successful, rehabilitation services must translate into practical benefits in the context of the home environment.

Families need clarification about what cognitive rehabilitation means and what it can offer. Questions that should be addressed with families include the following:
How do cognitive impairments relate to underlying brain functions?
How do cognitive impairments translate to everyday activities?
Do we remediate impairments or do we compensate for them?

What are the spared cognitive functions and strengths that can be used to compensate for losses?

What are the differences between remediation, compensation and functional skills training?

How do you accommodate to change and adjust interventions according to the natural history of the neurological condition?

What are good educational references and lists of community support services?

Impairment, disabilities and handicaps: an important distinction for families to understand

Clinical experience has shown that family members' anxieties and questions are alleviated when they are provided with a general theoretical framework that helps them to understand the links between pathology, issues of disability, and social handicaps. Education provides a way to untangle multiple compounding factors that can be very confusing. The terms impairment, disability and handicap are used by the World Health Organization (1980) to describe chronic conditions. They represent a useful method of characterizing the consequences of acquired brain dysfunction and are a good example of what should be taught to families.

Impairment: any loss or abnormality of psychological, physiological or anatomical structure or function.

Disability: any restriction or lack (resulting from an impairment) of ability to perform an activity in the manner or within the range considered normal for a human being.

Handicap: a disadvantage for a given individual resulting from an impairment or a disability that limits or prevents the fulfilment of a role that is normal (depending on age, sex, social and cultural factors for that individual).

In the context of brain injury, an amnestic disorder would be considered an *impairment*. At the *disability* level, the disorders would include: not being able to participate efficiently in a social interaction, not being able to discuss or recall what is watched on television or at the cinema, problems with reading newspapers or books, not being able to transmit a telephone message, to name but a few examples. These memory disorders create serious social *handicaps*. As a consequence of not being able to recall normally, individuals may be restricted in their ability to participate in a number of social roles: spouse, friend, coworker, volunteer. Any comprehensive rehabilitation intervention must address all three levels of function: impairment, disability and handicap.

Various professionals are more proficient at understanding and treating brain injury at different levels of function. Professionals with a restricted biological view of rehabilitation may have a poor appreciation of the progression from pathology to handicap and of the importance of external environmental factors in determining clinical outcome. Issues of pathology, clinical symptoms and signs (i.e. impairments) rarely have an analogue relation with issues of handicaps. Take, for example, two patients who have mild traumatic brain injury and attentional impairments; one, a young, highly skilled violin player, the other a high-school teacher near retirement. The patients may have dramatically different handicaps at discharge from hospital. The violin player, being a single mother at the beginning of her career, is the more functionally handicapped of the two. As handicaps relate to changes in social roles, level of independence and premorbidity issues, it is easy to understand how different psychosocial outcomes can result from similar impairments. It is wrong to try to force a linear fit between psychosocial outcomes and neuropsychological impairments. Dickmen et al. (1996) argued that, particularly when a brain injury is less severe, poor outcome often results from factors other than the impairment. They point out that the examination of the relationship between impairments and disabilities and of factors related to the individual's roles or environment (handicaps) that exacerbate or mitigate the impact of impairment on disability has the potential of improving our understanding of the mechanisms of disability and for reducing disability. Poor consideration of handicap issues results in well-intentioned rehabilitation efforts having minimal long-term impact.

Brain damage expresses itself through behaviour, and behaviour is highly dependent on the environment in which it occurs. Outcome is determined both by neurological damage and by consequent behaviour change, as well as by environmental support and the resources available to individuals and their families, a fact too often misunderstood by those who have a restricted view of brain function recovery. Unfortunately, lack of proper information and training still leads some health professionals and families to mislabel the behavioural consequences of various brain dysfunctions. For example, they may label a person with a cognitive impairment of reduced initiation, due to frontal lobe damage, as being lazy or uncooperative. The major challenge for professionals in such cases is to try to bridge the gap between the family's perception of the severity of the cognitive impairments and the patient's neuropsychologically based reduced self-perceptions. The wider the gap, the greater the possibility for excessive disability.

Preventive family interventions

An important contribution to the field of cognitive rehabilitation has been made by assimilating a variety of behaviour management techniques. We now recognize how some difficult and challenging behaviours can be evoked by the demands of daily living, and also how behaviour management techniques can be useful in minimizing excessive disability. Steele et al. (1990) found that patients with Alzheimer's disease placed in nursing homes were significantly more behaviourally disturbed than those cared for at home. They suggest that the severity of cognitive impairments per se might not be as important for the placement decision as difficult-to-manage behaviours. Two patients with equivalent cognitive impairments do not necessarily have equivalently difficult problem behaviours. Recent studies have shown how unobtrusive behaviour management techniques can be adapted to manage very difficult behaviours (Radebaugh, Buckholtz and Khachaturian, 1996).

Although behavioural management issues often predetermine the clinical course in cognitive rehabilitation, knowing what goes on in the brain is still essential to this endeavour. The following are ten general principles that families find useful in order to minimize the negative behavioural effects of cognitive disorders.

Problem behaviours are evoked by activities of daily living

In a classic Scandinavian study, Palmstierna and Wistedt (1987) found that 75 per cent of all aggressive behaviours in a group of institutionalized demented patients were triggered by demands of activities of daily living. In a control group of noninstitutionalized patients with schizophrenia, only 25 per cent of aggressive behaviours could be attributed to a trigger based in activities of daily living. Without any intervention, the problem behaviours receded quickly in the patients with dementia, whereas problems would escalate in the patients with schizophrenia, necessitating pharmacological interventions. In a follow-up study by Nilsson, Palmstierna and Wistedt (1988), the relevance and power of systematic observation and measurement of aggressive behaviours in institutionalized patients with dementia were shown. A six-week observation period of aggressive incidents, in the absence of any planned intervention, resulted in a dramatic decrease of aggressive behaviours from week one (91) to week six (16), a decrease of 82 per cent. These dramatic results give special meaning to the maxim in clinical psychology that 'observation is treatment'. Professional and family care providers realize that systematic observation alone, or even slight readjustments in their demands and expectations, can significantly reduce the frequency of challenging behaviours.

Learning can occur without awareness (implicit memory and automatic behaviour)

The knowledge that learning can still take place even if people are not aware (Jacoby and Witherspoon, 1982; Glisky, Schacter and Tulving, 1986) is having a major impact in the field of cognitive rehabilitation. As an example, Richards, Leach and Proulx (1990) have developed a prosthetic memory protocol that teaches patients with severe amnesia how to store information in a memory book and also how to retrieve the information in response to alarm cues. Although learning this new adaptive skill can take over 100 hours in some cases, the benefits have been dramatic for some clients and their families. The insight that learning can occur without awareness has not only been useful to tap into preserved memory functions to learn new skills that improve everyday functioning, but it has also helped families understand how previous skills, automatic behaviours and response styles can explain many adjustment difficulties. Patients with executive dysfunctions, for example, have behavioural adjustment problems that can be explained as 'excessive automaticity'. In other words, what has been learned premorbidly may lead to behavioural response styles that predominate and suffer from poor self-monitoring.

The importance of past memories and old knowledge

The fact that brain-injured individuals can remember events from long ago but have difficulty remembering recent events is often puzzling to families and other care providers. With proper education regarding the relative preservation of remote memories, families can utilize this knowledge to understand behaviour and defuse challenging situations.

Recently, for example, one of the author's elderly male residents with a severe cognitive impairment was taken to the washroom by a male nurse and had a catastrophic reaction. When this situation was presented to the family, they were quick to point out that their father, a holocaust survivor, had been sexually abused by male guards during his incarceration. The important lesson here was that this knowledge of a tragic past episode deeply engraved in this man's memory had an important impact on how care should be delivered. When dealing with severe cognitive impairments, we may be too quick to interpret patients' behaviours as 'difficult'.

Cognitive rehabilitation specialists are learning the importance of knowing patients' past experiences and making a careful inventory of salient past memories. This enterprise, however, cannot be done without the involvement of the family, particularly in the case of patients with dementia. At Baycrest Centre for Geriatric Care, a new home for the aged as well as a centre for cognitive disorders is being built. Families and the community are actively involved in this project. A good example of their input is that a curio cabinet will be built in a small alcove beside the door of each of the rooms. The cabinet will be used to display family photographs and a few salient personal possessions which will serve as cues to help residents locate their rooms.

The prevention of errors when learning

Amnesic patients learn better when prevented from making errors during the learning process (Baddeley, 1992; Hayman, Macdonald and Tulving, 1993; Baddeley and Wilson, 1994). Wilson et al. (1994) conducted a series of case studies applying this technique and obtained practical outcomes in patients with different aetiologies. When new clients with Alzheimer-type dementia join the respite day programmes, this insight is particularly important at the onset when, for example, they are taught to find the washroom.

Reducing interference by restructuring the environment

A common complaint of patients with cognitive impairments is their lack of efficiency with deliberate and effortful processing of information in everyday activities. Reducing distractions through a reorganization of the environment and readjusting previous habits goes a long way towards bypassing this problem. A typical example is the young student with a mild traumatic brain injury who used to enjoy studying with a radio on. By adjusting his habits to study in a quiet area, his grades began to improve. In the author's clinical experience, when patients are willing to make such adjustments, with the help of their families, they often report a reduction in mental fatigue.

Overlearning

Cognitive rehabilitation deals a lot with how learning is affected by brain dysfunctions. As things are remembered, things may be 'dismembered' with brain damage. Clients and families quickly appreciate how learning can still take place, although detours and practice through repetition are an important rule and the price to pay for successful rehabilitation. The word rehabilitation implies the importance of learning new 'habits' in order to adapt again to the demands of daily activities.

Structure, simplicity and familiarity

A great deal of confusion and anxiety can be eliminated with appropriate environmental adaptations. A primary goal for these supportive adjustments is to reduce the load on various memory systems. The Canada Mortgage and Housing Corporation has published a booklet (1995) on useful adaptations to the private home environment for patients with dementia and their caregivers.

Learning new communication skills and maximizing contextual support help families in their effort to eliminate confusing situations, especially with patients who have more severe cognitive impairments. Families are taught to avoid using analogies, metaphors or pronouns and to discard ambiguous communication. It is better to ask someone with symptoms of dementia to 'put on your blue shirt' rather than to say 'get dressed'. The more external referents the better; instead of saying 'which dress do you want to put on today?', it is better to actually show one dress, making the connection between the 'word' and the 'object' much easier. In short, confusing situations and disabling environments merit as much attention and professional intervention as the treatment of cognitive impairment itself.

The use of active strategies and scenarios that have real-life validity

Therapeutic interventions in psychology have been historically biased towards 'talking' therapies. This is not sufficient for clinicians involved in cognitive rehabilitation. Training programmes are most effective if the training involves tasks similar to those that are functionally important to patients (Park, Proulx and Towers, in press). In cognitive rehabilitation, 'knowing why' is only half the battle; 'doing it' is when new habits start to sink in.

The importance of various contexts for assessment and treatment

Carefully planned and monitored training in different settings is proving to be a key feature in any cognitive rehabilitation programme. This, of course, directly implies family involvement as soon as clients are referred for treatment. Observing an elderly woman with dementia in her own kitchen as opposed to being served dinner at the home of one of her children can present different scenarios in how memory disorders are expressed. The context and role of being a guest serve to inhibit perseverative inquiries of whether or not there is enough food for everyone, which becomes a major preoccupation when visitors show up in her own kitchen. Such context specificity is not only important to keep in mind when assessing challenging behaviours, it is also necessary to consider carefully when designing therapeutic interventions and ensuring generalization.

Maximizing 'control' for patients and families

In their study of cognitive function in relation to psychosocial variables in institutionalized elderly people, Winocur, Moscovitch and Freedman (1987) found that the more control elderly people feel they have, the better they do on tests measuring their memory for details and their decision-making skills. In addition, Winocur et al. found that the more active elderly people are, the better they will perform on tests measuring their cognitive skills. Clinical experience suggests that this is also the case with younger cognitively impaired individuals.

Conclusions

The goal of cognitive rehabilitation is to promote the autonomy and social integration of people with cognitive impairments. This chapter shows how this depends on successful family involvement. Clinical neuropsychology provides an important background in brain–behaviour relationships, and proper education of the client and family at this level is essential to any rehabilitation programming.

Cognitive rehabilitation is still mainly about compensation and palliative strategies to reduce symptoms and minimize the effects of disability. The chapter shows how appropriate compensation strategies can sometimes cause dramatic reductions in levels of disability. Compensation strategies should not be thought of as second best to direct remediation of impairments; both approaches are important and may complement each other. When someone has poor vision, for example, wearing glasses eliminates the disability without actually improving the visual impairment. Although research efforts in ophthalmology must continue, wearing glasses has been very useful for several hundred years.

Where things stop short in the field of cognitive rehabilitation is that our current model has too much of an exclusive focus on decrements. The chapter stresses not only how cognitive disabilities vary by the site of brain lesions or severity of cognitive impairment, but that the context in which these impairments are expressed represents practical challenges of independent living that need closer attention. This is important because family involvement occurs long before the admission of the elderly to institutions or long after discharge in the case of younger traumatic brain injury or stroke patients.

Insights from basic cognitive neurosciences have created an impetus for delivery of services as outlined in this chapter. Clearly, more research is needed to validate many of the clinical protocols currently being developed. Whether rehabilitation interventions use pharmacological manipulations, concepts from cognitive psychology, clinical neuropsychology, behavioural management techniques, or a combination of these, the evaluation of functional and psychosocial outcomes must also be included. Everyone agrees on the importance of the relationship between the characteristics of brain dysfunction and psychosocial outcomes, but limited empirical information stifles applications of these important relationships. Clinical enthusiasm must be submitted to the rigors of scientific methodologies, otherwise we may give people with cognitive impairments and their families false hope.

References

Abu-Zeid, H.A.H., Choi, N.W., Hsu, P.-H. and Maini, K.K. 1978. Prognostic factors in the survival of 1,484 stroke cases observed for 30 to 48 months. *Arch Neurol* **35**, 121–5.

Baddeley, A.D. 1992. Implicit memory and errorless learning: a link between cognitive theory and neuropsychological rehabilitation. In *Neuropsychology of Memory*, ed. L.K. Squire and N. Butters, pp. 309–14. New York: Guilford Press.

Baddeley, A.D. and Wilson, B.A. 1994. When implicit memory fails: amnesia and the problem error of elimination. *Neuropsychologia* **32**, 53–68.

Brodaty, H. and Gresham, M. 1989. Effect of a training programme to reduce stress in carers of patients with dementia. *BMJ* **299**, 1375–9.

Brodaty, H., McGilchrist, C., Harris, L. and Peters, F. 1993. Time until institutionalization and death in patients with dementia. *Arch Neurol* **50**, 643–50.

Brodaty, H. and Petes, K.E. 1991. Cost effectiveness of a training program for dementia carers. *Int Psychogeria* **3**(1), 11–22.

Canada Mortgage and Housing Corporation 1995. *At Home with Alzheimer's Disease: Useful Adaptations to the Home Environment*. Ottawa: CMHC, Government of Canada.

Dickmen, S., Machamer, J., Savoie, T. and Temkin, N. 1996. Life quality outcome in head injury. In *Neuropsychological Assessment of Neuropsychiatric Disorders*, ed. I. Grant and F. Adams, pp. 552–76. New York: Oxford University Press.

Evans, R.L., Pomoroy, S., Hammond, M.C. and Halar, E.M. 1985. The relationship between family function and treatment compliance after stroke. *VA Practitioner*, December, p. 10.

Gilchrist, E. and Wilkinson, M. 1979. Some factors determining prognosis in young people with severe head injuries. *Arch Neurol* **36**, 355–9.

Glisky, E.L., Schacter, D.L. and Tulving, E. 1986. Learning and retention of computer-related vocabulary in memory-impaired patients: method of vanishing cues. *J Clin Exp Neuropsychol* **8**, 292–312.

Hayman, C.A.G., Macdonald, C.A. and Tulving, E. 1993. The role of repetition and associative interference in new semantic learning in amnesia: a case experience. *J Cogn Neurosci* **5**, 375–89.

Henley, S., Pettit, S., Todd-Pokropek, A. and Tupper, A. 1985. Who goes home? Predictive factors in stroke recovery. *J Neurol Neurosurg Psychiatry* **48**, 1–6.

Jacoby, L.L. and Witherspoon, D. 1982. Remembering without awareness. *Can J Psychol* **36**, 300–24.

Kay, T. and Cavallo, M.M. 1994. The family system: impact, assessment and intervention. In *Neuropsychiatry of Traumatic Brain Injury*, ed. J.M. Silver, S.C. Yudofsky and R.E. Hales, pp. 533–67. Washington, DC: American Psychiatric Press.

Lehmann, J.T., DeLateur, B.J. and Fowler, R.S. Jr. et al. 1975. Stroke rehabilitation: outcome and prediction. *Arch Phys Med Rehabil* **56**, 383–9.

Lezak, M.D. 1978. Living with the characterologically altered brain injured patient. *J Clin Psychiatry* **39**, 592–8.

Lezak, M.D. 1988. Brain damage is a family affair. *J Clin Exp Neuropsychol* **10**, 111–23.

Nilsson, K., Palmstierna, T. and Wistedt, B. 1988. Aggressive behavior in hospitalized psychogeriatric patients. *Acta Psychiatr Scand* **78**, 172–5.

Novak, T.A., Bergquist, T.F. and Bennett, G. 1992. Family involvement in cognitive recovery following traumatic brain injury. In *Handbook of Head Trauma: Acute Care to Recovery*, ed. C.J. Long and L.K. Ross, pp. 327–65. New York: Plenum Press.

Palmstierna, T. and Wistedt, B. 1987. Staff observation aggression scale, SOAS; presentation and evaluation. *Acta Psychiatr Scand* **76**, 657–63.

Park, N.W., Proulx, G-B. and Towers, W.M. in press. Evaluation of the attention process training program. *Neuropsychol Rehabil*.

Radebaugh, T.S., Buckholtz, N. and Khachaturian, Z. 1996. Behavioral approaches to the treatment of Alzheimer's disease: research strategies. *Int Psychogeria* **8** (1), 7–12.

Richards, B., Leach, L. and Proulx, G-B. 1990. Training the use of external aids for selective memory disorders. Abstract presented at New York Academy of Science, Psychology Section, 11th Annual Conference, New York.

Smyth, S., Urman, S. and Nathanson, S. 1990. *Caring for the Caregivers: Final Report*. Toronto: Baycrest Centre for Geriatric Care.

Steele, C., Rovner, B., Chase, G.A. and Folstein, M. 1990. Psychiatric symptoms and nursing home placement of patients with Alzheimer's disease. *Am J Psychiatry* **147**, 1049–51.

Wagner, M.T. and Zacchigna, L.J. 1988. Comparison of cognitive versus physical disabilities on psychosocial functioning following stroke. Paper presented at the annual meeting of the American Academy of Physical Medicine and Rehabilitation/American Congress of Rehabilitation Medicine, Seattle, WA.

Wilson, B.A. 1986. *Rehabilitation of Memory*. New York: Guilford Press.

Wilson, B.A., Baddeley, A.D., Evans, J. and Shiel, A. 1994. Errorless learning in the rehabilitation of memory-impaired people. *Neuropsychol Rehabil* **4**, 307–26.

Winocur, G., Moscovitch, M. and Freedman, J. 1987. An investigation of cognitive function in relation to psychosocial variables in institutionalized old people. *Can J Psychol* **41**(2), 257–69.

World Health Organization 1980. *International Classification of Impairments, Disabilities, and Handicaps: a Manual of Classification Relating to the Consequences of Disease*. Geneva: WHO.

PART IV

Neurorehabilitation techniques

Introduction

Ian H. Robertson

What exactly is it that we are trying to do when we practise neurorehabilitation? Are we trying to reduce handicap, modify disability or – very ambitiously – reduce impairment? The chapters in this section show us that researchers in this field have been trying to do all three, though sometimes without being explicit about what it is they are precisely trying to do. We lack two major things in this field, namely, an agreed theoretical structure within which to embed our neurorehabilitation efforts, and a clear clinical context within which to position neuropsychological rehabilitation.

The first two chapters in this section deal elegantly with these issues. Wertz broods on the role of theory in aphasia therapy. He distinguishes between theory for and theory of neuropsychological rehabilitation in aphasia. Wertz makes the point that theories 'for' therapy try to predict how and why aphasic behaviours occur, but do not prescribe, specifically, how to correct these behaviours. Theories 'of' therapy may, on the other hand, fail to explain why and how aphasic behaviours occur, but make proposals for methods designed to remedy aphasic problems. Wertz makes the point that theories of both types – 'for' and 'of' – abound, but what is lacking is an integration of these theories with the known characteristics of the underlying neural structures and the mechanisms of plasticity and recovery.

Douglas Katz and Virginia Mills also make a plea for embedding rehabilitation within a good understanding of the biological constraints and characteristics in another very numerous client group – traumatic brain injury. They argue for an integration of the biological and learning models of recovery, and their rehabilita-

tion planning should take into account the pattern and time course of natural recovery. They point out that quite different learning strategies may be needed at different stages in the recovery process. Katz and Mills also show how little evidence there actually is for the effectiveness of cognitive rehabilitation, at least evidence based on randomized control trials as opposed to less rigorous forms of research.

They come out in favour of a functionally based treatment versus rehabilitation aimed at the basic cognitive processes themselves. Generally, the evidence favours an approach to rehabilitation which takes the real-life behaviours as the target of rehabilitation, rather than some cognitive abstraction. Furthermore, Katz and Mills argue that rehabilitation planning should recognize that problems may resolve without any intervention, and that rehabilitation resources should be appropriately targeted to those problems which are known not to resolve.

Robertson's chapter homes in on one particular type of cognitive deficit – attentional problems – and comes to the conclusion that it may indeed be possible to improve attentional functioning, mainly at the 'cognitive process' level of attack, as Katz and Mills would term it. However, this chapter does show that evidence for generalization is rather weak for some types of attentional rehabilitation, though somewhat stronger for others, such as limb activation training following neglect. Clearly, the type of approach outlined in this chapter must become integrated with the wider contexts provided by Katz, Mills and Wertz.

In her chapter, Catherine Mateer reviews rehabilitation strategies for executive problems which include both functionally oriented strategies as well as cognitive process-oriented strategies. She concludes that there is considerable evidence for the efficacy of such interventions, though again there is a very marked paucity of randomized control trials in this literature. Mateer argues that executive deficits can be modified using environmental manipulations, training of compensatory activities, as well as the application of procedures designed to improve the basic cognitive processes themselves. She also emphasizes problems of self-awareness and self-monitoring which are critical to rehabilitation, particularly rehabilitation of executive problems.

Barbara Wilson adopts a similar approach when considering the rehabilitation of memory problems. She emphasizes the compensatory or environmental manipulation approach to the rehabilitation of memory, although she provides intriguing evidence about the possible effectiveness of a somewhat less functionally oriented approach in the form of errorless learning. Errorless learning methods do, indeed, flow out of cognitive theory, and have been applied creatively to the practicalities of rehabilitation by Wilson.

A similar approach underpins Elizabeth and Martha Glisky's approach to memory rehabilitation for the elderly, though they review studies – for instance by Jacoby and colleagues and Neely and colleagues –

which suggest that for this particular client group, cognitive process-oriented therapies (as opposed to more functional approaches) may have promising effects on memory function.

Generally, however, functionally oriented rehabilitation procedures have their generalization measures built into the very therapy, and generalization is easier to demonstrate. Cognitive process-oriented therapies, on the other hand, usually have very limited measures of generalization, and where they do, generalization is often very hard to demonstrate.

What all of these chapters show us, however, is that there is a tremendous potential for extremely effective rehabilitation for a range of cognitive disorders, particularly memory, attention and aphasia. This currently is all at a very scattered and early stage of development, and Wertz, Katz and Mills throw down a challenge to Robertson, Wilson, Glisky and Glisky, and Mateer to integrate better our therapeutic approaches with underlying biological factors, as well as to consider more how practically and clinically our methods can become integrated into the wider clinical services as a whole. If these challenges can be met, then there can be little doubt that the next ten years will see the development of truly effective cognitive rehabilitation techniques.

17

The role of theory in aphasia therapy: art or science?

Robert T. Wertz

Introduction

When the author was at Stanford University's Graduate School, someone did an interesting piece of research with rabbits. Using electrodes implanted in auditory and visual cortex and paired auditory (click) and visual (light) stimuli, the investigator established that, over time, a response could be obtained from auditory cortex to a flash of light, and a response could be obtained from visual cortex to a click. The author has wondered about these results over the years when he sits knee to knee with an aphasic patient and pairs auditory and visual stimuli in an attempt to improve the patient's auditory comprehension or reading. Sometimes, this works, but, so far, the rabbits may be ahead.

Much of what clinicians do when they say they do therapy with aphasic people is fuelled by untested tenets (Rosenbek, 1979), and the role of theory in aphasia therapy is not, sometimes, stated explicitly (Horner and Loverso, 1991). However, theory does exist in many approaches to treating aphasia. Holland (1992) has divided these theories into those 'for' therapy – those that indicate what an aphasic patient's language deficits are and why they occur – and those 'of' therapy – those that prescribe how aphasic people should be treated. The former, typically, are guided by models of language processing. The latter, typically, result from clinical observation. Until recently (Gonzalez Rothi, 1992; Keefe, 1995), few theories either 'for' or 'of' aphasia therapy have considered advances in basic neuroscience, specifically brain plasticity and its influence on behaviour subsequent to cortical injury. This is surprising, given Kolb's (1992) suggestions, and

his observations in this volume, that the mechanisms used for plasticity are those used for recovery, and better treatments will result from better understanding and identification of the recovery process.

The purpose of this chapter is to examine the role of theory in aphasia therapy. Specifically, it discusses mutual concerns between those interested in the physiological basis of recovery and those who treat aphasic people; theory in aphasia therapy; and the potential for wedding theories of physiological recovery and theories 'for' and 'of' therapy into a 'neuro-behavioural' theory for and of therapy.

Mutual concerns

- Most improvement in aphasia occurs early postonset.
- If everything else is equal, age has no influence on improvement in aphasia.
- The size of the aphasia-producing lesion is related to severity but not to improvement.
- It is not known how the brain reacts to being aphasic.

Kolb (1992), discussing the mechanisms underlying recovery, listed three rules: the rules of time, size and reaction. Time, according to Kolb, may influence recovery in three ways: the amount of time since the injury; the age of the organism when injury occurs; and the effect of experience, over time, on recovery. The rule of size dictates the larger the lesion's size, the more severe the behavioural deficits. The rule of reaction involves the ways a damaged brain responds to being damaged.

Those who treat aphasic people have similar concerns. Time is assumed to influence the duration of physiological restitution – so-called 'spontaneous recovery'. In addition, the age of the aphasic person is assumed to influence recovery – younger aphasic people recover more, and older aphasic people recover less. The effect of experience – treatment, no treatment, type of treatment – is assumed to influence the amount of recovery obtained. Lesion size is also of concern to therapists: it is assumed that the larger the lesion, the more severe the aphasia and the less improvement one can expect. Finally, the role of reactive change in aphasia treatment is considered when specific treatments are selected for specific patients' levels of severity and patterns of language impairment. Again, an assumption is made: some treatments are more appropriate for specific levels of severity or patterns of impairment than other treatments. When these treatments result in improvement, we speculate why. Specifically, what has happened in the brain as a result of the treatment? Does return of function result from repair or reorganization in the damaged area? Or, does improvement result from other areas of the brain assuming functions previously served by the damaged area?

Rule of time

Time since onset

We believe that time since onset influences improvement in aphasia. For aphasia subsequent to ischaemic stroke, spontaneous recovery is limited to, at most, the first six months postonset (Wertz, 1983). Some aphasic people continue to improve spontaneously beyond six months postonset, but the available empirical evidence (Culton, 1969) suggests that improvement in language is not significant from one month to the next after three months postonset.

Figure 17.1 shows data for two groups of aphasic patients who suffered ischaemic strokes and participated in the first Veterans Administration Cooperative Study on Aphasia (Wertz et al., 1981). All patients were treated between four and 48 weeks postonset. Group A received individual treatment, and Group B received group treatment. Patients are divided into cohorts that represent the duration of the treatment received. For example, some received 11 weeks of treatment between four and 15 weeks postonset, and others received 22, 33

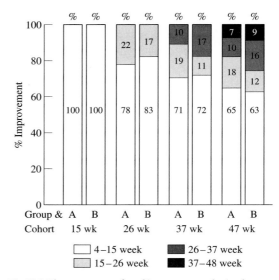

Fig. 17.1 The percentage of total improvement obtained during each 11-week treatment period by each treatment group (A, individual treatment; B, group treatment) in each cohort (4–15 weeks of treatment, 4–26 weeks of treatment, etc.) on the Porch Index of Communicative Ability (PICA) overall percentile score. (After Wertz et al., 1981. Reprinted with permission.)

and 44 weeks of treatment. If a patient is followed for only 15 weeks, all of the improvement observed occurs during that time period. However, if the patient is followed for longer, the amount of total improvement can be determined for specific time periods, for example between four and 15 weeks, 15 and 26 weeks, etc. In Fig. 17.1, notice that in the cohorts who received 26 or more weeks of treatment, most of the total improvement occurred early, between four and 15 weeks postonset. Because all of these patients were treated, it is not known how much of the improvement results from spontaneous recovery and how much results from treatment. Nevertheless, less and less improvement occurs, for what ever reason, as time passes.

Additional information has been provided by Basso, Capitani and Vignolo (1979). Treated aphasic patients were compared with self-selected no-treatment patients (those who rejected treatment, could not afford it, or lived where treatment was not available). Cohorts were established based on the time postonset when patients

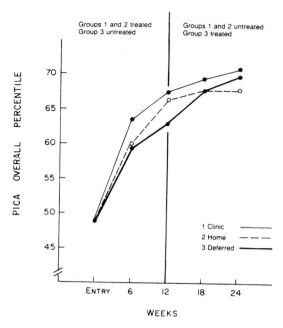

Fig. 17.2 Mean change in the Porch Index of Communicative Ability (PICA) overall percentile in each group during the 24-week treatment trial. The thin, solid line indicates Group 1 (treated by speech pathologists during the first 12 weeks); the dashed line indicates Group 2 (treated by trained volunteers during the first 12 weeks); and the thick, solid line indicates Group 3 (not treated during the first 12 weeks and treated by speech pathologists during the second 12 weeks). (After Wertz et al., 1986. Reprinted with permission.)

began treatment or elected not to be treated – before two months postonset, between two and six months postonset, and after six months postonset. Fewer untreated patients improved as time passed: 42 per cent of the cohort identified before two months postonset improved, 25 per cent improved in the two–six-month cohort, and 11 per cent improved in the six months or more cohort. This implies that if improvement occurs in untreated aphasic people, it is more likely to occur earlier postonset. Similarly, in Basso et al.'s treated cohorts, more patients (70 per cent) improved if they were treated early, before two months postonset, than those who were treated later – 51 per cent between two and six months postonset and 31 per cent after six months postonset.

The implication might be that treatment for aphasia should occur early postonset. However, contrast Basso et al.'s results with those obtained in the second Veterans Administration Cooperative Study on Aphasia (Wertz et al., 1986). As shown in Fig. 17.2, aphasic patients who had suffered a single, left hemisphere, ischaemic stroke and were two to 24 weeks postonset (mean = seven weeks postonset in all groups) were assigned randomly to three groups. Group I received 12 weeks of early treatment by speech pathologists. Group II received 12 weeks of early treatment by trained volunteers. Group III was followed, without treatment, for 12 weeks while Groups I and II were treated, and then received 12 weeks of treatment by speech pathologists while Groups I and II were followed, untreated, for 12 weeks. Weeks postonset and initial severity of aphasia were covaried in the analyses.

Group III (not treated during the first 12 weeks) showed significant improvement on the language outcome measure. What we call 'spontaneous recovery' exists. However, Group III does not improve as much as Group I (treated during the first 12 weeks by speech pathologists) or Group II (treated during the first 12 weeks by trained volunteers). Treatment appears to have an influence on improvement in aphasia.

Now, look at the crossover at 12 weeks. Groups I and II were no longer being treated, and Group III received treatment for 12 weeks. At 24 weeks, improvement in Group III caught up with improvement in Groups I and II, and there were no significant differences in improvement among groups at the 24-week endpoint. Thus, untreated aphasic people (Group III) improve early postonset, probably through the influence of spontaneous recovery. When treated, between 12 and 24 weeks, they continued to improve, probably through the influence of treatment. Conversely, Groups I and II improved when treated, during the first 12 weeks, probably from the combined influence of spontaneous recovery and treatment. Between 12 and 24 weeks, when they were no longer receiving treatment, improvement in Groups I and II waned.

What might we conclude from these results and those reported by others (Culton, 1969; Hartman, 1981; Lendrem and Lincoln, 1985)? First, it is apparent that untreated aphasic patients make significant improvement during an early period postonset. Second, significant improvement in untreated aphasic patients appears to end between three to, at most, six months postonset. Third, the amount and exact duration of what we call spontaneous recovery have not been determined precisely. Fourth, treatment appears to enhance improvement in aphasia. Fifth, unlike Basso et al.'s (1979) results that implied an advantage of early treatment, those in the second Veterans Administration cooperative study (Wertz et al., 1986) indicate that if treatment is going to last 12 weeks, it does not matter whether it is administered early, during the first 12 weeks, or later, during the second 12 weeks.

So, when should aphasic people be treated? The data do not provide a precise answer. The effects of early treatment are confounded by a cotherapist – spontaneous recovery. The amount of improvement seen in aphasic patients treated later postonset is typically less; however, later treatment may be essential in assisting aphasic people to obtain maximal, ultimate outcome.

Age at onset

Traditionally, we have believed that older aphasic patients have a poorer prognosis for improvement than younger aphasic patients. This position was based on clinical observation and a few longitudinal observations. Older patients differed from younger patients in the amount of improvement obtained. They also differed in general health, sensory deficits, number of strokes, and the possible presence of dementia. More recent reports (Lendrem and Lincoln, 1985; Kertesz, 1988; Wertz and Dronkers, 1990; Taylor-Sarno, 1992; Ogrezeanu et al., 1994) indicate, when everything else is equal, age does not influence improvement in aphasia. However, in age, everything, typically, is not equal, and older aphasic patients may not improve as much as younger aphasic patients. But that is not because they are aphasic. Probably, it is because they are old and suffer other sequelae of ageing.

Experience over time

Kolb (1992, p. 172) suggests 'there is now good evidence that environmental events can significantly ameliorate the effects of cortical injury'. In aphasia, the evidence concerning the influence of environment is limited to comparisons of aphasic people in natural (home) and custodial (nursing home) environments and, if treatment is considered to be an environmental event, comparisons of treated and untreated patients.

Holland (1980) reported that aphasic people in custodial environments (nursing homes) displayed more impairment in functional communication than aphasic people in noncustodial environments (their homes). However, she reported the same observation about nonaphasic people. Similarly, Lubinski (1981) reported the negative influence of a communication-impairing environment (nursing home) on communication in the normal elderly. In a setting in which no one talks or listens, the normal elderly abandon strategies they use to enhance comprehension and word finding.

When an aphasic person's environment is manipulated by treatment, clinical trials (Hagen, 1973; Basso et al., 1979; Shewan and Kertesz, 1984; Wertz et al., 1986; Poeck, Huber and Willmes, 1989; Katz and Wertz, 1997), with one exception (Lincoln et al., 1984), indicate treated aphasic people make significantly more improvement than aphasic people who receive no treatment. For example, Fig. 17.2 indicates that aphasic people treated by speech pathologists (Group I) made significantly more improvement than aphasic people who were not treated (Group III during the first 12 weeks of the treatment trial).

Whereas, an environment enriched by treatment appears to influence improvement in aphasia, care is necessary in interpreting the results of aphasia treatment trials. To demonstrate the efficacy of treatment for aphasia, study patients must meet the same selection criteria and be assigned randomly to treatment or no treatment. Only three investigations met these criteria. Wertz et al. (1986) and Katz and Wertz (1997) demonstrated that treated patients made significantly more improvement than untreated patients. Conversely, Lincoln et al. (1984) found no significant difference in improvement between treated and untreated aphasic patients. In the former two studies, aphasic subjects had suffered a single left hemisphere infarct, and all treated patients received the amount and duration of the treatment prescribed. In the latter investigation, aphasic subjects had suffered single or multiple, left and/or right hemisphere infarcts or haemorrhages, and only one-third of the treated patients received the amount and duration of the treatment prescribed. Thus, other variables may interact with and, perhaps, modify the influence of treatment as an environment.

Rule of size

It was believed that large lesions result in greater severity of aphasia and less improvement than small lesions (Kertesz, 1979). However, when the influence of the size of an aphasia-producing lesion on severity and improvement was examined (Wertz et al., 1992), mixed results were observed. The size of the lesion on computerized tomography and magnetic resonance imaging scans was determined and compared with severity and improvement on behavioural measures for aphasic patients who participated in a three-month treatment trial. Lesion size, among patients, ranged from small (14.4 cm) to large (148.9 cm). Pretreatment severity on two outcome measures, the *Porch Index of Communicative Ability* (Porch, 1967) and the *Western Aphasia Battery* (Kertesz, 1982), indicated a range from severe to mild aphasia. Comparison of pretreatment and posttreatment performance indicated a range of improvement from moderate to marked.

Relationships between lesion size and severity, both pretreatment and posttreatment, were significant. The size of the lesion predicted severity. Patients displayed significant improvement during the treatment trial, as indicated by significant change from pretreatment to posttreatment on both outcome measures. Correlations between lesion size and improvement were small and nonsignificant. These results imply that lesion size is significantly related to the severity of aphasia but not to improvement in aphasia.

To be precise about the influence of lesion size on improvement in aphasia, we may need to differentiate the amount of improvement from the ultimate outcome. For example, initially severe aphasic people may make more improvement than initially mild aphasic people, but they do not reach the ultimate outcome attained by initially mild aphasic people.

Moreover, the influence of lesion size may be confounded by the site of the lesion. For example, a small lesion in an important language area may have a stronger influence on severity and improvement than a large lesion that does not involve language areas.

Rule of reaction

Kolb (1992, p. 177) says 'When damaged, the brain changes in various ways that contribute both to the occurrence of recovery as well as to its failure to appear'. His examples from the animal literature – glial, axonal and dendritic reactions – permit no direct comparison with reports on aphasia. Speculation about how the human brain reacts subsequent to aphasia comes from electrophysiological, pharmacological, neuroradiological, and behavioural observations. For the most part, the inferences are intrahemispheric transfer – undamaged areas in the damaged hemisphere assume functions of damaged areas – or interhemispheric transfer – the undamaged, nondominant hemisphere assumes the function of the damaged dominant hemisphere. The following examples represent ways the brain may react to being aphasic.

Moore (1986), using electroencephalographic techniques, observed aphasic patients suppress alpha activity in the right hemisphere during language tasks, while normal subjects suppress alpha activity in the left hemisphere. Haaland and Wertz (1976) found aphasic patients who improved suppressed alpha activity in the right hemisphere, and patients who did not improve suppressed alpha activity in the left hemisphere. Moore's results imply aphasic people differ from normal subjects based on the hemisphere in which alpha activity is suppressed. The Holland and Wertz results imply possible interhemispheric transfer of function. Aphasic patients who improve may be using the right hemisphere – suppressing alpha activity – during language tasks, whereas aphasic patients who do not improve are not using the right hemisphere during language tasks.

Moore and Papanicolaou (1988), using dichotic listening tasks, found that aphasic patients displayed a left ear advantage, while normal subjects displayed the expected right ear advantage. Conversely, Niccum and colleagues (1986) found that dichotic listening in aphasic patients improved during the first six months postonset in both ears, and there was no definite ear advantage.

An early effort by Kinsbourne (1971), using the Wada technique with three aphasic patients, indicated no effects of left carotid injection on speech at six weeks postonset, but injection of the right carotid resulted in muteness.

Heiss et al. (1993), using positron emission tomography methodology, reported left hemisphere metabolism during rest predicted the severity and recovery of auditory comprehension in aphasic patients. During a speech activation task, metabolism in the area of the left hemisphere infarct, its mirror region in the right hemisphere, the left hemisphere Broca's area, and the entire left hemisphere predicted recovery from aphasia.

Mlcoch et al. (1994) conducted single photon emission tomography studies on nonfluent aphasic patients at 30 days and three months postonset. Initially, they noted hypoperfusion in the anterior and posterior regions of the basal ganglia, periventricular white matter, and inferior frontal regions. Only the inferior frontal regions were associated with the recovery of fluent speech. Four of five patients with inferior frontal hypoperfusion did not recover fluent speech. Eight of nine patients with no inferior frontal hypoperfusion recovered fluent speech.

What might we conclude from the limited evidence about how the damaged brain reacts to being aphasic? When aphasic people improve, it is not clear whether functions transfer to other areas within the damaged hemisphere or to the undamaged hemisphere. The most popular hypothesis has been the 'right hemisphere takes over'. But, the data are sparse and conflicting. Zaidel (1976) suggests the right hemisphere contributes to the recovery of comprehension but not of language production. Code (1997) argues that the right hemisphere is not mute and can support nonpropositional speech (automatic and familiar utterances). Gainotti's (1993) review provides some current conclusions. These include: the right hemisphere may play a role in improvement in aphasia in some patients, but a greater role is played by undamaged areas in the left hemisphere; the right hemisphere's contribution to recovery is more for comprehension than for expression; and the right hemisphere's contribution varies widely among individuals, probably because of differences in hemispheric representation of language among individuals.

Considerable caution is required when interpreting the limited evidence on how an aphasic brain reacts to being aphasic. Kolb (1992, p. 181) reports that 'training did not increase dendritic branching in the lesion animals' and 'if the brain changes in response to the injury it may not be capable of further change in response to other factors such as experience'. The data on physiological change in aphasic people come from, for the most part, treated aphasic people. Does behavioural intervention complement physiological change – increase it, hasten it? Or, does behavioural intervention combat physiological change – slow it, retard it? Some conditions require bed rest. Does aphasia require brain rest? The data, for example those presented in Fig. 17.2, imply improvement occurs in aphasic people with and without treatment, and significantly more improvement occurs in aphasic people who are treated than in those who are not treated. The relationship of this improvement in treated and untreated aphasic people with the brain's reaction to being damaged is not clear.

What might we conclude about the application of Kolb's (1992) rules of time, size and reaction to aphasic people? First, the amount of time since becoming aphasic appears to be related with improvement: more improvement occurs early in both treated and untreated aphasic people than later. The influence of age on improvement must be qualified. If older aphasic people display the same characteristics as younger aphasic people, age has no significant influence on improvement. However, older aphasic people typically do not display the same characteristics as younger aphasic people, and the sequelae that accompany ageing may influence the improvement of aphasia. Second, the size of an aphasia-producing lesion appears to influence severity, but it does not predict improvement. The problem may be in the way improvement is defined – amount or ultimate outcome. More severe aphasic people with larger lesions may improve more than milder aphasic people with smaller lesions. However, the initially severely aphasic person with a large lesion rarely attains the level of performance attained by the initially mildly aphasic person with a smaller lesion. In addition, the influence of the size of the aphasia-producing lesion probably interacts with the site of the aphasia-producing lesion. Third, it is not known how a damaged brain reacts to being aphasic. We speculate that language abilities may transfer to other areas within the damaged hemisphere or to the undamaged hemisphere. Neither speculation has been supported by acceptable empirical evidence. Aphasic brains do react, because most aphasic people improve, and treated aphasic people who meet specific selection criteria appear to improve more than untreated aphasic people who meet the same criteria. When treatment should occur, early or later postonset, and the most beneficial type of treatment have not been determined.

Theory in aphasia therapy

- Theories 'for' therapy are designed to address a theoretically specified impairment.
- Theories 'of' therapy are designed to evoke maximal improvement in aphasic behaviour.
- There is little evidence to demonstrate that a specific aphasic person requires a specific type of treatment.
- Both theories 'for' and 'of' therapy, for the most part, have ignored the aphasic brain's mechanisms for plasticity and recovery.

Horner and Loverso's (1991) review of 75 aphasia treatment studies indicated that less than 50 per cent applied an explicit theoretical model. Holland (1992, pp. 147–8) observed: 'If we are to serve aphasic patients better, provide useful information about restitution of cognitive functioning following brain damage, and turn clinical art into a science, we must develop explicit and falsifiable theories of treatment, test their assumptions, and compare and contrast various theoretically-driven forms of treatment'. Also, Caramazza (1989) argued that an informed choice of intervention cannot be made without a theory of the modifications a damaged cognitive system may undergo as a function of different forms of intervention.

Currently, theory in aphasia therapy has been divided, somewhat superficially, into theories 'for' therapy and theories 'of' therapy (Caramazza and Hillis, 1992; Holland, 1992). Theories 'for' therapy, generally, predict how and why aphasic behaviours occur, but

they do not prescribe, specifically, how to rectify aphasic behaviours. Theories 'of' therapy may neglect why and how aphasic behaviours occur, but they include methodology designed to remedy aphasic deficits.

Theories 'for' therapy

Howard and Hatfield (1987) criticised aphasia treatment studies because most asked 'Does therapy in general help aphasic people in general?'. Howard and Hatfield suggest that the question is not sensible, because most clinicians believe that different kinds of aphasia require different treatment. Although most clinicians may take this view, it has not been supported with empirical evidence. The efficacy of aphasia treatment studies discussed earlier demonstrates that therapy, in general, does help aphasic people, in general. Nevertheless, there has been considerable effort to combat the assumed methodological flaws (Coltheart, 1983) in aphasia treatment studies. These efforts are considered here as theories 'for' therapy.

Typically, theories 'for' therapy are based on cognitive neuropsychological theory. They employ a model of normal cognitive processes to identify an aphasic patient's specific impairment and to formulate a theoretical basis for hypothesizing about the underlying dysfunction. This approach, often described as 'theory-driven therapy', requires, according to Caramazza and Hillis (1992), a model of the cognitive processes to be treated, specific hypotheses about the nature of the damage to the processes in the patient to be treated, and hypotheses about how specific interventions may modify function in the damaged processes.

The early work in applying cognitive neuropsychological theory had two aims (Coltheart, 1985). First, models of cognitive processes were evaluated to determine their ability to explain impairment and preservation of abilities in people who displayed cognitive deficits subsequent to brain damage. Second, efforts were made to demonstrate that a brain-damaged person's deficits and retained abilities are exactly those that the cognitive model would predict.

More recently, cognitive neuropsychological remediation studies have begun to appear in the literature (de Partz, 1986; Behrmann, 1987; Byng, 1988; Berndt, 1992;

Mitchum, 1992; Saffran et al., 1992). Byng (1988) listed the requirements for conducting a cognitive neuro-psychological treatment study, essentially a test of a theory 'for' therapy. First, a cognitive disorder would be selected for treatment by specifying the nature of the disorder within the framework of a cognitive model. Second, it is necessary to demonstrate that the treatment of a damaged component in the model is successful and there is, or is not, an effect on other damaged components in the model, depending on the hypothesized relationship between or among components. Third, it is essential to demonstrate that improvement results, unequivocally, from the specific treatment and not from other, nonspecific factors.

Byng's (1988) carefully conducted treatment of two patients who displayed deficits in mapping thematic relations in sentence comprehension and production provided a test of the theory 'for' therapy approach. The therapy focused on the mapping disorder, and both patients improved in their abilities to comprehend and produce sentences. Both were five years or more postonset, challenging an explanation that improvement resulted from spontaneous recovery. Moreover, improvement occurred only on tasks that required mapping of thematic relations, and deficits unrelated to the mapping therapy did not improve.

Do Byng's results support the efficacy of her theory 'for' therapy? Certainly, she met the requirements: a damaged component in the model was treated, improvement occurred in the deficit that was treated and not in deficits that were not treated, and improvement did not appear to result from nonspecific factors. Thus, we might conclude that the treatment was efficacious. However, can we conclude that it was the treatment 'driven' by the theory 'for' therapy – the mapping hypothesis – that evoked the improvement? It is not certain that we can. A true test of the specific theory would require a comparison of treatments, one that is theory driven and one that is not. Utilizing an alternating treatments design – in some sessions the patient receives the theory-driven treatment (mapping therapy), and in other sessions, the patient receives another treatment (nonmapping therapy) – one could test the efficacy of the theory-driven treatment, for example improvement following sessions of mapping therapy and no improvement or less improvement following sessions of nonmapping therapy.

If theories 'for' therapy are to become theories 'of' therapy, Caramazza and Hillis (1992, p. 74) suggest the need for 'models of cognitive processes to drive rehabilitation and for rehabilitation studies to test models of cognitive processes'. Berndt (1992, p. 62), however, observed, 'In an attempt to describe modular systems, model-builders have ignored obvious interactions among cognitive operations from different domains', and 'these limitations are most apparent when approaching model-based interventions'. Finally, theories 'for' therapy are driven by detailed analyses of behaviour. Nowhere in the models of cognitive function is the nervous system represented, and nowhere in hypotheses for remediation are functional and structural substrates of neural plasticity considered. It seems necessary to incorporate the neurological bases of aphasia and the neural bases for recovery in aphasia into theories 'for' therapy or to demonstrate neither is applicable in planning treatment for and obtaining improvement in aphasia.

Theories 'of' therapy

Horner and Loverso (1991), in their review of theoretical models employed in aphasia therapy, observe that concerns in mending aphasia have been threefold: methodological, in which treatment employs sufficient controls to demonstrate therapy is efficacious; theoretical, in which there is an explicit rationale for the therapy administered; and clinical relevance, whether treatment evokes a useful change in an aphasic person's communication. Focusing on the theoretical concern, Horner and Loverso described six theoretical models they found in 75 treatment studies published between 1972 and 1988. Whereas a few models are similar to the theories 'for' therapy described above, all can be considered theories 'of' therapy because they are employed, primarily, to improve aphasic behaviour.

The models appear to be representative of what clinicians do when they say they do aphasia therapy. They include: a stimulation-facilitation model, a modality model, a linguistic model, a processing model, a minor-hemisphere mediation model, and a functional communication model. Each is based on a premise. For example, the stimulation-facilitation model posits that language is an integrative activity that is linked to sensory and motor modalities but cannot be considered bound to them (Schuell, Jenkins and Jimenez-Pabon, 1964; Duffy, 1986). Each provides a description of what aphasia might be. For example, the modality model takes the position that aphasia can be modality specific and may be characterized as a unimodality or multimodality performance deficit. Also, each advocates treatment principles. For example, the linguistic model applies treatment designed to restore language performance by organizing stimuli according to the linguistic system and to linguistic complexity.

All but one model, the functional communication model, intervene at the level of language impairment. Treatment tasks are designed to improve performance in specific modalities – auditory comprehension, reading, oral-expressive language, writing – or to mend a specific deficit – phonology, semantics, syntax. The linguistic and processing models are similar to the cognitive neuropsychology theories 'for' therapy in that treatment is designed to repair a specific disrupted performance in a linguistic or cognitive model. Only one model, the minor-hemisphere mediation model, addresses how recovery may occur in the brain: using minor-hemisphere abilities to facilitate communication through the use of imagery, drawing, melody, contextually rich stimuli, novel stimuli and humour.

The functional communication model differs from other models because therapy attempts to lessen disability. Its premise is that communication reflects the application of pragmatic rules, unconstrained by modality, linguistic or neurolinguistic considerations. Aphasia, in this model, is the ineffective use of language in natural communication contexts. Treatment is designed to improve communication by emphasizing pragmatic function over linguistic form; to enhance intermodality flexibility (speaking, gesturing, writing, drawing); and to develop strategies to avoid, circumvent or repair communication breakdown. This approach to treating aphasia (Davis and Wilcox, 1985) is important because it addresses the need to achieve 'functional outcomes' – reduction in disability – demanded by those who provide reimbursement for aphasia treatment.

Luria (1970) may have been the first to advocate treatment principles that relate to the brain's mechanisms used for recovery. His principles included disinhibition, intrasystemic reorganization, and intersystemic reorganization. Disinhibition postulated that an impaired behaviour was inhibited, because of brain damage, by another system. Treatment should be designed to inhibit the inhibitor. A behavioural example that received some early interest was the use of auditory stimulation to improve oral-expressive language. Assuming that a disrupted auditory system could inhibit speech, Birch and Lee (1955) stimulated aphasic people with noise and reported improved oral-expressive language. Weinstein's (1959) replication found that aphasic people performed worse when stimulated with noise. A third effort (Wertz and Porch, 1970) indicated that auditory stimulation resulted in improvement in some aphasic people, no change in some, and poorer performance in others.

Intrasystemic reorganization attempts to improve performance by moving it upwards or downwards within the defective system. For example, if oral-expressive language is impaired, one might employ singing or rhythmic chanting to improve speech. A treatment of this type is Melodic Intonation Therapy (Sparks, Helm and Albert, 1974), which is reported to improve oral expression in some patients who display Broca's aphasia.

Intersystemic treatment requires utilizing intact or less impaired performance to improve impaired performance. For example, if a patient has limited oral-expressive language but retains the ability to gesture, gestural performance is paired with attempts to speak. The gestures may be batons (taps with the hand) or meaningful gestures (using the fingers to make an 'okay' sign). The rationale is that successive pairing of gesture with attempts to speak will result in improved speech. A few single-case reports (Kearns, Simmons and Sisterhen, 1982; Wertz, LaPointe and Rosenbek, 1984; Rosenbek, LaPointe and Wertz, 1989) support the effectiveness of this method.

Theories 'of' therapy exist, and some therapists employ them. In fact, watch a treatment session and it is not difficult to identify what occurs as one of the therapeutic models listed by Horner and Loverso (1991).

However, unlike theories 'for' therapy, theories 'of' therapy place more emphasis on methods – how to fix aphasic deficits – and, perhaps, on clinical relevance – improved performance. Less attention is devoted to the theoretical rationale or cognitive model employed to 'drive' the therapy. Like theories 'for' therapy, theories 'of' therapy, with a few exceptions, devote little attention to the brain's mechanisms for plasticity and recovery.

Rosenzweig, Leiman and Breedlove (1996, p. 710) observed, 'For some people language recovery depends on specific forms of speech therapy. The exact forms of speech therapy are mainly improvisations supported by some degree of clinical success rather than being generated by theories'. A few pages later (p. 712), they continue: 'Therapy is a significant factor in the long-term recovery pattern of aphasia. As mentioned earlier, strategies employed by therapists tend to be improvised rather than based on knowledge of the brain mechanisms of speech'.

The author agrees that therapy influences recovery for some aphasic people. However, there is no empirical evidence to demonstrate that language recovery depends on specific forms of speech therapy. Except for the superiority of individual treatment over group treatment (Wertz et al., 1981), all comparisons of aphasia treatment studies have reported no significant difference in improvement between the treatments investigated (Wertz, 1993).

Claiming that speech therapy is not 'generated by theory' is incorrect. Theories 'for' and 'of' therapy abound. Thus, we do not lack theoretical principles. What is missing, as Rosenbek (1979, p. 164) observed, is that the principles 'have escaped rigorous testing'. Moreover, it is not that treatment ignores 'knowledge of the brain mechanisms of speech'. It ignores the damaged brain's mechanisms for plasticity and recovery.

Neurobehavioural theory 'for' and 'of' therapy

- A neurobehavioural theory of therapy would require different treatments at different points in time post-onset.
- Early treatment would be restorative and designed to enhance physiological recovery at or around the site of the lesion.

- Later treatment would be substitution and designed to enhance intrahemispheric or interhemispheric transfer of function.
- Neurobehavioural theory is a speculation in search of empirical support.

If Kolb (1992) is correct – a damaged brain's mechanisms used for plasticity are those used for recovery – then his suggestion that better treatments will result from better understanding and identification of the recovery process is sound. Moreover, behavioural treatments should enhance the damaged brain's mechanisms for recovery and not combat or ignore them. Until recently (Gonzalez Rothi, 1992; Keefe, 1995), theory in aphasia therapy has, for the most part, ignored advances in basic neuroscience that address plasticity in the adult mammalian brain and cortical reorganization that occurs in response to cortical injury and environmental demands.

Gonzalez Rothi (1992) proposed a neurobehavioural theory 'for' and 'of' therapy. This theory employs two concepts from the brain plasticity literature – restoration and substitution (Lawrence and Stein, 1978). Treatment techniques designed to enhance restoration – physiological recovery at or around the site of the lesion and the removal of functional influences a lesion might have on other areas of the brain – would be employed early, within the first three to six months postonset, when restoration is assumed to occur. Treatment techniques designed to enhance substitution – intrahemispheric and/or interhemispheric transfer of function – would be employed later, after three to six months postonset. Specific restoration techniques would be aimed at reducing impairment. They would be stimulus–response activities designed to restore auditory comprehension, reading, oral-expressive language, and writing. Emphasis would be placed on massed practice. Specific substitution techniques would be aimed at reducing impairment and disability. Intrahemispheric and interhemispheric reorganization to reduce impairment would be sought, for example through Luria's (1970) intrasystemic reorganization, Melodic Intonation Therapy (Sparks et al., 1974), and intersystemic reorganization, pairing intact gesture with impaired oral-expression (Rosenbek et al., 1989). To reduce disability, intrahemispheric and interhemispheric reorganization would be sought by employing pragmatic methods, for example promoting aphasics' communicative effectiveness (Davis and Wilcox, 1985) that encourages the use of all modalities – speech, gesture, writing, drawing – to achieve communication.

This neurobehavioural theory meets the requirements of a theory 'for' therapy. First, it employs a model of the processes to be treated – auditory comprehension, reading, oral-expressive language, and writing. Although the model is based on cortical plasticity and recovery rather than on cognitive processes, it could incorporate a model of cognitive processes, and careful appraisal would determine which processes were defective. Second, it permits specifying hypotheses about the nature of the damage in the processes to be treated. The hypotheses could be neurologically based – damage in primary auditory cortex results in impaired auditory comprehension – or cognitively based – impairment in the phonological input lexicon – or both. Third, it permits hypotheses about how specific interventions may modify the functioning of the damaged processes. For example, in a patient who is one week postonset and displays damage in the phonological input lexicon, restorative drill on discriminating among and assigning meaning to phonemes will improve the use of the phonological input lexicon. Also, it provides the additional requirement for a theory 'of' therapy by prescribing the methodology to be employed in treatment. For example, for a patient who is six months postonset and displays intact gestures and impaired oral-expressive word finding, substitution treatment would pair meaningful gestures that represent words with attempts to say the words represented by the gestures.

If we believe a neurobehavioural theory 'of' and 'for' therapy will benefit aphasic people, we need to prove it. This could be accomplished with single-case, group, or combined single-case and group designs (Wertz, 1992). For example, to test the theory proposed by Gonzalez Rothi (1992), we might assign acutely aphasic people, less than three months postonset, who meet additional selection criteria (Wertz, 1992) to three groups: Group I, restoration treatment; Group II, substitution treatment; and Group III, deferred treatment. Groups I and II would be treated with the prescribed treatment for three months, and Group III would be followed, untreated. After three months of treatment, our theory would predict that Group I (restoration treatment) would display significantly more improvement than Groups II and III, and there would be no significant difference in improvement between Groups II and III. Improvement would be determined by change between pretreatment and posttreatment performance on standardized measures of aphasia. In addition, to test hypotheses based on cognitive neuropsychological models, each study patient in Groups I and II would be placed in a single-case, multiple baseline design to test theory-driven remediation of a specific cognitive deficit. Restrictions would be that Group I theory-driven treatment would follow the restoration model and Group II theory-driven treatment would follow the substitution model.

To test the temporal implication in the theory – restoration therapy early and substitution therapy later – treatment would 'cross-over' after the early three-month trial, when the study patients were six months postonset. Group I would receive substitution treatment, Group II would receive restorative treatment, and Group III would continue untreated. After an additional three months of treatment, we would predict continued, significant improvement in Group I and less or no improvement in Groups II and III. Finally, after the completion of the six-month treatment trial, therapy would continue with Group II and be offered to Group III. If supported by data from the treatment trial, the treatment would be substitution therapy, because subjects in these groups would be beyond six months postonset.

If we believe that the type of treatment – restorative or substitution – at specific points in time postonset – before and after six months – influences the brain's mechanisms for recovery, we need to verify changes that occur in the brain. For example, serial positron emission tomography scans could be obtained pretreatment and after three and six months of treatment. The theory predicts that Group I (restorative therapy during the first three months) would display increased metabolism in the area of the lesion, and Groups II and III would not. After Group I receives substitution treatment, during the second three months of the treatment trial, the theory predicts Group I subjects would display increased metabolism in areas of the damaged hemisphere different from the site of the lesion (intrahemispheric transfer) or areas in the other hemisphere (interhemispheric transfer). Group II (restorative treatment during the second three months) and Group III (no treatment) would not display increased metabolism intrahemispherically or interhemispherically.

Few theories 'for' or 'of' therapy consider how a damaged brain attempts to restore function. Speculations by Gonzalez Rothi (1992) and Keefe (1995) permit the development of a neurobehavioural theory 'for' and 'of' therapy. The theory is 'driven' by the type of therapy – restorative or substitution – provided at specific points in time postonset – early, within the first three to six months, or later, within the second three to six months. A potential treatment trial was outlined to test the theory. Like existing theories 'of' and 'for' therapy, a neurobehavioural theory 'for' and 'of' therapy is a speculation in search of empirical support.

Conclusions

Much of what occurs in recovery from aphasia appears to parallel observations in the basic neuroscience literature about the brain's plasticity and recovery mechanisms. Most aphasic people improve in their communicative abilities. This improvement occurs without treatment (spontaneous recovery) and with treatment. The duration of spontaneous recovery and the amount of improvement that occurs during this period have not been specified precisely. For aphasic people who meet specific selection criteria, treatment appears to result in more improvement than that obtained from spontaneous recovery alone.

Additional observations in the basic neuroscience literature on the brain's mechanisms for recovery remain speculative in aphasia, for example age at onset of brain damage; amount of time since injury; the effect of experience over time; the size of the lesion; and the reaction of the brain to being damaged. Generally, if everything else is equal, age has no significant influence on recovery in aphasia. More improvement in aphasia occurs early postonset, within the first three months, than later postonset. The presence or absence of experience

(treatment) influences improvement. Treated aphasic people improve more than untreated aphasic people. However, the kind of experience (treatment) and when that experience should occur has not been determined. The size of the aphasia-producing lesion appears to be related to the severity of aphasia, but the influence of lesion size on improvement is debatable. Probably, site of lesion interacts with lesion size to influence improvement. Finally, how the aphasic person's brain reacts to being aphasic is essentially unknown.

Theory in aphasia therapy is not lacking. Theories can be divided into those 'for' therapy, dictated by cognitive neuropsychological models, and those 'of' therapy, 'driven' by methods designed to improve aphasic deficits. Neither includes specific attention to plasticity in the aphasic brain or deals with how that brain attempts to recover from aphasia. This chapter describes a neurobehavioural theory 'for' and 'of' therapy and a means for testing that theory. Data to support the superiority of any one theory for treating aphasia over the others, including the proposed neurobehavioural theory, do not exist.

Young investigators need not worry that all of the questions about the role of theory in aphasia therapy have been answered. Specifically, there is a need to develop and test a theory that indicates and explains what kind of therapy is most beneficial for what kind of aphasic patient at which point in time postonset. These efforts should be designed to explain how an aphasic brain reacts to and attempts to recover from being aphasic. This is, at least, a portion of the work that remains undone.

References

Basso, A., Capitani, E. and Vignolo, L. 1979. Influence of rehabilitation of language skills in aphasic patients: a controlled study. *Arch Neurol* 36, 190–6.

Behrmann, M. 1987. The rites of righting writing: homophone remediation in acquired dysgraphia. *Cogn Neuropsychol* 4, 365–84.

Berndt, R.S. 1992. Using data from treatment studies to elaborate cognitive models: non-lexical reading, an example. *National Institute on Deafness and Other Communication Disorders Monograph* 2, 47–64.

Birch, H.G. and Lee, J. 1955. Cortical inhibition in expressive aphasia. *Am Med Assoc Arch Neurol Psychiatry* **74**, 514–17.

Byng, S. 1988. Sentence processing deficits: theory and therapy. *Cogn Neuropsychol* **5**, 629–76.

Caramazza, A. 1989. Cognitive neuropsychology and rehabilitation: an unfulfilled promise? In *Cognitive Approaches in Neuropsychological Rehabilitation*, ed. X. Seron and G. Deloche, pp. 383–98. Hillsdale, NJ: Lawrence Erlbaum.

Caramazza, A. and Hillis, A.E. 1992. For a theory of remediation of cognitive deficits. *National Institute on Deafness and Other Communication Disorders Monograph* **2**, 65–75.

Code, C. 1997. Can the right hemisphere speak? *Brain Lang* **57**, 38–59.

Coltheart, M. 1983. Aphasia therapy research: a single case study approach. In *Aphasia Therapy*, ed. C. Code and D. Muller, pp. 193–202. London: Edward Arnold.

Coltheart, M. 1985. Cognitive neuropsychology and the study of reading. In *Attention and Performance XI*, ed. M.I. Posner and O.S.M. Marin, pp. 3–37. Hillsdale, NJ: Lawrence Erlbaum.

Culton, J.L. 1969. Spontaneous recovery from aphasia. *J Speech Hear Res* **12**, 825–32.

Davis, G.A. and Wilcox, M.J. 1985. *Adult Aphasia Rehabilitation: Applied Pragmatics.* San Diego: College-Hill Press.

de Partz, M.P. 1986. Re-education of a deep dyslexic patient: rationale of the methods and results. *Cogn Neuropsychol* **3**, 149–77.

Duffy, J.R. 1986. Schuell's stimulation approach to rehabilitation. In *Language Intervention Strategies in Adult Aphasia*, 2nd edn, ed. R. Chapey, pp. 187–214. Baltimore: Williams and Wilkins.

Gainotti, G. 1993. The role of the right hemisphere in recovery from aphasia. *Eur J Dis Comm* **28**, 227–46.

Gonzalez Rothi, L.J. 1992. Theory and clinical intervention: one clinician's view. *National Institute on Deafness and Other Communication Disorders Monograph*, **2**, 91–8.

Haaland, K.Y. and Wertz, R.T. 1976. Interhemispheric EEG activity in normal and aphasic adults. *Percept Mot Skills* **42**, 827–33.

Hagen, C. 1973. Communication abilities in hemiplegia: effects of speech therapy. *Arch Phys Med Rehabil* **54**, 454–63.

Hartman, J. 1981. Measurement of early spontaneous recovery of aphasia with stroke. *Ann Neurol* **9**, 89–91.

Heiss, W.D., Kessler, J., Karbe, H., Fink, G.R. and Pawlik, G. 1993. Cerebral glucose metabolism as a predictor of recovery from aphasia in ischemic stroke. *Arch Neurol* **50**, 958–64.

Holland, A.L. 1980. *Communicative Abilities in Daily Living.* Baltimore: University Park Press.

Holland, A.L. 1992. Some thoughts on future needs and directions for research and treatment of aphasia. *National Institute on Deafness and Other Communication Disorders Monograph* **2**, 147–52.

Horner, J. and Loverso, F.L. 1991. Models of aphasia treatment in clinical aphasiology 1972–1988. In *Clinical Aphasiology*, Vol. 20, ed. T.E. Prescott, pp. 61–75. Austin, TX: Pro-Ed.

Howard, D. and Hatfield, F.M. 1987. *Aphasia Therapy: Historical and Contemporary Issues.* London: Lawrence Erlbaum.

Katz, R.C. and Wertz, R.T. 1997. The efficacy of computer-provided reading treatment for chronic aphasic adults. *J Speech Lang Hear Res* **40**, 493–507.

Kearns, K.P., Simmons, N.N. and Sisterhen, C. 1982. Gestural sign (Amer–Ind) as a facilitator of verbalization of patients with aphasia. In *Clinical Aphasiology*, Vol. 12, ed. R.H. Brookshire, pp. 183–91. Minneapolis, MN: BRK Publishers.

Keefe, K.A. 1995. Applying basic neuroscience to aphasia therapy: what the animals are telling us. *Am J Speech Lang Pathol* **4**, 88–93.

Kertesz, A. 1979. *Aphasia and Associated Disorders: Taxonomy, Localization, and Recovery.* New York: Grune & Stratton.

Kertesz, A. 1982. *Western Aphasia Battery.* New York: Grune & Stratton.

Kertesz, A. 1988. What do we learn from recovery from aphasia? *Adv Neurol* **47**, 277–92.

Kinsbourne, M. 1971. The minor cerebral hemisphere as a source of aphasic speech. *Arch Neurol* **25**, 302–6.

Kolb, B. 1992. Mechanisms underlying recovery from cortical injury: reflections on progress and directions for the future. In *Recovery from Brain Damage*, ed. F.D. Rose and D.A. Johnson, pp. 169–86. New York: Plenum Press.

Lawrence, S. and Stein, D. (1978). Recovery after brain damage and the concept of localization of function. In *Recovery from Brain Damage: Research and Theory*, ed. S. Finger, pp. 369–407. New York: Plenum Press.

Lendrem, W. and Lincoln, N.B. 1985. Spontaneous recovery of language in patients with aphasia between 4 and 34 weeks after stroke. *J Neurol Neurosurg Psychiatry* **48**, 743–8.

Lincoln, N.B., McGuirk, E., Mulley, G.P., Lendrem, W., Jones, A.C. and Mitchell, J.R.A. 1984. Effectiveness of speech therapy for aphasic stroke patients: a randomized controlled trial. *Lancet* **1**, 1197–200.

Lubinski, R. 1981. Speech language and audiology programs in home health care agencies and nursing homes. In *Aging: Communication Processes and Disorders*, ed. D.S. Beasley and G.A. Davis, pp. 339–56. New York: Grune & Stratton.

Luria, A.R. 1970. *Traumatic Aphasia: Its Syndromes, Psychology, and Treatment.* The Hague: Mouton.

Mitchum, C.C. 1992. Treatment generalization and the application of cognitive neuropsychological models in aphasia therapy. *National Institute on Deafness and Other Communication Disorders Monograph* **2**, 99–116.

Mlcoch, A.G., Bushnell, D.L., Gupta, S. and Milo, T.J. 1994. Speech fluency in aphasia. Regional cerebral blood flow correlates of recovery using single-photon emission computed tomography. *J Neuroimaging* **4**, 6–10.

Moore, B.D. and Papanicolaou, A.C. 1988. Dichotic-listening evidence of right-hemisphere involvement in recovery from aphasia following stroke. *J Clin Exp Neuropsychol* **10**, 380–6.

Moore, W.H. 1986. Hemispheric alpha asymmetries and behavioral responses of aphasic and normal subjects for the recall and recognition of active, passive, and negative sentences. *Brain Lang* **29**, 286–300.

Niccum, N., Selnes, O.A., Speaks, C., Risse, G.L. and Rubens, A.B. 1986. Longitudinal dichotic listening patterns for aphasic patients. III. Relationship to language and memory variables. *Brain Lang* **28**, 303–17.

Ogrezeanu, V., Voinescu, I., Mihailescu, L. and Jipescu, I. 1994. 'Spontaneous' recovery in aphasics after single ischemic stroke. *Romanian J Neurol Psychiatry* **32**, 77–90.

Poeck, K., Huber, W. and Willmes, K. 1989. Outcome of intensive language treatment in aphasia. *J Speech Hear Disord* **54**, 471–9.

Porch, B.E. 1967. *Porch Index of Communicative Ability.* Palo Alto, CA: Consulting Psychologists Press.

Rosenbek, J.C. 1979. Wrinkled feet. In *Clinical Aphasiology*, Vol. 9, ed. R.H. Brookshire, pp. 163–76. Minneapolis, MN: BRK Publishers.

Rosenbek, J.C., LaPointe, L.L. and Wertz, R.T. 1989. *Aphasia: a Clinical Approach.* Austin, TX: Pro Ed.

Rosenzweig, M.R., Leiman, A.L. and Breedlove, S.M. 1996. *Biological Psychology.* Boston: Sinauer Associates.

Saffran, E.M., Schwartz, M.F., Fink, R., Myers, J. and Martin, N. 1992. Mapping therapy: an approach to remediating agrammatic sentence comprehension and production. *National Institute on Deafness and Other Communication Disorders Monograph* **2**, 77–90.

Schuell, H., Jenkins, J.J. and Jimenez-Pabon, E. 1964. *Aphasia in Adults.* New York: Harper and Row.

Shewan, C.M. and Kertesz, A. 1984. Effects of speech and language treatment on recovery from aphasia. *Brain Lang* **23**, 272–99.

Sparks, R., Helm, N. and Albert, M. 1974. Aphasia rehabilitation resulting from melodic intonation therapy. *Cortex* **10**, 303–16.

Taylor-Sarno, M. 1992. Preliminary findings in a study of age, linguistic evolution and quality of life in recovery from aphasia. *Scand J Rehabil Med Suppl* **26**, 43–59.

Weinstein, S. 1959. Experimental analysis of an attempt to improve speech in cases of expressive aphasia. *Neurology* **9**, 632–5.

Wertz, R.T. 1983. Language intervention context and setting for the aphasic adult: when? In *Contemporary Issues in Language Intervention, ASHA Reports 12*, ed. J. Miller, D.E. Yoder and R. Schiefelbusch, pp. 196–220. Rockville, MD: American Speech–Language–Hearing Association.

Wertz, R.T. 1992. A single case for group treatment studies in aphasia. *National Institute on Deafness and Other Communication Disorders Monograph* **2**, 25–36.

Wertz, R.T. 1993. Efficacy of various methods of therapy. In *Foundations of Aphasia Rehabilitation*, ed. M. Paradis, pp. 61–75. Oxford: Pergamon Press.

Wertz, R.T., Collins, M.J., Weiss, D. et al. 1981. Veterans Administration Cooperative Study on Aphasia: a comparison of individual and group treatment. *J Speech Hear Res* **24**, 580–94.

Wertz, R.T. and Dronkers, N.F. 1990. Effects of age on aphasia. In *Proceedings of the Research Symposium on Communication Sciences and Disorders and Aging, ASHA Reports 19*, ed. E. Cherow, pp. 88–98. Rockville, MD: American Speech–Language–Hearing Association.

Wertz, R.T., Dronkers, N.F., Shapiro, J.K. and Knight, R.T. 1992. Lesion size, severity, and improvement in aphasia. Paper presented to the Fifth International Aphasia Rehabilitation Conference, Zurich, Switzerland.

Wertz, R.T., LaPointe, L.L. and Rosenbek, J.C. 1984. *Apraxia of Speech in Adults: the Disorder and Its Management.* San Diego: Singular Publishing Group.

Wertz, R.T. and Porch, B.E. 1970. Effects of masking noise on the verbal performance of adult aphasics. *Cortex* **6**, 399–409.

Wertz, R.T., Weiss, D.G., Aten, J.L. et al. 1986. Comparison of clinic, home, and deferred language treatment for aphasia: a Veterans Administration Cooperative Study. *Arch Neurol* **43**, 653–8.

Zaidel, E. 1976. Auditory vocabulary of the right hemisphere after brain bisection or hemidecortication. *Cortex* **12**, 191–211.

18

Traumatic brain injury: natural history and efficacy of cognitive rehabilitation

Douglas I. Katz and Virginia M. Mills

Introduction

- Rehabilitation is expensive and the actual benefit in terms of reducing impairment, disability and handicap in individuals with brain injury is uncertain.
- There is no class I evidence (randomized control studies), only class II and III evidence supporting the efficacy of cognitive rehabilitation.
- In the absence of strong evidence and guidelines for cognitive rehabilitation, health care payers, aiming to minimize costs, may not support this treatment.
- Some clinically principled recommendations can be made based on presently available evidence of the effectiveness of cognitive rehabilitation and an understanding of the interaction of natural history and rehabilitation.
- This chapter emphasizes two major themes: (1) different rehabilitation strategies may be effective at different stages of recovery after traumatic brain injury; and (2) formulations of diagnosis and projections of prognosis and natural history in a particular patient should suggest treatments that may or may not be effective or necessary.

The direct cost of rehabilitation for catastrophic neurological injuries (brain and spinal cord) in the USA is $4 billion yearly (Cope and O'Lear, 1993). Traumatic brain injury accounts for the overwhelming bulk of that cost. The annual total cost of traumatic brain injury in the USA, including both direct and indirect costs, was calculated at $44 billion (1988 dollars) (Max, Mackenzie and Rice, 1991). In a cost analysis of 550 survivors of traumatic brain injury in Colorado (1989–90), rehabilitation made up nearly one-quarter of direct medical costs per case ($48K/$196K) over a four-year period (acute care = $66K) (Brooks et al., 1995). A major focus of the rehabilitative effort for patients with traumatic brain injury is cognitive rehabilitation. The treatment of cognitive and behavioural disorders after traumatic brain injury usually extends long after the treatment of physical problems has been completed. Although a general benefit of rehabilitation, including cognitive rehabilitation, for these patients has been a tacit conclusion, the actual impact of rehabilitation on reducing impairment, disability or handicap for the individual or on cost savings for society is still in question. The overall question is 'does rehabilitation work?' for patients with traumatic brain injury, and if it does work, specifically, 'what works?', 'when does it work?' and 'for whom does it work?'

The evidence to answer these questions is still limited and especially controversial for cognitive rehabilitation. With the growing interest in the USA in clinical practice guideline development to make more effective and efficient use of scarce medical resources, systems have been developed to assess research evidence (Institute of Medicine, 1992). Research evidence is often categorized as class I (randomized, controlled trials), class II (well-designed prospective and retrospective analyses, including cohort, observational and case control studies), and class III (retrospective and prospectively collected case series, unmatched or nonrandomized controls, case reviews, case reports, expert opinion). Based on such a system, there is no class I evidence to support the overall efficacy of rehabilitation for patients with traumatic brain injury. There will obviously never be the highest level of class I evidence for treatment effect – the double-blind, randomized trial – because of the public nature of rehabilitative treatment. Even single-blind, randomized, no-treatment comparisons are unlikely because of the perception that it is unethical to withhold possibly effective treatment. Randomized studies comparing different treatment modalities can be performed and should further the evidence for the benefits of rehabilitation in the future. Some class II and mostly class III evidence supplies the present support for rehabilitation efficacy.

Given the evidence available, standards for cognitive rehabilitation of patients with traumatic brain injury, implying a high degree of clinical certainty, cannot yet be applied. Some rehabilitation treatment guidelines could be recommended based on the bulk of the evidence (class II and III) with regard to overall benefits of some types of rehabilitation services at different points postinjury. However, there is not even moderate clinical certainty regarding the specific questions related to the efficacy of specific treatment modalities, the response of particular injury types or severity, the response of particular clinical problems, or the period of recovery for which particular treatments are effective. It is clear that any guidelines for cognitive rehabilitation will need to consider at least three factors: the nature of the treatment, the nature of the patient's injury, and the patient's stage of recovery.

Therefore, given the lack of complete information, how should rehabilitation treatment choices be made for patients with traumatic brain injury? In the USA, these decisions have largely been driven by the availability of services and the willingness of payers to support these services, two highly interdependent factors. Clinical need and demonstrated efficacy have been secondary or nonexistent criteria. Cost is increasingly becoming the driving factor. Payers are increasingly demanding cost efficiency, and the clarity of demonstrated efficacy is becoming a prerequisite for the continued unquestioned support of rehabilitation services. Without this support or adequate clinical standards and guidelines, cost criteria may dominate. For instance, although it is well known that the natural course of recovery of severe traumatic brain injury typically extends for more than a year, and that later postacute interventions may be crucial for the return of

some patients to productive roles, many managed care plans in the USA limit rehabilitation services to a total of 60 or 90 days.

It seems clear that physicians and rehabilitation clinicians must advise on rehabilitation decision making to help guide choices within these economic constraints. This advice should be informed by an understanding of natural recovery and an appreciation of the possible effectiveness of cognitive rehabilitation at different phases of recovery, based on the available research evidence. Even with the paucity of standards and class I evidence, clinicians should be able to provide some evidence-based and clinically principled recommendations for rehabilitative treatment. These recommendations should include consideration of the constraints of cost reduction and resource limitations.

Neurologically guided diagnosis and prognosis can provide a framework for appropriate treatment planning in cognitive rehabilitation for patients with traumatic brain injury. (See Mills, Cassidy and Katz, 1997, for a complete discussion of this approach.) The treatment plan must respect the natural history of this disorder just as any treatment plan should take into account the natural course of any medical disorder. However, measurement of the treatment effects of cognitive rehabilitation is distinct from other, more physical, medical disorders because it is not described simply by the reduction of a specific pathophysiology or symptom but by improved social functioning or reduced disability. Measures of cognitive rehabilitation results are therefore more diffuse and multifactorial. The treatments are also difficult to specify, entailing multiple interventions, formal and informal, performed by a variety of clinicians, often using nonstandardized methods.

The following sections elaborate several issues necessary for cognitive rehabilitation treatment planning for patients with traumatic brain injury: (1) clinical diagnosis and prognosis, including appreciation of the pathophysiology, natural history and outcome after injury; (2) the interaction of natural history and rehabilitation in terms of biological versus learning models of recovery; (3) types of cognitive rehabilitation interventions and treatment settings; (4) summary of available evidence for efficacy (process specific, functionally based and overall effectiveness at different treatment stages); and (5) recommendations for cognitive rehabilitation planning in the context of natural history. This chapter emphasizes the fact that the effectiveness of specific cognitive rehabilitative treatments may differ depending on the stage of recovery and that the expected natural course of recovery should help determine what treatments may or may not be necessary or effective.

Diagnosis and prognosis

- Pathophysiologically based diagnosis and prognosis aid rehabilitation planning by promoting understanding of clinical problems in terms of neurological syndromes, stage of recovery, projected outcome, and interacting noninjury factors.
- The multiple pathological consequences of traumatic brain injury can be defined according to focal and diffuse as well as primary and secondary causes of brain damage.
- Diffuse axonal injury is the principal, primary diffuse pathology and is associated with a predictable pattern of recovery from unconsciousness, through confusion with posttraumatic amnesia, through a postconfusional residual phase. The durations of the stages of recovery are proportional to injury severity and are influenced by other factors such as age and secondary hypoxic–ischaemic injury.
- Focal cortical contusions are the principal, primary focal pathology. Clinical consequences relate to lesion characteristics, including location (typically frontal and temporal), size, laterality and secondary effects. When combined with diffuse axonal injury, the clinical effects are embedded in the evolving clinical pattern of recovery of the injury.
- Important clinical predictors of outcome from diffuse injury include Glasgow Coma Scale scores, duration of unconsciousness, and duration of posttraumatic amnesia. Other injury and noninjury factors may have important interactions with these predictors in determining prognosis.

Diagnosis that is useful for rehabilitation planning should incorporate several elements that go beyond the diagnostic label alone or the list of functional deficits

Table 18.1 Types of focal and diffuse neuropathology after traumatic brain injury

	Focal	Diffuse
Primary injury	Focal cortical contusion	Diffuse axonal injury
	Deep cerebral haemorrhage	Petechial white matter haemorrhage
	(Extracerebral haemorrhage)	
Secondary injury	Delayed neuronal injury	Delayed neuronal injury
	Microvascular injury	Microvascular injury
	Focal hypoxic–ischaemic injury	Diffuse hypoxic–ischaemic injury
	Herniation	

that typifies the traditional rehabilitation diagnosis. For traumatic brain injury, this includes: (1) a pathophysiologically based diagnosis; (2) an assessment of the patients' clinical problems (impairments and disabilities) in the context of pathophysiology, corresponding neurological syndromes, and natural history; (3) the projected time course of recovery, prognosis of various problems and probability of overall social outcome; and (4) an account of non-injury factors that impact recovery such as age, premorbid status, family and social supports, home environment and comorbidities.

Pathophysiology of traumatic brain injury

For clinical purposes, it is useful to divide the pathological consequences of traumatic brain injury into diffuse and focal categories. There are several possible primary and secondary pathophysiological events in each category (Table 18.1).

Diffuse injury

The principal diffuse pathology is diffuse axonal injury, which results from inertial forces, usually produced by rapid deceleration such as occurs in motor vehicle accidents. These forces produce deformation or strains (particularly shear and tensile) that cause microscopic damage to axons. Although axonal damage is the defining injury, the complete picture of diffuse axonal injury involves a number of related phenomena, including: rupture of capillaries or small blood vessels to produce petechial white matter haemorrhages or small subarachnoid or intraventricular haemorrhage; loss of vasoregulation causing vascular engorgement and intracellular and interstitial oedema (Clasen and Penn, 1987); breakdown of the blood–brain barrier (Povlishock, 1985); and surges of excitatory neurotransmitters that may lead to delayed neuronal death (Hayes et al., 1986; Hayes, Jenkins and Lyeth, 1992). The clinical diagnosis rests largely on the mechanical and clinical phenomena, and on supportive findings on neuroimaging. Severe diffuse axonal injury requires significant inertial forces, such as those produced in motor vehicle accidents or falls of greater than 2 metres. The clinical profile of severe diffuse axonal injury includes *immediate* loss of consciousness (Adams et al., 1982, 1991). Acute neuroimaging may show the petechial haemorrhages or small subarachnoid or intraventricular haemorrhages noted above, or signs of diffuse swelling; computerized tomography may also be relatively negative, even in the setting of severe axonal disruption (Lobato et al., 1983; Marshall et al., 1991b). A major point from the animal models of diffuse axonal injury is that the clinical effects of the injury are proportional to the amount of axonal disruption (Ommaya and Gennarelli, 1974; Gennarelli et al., 1982). For instance, coma duration may range from seconds in the least severe, mild concussive injuries to weeks in the most severe injuries.

The severity of associated vascular and excitotoxic phenomena, although relatively proportional to the amount of axonal disruption, probably accounts for some variability in recovery. Excitotoxicity may contribute to the pathophysiology of coma and posttraumatic amnesia (Dixon, Taft and Hayes, 1993). Secondary injury, such as delayed neuronal injury, microvascular injury and diffuse hypoxic–ischaemic injury, certainly affects overall outcome. Diffuse hypoxic–ischaemic injury is common in more severe injuries, especially in cases of systemic hypotension, respiratory compromise and severe intracranial hypertension (Graham, Adams

and Doyle, 1979). Diagnosis is difficult because there are no specific diagnostic markers of diffuse hypoxic–ischaemic injury; the diagnosis is suspected on clinical grounds such as with the occurrence of sustained systemic hypotension <90 mmHg or intracranial hypertension >20 mmHg, or clinical signs compatible with particular distributions of diffuse hypoxic–ischaemic injury in susceptible areas – hippocampi, basal ganglia, borderzone areas, cerebellum. Preventing the second wave of injury, including excitotoxicity, and diffuse hypoxic–ischaemic injury is becoming an important target of early intervention.

Focal injury

The principal focal pathology after traumatic brain injury is focal cortical contusion. Focal cortical contusion results from either contact forces, such as from a blow to the head, causing direct localized damage to the brain underneath, or inertial forces causing localized damage in areas where the brain is relatively confined, such as the anterior and middle fossae, producing excessive localized strain. This predisposes the anterior and inferior frontal and temporal areas to this injury. Focal cortical contusion consists of localized cortical damage, rupture of surface vessels with haemorrhage of varying depth and secondary reactive changes, including mass effect, both locally and distally. Another form of focal vascular injury occurs deep in the brain, without cortical involvement, and is probably related to rupture of deep penetrating arteries (Katz et al., 1989). Focal cortical contusion and deep haemorrhages are diagnosed entirely by neuroimaging. They are not directly associated with loss of consciousness, although the reactive and secondary effects might contribute to altered consciousness.

Focal hypoxic–ischaemic injury results from compromise of a local vascular bed territory near regions of high localized pressure gradients from mass lesions or in a large artery territory, most commonly the posterior cerebral artery following temporal herniation. Neuroimaging confirms the diagnosis.

Herniation causes clinical effects by way of compression of vascular and neural structures. Large vessel strokes (focal hypoxic–ischaemic injury) have already

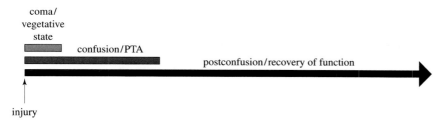

Fig. 18.1 Epochs of recovery following traumatic brain injury with diffuse pathology. PTA = posttraumatic amnesia.

been mentioned; small haemorrhages or infarctions in the brainstem and diencephalon and direct damage to basal neural tissues such as midbrain, hypothalamus, medial temporal lobe and third cranial nerve are typical of temporal and transtentorial herniations (Plum and Posner, 1980). The acute effects of herniation are well described but the natural history and longer term effects have not been well studied.

Natural history and outcome

Diffuse injury

Patients with diffuse pathology (diffuse axonal injury and associated secondary injury) follow a fairly stereotypical pattern of natural recovery that is discernible across the range of severities. The pattern may be defined according to three main epochs of recovery (Fig. 18.1). The first epoch is immediate unconsciousness, without lucid interval, followed by a proportionally longer period of confusion, closely tied to dense anterograde amnesia (posttraumatic amnesia), followed by an even longer period of residual recovery. The duration of these epochs corresponds to injury severity and forms a basis for predicting time course and outcome. The length of unconsciousness and duration of posttraumatic amnesia are commonly used indices of severity and outcome predictors, particularly for patients with primarily diffuse injury. Of course, outcome is influenced by a multiplicity of injury and noninjury factors.

These stages have been further described in various ways, such as the Rancho Los Amigos levels of cognitive functioning (Hagen et al., 1972; Table 18.2). The schema described here conforms to more conventional neuro-

logical nomenclature (Alexander, 1982; Katz, 1992, 1997; Katz and Alexander, 1994b; Table 18.3). The corresponding Rancho Los Amigos level is placed in parethesis for comparison. Coma (Rancho level 1), the first stage, occurs immediately, without lucid interval. The depth of coma in the first few hours (as measured by the Glasgow Coma Score) is an important index of severity and outcome. All survivors eventually open their eyes and appear wakeful but have no purposeful attention or cognitive responsiveness – vegetative state/wakeful unconsciousness (Rancho level 2). A small proportion of very severely injured patients remain *permanently vegetative*; the vast majority progress to a state of erratic, directed responsiveness, often mute or hypoverbal, referred to as minimally conscious state (Rancho level 3). Ability to follow commands is the usual marker of this stage, and duration of coma is most often defined by the time to the onset of this stage. This is another important index of severity and an outcome predictor. As patients begin to respond more reliably and speak more consistently, they emerge into the next stage, defined by severe attentional disturbance and dense anterograde (posttraumatic) amnesia – confusional state (Rancho level 4, 5 to 6). Agitated, poorly modulated or, less commonly, hypokinetic behavioural disturbances are common. Vast improvements in directed and sustained attention, restoration of continuous day-to-day memory and orientation mark the end of this stage. The duration of posttraumatic amnesia is the last important clinical index of severity of diffuse axonal injury. In the postconfusional/evolving independence (Rancho levels 6 to 7) stage, patients begin to show functional independence; however, they still have cognitive problems, particularly in higher level attention, memory and executive function. Most hospital-

Table 18.2 Rancho Los Amigos levels of cognitive functioning

I	No response
II	Generalized responses
III	Localized responses
IV	Confused – agitated
V	Confused – inappropriate
VI	Confused – appropriate
VII	Automatic – appropriate
VIII	Purposeful and appropriate

Table 18.3 Stages of recovery from diffuse axonal injury

1. Coma: unresponsive, eyes closed

2. Vegetative state/wakeful unconsciousness: no cognitive responsiveness, gross wakefulness, sleep–wake cycles

3. Minimally conscious state: purposeful wakefulness, responds to some commands, often mute

4. Confusional state: recovered speech, amnesic (posttraumatic amnesia), severe attentional deficits, agitated, hypoaroused or labile behaviour

5. Postconfusional/evolving independence: resolution of posttraumatic amnesia, cognitive improvement, achieving independence in daily self-care, improving social interaction, developing independence at home

6. Social competence/community re-entry: recovering cognitive abilities, goal-directed behaviours, social skills, personality, developing independence in the community, returning to academic or vocational pursuits

ized rehabilitation patients go home at this stage. Later recovery, termed social competence/community re-entry (Rancho level 7 to 8), mainly involves the restoration of previous capacities of cognitive and social functioning.

Several points regarding this process of recovery deserve emphasis. The duration of these stages is proportional to injury severity. Most patients with diffuse axonal injury, from the least severe to the most severe injuries, pass through these stages; in the least severe (mild concussions) the transition through earlier stages may be brief (seconds to minutes) and unwitnessed, and in the most severe, recovery may stall at one or another stage (Fig. 18.2). Although for some patients distinct stages may not be clinically identifiable, some stages are probably obligatory. For instance, patients who experience coma must evolve through a confusional state and posttraumatic amnesia to the later stages. Finally, these stages are proportionally related in duration, although exceptions do occur. Each subsequent pair of stages – coma/vegetative state, mute responsiveness/confusional state, evolving independence/competence – is usually several fold longer than the previous pair. This proportionality is useful in predicting the time course of recovery from diffuse axonal injury (Katz and Alexander, 1994a, 1994b; see below).

This discussion has centred around the cognitive and behavioural aspects of recovery, the most consistent manifestations. Diffuse axonal injury frequently produces motor deficits, often a mix of different problems. Cerebellar, vestibular and postural deficits are common.

Spastic paresis frequently occurs, often combined with the other signs. Hypokinesia is another common early sign, perhaps due to the high incidence of diffuse axonal injury lesions in frontal parasagittal areas. The recovery of motor problems generally evolves over a longer period of time than similar problems seen in focal ischaemic damage (stroke). Nevertheless, the recovery of physical problems evolves more rapidly than the recovery of psychosocial problems (McLean, Dikmen and Temkin, 1993).

Predicting the outcome of diffuse axonal injury

Three clinical indices of severity are the best available predictors of outcome of diffuse axonal injury: Glasgow Coma Score, duration of coma, and duration of anterograde amnesia. These severity measures have a strong relationship to each other and this relationship can help predict the early course of recovery. Recognizing the necessary proportional relationship between the stages of recovery from diffuse axonal injury, a regression model was derived to predict roughly posttraumatic

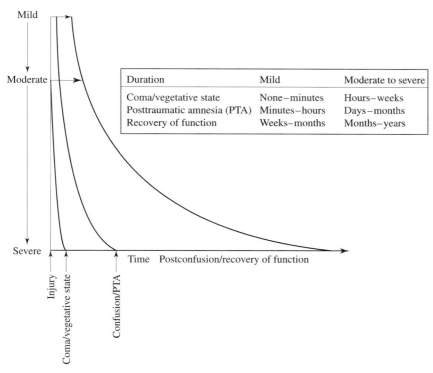

Duration	Mild	Moderate to severe
Coma/vegetative state	None–minutes	Hours–weeks
Posttraumatic amnesia (PTA)	Minutes–hours	Days–months
Recovery of function	Weeks–months	Months–years

Fig. 18.2 The pattern of recovery following diffuse traumatic brain injury across a range of severity from mild to severe. This illustrates the relative duration and proportionality of epochs of recovery at different injury severities.

amnesia duration (PTA) from coma duration (loss of consciousness, LOC): PTA (weeks) = 0.4 x LOC (days) + 3.6 (Katz and Alexander, 1994a). Such a prediction can be especially valuable in clinical planning and in projecting the length of hospitalization for patients in rehabilitation.

Glasgow Coma Score in the first few hours, particularly the lowest postresuscitation score (Levin, Gary and Eisenberg, 1990), has a strong relationship to outcome. Factors other than diffuse axonal injury that may depress the Glasgow Coma Score should be distinguished because they may confound the predictive value of the score. Prognosis is much worse with a Glasgow Coma Score below 6. The Traumatic Coma Data Bank study reported only 16 per cent *moderate disability* or *good recovery* in patients with a score of less than 6, but up to 63 per cent *moderate disability* or *good*

recovery in those with scores between 6 and 8 (Marshall et al., 1991a). In a rehabilitation population of survivors with a diagnosis of moderate to severe diffuse axonal injury, 21 per cent achieved *good recovery* and 26 per cent *severe disability* at one year with scores less than 6, and 37 per cent achieved *good recovery* and 15 per cent *severe disability* with scores of 6 to 8 (Fig. 18.3).

Coma duration and posttraumatic amnesia have an even stronger relationship to outcome. In rehabilitation populations, they had a fairly strong relationship to Glasgow Outcome Scale scores (Katz, 1992; Katz and Alexander, 1994a) and Disability Rating Scale and Functional Independence Measure scores (Hall et al., 1993). As examples, in the authors' series (rehabilitation population) of patients with diffuse axonal injury, of those with coma duration between one day and one week, 49 per cent had a good recovery at one year; no

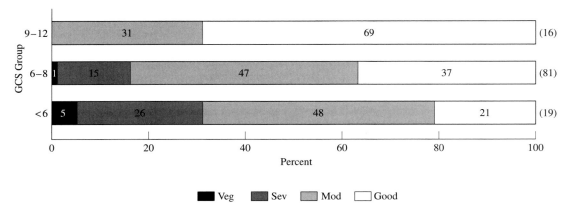

Fig. 18.3 Outcome probability at one year postinjury in a group of patients ($n=116$) admitted to inpatient rehabilitation with moderate to severe traumatic brain injury classified by acute admission Glascow Coma Scores (GCS). Outcomes are categorized by the Glasgow Outcome Scale (veg, vegetative state; sev, severe disability; mod, moderate disability; good, good recovery).

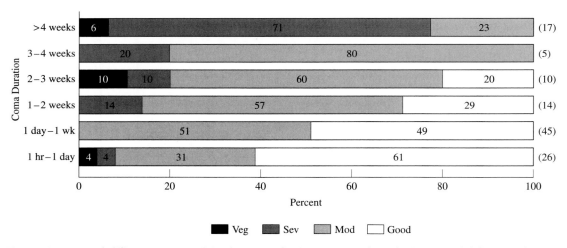

Fig. 18.4 Outcome probability at one year postinjury in a group of patients ($n=117$) admitted to inpatient rehabilitation with moderate to severe traumatic brain injury classified by duration of unconsciousness (coma + vegetative state). Outcomes are categorized by the Glascow Outcome Scale (veg, vegetative state; sev, severe disability; mod, moderate disability; good, good recovery).

patient with over three weeks' coma made a good recovery, whereas 64 per cent were severely disabled or vegetative (Fig. 18.4). Of those with posttraumatic amnesia duration less than two weeks, 76 per cent achieved a good recovery, 22 per cent were moderately disabled and 2 per cent severely disabled at one year; with 8–12 weeks' posttraumatic amnesia, outcome worsened to

12 per cent good recovery, 75 per cent moderate disability and 13 per cent severe disability. Nobody with over 12 weeks posttraumatic amnesia achieved a good recovery (Fig. 18.5). The data provided in Figs. 18.3, 18.4 and 18.5 for coma and posttraumatic amnesia can therefore provide estimates of outcome for survivors of traumatic brain injury with diffuse axonal injury.

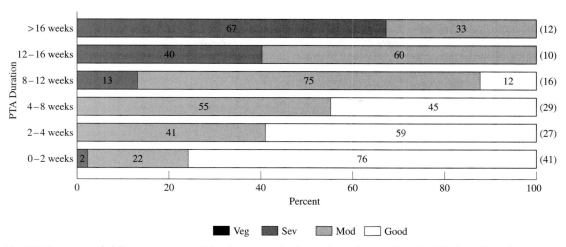

Fig. 18.5 Outcome probability at one year postinjury in a group of patients admitted to inpatient rehabilitation with moderate to severe traumatic brain injury classified by duration of posttraumatic amnesia (PTA). Outcomes are categorized by the Glascow Outcome Scale (veg, vegetative state; sev, severe disability; mod, moderate disability; good, good recovery).

Age appears to have a complex effect on recovery from diffuse axonal injury. For any severity, posttraumatic amnesia is prolonged with advancing age, especially over the age of 40 (Fig. 18.6). Quality of functional outcome also worsens above the age of 40 (Jennett and Teasdale, 1981; Narayan et al., 1981; Katz and Alexander, 1994a). No patient over the age of 40 who was comatose for over one hour achieved a good recovery by one year after injury, whereas nearly 50 per cent of those under 40 achieved a good recovery (Fig. 18.7; Katz and Alexander, 1994a).

In summary, outcome of diffuse axonal injury is best predicted by severity measures and the best predictions are achieved by posttraumatic amnesia duration, followed by coma duration, followed by Glasgow Coma Score. Posttraumatic amnesia explained nearly half the variance of one-year outcome in a group of patients with diffuse axonal injury (Katz and Alexander, 1994a). These predictors are most meaningful when applied to patients with diffuse axonal injury and do not significantly predict outcome for patients with focal pathology (Katz and Alexander, 1994a). The interrelationship of severity variables is also useful in predicting the duration of posttraumatic amnesia from coma duration.

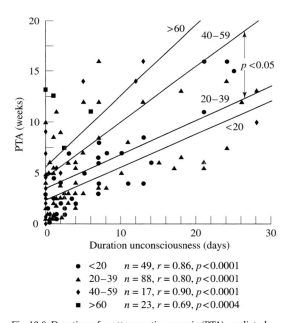

$\bullet$ <20 $n = 49, r = 0.86, p < 0.0001$
$\blacktriangle$ 20–39 $n = 88, r = 0.80, p < 0.0001$
$\blacklozenge$ 40–59 $n = 17, r = 0.90, p < 0.0001$
$\blacksquare$ >60 $n = 23, r = 0.69, p < 0.0004$

Fig. 18.6 Duration of posttraumatic amnesia (PTA) predicted by the duration of unconsciousness in a group of patients with diffuse axonal brain injury at different age groups. For any duration of unconsciousness, the predicted duration of posttraumatic amnesia was longer in the older age groups. The effect was significant ($p < 0.05$) over the age of 40.

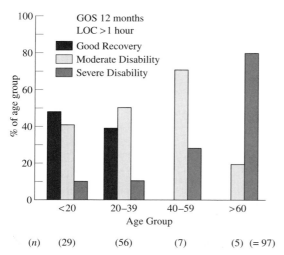

(*n*)   (29)   (56)   (7)   (5) (= 97)

Fig. 18.7 Outcome probability at one year postinjury in a group of patients admitted to inpatient rehabilitation with moderate to severe diffuse axonal brain injury for different age groups. Outcomes are categorized by the Glasgow Outcome Scale (GOS). Outcome was worse for older age groups. No person over 40 who was unconscious for more than one hour achieved a good recovery at one year.

Focal injury

The natural history of focal cortical contusion after the acute phase of recovery is largely dependent on the location of the lesion. The usual location of focal cortical contusion in limbic and heteromodal association areas of the frontal and temporal lobes defines its typical cognitive and behavioural effects. Residual problems in executive functioning or behaviour modulation are well-recognized residual sequelae of focal cortical contusion. Other locations may produce different problems; for instance, lesions extending more posteriorly in the left temporal association area may cause language problems, characteristically anomic or transcortical sensory aphasia.

Several other dimensions are important in determining the outcome of focal cortical contusion: (1) the size and, particularly, the depth of the lesion; (2) bilaterality, especially involving homologous areas; and (3) distal secondary damage. Small, superficial focal cortical contusions may have few, if any, late clinical consequences. Differences in lesion depth, involving greater or lesser

Focal vs. diffuse

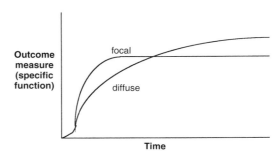

Fig. 18.8 Recovery curves comparing the typical course for focal versus diffuse traumatic brain injury pathology. A particular impairment of similar severity will generally recover over a more protracted period after diffuse injury than after focal injury.

quantities of white matter pathways, can make enormous differences in clinical recovery, depending on the amount of disrupted cortical–cortical and cortical–subcortical connectivity. Bilateral involvement may portend a much worse prognosis and, conversely, patients with unilateral lesions, particularly involving less lateralized systems (e.g. prefrontal), can have considerable recovery.

The time course of recovery from focal cortical contusion is probably identical to that of focal haemorrhagic lesions of other aetiologies. The main point is that problems related to focal cortical contusion recover on a more rapidly evolving recovery curve than similar problems, of similar severity, related to diffuse axonal injury (e.g. executive functions: Fig. 18.8). It also deserves emphasis that the specific residual problems associated with focal cortical contusion can usually be clarified only after the resolution of acute and subacute secondary reactive processes (e.g. mass effect, oedema).

The clinical effects of focal pathology are often embedded in the evolving clinical process of diffuse injuries. The detection of particular localizing syndromes may be difficult until unmasked with the resolution of attention problems as confusion clears. Furthermore, the typical cognitive and behavioural effects of focal injury (frontal and temporal) are often indistinguishable from the later stage effects of diffuse pathology, which must also affect 'frontal' systems.

Interaction of natural history and rehabilitation: biological versus learning models of recovery

- The *biological* model and the *learning* model of recovery emphasize differently the factors that may influence recovery. The biological model emphasizes pathophysiological events and brain plasticity, and the learning model emphasizes the role of experience, practice and the environment in producing functional recovery.
- There is a complex interaction between the biological recovery process and experience, which is supported by animal models of recovery that demonstrate environmental and learning effects on brain plasticity.
- The relative influence of interacting biological and environmental factors probably varies at different times postinjury. At earlier stages of recovery after traumatic brain injury, the relative influence of biological factors is probably much greater, and at later stages learning, experience and other noninjury factors (psychological, social, environmental) probably play a much larger role in shaping recovery.

The central premise of rehabilitation is that an intervention will produce some change in a person's functioning that would not occur as well, as quickly, or at all on its own. How a person with an injured brain improves and learns to function better is a complex and controversial question (Levin, 1990; Volpe and McDowell, 1990). The arguments often divide along the lines of two disparate models of recovery – one more biologically centred, the other centred on learning, experience and psychological processes (Ben Yishay and Diller, 1993). The biological models emphasize the pathophysiological events and brain plasticity as the main constraints on functioning and recovery. Learning and adaptation secondarily interact with biological systems in the recovery process. Advocates of this model tend to be more critical and sceptical about the effectiveness of rehabilitation, especially cognitive rehabilitation. The learning model emphasizes the role of experience, practice and the environment in producing functional changes by way of the restoration of impaired capacities or substitution of new means of functioning. This model renders the role of natural history to the background and is generally more optimistic about the role of rehabilitation in promoting recovery (Berrol, 1990; Ben Yishay and Diller, 1993). Advocates of the biological model often relegate therapy and rehabilitation to the realm of insignificant background noise in studying the process of recovery and outcome; advocates of the learning model often view natural history and spontaneous recovery as merely confounding factors in assessing the effects of rehabilitation.

It is generally agreed that there is a complex interaction between the biological recovery process and experience (Bach-y-Rita and Wicab Bach-y-Rita, 1990; Bach-y-Rita, 1992). The nature of this interaction is poorly understood, although the two extreme sides of the questions are relatively uncontroversial. On one side, it is clear that brain-injured patients can learn, using one or another type of learning (see below), and learning facilitates successful functional substitution (compensation). On the other extreme, it is clear that neurological functional reorganization occurs by way of a number of biological processes that evolve independently of any specific intervention or experience. These processes include the resolution of early postinjury pathophysiological phenomena (e.g. brain oedema), vicariation or redistribution of a particular function to other parts of the brain and, to some extent, reactive synaptogenesis and new receptor formation (see Almli and Finger, 1988; Bach-y-Rita, 1992, for a review). The core question concerning these two extremes is whether specific therapeutic interactions affect brain plasticity and reorganization in ways that would have not passively occurred. Evidence from animal models is available. For example, brain-damaged animals which were trained showed both performance improvement and corresponding increase in dendritic branching associated with training compared to animals which were restricted from training or environmental enrichment (Kolb and Gibb, 1991, 1993).

Accepting the premise that there is an interaction between natural recovery and experience begs the questions of up to what time postinjury can this interaction occur and how does the proportional contribution of learning versus biological recovery change over time. It is evident that biological factors are more important and less alterable earlier in recovery and that their proportional contribution decreases at longer times postinjury. Even after spontaneous biological recovery plateaus, the effects of learning, environment and psychological factors may have specific physiological effects (Bach-y-Rita, 1992). Neurophysiological events, however, are much more important in determining the earlier stages of recovery. For traumatic brain injury, learning and experience probably have little or no effect on altering the time course of coma, vegetative or confusional stages of recovery. Paradoxically, this is when much intense rehabilitation effort is applied in inpatient acute rehabilitation facilities. There is not convincing evidence that interventions such as sensory stimulation or reality orientation groups have any effect on the resolution of unconsciousness or posttraumatic amnesia, respectively. For example, of more than ten representative studies on sensory stimulation, the majority show some transient improvement in gross wakefulness (see Giacino, 1996, for a review), but only one claims shorter unconsciousness (Mitchell et al., 1990). This may simply indicate injury of lesser severity rather than a direct effect of stimulation. Novack and colleagues (1996) found that patients in the earlier stages of recovery during inpatient rehabilitation (probably most were in confusional states, but this was not specified) improved in attention and functional measures at the same rate whether or not they received specific structured attentional treatment. This indicates that the early stages of recovery after traumatic brain injury probably evolve on a biologically driven time course independent of any intervention that can accelerate recovery (although some interventions may retard recovery).

Nevertheless, rehabilitation efforts can be important at these stages. Efforts at supportive nursing care, appropriate nutritional support, the maintenance of range of motion, proper bed and chair positioning, and the treatment of medical complications are among the important measures to maintain optimum natural recovery and prepare a patient for more active rehabilitative efforts at later stages. Rather than attempting to modify the rate of recovery, rehabilitative strategies during the confusional stage can concentrate on managing symptoms (i.e. cognitive and behavioural problems) through environmental manipulation and appropriate types of interaction and stimulation. The overall goal would be to allow a patient to recover through this stage as easily as possible, avoiding factors that may worsen symptoms or slow recovery (e.g. some sedating medications). At later stages of recovery, postconfusion and beyond, learning, experience and a host of noninjury factors (e.g. psychological, social, environmental) seem to play a much larger role in shaping recovery. It would therefore appear that there is validity in both biological and learning models of recovery. There is a dynamic interaction of various influences, including pathophysiological, environmental, new learning, and previous behaviour patterns, that varies in proportion over time.

Rehabilitation interventions and treatment settings

- Rehabilitation strategies generally fall into the categories of restorative or compensatory interventions. Cognitive rehabilitation divides along two general strategies: process-specific cognitive rehabilitation and functional skills training.

- Rehabilitation for patients with traumatic brain injury is provided in a number of settings, including the acute hospital, inpatient rehabilitation hospital unit, subacute or skilled nursing facility, outpatient programme, day programme, home therapies, transitional living programme, and vocational rehabilitation programme. The choice of settings is guided by injury severity, stage of recovery, prognosis, progress rate, local availability and payer support.

Cope (1995) has outlined the elements of comprehensive traumatic brain injury rehabilitation. These elements include: (1) rehabilitative medical and nursing care; (2) prevention of secondary deterioration; (3) maximization of the natural recovery process; (4) facilitating incremental functional gains through specific interventions (mobility, self-care, communication); (5) providing the optimal environment for neurological recovery (e.g. drugs, environment, experience); (6) compensatory techniques for areas of poor recovery; (7) provision of appropriate equipment (wheelchairs, orthoses); and (8) environmental modifications (architectural, transportation, social).

Rehabilitation strategies generally fall within the realm of restorative versus compensatory interventions. Restorative strategies tend to be more controversial because there is a limited amount of supportive research evidence and it is often difficult to separate treatment effects from spontaneous recovery. Strategies of cognitive rehabilitation divide along similar lines: direct treatment of cognitive processes versus functional skills training. On the surface, functional skills training, when targeting real-world activities, seems more direct, practical and, perhaps, less costly. Direct treatment of cognitive processes is appealing because treatment of the underlying process should allow generalization of improvement to a variety of tasks and situations; however, the efficacy of rehabilitative treatment aimed at restoring specific cognitive processes remains largely unproven.

In the USA, rehabilitation is provided in a number of settings, guided by severity, stage of recovery, rate of progress and prognosis, local availability, and payer support. The provision of rehabilitation services begins in the acute hospital setting for moderate to severe traumatic brain injury patients, focusing mainly on preventative aspects of care during coma through minimally conscious stages. Transfer to acute rehabilitation usually occurs during the minimally conscious or confusional stages for patients with severe traumatic brain injury. Patients who are less severely injured are either discharged home from the emergency room or after a stay in an acute hospital. They may be referred to some outpatient rehabilitation services. The most severe, 'slow to recover' patients may move from the acute hospital to subacute or skilled nursing facilities; they may, however, also be admitted to an acute rehabilitation facility for a period of time. After acute rehabilitation most patients go home, usually some time after resolution of confusion and posttraumatic amnesia. Outpatient services are provided through outpatient programmes, day programmes or home therapies. Postacute rehabilitation may also entail residential treatment in a transitional living programme. At later stages of recovery (social competence), outpatient therapies or transitional living programmes may focus on community re-entry, working on functional tasks for home and community independence. Some pro-grammes incorporate process-specific cognitive rehabilitation (e.g. computer modules), various forms of psychological support, and awareness training in addition to functionally based treatment (Prigatano, 1986; Rattok et al., 1992; Ben-Yishay and Diller, 1993). Still later, for those who recover adequately, specific vocational rehabilitation services may be rendered to facilitate a return to work. Patients with less complete recovery may require long-term residential or institutional care, daily assistance and supervision by family and others at home, or assistance from personal care attendants. Again, the path through the system varies based on severity, levels of recovery and availability of resources (Peters and McLean, 1995).

Efficacy of rehabilitation after traumatic brain injury

- Process-specific rehabilitation strategies for patients with traumatic brain injury have largely been aimed at attention, memory and executive functions.
- Findings supporting a hierarchical programme for attention remediation have been mixed. There is little support for specific memory remediation but there has been success reported with memory compensatory strategies and the use of procedural learning strategies. There is modest support for the effectiveness of compensatory strategies for executive functions.
- Lasting improvements have been reported in patients receiving primarily functionally based cognitive rehabilitation, which may be a more direct, cost-effective form of treatment than process-specific cognitive rehabilitation.
- In reviewing studies of the overall effectiveness of cognitive rehabilitation, the preponderance of evidence indicates some benefit across the continuum of services. Most studies look at postacute rehabilitation populations in pretreatment versus posttreatment designs; there are a few controlled studies, none randomly assigned.
- No studies delineate the critical factors for treatment success. There is no apparent superiority of one method over another when compared.

Process-specific rehabilitation strategies

A complete discussion of the efficacy of specific strategies of cognitive rehabilitation is beyond the realm of this chapter (See Robertson, 1993, for a more complete review). There are very few well-designed studies of rehabilitation in patients with traumatic brain injury.

Process-specific cognitive rehabilitation for patients with traumatic brain injury usually targets three areas: attention, memory and executive function. Sohlberg and Mateer (1987) evaluated a hierarchical treatment programme designed to remediate attention. Using a single-subject, multiple-baseline design, they found improvement in attention in four patients that appeared to be specific to attentional processes and not to other cognitive functions (e.g. visual processing). The sample was small, and chronicity and aetiology varied. Another single-subject, multiple-baseline study of attention training failed to show any benefit beyond spontaneous recovery and practice effects using a computer training module (Ponsford and Kinsella, 1988). As previously cited, Novack and colleagues (1996) demonstrated no difference in posttreatment attention scores (digit span forwards and backwards, mental control, simple and choice reaction times) or functional measures (Functional Independence Measure scores) in a group of patients on an inpatient rehabilitation unit receiving focused attention training (Sohlberg and Mateer's method) compared to a matched control group receiving unstructured interventions. It remains uncertain whether specific attention training can improve any aspect of attention and, if attention is improved, whether it will remain improved and generalize to functioning outside the area of training or to the real world. The findings of the Sohlberg and Mateer study are compelling, and single-case design studies such as these can provide evidence for treatment effects without the necessity for large group studies that inevitably introduce heterogeneity. However, because the number of patients in this study is small and the patient group is heterogeneous, it is difficult to know how broadly applicable the findings are.

The case for specific process remediation for memory is less compelling. There is no convincing evidence that memory functioning can be improved by 'exercise' or practice. Compensatory strategies, especially those using memory aids, are helpful in improving function. Wilson (1992) followed up 26/29 patients who had been taught compensations five to ten years earlier and found that the majority was still using these strategies, and to a greater extent than at the time of rehabilitation.

Implicit memory strategies have been successful in traumatic brain injury patients with severe declarative memory deficits. Procedural learning is often preserved even when declarative memory is severity effected. Giles and Shore (1989) demonstrated successful learning of compensatory strategies for activities of daily living in a patient with very severe memory problems who had been unable to master basic activities of daily living after more than five months of therapy. The strategies included incorporation of as many premorbidly proceduralized routines as possible, combined with breakdown of new compensations into steps that were practised repeatedly. The patient learned and maintained independence in washing and dressing after just 12 sessions, probably because the strategies largely exploited procedural learning capacities. In an often-cited case report, Glisky and coworkers (1984) taught a brain-injured person with dense anterograde memory deficits to learn a complex new job task using an implicit memory system of 'vanishing cues' and procedural memory. The patient was able to perform the job successfully despite continuing severe memory loss. Although a good demonstration of the use of an implicit memory system to facilitate learning, this model is not applicable to most patients with traumatic brain injury because the patient had persistently severe declarative memory loss, more severe than typically observed in patients with severe traumatic brain injury. Furthermore, the labour intensity of such a procedure is not practical for most patients. Kime, Lamb and Wilson (1996) demonstrated the use of procedural memory in acquiring a compensatory strategy (use of datebook and calendar) in a patient with persistent dense amnesia after traumatic brain injury complicated by status epilepticus. The patient even generalized the strategy beyond the datebook and calendar to related tasks. This learning occurred despite very poor performance on standardized declarative memory evaluations.

Evidence regarding the training of executive functions is limited. Training of task specific routines is fairly well accepted; but this proceduralization of particular tasks, even complex tasks, is specific to the task and does not necessarily improve the execution of other related tasks. Attempts to train executive strategies have had some modest success. Von Cramon and Matthes-von Cramon (1990) trained problem-solving techniques and found improvement on psychometric evaluations and functional problem solving compared to controls. Cicerone and Wood (1987) trained a self-instructional strategy to solve a Tower of London type task and found some generalization to another problem-solving task, but only after further direct training in real-life situations.

Comparisons of specific strategies to treat motor problems have rarely been studied in patients with traumatic brain injury. A number of studies have compared different techniques in stroke patients (e.g. Bobath neurodevelopmental therapy, Rood approach, Brunnstrom movement therapy, Carr and Sheppard motor relearning, biofeedback, electrical stimulation, forced use). In general, no approach has stood out as better than any other. A few studies have shown some advantage of 'forced use' techniques (Russo, 1995), but these procedures are often quite disturbing to patients. Some techniques are more time consuming (e.g. neuro-developmental) than others, so economic pressures may guide treatment choices.

Functionally based treatment: skills training

Functionally based treatment was defined by Mateer as therapy carried out in a wholly functional context (Sohlberg and Mateer, 1989). This treatment method aims at improving performance on specific skills by directly training those skills in as natural a situation as possible. The skills might range from a specific activities of daily living task to a compensatory strategy (e.g. the use of a calendar book). Functionally based treatment may incorporate a number of specific treatment elements, such as: (1) procedural learning, (2) training in the use of memory aids and time planners, (3) repeated practice, (4) teaching subroutines of an activity and then chaining together the subroutines (such as

cooking), (5) patient education about brain injury, and (6) psychological support to patients and their families.

This method is widely used by rehabilitation clinicians, either combined with or exclusive of cognitive process training methods. Patients treated with primarily functionally based treatment have demonstrated lasting improvements in performance in the home, community, recreational activities, school and work settings, even years after their injury (Fryer and Haffey, 1987; Ruff and Neimann, 1990; Mills et al., 1992). As mentioned earlier, functionally based treatment is probably a more efficient and cost-effective method than process-specific rehabilitation because it aims directly at performance improvement in a real-life, functional activity. A theoretical downside of functionally based methods compared to cognitive process training is that improvement is skill specific and less generalizable than might be expected from improvement in cognitive processes. These conclusions are as yet tentative, deriving from the few studies that compare these methods (Ruff and Neimann, 1990; Mills et al., 1992). It is impossible adequately to tease out the effects of the specific treatment methods on patient improvement to show an advantage of one method over the other. In general, improvement is reported no matter which method is emphasized.

Overall effectiveness of traumatic brain injury rehabilitation along the treatment continuum

A number of studies have been reported using quasi-experimental designs (see Cope, 1995, for a more extensive review). These studies look at the overall, 'black box' effects of the particular rehabilitation programmes reported, and the critical, 'active' components cannot be specified. The studies use one of several methodologies: (1) comparison with historic controls; (2) before/after treatment, usually including a 'stable' group after the recovery plateau; (3) comparing groups receiving earlier versus later or higher versus lower intensity rehabilitation; and (4) comparison with matched controls (rare). Again, there are no prospective, randomly assigned controlled studies and certainly no blinded studies. The evidence is reviewed according to treatment setting.

Acute hospital/neurosurgical intensive care unit

It is clear at this early stage of treatment, as well as in the acute inpatient rehabilitation setting, that good medical, nursing and preventative care, such as range of motion and skin protection, are important rehabilitation measures. One has only to look at reports before these measures became the standard of care to understand the prevalence of complications resulting from the lack of such care. Rusk et al. (Rusk, Lowman and Block, 1966; Rusk, Block and Lowman, 1969) reported a high prevalence of frozen shoulders, decubiti, major joint deformities, contractures ('fixed in sitting'), and urinary tract infections among 127 traumatic brain injury patients who received limited rehabilitation treatments. One study looked at the effect of early rehabilitation efforts, including prevention, sensory stimulation, mobilization and family involvement, compared to a control group receiving treatment after a delay (MacKay et al., 1992). The study reported a shorter length of stay and greater home discharge for the early treatment group compared to controls. The results are difficult to interpret because the delayed treatment control group was much more severely injured than the early treatment group (coma 53.8 days versus 18.9 days for the experimental group).

Acute inpatient rehabilitation

Some studies report improvement in a functional measure but do not control for spontaneous improvement to substantiate the treatment effect. There are also group studies that compare outcome at different intensities of intervention or based on early versus late admission to rehabilitation. Two studies looked at differences in treatment intensities and claimed shorter rehabilitation hospitalization and better function for the group receiving more intense treatment; however, differences were not significant in one study (Blackerby, 1990) and injury severity was not well controlled in the other (Spivack et al., 1992). The evaluation of early versus late admission to rehabilitation in groups matched for severity by coma duration indicated a reduced length of stay and significantly better functioning at follow-up at least two years later for the group that received earlier intervention (Cope and Hall, 1982). Closer examination indicates some possibly important differences between the groups. The delayed treatment group had a greater incidence of comorbidities (surgeries, seizures, tracheostomies) and more frequent bilateral focal lesions (an unfavourable prognostic sign) than the earlier intervention group. One of the few studies with an untreated control group showed less dependency, better functioning, better vocational status and reduced overall cost for the treated group compared to the untreated controls (Aronow, 1987). The analysis was covaried for severity (by posttraumatic amnesia duration), but when all variables were considered, age and days in acute hospital predicted a greater amount of the variance of outcome than rehabilitation treatment. This points out that there is a multiplicity of factors that may contribute to outcome prediction and improvement. One must always consider these factors and their interaction when comparing different treatment groups, and the contribution of a particular treatment to a patient's improvement.

Postacute rehabilitation

Most efficacy studies have been performed on postacute populations, in whom some stability of biological recovery is assumed. All of the studies of postacute outpatient and residential rehabilitation involved preprogramme versus postprogramme measurement to demonstrate efficacy (Prigatano, et al., 1984; Scherzer, 1986; Ben-Yishay et al., 1987; Fryer and Haffey, 1987; Ruff and Neimann, 1990; Cope et al., 1991; Johnston, 1991; Johnston and Lewis, 1991; Rattok et al., 1992; Mills et al., 1992; Malec et al., 1993). All studies show improvement in one or another outcome measure. Three of the studies contrasted different treatment methods, including a general day treatment programme or a community re-entry model, versus formal cognitive rehabilitation (Fryer and Haffey, 1987; Ruff and Neimann, 1990). Rattok and coauthors compared three treatment mixes, variously emphasizing social skills versus cognitive remediation versus both. All of these studies found benefit no matter what method was used. Rattok claimed that the groups incorporating a balance of all treatment components did better than the group for which a component was withheld, but the results do not substantiate this claim.

There have been some studies using a comparison group of controls receiving no rehabilitation or an unspecified alternative treatment. Prigatano and colleagues (1984), using matched, untreated controls, showed that a group treated in a postacute programme with emphasis on psychological adjustment and awareness in addition to cognitive improvement had significant reductions in emotional distress and higher levels of employment (50 per cent versus vs. 36 per cent) than the untreated controls. The study was later replicated (Prigatano et al., 1994) with a larger sample of patients and again showed better rates of return to employment in the treated group versus controls (79 per cent versus 50 per cent). Despite these improvements, neuropsychological test measures did not significantly improve in the treated group compared to the controls. In addition to the positive effects of postacute rehabilitation, this study points out the possibility of functional gains in the absence of psychometric improvement.

Two programmes specifically for vocational and cognitive treatment demonstrated significant success (Wehman et al., 1990; Haffey and Abrams, 1991). Haffey and Abrams used a nontreated control group matched by severity (coma) and found 71 per cent employment in the treated group versus 40 per cent in controls.

In an extension of findings from a previously described postacute programme which emphasizes functionally based treatment over process-specific methods (Mills et al., 1992), outcomes were analysed of 147 patients with traumatic brain injury compared to a small control group. The control group comprised eight patients who had been assessed and accepted into the programme but were unable to receive treatment due to financial reasons. Both the treatment group and the control group had treatment goals formulated at the time of their initial assessment. The control group was a little older, better educated and less severely injured than the treatment group (Table 18.4). On follow-up interviews several months to a few years after their programme assessment, it was determined that the control group had only achieved 17 per cent of the targeted outcome goals, compared to a 76 per cent completion

Table 18.4 Comparison of treatment group and control group: postacute, functionally based treatment programme

	Treatment group	Nontreatment control group
Number of patients with traumatic brain injury	147	8
Gender	105 male, 42 female	7 male, 1 female
Mean age (years)	31.5	37
Mean education (years)	11.8	13.0
Median duration unconsciousness (days)	12	0.04
Median duration posttraumatic amnesia (weeks)	8	4.3
Median time postinjury (months)	23	11

rate for the treated group. In addition to further evidence for the efficacy of postacute cognitive rehabilitation, this study lends support to the assertion that functionally based treatment in the absence of specific cognitive process rehabilitation can lead to sustained improvement in real-world functioning.

In a meta-analysis of postacute cognitive rehabilitation compared to unspecified treatment (referred to as 'natural recovery'), Malec and Basford (1996) showed a general benefit of postacute traumatic brain injury cognitive rehabilitation increasing the chances of return to independent work, training or homemaking (56 per cent for those treated in postacute rehabilitation versus 43 per cent in unspecified or no treatment; $p < 0.001$). They concluded that more intensive programmes were even better (60–80 per cent return to work, training or homemaking). There was no consistent relationship of outcome predictors such as injury severity, chronicity, cognitive status, age, education or length of stay with success in postacute rehabilitation.

The preponderance of evidence appears to indicate some benefit of rehabilitation across the continuum of acute and postacute services. All studies have their weaknesses and as yet no randomized, controlled trials have been performed. The strongest arguments for the benefit of rehabilitation come from the few matched control studies and the postacute studies including patients at a relatively stable point in recovery. None of the studies can delineate the critical factors that may promote recovery; indeed, comparisons of different overall treatment approaches fail to indicate the superiority of any one method. As economic pressures and demands for evidence of efficacy increase, better studies using randomized controls, comparing different treatment approaches, different treatment settings or treatment at different times postinjury will be needed.

Recommendations: rehabilitation planning in the context of the natural history of traumatic brain injury

- Rehabilitation planning in the context of natural history should recognize the pattern and time course of natural recovery after traumatic brain injury, the problems that define and limit each stage of recovery, as well as the most effective learning strategies (e.g. declarative versus procedural) at different stages.
- Planning and goal setting should also consider that some problems recover without treatment and some problems will not recover with any treatment.
- Deviations from expected natural history should trigger a search for reversible complications of recovery.
- In the earliest stages of recovery, when arousal is the limiting problem, the maintenance of optimum health and preventing early complications should be the primary rehabilitation focus. In the confusional stage, when attention and anterograde amnesia are main constraints, managing confusion as safely and easily as possible is the primary goal.
- In later stages of recovery, cognitive rehabilitation goals should focus on proceduralizing and reproceduralizing the tasks of everyday life, including social skills, and moving to more complex daily activities and decision making as appropriate.
- Emphasis should always be on improving people's functioning in real-world activities and in areas that are personally relevant to the needs, capabilities and constraints of their environment.

Several principles should be considered in applying cognitive rehabilitation within the context of the natural history of traumatic brain injury. First, as discussed above, the rehabilitation should recognize the obligatory pattern and time course of recovery, especially of the early stages of recovery. Second, rehabilitation planning should recognize the problems that define each stage of recovery to develop appropriate strategies and targets of management. A corollary of this is that different modes of learning (e.g. procedural versus declarative) are more or less effective at different stages of recovery. Third, rehabilitation planning should appreciate that some problems recover without direct treatment (e.g. confusion), and some problems with a poor neurological prognosis will not recover with any treatment. Finally, deviations from expected natural history should suggest a search for treatable problems that may be disrupting recovery (e.g. hydrocephalus, depression, substance abuse).

Table 18.5 summarizes cognitive treatment strategies and their possible effectiveness at different stages of recovery. During coma and vegetative state, treatments aimed at improving arousal include sensory stimulation programmes and the use of pharmacological stimulants and dopamine agonists. Neither has been clearly shown to alter the course of unconsciousness, though enhancement in arousal is typically observed. In a small pilot study, four patients receiving an organized sensory stimulation protocol showed higher cognitive functioning and shorter length of stay compared to four retrospectively matched controls (Wood et al., 1992). The sample was too small to be conclusive and patients were not randomly assigned. The main goals of rehabilitation at this stage are assuring optimum health, nutrition, medical and nursing care and preventing complications that will make later interventions more difficult. Emphases include range of motion and tone management, avoiding pressure sores and preventing aspiration. The evidence supporting this form of rehabilitation is relatively uncontroversial. The case for early rehabilitation efforts directed at accelerating the return of conscious behaviour is much weaker and there is little support for elaborate sensory stimulation programmes.

At the minimally conscious and confusional state stages, the main rehabilitation strategies should be managing confusion, largely through manipulation of

Table 18.5 Cognitive rehabilitation strategies at different stages of recovery after traumatic brain injury

Description	Cognitive problems	Treatment strategies	Effective?
Coma/vegetative state			
Unawareness, eyes closed/	arousal, consciousness	Sensory stimulation	Unlikely
unawareness, sleep–wake cycles		Pharmacological (stimulants)	Possibly
Minimally conscious state/confusional state			
Purposeful wakefulness,	Focused and sustained	Environmental and symptom management	Yes
follows commands (agitated or	attention, amnesia	Declarative learning	No
hypoaroused)	(posttraumatic amnesia)	Procedural learning	Yes
		Restorative techniques	Unlikely
		Pharmacological	Possibly
Postconfusion/social competence			
Resolution of posttraumatic	Divided attention, difficult	Declarative learning	Yes
amnesia and basic attention/	memory tasks, executive	Procedural learning (complex skills)	Yes
recovering higher cognitive	functions	Structure and compensation	Yes
and social abilities		Restorative techniques	Possibly

the environment. Recognizing that confusion will evolve on its own and that treatment cannot make somebody 'unconfused', the goal should be to enable patients to pass through the stage of confusion as safely and easily as possible.

Pharmacological strategies are yet to be proven. There is some evidence that dopamine agonists and stimulants can help focus attention and improve behaviour, but there is no evidence that they change the time course of confusion (Chandler, Barnhill and Gualtieri, 1988; Gualtieri and Evans, 1990). One double blind study of methylphenidate failed to show effects in a more chronic group of patients (Speech et al., 1993; Table 18.6).

Because dense anterograde memory deficits characterize these stages, strategies that depend on declarative learning are ineffective. Although patients in confusional states cannot recall episodic information or explicitly learn recently presented information, there is evidence that procedural learning can occur. Ewart and coworkers (1989) demonstrated that procedural memory was preserved during posttraumatic amnesia. They found that patients could learn to mirror read and improve rotary pursuit motor performance even though they had no explicit recall of words read or performing the tasks. This preserved capacity can be exploited to teach patients skills and procedures despite severely impaired declarative memory. Patients can learn, for instance, compensatory strategies for transfers though they have no explicit knowledge of the steps of the task.

In summary, rehabilitation during confusion should consist of: (1) regulating the patient's environment to assure appropriate levels of stimulation; (2) resetting sleep/wake cycles; (3) adjusting the timing and duration of interactions to the patient's attention span; (4) assuring patient, family and staff safety; (5) removing environmental triggers of agitation; (6) exploiting preserved procedural memory capacity; (7) using familiar objects and routines; (8) using medications, (e.g. sedatives, tranquillizers) judiciously; and (9) recognizing and treating secondary and iatrogenic problems. Treatment during this epoch should occur in an acute rehabilitation setting with staff with the experience and expertise to manage these cognitive and behaviour problems. The need for a safe, protective environment is reason enough to justify this level of rehabilitation, although evidence for direct effects of rehabilitation on the rate of recovery is lacking.

During the postconfusional/residual recovery stages, declarative memory strategies are once again effective, together with procedural strategies, although new

Table 18.6 Pharmacology and traumatic brain injury rehabilitation

Indication	Medication class	Evidence
Arousal/attention/ initiation	Stimulants	Multiple case reports/series improved arousal, attention and intention
	Dopamine agonist	Double-blind, controlled study measles encephalitis showed benefit L-dopa
	Tricyclics	Two double-blind studies of methylphenidate, equivocal neuropsychological
	SSRIs	improvement
Memory	Cholinergic physostigmine	Three double-blind studies (physostigmine), two equivocal improvement (attention better), one showed benefit
	tacrine	One double-blind study of methylphenidate and amphetamine had benefit
	Stimulants	
	Tricyclics	
	Dopamine agonists	

Notes:
SSRIs, selective serotonin reuptake inhibitors.

learning may remain inefficient. Goals should be centred around the tasks of everyday life. Patients should first develop a routine for basic self-care activities and then learn or relearn the schemas and contingencies of increasingly complex daily activities and decision making. They may need to be trained to use new compensatory strategies such as memory aids or to reproceduralize premorbid capacities such as social skills. Even the small proportion of patients who have dense amnesia persisting in the postconfusional phase of recovery can benefit from procedural learning of compensatory strategies to enhance functional independence (Glisky et al., 1984; Kime et al., 1996). Learning and improvement in one or another schema or skill are probably specific to that activity and do not generalize well to other skills. This rehabilitation is best performed in as close to a real-world context as possible. Interventions aimed at compensating for degraded executive functions include: environmental modifications to provide cues and structure; training task-specific routines; the use of external compensatory systems; and behavioural modification, pragmatic and social skills training (see Sohlberg, Mateer and Stuss, 1993, for a complete discussion of these approaches). Psychological and social supports are extremely important at these stages. Special interventions may be needed to treat depression or promote awareness and adjustment to a new level of functioning.

Treatment at these stages should begin at the tran-sition from acute inpatient rehabilitation to outpatient or residential postacute services. The later stages may occur in more specialized community re-entry and vocational programmes. Again, the evidence for the efficacy of these re-entry programmes is not conclusive, but highly suggestive. The issue of what treatment methods or strategies work best is not at all conclusive; there can be no specific guidelines at this point. Present evidence indicates that different methods are successful and the critical elements or advantage of one over another have yet to be determined. It is clear, however, that some methods are more labour intensive and costly than others. In general, functionally based treatments are more direct and practical than programmes that include elaborate, process-oriented cognitive rehabilitation. In any case, rehabilitation should ultimately be personally relevant to the immediate needs and capabilities of the patients and their families and to the constraints of the patients' environment.

Conclusions

This chapter attempts to highlight the interaction of natural history and therapy interventions in the recovery of patients with traumatic brain injury. It notes that the relative influence of biological, learning and environmental factors probably changes over time in that the influence of biological factors predominates in the early stages of recovery and lessens in later stages.

Learning and experience can have physiological effects, but the specific effects on plasticity and neural reorganization are not certain.

The chapter presents systems of diagnosis and prognosis that help in the understanding and prediction of the process of recovery in individual patients. It emphasizes the themes that the effectiveness of some forms of cognitive rehabilitation may differ at various stages of recovery and that understanding where a patient is in the natural process of recovery should help in the selection of appropriate and effective treatment targets and strategies for that stage. Rehabilitation strategies and goals should respect natural recovery and prognosis, and be consistent with problems and capacities at different stages of recovery. Rehabilitation planning should recognize that problems may evolve without any specific intervention or may not recover even with intervention.

In reviewing the evidence for the efficacy of cognitive rehabilitation, the preponderance of class III and a more limited amount of class II evidence probably does not provide enough clinical certainty in most areas to support extensive guidelines for cognitive rehabilitation. Overall, the research evidence does support that at least some efforts at cognitive rehabilitation are effective in promoting functional recovery. The critical elements and critical periods for effectiveness are not known. Some methods appear more effective than others. Some methods are probably more direct, practical and economic than others (e.g. functionally based treatment). However, cognitive rehabilitation should aim at goals that are personally relevant to the patient's immediate needs, capabilities and environmental constraints.

References

Adams, J.H., Graham, D.I., Gennarelli, T.A. and Maxwell, W.L. 1991. Diffuse axonal injury in non-missile head injury. *J Neurol Neurosurg Psychiatry* **54**, 481–3.

Adams, J.H., Graham, D.I., Murray, L.S. and Scott, G. 1982. Diffuse axonal injury due to nonmissile head injury in humans: an analysis of 45 cases. *Ann Neurol* **12**, 557–63.

Alexander, M.P. 1982. Traumatic brain injury. In *Psychiatric Aspects of Neurological Disease*, ed. D.F. Benson and D. Blumer, pp. 251–78. New York: Grune and Stratton.

Almli, C. and Finger, S. 1988. Brain injury and recovery: theoretical and controversial issues. In *Toward a Definition of Recovery of Function*, ed. S. Finger, T. LeVere, C. Almli and D. Stein. New York: Plenum Press.

Aronow, H.U. 1987. Rehabilitation effectiveness with severe brain injury: translating research into policy. *J Head Trauma Rehabil* **2**, 24–36.

Bach-y-Rita, P. 1992. Recovery from brain damage. *J Neurol Rehabil* **6**, 191–9.

Bach-y-Rita, P. and Wicab Bach-y-Rita, E. 1990. Biological and psychosocial factors in recovery from brain damage in humans. *Can J Psychol* **44**, 148–65.

Ben-Yishay, Y. and Diller, L. 1993. Cognitive remediation in traumatic brain injury: update and issues. *Arch Phys Med Rehabil* **74**, 204–13.

Ben-Yishay, Y., Silver, S.M., Piasetsky, E. et al. 1987. Relationship between employability and vocational outcome after intensive holistic cognitive rehabilitation. *J Head Trauma Rehabil* **2**, 35–48.

Berrol, S. 1990. Issues in cognitive rehabilitation. *Arch Neurol* **47**, 219–20.

Blackerby, W.F. 1990. Intensity of rehabilitation and length of stay. *Brain Inj* **4**, 167–73.

Brooks, C.A., Lindstrom, J., McCray, J. and Whiteneck, G.G. 1995. Cost of medical care for a population-based sample of persons surviving traumatic brain injury. *J Head Trauma Rehabil* **10**, 1–13.

Chandler, M.C., Barnhill, J.L. and Gualtieri, C.T. 1988. Amantadine for the agitated head injury patient. *Brain In* **2**, 309–11.

Cicerone, K.D. and Wood, J.C. 1987. Planning disorder after closed head injury. *Arch Phys Med Rehabil* **68**, 111–15.

Clasen, R.A. and Penn, R.D. 1987. Traumatic brain swelling and edema. In *Head Injury*, ed. P.R. Cooper, pp. 285–312. Baltimore: Williams & Wilkins.

Cope, D.N. 1995. The effectiveness of traumatic brain injury rehabilitation: a review. *Brain Inj* **9**, 649–70.

Cope, D.N., Cole, J.R., Hall, K.M. et al. 1991. Brain injury: analysis of outcomes in a post-acute rehabilitation system. Part 1: General analysis. *Brain Inj* **5**, 111–25.

Cope, D.N. and Hall, K. 1982. Head injury rehabilitation: benefit of early intervention. *Arch Phys Med Rehabil* **63**, 433–7.

Cope. D.N. and O'Lear, J. 1993. A clinical and economic perspective on head injury rehabilitation. *J Head Trauma Rehabil* **8**, 1–14.

Dixon, C.I., Taft, W.C. and Hayes, R.L. 1993. Mechanism of mild traumatic brain injury. *J Head Trauma Rehabil* **8**, 1–12.

Ewart, J., Levin, H.S., Watson, M.G. and Kalisky, Z. 1989. Procedural memory during post-traumatic amnesia in survivors of closed head injury: implications for rehabilitation. *Arch Neurol* **46**, 911–16.

Fryer, L.J. and Haffey, W.J. 1987. Cognitive rehabilitation and community readaptation: outcomes from two model programs. *J Head Trauma Rehabil* **2**, 51–63.

Gennarelli, T.A., Spielman, G.M., Langfitt, T.W. et al. 1982. Influence of type of intracranial lesion on outcome from severe head injury. *J Neurosurg* **56**, 26–32.

Giacino, J.T. 1996. Sensory stimulation: theoretical perspectives and the evidence for effectiveness. *NeuroRehabil* **6**, 69–78.

Giles, G.M. and Shore, M. 1989. A rapid method for teaching severely brain-injured adults how to wash and dress. *Arch Phys Med Rehabil* **70**, 156–8.

Glisky, E.L., Schacter, D.L. and Tulving, E. 1984. Computer learning by memory-impaired patients: acquisition and retention of complex knowledge. *Neuropsychologia* **24**, 313–28.

Graham, D.I., Adams, J.H. and Doyle, D. 1979. Ischemic brain damage in fatal nonmissile head injuries. *J Neurosci* **39**, 213–34.

Gualtieri, C.T. and Evans, R.W. 1990. Stimulant treatment for the neurobehavioral sequelae of traumatic brain injury. *Brain Inj* **4**, 339–47.

Haffey, W.J. and Abrams, D.L. 1991. Employment outcomes for participants in a brain injury work reentry program: preliminary findings. *J Head Trauma Rehabil* **6**, 24–34.

Hagen, C., Malkmus, D. and Durham, P. 1972. *Levels of Cognitive Functioning.* Downey, CA: Ranchos Los Amigos Hospital.

Hall, K.M., Hamilton, B.B., Gordon, W.A. and Zasler, N.D. 1993. Characteristics and comparisons of functional assessment indices: Disability Rating Scale, Functional Independence Measure and Functional Assessment Measure. *J Head Trauma Rehabil* **8**, 60–74.

Hayes, R.L., Jenkins, L.W. and Lyeth, B.G. 1992. Neurochemical aspects of head injury: role of excitatory neurotransmission. *J Head Trauma Rehabil* **7**, 16–28.

Hayes, R.L., Stonnington, H.H., Lyeth, B.G., Dixon, C.F. and Yamamoto, T. 1986. Metabolic and neurophysiologic sequelae of brain injury: a cholinergic hypothesis. *J Cent Nerv Sys Trauma* **3**, 163–73.

Institute of Medicine 1992. *Committee on Clinical Practice Guidelines: Guidelines for Clinical Practice: from Development to Use,* ed. M.J. Field and K.N. Lohr. Washington, DC: National Academy Press.

Jennett, B. and Teasdale, G. 1981. *Management of Head Injuries.* Philadelphia: F.A. Davis.

Johnston, M.V. 1991. Outcomes of community re-entry programmes for brain injury survivors. Part 2: Further investigations. *Brain Inj* **5**, 155–68.

Johnston, M.V. and Lewis, F.D. 1991. Outcomes of community re-entry programmes for brain injury survivors. Parts 1: Independent living and productive activities. *Brain Inj* **5**, 141–54.

Katz, D.I. 1992. Neuropathology and neurobehavioral recovery from closed head injury. *J Head Trauma Rehabil* **7**, 1–15.

Katz, D.I. 1997. Traumatic brain injury. In *Neurologic Rehabilitation: a Guide to Diagnosis, Prognosis and Treatment Planning,* ed. V.M. Mills, J.W. Cassidy and D.I. Katz, pp. 105-43. Cambridge: Blackwell Science Publishers.

Katz, D.I. and Alexander, M.P. 1994a. Predicting outcome and course of recovery in patients admitted to rehabilitation. *Arch Neurol* **51**, 661–70.

Katz, D.I. and Alexander, M.P. 1994b. Traumatic brain injury. In *The Handbook of Neurorehabilitation,* ed. J.R. Couch and D.C. Good, pp. 493–549. New York: Marcel Dekker.

Katz, D.I., Alexander, M.P., Seliger, G.M. and Bellas, D.N. 1989. Traumatic basal ganglia hemorrhage: clinicopathologic features and outcome. *Neurology* **39**, 897–904.

Kime, S.K., Lamb, D.G. and Wilson, B.A. 1996. Use of a comprehensive programme of external cueing to enhance procedural memory in a patient with dense amnesia. *Brain Inj* **10**, 17–26.

Kolb, B. and Gibb, R. 1991. Environmental enrichment and cortical injury: behavioral and anatomical consequences of frontal cortex lesions. *Cereb Cortex* **1**, 189–98.

Kolb, B. and Gibb, R. 1993. Possible anatomic basis of recovery of function after neonatal frontal lesions in rats. *Behav Neurol* **107**, 799–811.

Levin, H.S. 1990. Cognitive rehabilitation, unproven but promising. *Arch Neurol* **47**, 223–4.

Levin, H.S., Gary, H.E. and Eisenberg, H.M. 1990. Neurobehavioral outcome one year after severe head injury: experience of the traumatic coma databank. *J Neurosurg* **73**, 699–709.

Lobato, R.D., Cordobes, F., Rivas, J.J. et al. 1983. Outcome from severe head injury related to the type of intracranial lesion: a computerized tomography study. *J Neurosurg* **59**, 762–74.

MacKay, L.E., Bernstein, B.A., Chapman, P.E. et al. 1992. Early intervention in severe head injury: long-term benefits of a formalized program. *Arch Phy Med Rehabil* **73**, 635–41.

Malec, J.F. and Basford, J.S. 1996. Postacute brain injury rehabilitation. *Arch Phys Med Rehabil* **77**, 198–207.

Malec, J.F., Smigielski, J.S., DePompolo, R.W. et al. 1993. Outcome evaluation and prediction in a comprehensive-integrated post-acute outpatient brain injury rehabilitation programme. *Brain Inj* **7**, 15–29.

Marshall, L.F., Gautille, T., Klauber, M.R. et al. 1991a. The outcome of severe closed head injury. *Neurosurgery* **75** (Suppl.), 28–36.

Marshall, L.F., Marshall, S.B., Klauber, M.R. et al. 1991b. A new classification of head injury based on computer tomography. *Neurosurgery* **75** (Suppl.), 14–17.

Max, W., MacKenzie, E.J. and Rice, D.P. 1991. Head injuries: costs and consequences. *J Head Trauma Rehabil* **6**, 76–91.

McLean, A., Dikmen, S.S. and Temkin, N.R. 1993. Psychosocial recovery after head injury. *Arch Phys Med Rehabil* **74**, 1041–6.

Mills, V.M., Cassidy, J.W. and Katz, D.I., eds. 1997. *Neurologic Rehabilitation: a Guide to Diagnosis, Prognosis and Treatment Planning.* Cambridge: Blackwell Science.

Mills, V.M., Nesbeda, T., Katz, D.I. et al. 1992. Outcomes for traumatically brain-injured patients following post-acute rehabilitation programmes. *Brain Inj* **6**, 219–28.

Mitchell, S., Bradley, V.A., Welch, J.L. et al. 1990. Coma arousal procedure: a therapeutic intervention in the treatment of head injury. *Brain Inj* **3**, 273–9.

Narayan, R.K., Greenberg, R.P., Miller, J.D. et al. 1981. Improved confidence of outcome prediction in severe head injury. *J Neurosurg* **54**, 751–62.

Novack, T.A., Caldwell, S.G., Duke, L.W., Bergquist, T.F. and Gage, R.J. 1996. Focused versus unstructured intervention for attention deficits after traumatic brain injury. *J Head Trauma Rehabil* **11**, 52–60.

Ommaya, A.K. and Gennarelli, T.A. 1974. Cerebral concussion and traumatic unconsciousness: correlations of experimental and clinical observations on blunt head injuries. *Brain* **97**, 633–54.

Peters, M.D. and McLean, A. 1995. The evolution of the clinical–scientific model of neurologic rehabilitation. *Brain Inj* **9**, 543–52.

Plum, F. and Posner, J.B. 1980. *The Diagnosis of Stupor and Coma.* Philadelphia: F.A. Davis.

Ponsford, J.L. and Kinsella, G. 1988. Evaluation of a remedial programme for attentional deficits following closed head injury. *J Clin Exp Neuropsychol* **10**, 693–708.

Povlishock, J. 1985. The morphopathologic responses to experimental head injuries of varying severity. In *Central Nervous System Status Report*, ed. D. Beck and J. Povlishock, pp. 443–52. Richmond, VA: Byrd Press.

Prigatano, G. 1986. *Neuropsychological Rehabilitation.* Baltimore, MD: Johns Hopkins University Press.

Prigatano, G.P., Fordyce, D.J., Zeiner, H.K. et al. 1984. Neuropsychological rehabilitation after closed head injury in young adults. *J Neurol Neurosurg Psychiatry* **47**, 505–13.

Prigatano, G.P., Klonoff, P.S., O'Brien, K.P. et al. 1994. Productivity after neuropsychologically oriented milieu rehabilitation. *J Head Trauma Rehabil* **9**, 91–102.

Rattok, J., Ben-Yishay, Y., Ezrachi, O. et al. 1992. Outcome of different treatment mixes in a multidimensional neuropsychological rehabilitation program. *Neuropsychology* **6**, 395–415.

Robertson, I.H. 1993. Cognitive rehabilitation in neurologic disease. *Curr Opin Neurol* **6**, 756–60.

Ruff, R.M. and Neimann, H. 1990. Cognitive rehabilitation versus day treatment in head-injured adults: is there an impact on emotional and psychosocial adjustment? *Brain Inj* **4**, 339–47.

Rusk, H.A., Block, J.M. and Lowman, E.W. 1969. Rehabilitation following traumatic brain damage. *Med Clin N Am* **53**, 677–84.

Rusk, H.A., Lowman, E.W. and Block, J.M. 1966. Rehabilitation for the patient with head injuries. *Clin Neurosurg* **12**, 312–23.

Russo, S.G. 1995. Hemiplegic upper extremity rehabilitation: a review of the forced-use paradym. *Neurol Rep* **19**, 17–22.

Scherzer, B.P. 1986. Rehabilitation following severe head trauma. Results of a three-year program. *Arch Phys Med Rehabil* **67**, 366–74.

Sohlberg, M.M. and Mateer, C.A. 1987. Effectiveness of attention training program. *J Clin Exp Neuropsychol* **9**, 117–30.

Sohlberg, M.M. and Mateer, C.A. 1989. *Introduction to Cognitive Rehabilitation: Theory and Practice.* New York: Guilford Press.

Sohlberg, M.M., Mateer, C.A. and Stuss, D.T. 1993. Contemporary approaches to the management of executive control dysfunction. *J Head Trauma Rehabil* **8**, 45–58.

Speech, T.J., Rao, S.M., Osmon, D.C. and Sperry, L.T. 1993. A double-blind controlled study of methylphenidate treatment in closed head injury. *Brain Inj* **7**, 333–8.

Spivack, G., Spettle, C.M., Ellis, D.W. et al. 1992. Effects of intensity of treatment and lengths of stay on rehabilitation outcomes. *Brain Inj* **6**, 419–34.

Volpe, B.T. and McDowell, F.H. 1990. The efficacy of cognitive rehabilitation in patients with traumatic brain injury. *Arch Neurol* **47**, 220–2.

von Cramon, D.Y. and Matthes-von Cramon, G. 1990. Frontal lobe dysfunction in patients – theoretical approaches. In *Cognitive Rehabilitation in Perspective*, ed. R.L. Wood and I. Fussey, pp. 164–79. London: Taylor & Francis.

Wehman, P.H., Kreuizer, J.S., West, M.D. et al. 1990. Return to work for persons with traumatic brain injury: a supported employment approach. *Arch Phys Med Rehabil* **71**, 1047–52.

Wilson, B. 1992. Recovery and compensatory strategies in head injured memory impaired people several years after insult. *J Neurol Neursurg Psychiatry* **55**, 177–80.

Wood, R.L., Winkowski, T.B., Miller, J.L. et al. 1992. Evaluating sensory regulation as a method to improve awareness in patients with altered states of consciousness: a pilot study. *Brain Inj* **6**, 411–18.

19

The rehabilitation of attention

Ian H. Robertson

Introduction

- Adequate attention is critical for many types of learning.
- Learning underpins much recovery after brain damage.
- Attention consists of a number of different subsystems, including those for selective, sustained and spatial attention.

Just as learning is likely to be a central mechanism in the recovery of function following stroke, so attention is the prerequisite for adequate learning (Moscovitch, 1994). Recent evidence shows that separable attentional circuits for sustained attention, selective attention and spatial orientation exist in the brain (Posner and Peterson, 1990), with specialized function and distinct neuroanatomical organization, including a strong right hemisphere specialization for sustained attention. It is likely that the abilities endogenously to select, sustain and orient attention are critical in the process of learning underlying the recovery of motor and other functions following brain damage (Robertson, 1999, in press), and, indeed, there is evidence to suggest that sustained attention capacity predicts recovery of function over time following stroke (Ben-Yishay et al., 1968; Blanc-Garin, 1994; Robertson et al., 1997c).

Put simply, if a brain-injured patient cannot deploy attention in a selective, sustained or spatially appropriate way, then he or she will not be able to attend to the relevant external and internal stimuli sufficiently to relearn cognitive, motor, perceptual and other skills. Previous studies have shown that lateralized spatial attention (spatial neglect) predicts the recovery of func-

tion following stroke (Denes et al., 1982; Fullerton, McSherry and Stout, 1986). Furthermore, a number of studies have shown that apparently primary sensory and motor problems are actually attributable to attentional factors. For instance, one study (Sterzi et al., 1993) found that the incidence of apparently primary deficits in visual, tactile, proprioceptive and motor functions is higher in patients who have suffered right hemisphere strokes compared to carefully matched patients with equivalent left hemisphere damage. A recent positron emission tomography study of normals demonstrated that blood flow to the primary sensory cortex can be modified by attentional/expectancy variables, such that it decreases in those somatic areas where stimulation is not expected (Drevets et al., 1995). This gives support to the view that attention can have a major role in influencing the function of primary sensory and motor circuits, and therefore in recovering function within these circuits following brain lesion. Attentional deficits have also been identified as a factor mediating poor awareness of output in jargon aphasia (Shuren et al., 1995).

Attentional deficits following brain damage or disease are, of course, also important in themselves in terms of the direct effects they can have on contemporary behaviour, and not just in terms of their effects on long-term learning. Following traumatic brain injury, for instance, reports by relatives emphasize difficulties in concentration (McKinlay, 1981) and, indeed, neuropsychologically measured attentional impairment predicts return to work after head injury (Brooks and McKinlay, 1987). Furthermore, certain performance measures of attention have been shown to predict everyday attentional failures and absent-mindedness in both normals and traumatic brain-injured subjects (Robertson et al., 1997a). The spatial attentional deficits following unilateral neglect are also manifestly disabling in themselves, even setting aside any effects they have on long-term motor and other recovery (Sea, Henderson and Cermack, 1993).

There is also compelling evidence that different attentional systems may interact in important ways, and this can have important rehabilitation implications. For instance positron emission tomography scan evidence suggests that the right hemisphere alertness system may have a reciprocal relationship with the putatively anterior cingulate-based selection system (Cohen et al., 1988). To give another example, there may be strong facilitatory relationships between the right hemisphere alertness system on the one hand, and the posterior spatial orientation system on the other, as predicted by Posner (1993) and as demonstrated empirically by Robertson and colleagues (1995, 1998b). The nature of these interactions may have an important bearing on the rehabilitation of attention, as will become obvious later in this chapter.

A comment on the relationship between attentional and executive processes is also required at this juncture (see Chapter 20 for a discussion of the rehabilitation of executive functions). Both types of process are to a considerable extent frontally based, and the terms are sometimes used interchangeably: indeed, one of the key current goals of cognitive science is to create a satisfactory theoretical rubric within which both types of phenomena can be accommodated (Stuss et al., 1995).

In practical terms, however, rehabilitation studies of attention and executive functions have fallen into two reasonably distinct camps, with three main dimensions of difference, namely time course, complexity and structure. With respect to time course, attentional rehabilitation has usually, but not always, used time-constrained, usually computerized paradigms; whereas executive function retraining (for example von Cramon, von Cramon and Mai, 1991; von Cramon and von Cramon, 1992) has usually used nontime-constrained paradigms. Regarding complexity, attentional training has usually focused on relatively simple tasks; while executive programmes have focused on more complex tasks

such as problem solving. Finally, regarding structure, attentional training has involved a large amount of external structure and a relatively low demand for initiative in doing the tasks; whereas executive training has typically used tasks requiring the subject to impose structure on ambiguous situations and to choose and self-initiate various behavioural and cognitive routines. It is likely that these distinctions are somewhat superficial and a coherent theory will amalgamate these two types of paradigm; for the time being, however, pragmatism constrains us to examine these two literatures independently.

Rehabilitation of attentional deficits

- Nonspecific attentional training has yielded very mixed results; generalization to everyday life functions has not been demonstrated.
- Training of sustained attention appears to be possible; generalization to everyday life functions has been demonstrated in one study.
- Sustained attention training has, however, been shown to generalize in a theoretically predictable way to unilateral left inattention.

Given the important direct and indirect detrimental effects on behaviour of attentional deficits identified above, it is clear that the rehabilitation of such deficits should be a priority. But is it, in fact, possible to rehabilitate attention? Before answering this question, it should be pointed out that most published studies on the rehabilitation of attention have been carried out largely in a theoretical vacuum, i.e. without clarifying which aspect of attention they are targeting. Relatively few studies have targeted specific subtypes of attention, a notable exception being studies aimed at unilateral inattention, in which the spatial deficit predominates. Studies evaluating (a) nonspecific attentional deficits, (b) specific subtypes of nonlateralized attention, and (c) spatial inattention are therefore dealt with in turn. The question as to whether the rehabilitation of attentional deficits is possible is then returned to.

Nonspecific rehabilitation of attention

Attentional training is to a large extent the child of the personal, desktop computer. The capacity of computers to present precisely timed stimuli and measure response times accurately has led researchers to ask the question as to whether providing attentionally demanding exercises on computer can provoke improvements in attentional function. Hence, most of the studies in this section concern attempts at computerized attentional rehabilitation.

One of the earliest published studies (Malec et al., 1984) looked at the effect of videogame attentional training. It compared the performance of ten head-injured patients a mean of 80 days postinjury using a randomized, double-crossover study design. The subjects were randomly assigned to four weeks following the ABAB or BABA patterns (A = one week of videogame training; B = one week of no training), being assessed on a number of tests of attention at the end of each of the four weeks. Whereas substantial improvements on attentional tests were found over the four weeks, there was no significant difference after training versus non-training weeks, leading to the conclusion that the observed improvements had nothing to do with the training given. This well-conducted study illustrates well the pitfalls of relying on simple before–after data, as occurs in several early studies not reviewed in this chapter.

Ponsford and Kinsella (1988) carried out a series of single-case studies using a rigorous methodology which stands in sharp contrast to the majority of very weak studies in the computer-rehabilitation literature. Ten severely head-injured patients (aged 17–38 years; 6 to 34 weeks postinjury) were exposed to a no-training condition, a computerized attentional training condition, a condition of the latter plus therapist feedback and reinforcement, and a return to baseline condition in the context of a multiple-baseline-by-subjects design, with two baseline lengths, three and six weeks respectively. In addition, a matched control group of nonhead-injured orthopaedic cases was assessed on the test variables.

Training included simple reaction-time training, a visual search/matching task, choice/go–no go reaction time, vigilance ('spot the (target) letter' of a series of random letters appearing on the screen), and a number-detection task ('spot the numbers which are either even or a multiple of five'). Tests given over the

various training and baseline phases were a four-choice reaction-time task, a symbol–digit modalities test, and a letter-cancellation test. In addition, a similarities subtest of a version of the Wechsler Adult Intelligence Scale (WAIS) was given at the end of each phase of training. Finally, a rating scale was given by occupational therapists of the patient's attentional behaviour in day-to-day activities, as well as a video of performance on a clerical task which was assessed at the beginning and end of each phase.

Though there were steady improvements in time on performance of these measures for the ten subjects, this improvement bore no significant relationship to the training offered, as assessed by (group) analyses of variance using regression analysis-determined slopes of lines within each phase as the dependent variable. Interrupted time–series analysis of each individual case yielded similarly negative results. In conclusion, this study found no training effects of computerized attentional training.

Sohlberg and Mateer (1987) carried out four single-case studies with two closed head-injury patients, one open head-injury case, and one person who had suffered an aneurysm. The studies ranged from 12 to 72 months postonset of injury. The authors used as their treatment computer-based procedures including simple reaction time, choice reaction time, 'alternating attention' tasks, which included arithmetical exercises, and divided attention tasks.

A multiple-baseline-by-function design was used in the study. The measure of attention used was the Paced Auditory Serial Addition Test (PASAT) and a test of spatial relations was used as the measure of visual information processing. A baseline measure on these two measures was obtained on between one and three occasions. Attention training was implemented first with three cases, and between two and three measures of PASAT were taken. The trainees received seven to nine sessions of attentional training per week for between four and eight weeks. It was over this period that the two to three measures of attention and of visual functioning were taken. All subjects showed an increase in PASAT scores from baseline to training phase, and it is interesting to note that the fourth person, who received visual processing training first, also showed an increase in

PASAT performance in the absence of attentional training. Thus, the possibility arises that the improvements in the other cases were due to practice effects in the PASAT. In the latter case, however, further improvements in PASAT were noted following the onset of attentional training. The fact that improvements in visual functioning were only noted in one case in association with attentional training argues for a specific training effect, but it may simply represent a greater susceptibility to practice effects of one test over the other.

This study represented a good attempt at a well-controlled, multiple-baseline study, but suffered from having over-short baselines, thus preventing the 'ironing-out' of practice effects, or at least allowing a stable phase to be achieved. The reliance on just one test of attention was also problematic, particularly when the test is one in which practice effects are found in clinical observation. Nevertheless, in one of the cases, a dramatic improvement in PASAT followed the instigation of training, and this was arguably too great to be attributed to a practice effect. Thus, this study suggests that attentional training may have positive effects, at least in the short term, though there is no evidence that these effects in any way affect either the real-life functioning of patients or their performance on other types of psychological tests.

Sturm et al. (1983) matched two groups each of 15 mixed head-injured and stroke patients, testing them on a comprehensive neuropsychological battery of 16 tests at intake, at four weeks and then at eight weeks. The first group received 14 training sessions of mean length 15 minutes for the first four weeks, and nothing for the second four weeks. The reverse was true for the second group. Test scores were compared in this crossover design at both four and eight weeks.

Seventeen of the 30 men had suffered vascular accidents (9 right hemisphere, 13 left hemisphere), ten had suffered traumatic brain injury, and three had suffered injuries of other types; the mean time since onset of injury was 10.2 and 9.5 months respectively.

Training took place on the Vienna Test System, consisting of a range of attention and perceptual speed tasks, including simple and choice reaction time to visual and acoustic stimuli and reaction to target pictorial stimuli embedded within several similar stimuli.

The difficulty of these tasks was steadily increased, for example requiring different reactions to different and complex combinations of stimuli in various modalities.

Two control groups of matched nonbrain-damaged patients underwent a procedure identical to that of the brain-damaged patients in order to control for practice effects. The results were impressive. Significant improvements in test scores were observed following training but not following the nontraining period in both groups. These improvements were particularly evident on tests which were similar in form to the training tests (e.g. reaction-time and perceptual discrimination tasks), but they were also apparent on a wide range of less closely related tests of psychomotor function, logical thinking, word fluency and spatial reasoning. These effects were stable for at least four weeks following the cessation of training, and no comparable effects were obtained for the control groups. Though the study was not without methodological flaws (e.g. lack of blind assessment, use of matching rather than randomization), and though no generalization to everyday life was sought or demonstrated, the results suggested that computerized attentional training may produce changes in unrelated cognitive function.

Gray and Robertson (1989) carried out three multiple-baseline, single-case studies with three men following severe closed head injury (ages 20, 30 and 19, respectively; time postinjury 12, 36 and 6 months, respectively). In all cases, repeated measures at baseline and then training were taken of at least one function which was expected to improve with training, and of at least one which was not expected to improve. In the first case, no significant changes on discrimination reaction time were found over six weeks' baseline and nine weeks' training, while a relatively stable baseline on a combined score of digit span forward, digit span backward and arithmetic was followed by a statistically significant increase in this compound score during the training phase.

The training consisted of a rapid number-calculation training task (simultaneous presentation of four numbers, one of which is repeated) and a digit–symbol transfer task (matching numbers with symbols). Neither of these involved standard reaction-time components. Thus, it was predicted that effects would be found on 'working memory'-type tasks and not on reaction-time tasks, as indeed proved to be the case.

The second case was trained using a 'Stroop' training programme in which subjects are required to press coloured buttons on the computer in response to colour names presented on the screen according to one of two rules: the rules were pressing according to the colour the word spelled or to the colour in which it was written. A structured cueing system was built into the training, based on a verbal self-regulation strategy, and eventually the rules changed without cueing or warning in the advanced stages of therapy.

Over a three-week baseline, followed by a seven-week training phase, scores on a memory test did not change, whereas scores on the compound working memory tests improved significantly over the training phase.

In the third case, training was based on Digit Symbol Transfer, Stroop and an arcade-type reaction-time-type game. Over a baseline of five weeks and over a training phase of eight weeks, no improvements in a control measure – delayed recall from verbal memory – were found. However, statistically significant improvements in the working memory target scores were found (i.e. digit span and arithmetic).

These case studies did not attempt to show generalization over time or to everyday life. Nor was there blind assessment. Nevertheless, the studies do support the conclusions of both Sohlberg and Mateer and Sturm et al. described above.

Gray et al. (1992) reported a randomized controlled trial of computerized attentional rehabilitation. Thirty-one patients showing attentional problems following brain damage (17 closed head injury; 14 other types of injury) were randomly allocated to an experimental group ($n = 17$; mean age 26.2 years) and a control group ($n = 14$; mean age 34.1 years), and then followed up posttraining and at six months by a researcher blind to group allocation.

Training consisted of a mean of 15.3 hours of computerized training on reaction-time tasks, rapid number comparison, digit–symbol transfer, Stroop (see the details of the previous study for a description of these), as well as on a number of 'arcade'-type divided reaction-time tasks, some of which had been specially written for brain-injured patients.

The control group received a mean of 12.7 hours of recreational computing, consisting of computer quizzes and games which the authors judged made few attentional demands on the patients.

Immediately posttraining, no significant difference between the two groups emerged once a number of pre-training variables were entered into a covariance analysis. At six-month follow-up, on the other hand, clear improvements for the experimental group were found on PASAT and on the Arithmetic Subtest of the WAIS (Revised) after covariance of relevant pretreatment variables.

No improvements of the experimental group versus the control group were found on emotional and behavioural variables assessed by rating scales and questionnaires given to subjects and relatives, though these scales were not specifically designed for brain-damaged patients and may have been insufficiently sensitive to show any changes, if indeed any existed. The authors were unable to explain the 'sleeper effect' of the obtained results.

Niemann, Ruff and Baser (1990) evaluated the efficacy of a computer-assisted attention-retraining programme; 29 subjects, at least 12 months postinjury, who were suffering from moderate to severe traumatic brain injury were studied. The subjects were randomly assigned to attention training versus a control memory training, with training lasting nine weeks with two two-hour sessions per week for both groups. The experimental design consisted of a multiple-baseline procedure which showed that the experimental group improved significantly in comparison with the control group on measures of attention, with the reversed pattern for the memory measures not being observed. However, none of the treatment effects generalized to a second group of attentional measures.

Overview of nonspecific attention rehabilitation studies

Whereas some of the above studies showed some limited effects of nonspecific attentional training to other laboratory-based measures of attention, several failed to show any such effects, and none demonstrated generalization to everyday functioning. Nevertheless, the limited positive findings of some studies suggest that further investigation of this phenomenon is warranted. However, the fate of attentional training for schizophrenia should be borne in mind here, for which the familiar story of failure of generalization of computer-based rehabilitation has been told (Benedict et al., 1994).

How might any effects – assuming that there are any – be obtained? One possibility is that the observed improvements were based on the learning of a strategy for regulating attention and arousal. Other studies have more directly targeted this aspect of self-sustained alertness, rather than using the 'scattergun' attentional training approach of the studies just described.

Rehabilitation of specific nonlateralized attentional deficits

The few studies which have been specifically targeted have largely been aimed at problems of alertness and sustained attention. Only one study has systematically tackled separate types of attention, namely that by Sturm et al., which is described at the end of this section.

Wood and Fussey (1987) trained ten severely brain-injured patients using a vigilance task requiring the patients to monitor a line of symbols moving left to right across the computer screen, and requiring a rapid response when a prescribed match occurred between the symbol in a 'window' through which the string passed and one of a number of symbols on the bottom half of the screen. Training lasted for four weeks, a total of 20 one-hour sessions.

The control group of brain-injured patients was not randomly allocated to no-treatment, but rather was matched, a weaker strategy. Baseline, posttraining and 20-day follow-up data were collected on pursuit rotor, digit–symbol, choice and simple reaction time, visual vigilance tasks, and two ratings of behavioural ratings carried out at unspecified times and under unspecified conditions 'hourly over five days' (Wood and Fussey, 1987, p. 151).

No significant differences emerged between groups except for a delayed improvement on choice reaction time in the experimental group, which was apparent only at second follow-up, and on the behavioural

recordings, on both of which there appeared to be a significantly greater improvement by the trained compared with the untrained group.

Such differences are, however, difficult to assess when no reliability measures for the tests used are given. One of these measures was a nurse/therapist rating made by marking on a horizontal line with 'poor attention in therapy' at one end and 'good attention in therapy' at the other. The other measure involved recordings being made every two minutes in a one-hour session by the therapist stating whether the subject was or was not attending at the specified time.

These results are uninterpretable in the absence of information about the reliability of such subjective and difficult-to-carry-out ratings, particularly when the raters were not blind as to treatment condition and when the groups were not randomly allocated. The lack of an effect of training on cognitive tasks, on the other hand, adds another negative finding about computerized training to those already cited above.

Wilson and Robertson (1992) treated reading difficulties caused by attentional problems in a traumatically brain-injured person. The training consisted of a behavioural goal-setting/shaping method, aimed at gradually increasing the length of time for which the subject could concentrate on reading before his attention slipped. The effective period for which concentration on reading could be sustained rose from two minutes to five minutes over the course of the study. However, generalization to untrained reading material was not obtained through this goal-setting procedure, except when the procedure was repeated under conditions of auditory distraction (secondary spoken text during reading exercises).

Sturm and his colleagues in Aachen, Germany, carried out the first study of attentional training which independently targeted distinct aspects of attention (Sturm et al., 1997). They used computerized training procedures which targeted alertness, vigilance, selective and divided attention with 38 stroke patients (22 left hemisphere and 16 right hemisphere) who were a median 5.5 months poststroke. Fourteen one-hour sessions of training aimed at one of two attentional deficits on which they were most impaired was carried out, and changes in attention were measured on an independent set of computerized attentional tests. The authors compared changes in the type of attention which was specifically targeted with changes on the other impaired attentional measure which was not specifically targeted. Significantly greater changes were observed on the specifically targeted attentional measure. However, no evidence of generalization beyond a second set of computerized attentional measures was obtained.

A further study, which aimed to improve both sustained attention and unilateral inattention, is the subject of the next section of this chapter (Robertson et al., 1995). This study was based on the view that sustained attention refers to the ability to maintain alertness in circumstances in which there is little change or novelty in the environment. While a loud noise or unexpected sight draws our attention from the outside – that is, *exogenously* – we also need the additional capacity to maintain attention from internal sources – that is, *endogenously*. We need this capacity when driving along a straight and unchanging road at night or when listening to a long lecture.

This ability to sustain a state of alertness is more strongly represented in the right hemisphere of the brain than in the left, and in particular in the right frontal lobe. This has been recently shown in a study investigating the blood flow changes that take place when normal subjects sustain a state of alertness (Pardo, Fox and Raichle, 1991). Subjects were asked to count the number of times they were touched on their foot over a 40-second period while their regional cerebral blood flow was charted using positron emission tomography. Irrespective of which toe was stimulated, the right frontoparietal areas were significantly more activated in this task of sustained attention to parts of the body. A similar finding was obtained when the subjects had to look at a computer screen to detect brief dimmings of a central stimulus.

Posner (1993) argues that the ability to shift attention to the left or right is controlled by a spatial orientation system, partly located in the inferior parietal lobes of the brain. This is one of the areas thought to be impaired in spatial neglect. A second attention system modulates the efficiency with which this spatial orientation system works; this is the right hemisphere sustained attention system described above. The effects of increasing sustained attention, therefore, may consequently provide a secondary modulation of the primary orientation system. If this is so, then such modulation may provide another approach for influencing neglect that bypasses the problems of the lack of awareness so characteristic of neglect. This impairment of sustained attention can be manifested in patients' tendency easily to lose concentration during therapy. Relatives also comment that stroke patients 'drift off' and appear not to be listening while they are talking to them.

Impairments of sustained attention can be assessed using tone-counting tasks (Wilkins, Shallice and McCarthy, 1987; Robertson et al., 1996). The question posed was whether lateralized neglect performance could be improved by directing treatment resources to sustained attention systems which are presumed to modulate spatial orientation, an assertion for which there is strong experimental evidence (Robertson et al., 1998b).

The first research to suggest a method for training sustained attention was carried out in Canada by Meichenbaum and Goodman (1971) with impulsive children. These studies showed that attention could be brought under voluntary control by 'self-instructional' procedures. The results suggest that it may be possible to train neglect patients who have sustained attention problems to improve their alertness by training them endogenously to 'switch on' their sustained attention system using the types of learned verbal self-instructions used by Meichenbaum. If Posner's account is right, then such training should not only improve sustained attention, but should also improve orientation to the left side of space, because of the close connections between the sustained attention and the spatial orientation systems.

The Robertson et al. (1997b) study employed a related approach with a number of patients suffering from long-standing unilateral neglect. Most patients with severe unilateral neglect also have problems with sustained attention. The procedures involved training subjects to improve their internal (endogenous) control of attention of 'talking themselves through it' in a fixed series of stages. The aim of this treatment was to bring attention to task under voluntary verbal control, and thereby reduce distractibility and improve the length of concentration.

In the Sustained Attention Training procedure used, patients were trained while doing a variety of tasks which did not emphasize lateralized scanning: periodically, the patients had their attention drawn to the task by the combination of a loud noise and an instruction to attend. Patients were then gradually taught to 'take over' this alerting procedure, so that eventually it became a self-alerting procedure.

The results of this training with eight patients were very encouraging. Not only were there improvements in sustained attention, but there were also improvements in spatial neglect over and above those expected with natural recovery. One possible explanation for this is that many patients show greater awareness of their difficulties sustaining attention than of their tendency to neglect the left side of space. If this is true, then such patients may be more likely to implement the training procedure and to employ it in everyday life.

Again, however, the generalizability of these findings for more than 24 hours beyond the experimental setting or to everyday life activities was not tested. Nevertheless, the results were encouraging in terms of rehabilitating both sustained attention and spatial inattention, which is the subject of the next section of this chapter.

Rehabilitation of spatial inattention

- Rehabilitation of unilateral left inattention appears to be possible.
- Some generalization to everyday life functions has been demonstrated.
- The three methods for which some clinical efficacy has been demonstrated are scanning training, limb activation training, and sustained attention training.

Visual scanning training for neglect

A straightforward behavioural approach to the phenomenon of inattention to the left side of space is to try to train patients to engage in voluntary scanning to the left side of space. There is some evidence (a) that spontaneous recovery from neglect may occur through this type of mechanism (Goodale et al., 1990; Robertson et al., 1994), and (b) that such compensatory scanning may be disrupted by secondary nonvisual tasks (Robertson and Frasca, 1992). Such a view is compatible with evidence that voluntary and automatic spatial orientation of attention may be subserved by neural circuits different from those controlling automatic, exogenously elicited attentional shifts (Henik, Rafal and Rhodes, 1994). In other words, scanning could work by training patients to use the frontal-based voluntary (endogenous) spatial attentional system to compensate for a malfunctioning automatic system. This view would also be compatible with the evidence cited above that secondary tasks can disrupt spatial processing on the left side in patients who are partially or completely intact on particular spatial tasks.

However, the evidence on the effectiveness of scanning training is mixed, and generally the finding is that, while patients can be trained to scan to the left in particular situations, it is very difficult to show evidence of generalization of this voluntary scanning beyond the trained situations. For example, Wagenaar et al. (1992) carried out five single-case studies of the effectiveness of the sorts of scanning training used by Weinberg and colleagues in New York (Weinberg et al., 1977) and found, as had Gouvier et al. (1987) before them, no evidence of generalization of training to nontrained test situations.

In contrast to the above negative results are two recent studies which suggest that positive effects of scanning-type training may be observed under certain circumstances. Pizzamiglio et al. (1992) trained 13 stroke patients showing chronic unilateral left neglect using scanning-training methods derived from Weinberg and Diller's pioneering work. They found that 40 hours of therapy produced improvements on conventional tests of neglect as well as on a semistructured scale of neglect behaviour. However, the design was of a single group before–after type, and there was no blind assessment, although the improvements were confined to neglect measures and not to other visuoperceptual functions. Nevertheless, a randomized group study by the same group also found positive results (Antonucci et al., 1995), and so it seems likely that scanning training should have a place in the rehabilitation of unilateral inattention.

Limb activation treatments for neglect

Limb movements on the side contralateral to a lesion may cause improvements in visual attention to the left side of extrapersonal space in neglect patients, and it appears that, to be effective, these movements must be (a) willed rather than passive, and (b) carried out in left hemispace (Robertson and North, 1992; Robertson, North and Geggie, 1992). These effects have been interpreted in terms of Rizzolatti's model of attentional–motor integration (Rizzolatti and Berti, 1990).

Robertson et al. (1992, 1998a), using single-case experimental design methodology, have shown that limb activation methods improve not only test performance but also observed difficulties in everyday life function, and this effect was confirmed by blind assessment in one of the three cases reported. The use of a simple Neglect Alert Device attached to a patient's left side, which emits randomly spaced buzzes to which the patient must respond by pressing with some part of the affected side, makes this treatment more cost effective and practicable in everyday clinical situations than most scanning training procedures, though it may prove to be necessary for both types of treatment to be carried out in tandem, especially in more severe cases of neglect. It is also likely that this training may only be effective with neglect patients suffering from personal (body) as well as extrapersonal neglect.

Worthington (1996) carried out a single-case study of a patient with left neglect dyslexia after a right hemisphere stroke. He compared limb activation with limb activation plus visual cueing and demonstrated the success of both strategies in reducing neglect dyslexic errors, but showed that the combined strategy had longer lasting effects, reducing the neglect dyslexia up to 18 months posttraining.

Many other types of method have been shown to produce temporary changes in unilateral neglect, but controlled clinical studies of the effects of training beyond these immediate effects have only been carried out in the areas reviewed above, namely scanning training, limb activation training, and sustained attention training. In general, the results of these studies give some grounds for optimism that the rehabilitation of lateralized inattentional disorders may be effective under some circumstances and to a limited degree.

Can attentional deficits be rehabilitated?

- Attentional rehabilitation shows promise for future clinical research.
- New attempts to demonstrate generalization to everyday life are needed.
- All future rehabilitation strategies should target specific subtypes of attention, and nonspecific training of attention should be abandoned.

There are grounds for optimism that certain types of attentional deficit may be amenable to a certain degree of rehabilitation. The evidence is strongest for unilateral left inattention (left visuospatial neglect), though there is some evidence for effects of sustained attention training. Mixed, nontheoretically based attentional rehabilitation procedures have yielded very variable results. Other types of attention, such as selective attention, have not been targeted, except in one study which showed promising results, albeit only to computerized tests of attention which were not sufficiently dissimilar from the training materials to allow conclusions to be drawn about generalizability to everyday life (Sturm et al., 1997).

It seems clear that this area warrants further research, but that there is no longer any justification for carrying out rehabilitation studies without being clear as to what aspect of attention is being trained. Finally, while attentional deficits seem to be important in the recovery of other types of cognitive function after brain damage, as yet we have no information to tell us whether attentional rehabilitation can influence the course of recovery of these other functions.

Future research should also attempt to evaluate the effects of attentional training on everyday life functions, and the combination of such an approach with theoretically oriented rehabilitation should produce advances of both clinical and theoretical importance. It is likely that these rehabilitation advances will go hand in hand with the evolution of better integrated theories of executive and attentional function. It may also be the case that the optimal approach for attentional rehabilitation will involve the combination of behavioural and pharmacological interventions. Functional imaging may also help determine the mechanisms of any observed recovery, and will allow us to determine the interaction between attentional systems and other networks in the brain whose functioning may partially depend on intact attentional capacity. A final consideration in planning rehabilitation studies is to consider the practicalities of delivering particular rehabilitation procedures. With the increasing constriction of the amount of time and labour available for rehabilitation, questions of cost effectiveness and acceptability to clients should also figure in the design and evaluation of particular therapeutic strategies.

Conclusions

Just as learning is likely to be a central mechanism in the recovery of function following stroke, so attention is the prerequisite for adequate learning and, indeed, attentional deficits do predict motor and other recovery following brain damage. Attention consists of a number of different subsystems, including those for selective, sustained and spatial attention. Nonspecific attentional training has yielded very mixed results, and generalization to everyday life functions has not been demonstrated. On the other hand, training of sustained attention appears to be possible, though again generalization to everyday life functions has not been demonstrated; sustained attention training has, however, been shown to generalize in a theoretically predictable way to improve unilateral left inattention. The rehabilitation of unilateral left inattention appears to be possible, with some generalization to everyday life functions having been demonstrated. The three methods for which some clinical efficacy has been shown are scanning training, limb activation training, and sustained attention training. Therefore, attentional rehabilitation shows promise for future clinical research, though improved attempts to demonstrate generalization to everyday life are needed and all future rehabilitation strategies should target specific subtypes of attention.

References

Antonucci, G., Guariglia, C., Judica, A. et al. 1995. Effectiveness of neglect rehabilitation in a randomized group study. *J Clin Exp Neuropsychol* 17, 383–9

Ben-Yishay, Y., Diller, L., Gerstman, L. and Haas, A. 1968. The relationship between impersistence, intellectual function and outcome of rehabilitation in patients with left hemiplegia. *Neurology* 18, 852–61.

Benedict, R.H.B., Harris, A.E., Markow, T., McCormick, J.A., Nuechterlein, K.H. and Asarnow, R.F. 1994. Effects of attention training on information processing in schizophrenia. *Schizophr Bull* 20, 537–46.

Blanc-Garin, J. 1994. Patterns of recovery from hemiplegia following stroke. *Neuropsychol Rehabil* 4, 359–85.

Brooks, D.N. and McKinlay, W. 1987. Return to work within the first seven years of severe head injury. *Brain Inj* 1, 5–15.

Cohen, R.M., Semple, W.E., Gross, M., Holcomb, H.J., Dowling, S. and Nordahl, T.E. 1988. Functional localization of sustained attention. *Neuropsychiatry Neuropsychol Behav Neurol* 1, 3–20.

Denes, G., Semenza, C., Stoppa, E. and Lis, A. 1982. Unilateral spatial neglect and recovery from hemiplegia. A follow-up study. *Brain* 105, 543–52.

Drevets, W.C., Burton, H., Videen, T.O., Snyder, A.Z., Simpson, J.R. and Raichle, M.E. 1995. Blood flow changes in human somatosensory cortex during anticipated stimulation. *Nature* 373, 249–52.

Fullerton, K.J., McSherry, P. and Stout, M. 1986. Albert's Test: a neglected test of perceptual neglect. *Lancet* 1, 430–2.

Goodale, M.A., Milner, A.D., Jakobson, L.S. and Carey, D.P. 1990. Kinematic analysis of limb movements in neuropsychological research: subtle deficits and recovery of function. *Can J Psychol* 44, 180–95.

Gouvier, W., Bua, B., Blanton, P. and Urey, J. 1987. Behavioural changes following visual scanning training: observation of five cases. *Int J Clin Neuropsychol* 9, 74–80.

Gray, J. and Robertson, I. 1989. Remediation of attentional difficulties following brain injury: three experimental single case studies. *Brain Inj* 3, 163–70.

Gray, J.M., Robertson, I.H., Pentland, B. and Anderson, S.I. 1992). Microcomputer based cognitive rehabilitation for brain damage: a randomised group controlled trial. *Neuropsychol Rehabil* 2, 97–116.

Henik, A., Rafal, R. and Rhodes, D. 1994. Visually guided saccades after lesions of the human frontal eye fields. *J Cogn Neurosci* 6, 400–11.

Malec, J., Jones, R., Rao, N. and Stubbs, K. 1984. Video-game practise effect on sustained attention in patients with craniocerebral trauma. *Cogn Rehabil* 2, 18–23.

McKinlay, W.M. 1981. The short-term outcome of severe blunt head injury as reported by relatives of the injured persons. *J Neurol Neurosurg Psychiatry* 44, 527–33.

Meichenbaum, D. and Goodman, J. 1971. Training impulsive children to talk to themselves: a means of developing control. *J Abnorm Psychol* 77, 115–26.

Moscovitch, M. 1994. Cognitive resources and dual-task interference effects at retrieval in normal people: the role of the frontal lobes and medial temporal cortex. *Neuropsychology* 8, 524–34.

Niemann, H., Ruff, R.M. and Baser, C.A. 1990. Computer-assisted attention retraining in head injured individuals: a controlled efficacy study of an outpatient program. *J Consult Clin Psychol* 38, 811–17.

Pardo, J.V., Fox, P.T. and Raichle, M.E. 1991. Localization of a human system for sustained attention by positron emission tomography. *Nature* 349, 61–4.

Pizzamiglio, L., Antonucci, G., Judica, A., Montenero, P., Razzano, C. and Zoccolotti, P. 1992. Cognitive rehabilitation of the hemineglect disorder in chronic patients with unilateral right brain damage. *J Clin Exp Neuropsychol* 14, 901–23.

Ponsford, J. and Kinsella, G. 1988. Evaluation of a remedial programme for attentional deficits following closed head-injury. *J Clin Exp Neuropsychol* 10, 693–708.

Posner, M.I. 1993. Interaction of arousal and selection in the posterior attention network. In *Attention: Selection, Awareness and Control*, ed. A. Baddeley and L. Weiskrantz, pp. 390–405. Oxford: Clarendon Press.

Posner, M.I. and Peterson, S.E. 1990. The attention system of the human brain. *Ann Rev Neurosci* 13, 25–42.

Rizzolatti, G. and Berti, A. 1990. Neglect as neural representation deficit. *Rev Neurol (Paris)* 146, 626–34.

Robertson, I.H. (1999). Theory-driven neuropsychological rehabilitation: the role of attention and competition in recovery of function after brain damage. In *Attention and Performance XVII*, ed. D. Gopher and A. Koriat, Cambridge, MA: MIT Press.

Robertson, I.H. (in press). Rehabilitation of brain damage: brain plasticity and principles of guided recovery. *Psych Bull.*

Robertson, I.H. and Frasca, R. 1992. Attentional load and visual neglect. *Int J Neurosci* 62, 45–56.

Robertson, I.H., Halligan, P.W., Bergego, C. et al. 1994. Right neglect after right brain damage? *Cortex* 30, 199–214.

Robertson, I.H., Hogg, K. and McMillan, T.M. 1998a. Rehabilitation of unilateral neglect: reducing inhibitory competition by contralesional limb activation. *Neuropsychol Rehabil* 8, 19–30.

Robertson, I.H., Manly, T., Andrade, J., Baddeley, B.T. and Yiend, J. 1997a. Oops!: performance correlates of everyday attentional failures: the Sustained Attention to Response Task (SART). *Neuropsychologia* 35, 747–58.

Robertson, I.H., Manly, T., et al. 1997b. Auditory sustained attention is a marker of unilateral spatial neglect. *Neuropsychologia* 35, 1527–32.

Robertson, I.H., Mattingley, J.B., Rorden, C. and Driver, J. 1998b.

Phasic alerting of right hemisphere neglect patients overcomes their spatial deficit in visual awareness. *Nature* 395, 169–72.

Robertson, I.H. and North, N. 1992. Spatio-motor cueing in unilateral neglect: the role of hemispace, hand and motor activation. *Neuropsychologia* 30, 553–63.

Robertson, I.H., North, N. and Geggie, C. 1992. Spatio-motor cueing in unilateral neglect: three single case studies of its therapeutic effectiveness. *J Neurol Neurosurg Psychiatry* 55, 799–805.

Robertson, I.H., Ridgeway, V., Greenfield, E. and Parr, A. 1997c. Motor recovery after stroke depends on intact sustained attention: a two-year follow-up study. *Neuropsychology* 11, 290–5.

Robertson, I.H., Tegnér, R., Tham, K., Lo, A. and Nimmo-Smith, I. 1995. Sustained attention training for unilateral neglect: theoretical and rehabilitation implications. *J Clin Exp Neuropsychol* 17, 416–30.

Robertson, I.H., Ward, T., Ridgeway, V. and Nimmo-Smith, I. 1996. The structure of normal human attention: the Test of Everyday Attention. *J Int Neuropsychol Soc* 2, 525–34.

Sea, M.C., Henderson, A. and Cermack, S.A. 1993. Patterns of visual spatial inattention and their functional significance in stroke patients. *Arch Phys Med Rehabil* 74, 355–61.

Shuren, J.E., Hammond, C.S., Maher, L.M., Rothi, L.J.G. and Heilman, K.M. 1995. Attention and anosognosia: the case of a jargonaphasic patient with unawareness of language deficit. *Neurology* 45, 376–78.

Sohlberg, M. and Mateer, C. 1987. Effectiveness of an attention-training programme. *J Clin Exp Neuropsychol* 9, 117–30.

Sterzi, R., Bottini, G., Celani, M. et al. 1993. Hemianopia, hemianaesthesia and hemiplegia after right and left hemisphere damage. A hemispheric difference. *J Neurol Neurosurg Psychiatry* 56, 308–10.

Sturm, W., Dahmen, W., Hartje, W. and Willmes, K. 1983. Ergebnisse eines Trainingsprogramms zur Verbesserung der visuellen Auffassungsshnelligkeit und Konzentrationsfahigkeit bei Hirngeschaditgten. *Arch Psychiatrie Nerven* 233, 9–22.

Sturm, W., Willmes, K., Orgass, B. and Hartje, W. 1997. Do specific attention deficits need specific training. *Neuropsychol Rehabil* 7, 81–176.

Stuss, D.T., Shallice, T., Alexander, M.P. and Picton, T.W. 1995. A multidisciplinary approach to anterior attentional functions. *Ann NY Acad Sci* 769, 191–211.

von Cramon, D.Y.V. and von Cramon, G.M. 1992. Reflections on the treatment of brain-injured patients suffering from problem-solving disorders. *Neuropsychol Rehabil* 2, 207–30.

von Cramon, D.Y.V., von Cramon, G.M. and Mai, N. 1991.

Problem-solving deficits in brain-injured patients: a therapeutic approach. *Neuropsychol Rehabil* 1, 45–64.

Wagenaar, R.C., Wieringen, P.C.W.V., Netelenbos, J.B., Meijer, O.G. and Kuik, D.J. 1992. The transfer of scanning training effects in visual attention after stroke: five single case studies. *Disabil Rehabil* 14, 51–60.

Weinberg, J., Diller, L., Gordon, W. et al. 1977. Visual scanning training effect on reading-related tasks in acquired right brain damage. *Arch Phys Med Rehabil* 58, 479–86.

Wilkins, A.J., Shallice, T. and McCarthy, R. 1987. Frontal lesions and sustained attention. *Neuropsychologia* 25, 359–65.

Wilson, C. and Robertson, I.H. 1992. A home-based intervention for attentional slips during reading following head injury: a single case study. *Neuropsychol Rehabil* 2, 193–205.

Wood, R.L.I. and Fussey, I. 1987. Computer-based cognitive retraining: a controlled study. *Int Disabil Stud* 9, 149–53.

Worthington, A.D. 1996. Cueing strategies in neglect dyslexia. *Neuropsychol Rehabil* 6, 1–17.

20

The rehabilitation of executive disorders

Catherine A. Mateer

Introduction

- Individuals with executive function impairments display problems in starting and stopping, making mental and behavioural shifts, with attention, and with awareness of self and others.
- Component processes hypothesized to support executive control include activation/drive systems, inhibitory control, working memory, interference control, prospective memory, and self-monitoring/regulation.

This chapter deals with the rehabilitation of individuals who demonstrate disorders of executive function. Executive functions have long been thought to be dependent on the integrity of the frontal lobes. Goldstein, Kleist, Hebb, Benton and a number of other early and influential theorists of this century discussed the nature of frontal lobe functions. It was Luria, however, who proposed that the prefrontal cortex supported the highest levels of cognitive organization and who described this area as the 'central executive' of the brain. In his model, the frontal lobes were responsible for planning, initiating, regulating and verifying a sequence of actions (Luria, 1966). Interest in and examination of so-called executive functioning have increased exponentially over the last two decades, although a coherent structure and taxonomy in which to conceptualize the myriad of functions this concept includes are still elusive (Tranel, Anderson and Benton, 1994).

From a clinical and rehabilitation perspective, the challenges faced in attempting to deal with executive disorders are enormous. Individuals with these disorders demonstrate a wide variety of cognitive and behavioural disorders and difficulties. Some of the more prominent problems commonly demonstrated by individuals with frontal involvement are listed below.

1. Problems of 'starting'. Individuals may demonstrate markedly reduced initiation and spontaneity of behaviour. In many cases, they may verbalize an intent to act, but fail to follow through. With cues, prompts or assists, the patient may be able to engage in the behaviour, but does not do so in the absence of such cues.

2. Problems with 'stopping'. Individuals may demonstrate disinhibition, impulsivity, and quick shifts in behaviour and emotional tone.

3. Difficulties in making mental or behavioural shifts. Individuals may demonstrate rigid, inflexible or perseverative behaviour, seemingly becoming fixed in a response set that is no longer appropriate or productive.

4. Problems with attention. Individuals with frontal dysfunction are often distractible and display poor selective and divided attention.

5. Problems with awareness of self and others. Individuals may display very limited or no apparent understanding and appreciation with regard to the nature of their difficulties or the impact these difficulties have on everyday functioning; they may also have a limited appreciation of their impact on others, or on the feelings, motivations or intentions of others.

Deficits in these areas are common in many of the neurological conditions in which frontal functions are known to be affected, including traumatic brain injury, frontal dementias, schizophrenia and Parkinson's disease.

A conceptualization of executive functions

This chapter describes techniques for managing the cognitive and behavioural sequelae of frontal lobe injury and treatment strategies designed to address executive function impairments.

Anatomically, the frontal lobes are large, complex and heterogeneous (Jouandet and Gazzaniga, 1979; Fuster, 1989). Correspondingly, there is great variation in the functional consequences of frontal lobe damage. In an attempt to integrate the range of cognitive and behavioural dysfunctions observed following injury to this system, a variety of hierarchical models of frontal function has been proposed. At a global level, the primary function of the prefrontal cortex is the temporal organization, integration, formulation and execution of novel behavioural sequences that are responsive to environmental demands and constraints and to internal motivations and drives, and contribute to orderly, purposive behaviour. Damage to the system globally results in a fragmentation of complex action sequences. Whereas individual actions are possible, they may lack goal directedness, structure and/or temporal organization.

In order to demonstrate flexible goal-directed behaviour, however, a number of what West (1996) called 'subservient' or component processes are necessary. The following are hypothesized as necessary component processes.

1. The system must be 'activated'. Initiation and drive appear primarily dependent on mesial frontal structures. Duffy and Campbell (1994) described three prefrontal syndromes: the dysexecutive type (dorsolateral convexity), the disinhibited type (orbitofrontal), and the apathetic type (mesial frontal lobe). The last-mentioned is thought to reflect an imbalance between the cingulum and the supplementary motor area. Stimulation of the cingulum has been found to cause arousal, whereas stimulation of the supplementary motor area has been found to result in cessation of volitional activity, with a subjective sense of the absence of the will to move. It has been hypothesized that disconnection of cingulum input to the supplementary motor area may result in varying degrees of release of supplementary motor area activity, leading to problems with initiation and volition (Stuss and Benson, 1986; Duffy and Campbell, 1994). Several researchers have documented problems with volition and motivated behaviour following anterior cingulate damage or disruption (Ishii, Nishihara and Imamura, 1986; Frith et al., 1991).

2. The individual must have a mechanism for inhibiting prepotent response tendencies. The responses cued by stimuli in the environment or emerging from within the organism need to be inhibited if they are inappropriate to the setting or to the long-term goals of the individual. Individuals with frontal involvement are often overresponsive to environmental cues and appear to be easily distracted. They may also appear inflexible and respond with familiar or previously rewarded behaviour patterns even when such behaviour is no longer successful (Dempster, 1991, 1993). The prefrontal cortex is hypothesized to inhibit prepotent responses from gaining control of the action and to help sustain attention to task despite distraction or the waning of attention over time. The problems with inhibition are most obvious on nonroutine or novel tasks or when a prepotent response must be inhibited (Stuss and Benson, 1987; Diamond, 1988; Fuster, 1989; Knight and Grabowecky, 1995).

3. Extensive literature suggests that the prefrontal cortex plays an important role in the on-line maintenance of representational memory during task-related processing (Goldman-Rakic, 1987; Fuster, 1989). The capacity for 'working memory' is necessary to maintain on-line task-relevant information in order to guide behaviour in the absence of external cues. Without such an internalized representation to guide behaviour, the individual is likely to resort to a prepotent response leading to perseveration or to stimulus-bound behaviour that is manifest as distractibility or impulsivity. Behaviour may then be guided by dominant but inappropriate sources of internal or external information.

4. The frontal cortex appears to be involved in 'interference control'. It functions to clear task-irrelevant

information from working memory, and to suppress interfering stimuli from the external environment or arising from internal sources (West, 1996).

5. The capacity for 'prospective memory' allows the individual to act on a prior intent. It can operate to prepare for and initiate the execution of an action in response to internal or external cues. Prospective memory appears to be separable from retrospective memory and to rely heavily on frontal systems (Sohlberg and Mateer, 1989a, 1989b; Shallice and Burgess, 1991a; Cockburn, 1996).

6. The frontal lobes play an important role in self-awareness, and disruption of this system may result in a lack of awareness either for specific errors or for major changes in behaviour and function. In some instances, individuals may demonstrate an intellectual awareness of errors or difficulties, but are unable to modify their behaviour based on this knowledge (Stuss and Benson, 1987; Stuss, 1991a; Duncan, 1995).

These various components of executive function can fractionate and interact in complex ways. Given the complexities of this system, and the fact that individuals with frontal involvement are likely to demonstrate differing patterns of strengths and weaknesses, it is challenging to develop effective intervention strategies. Should rehabilitation specialists look globally at behaviour and try to improve functioning in particular settings at that level, or should they try to understand and improve the functioning of the various cognitive processes contributing to the global behaviour in the hope that this will lead to more general improvements in function across a multitude of settings? Some researchers and clinicians have argued for a solely functional approach to skill and task development, whereas others have argued that rehabilitation methods precisely targeted to the particular type of frontal impairment must be developed and implemented (Mateer, 1997; Robertson, 1999).

Assessment of executive control functions

- A comprehensive assessment of frontal and executive control functions is essential for treatment planning.
- Although one must be aware of potential problems

with the sensitivity and specificity of psychometric measures of frontal functioning, a number of tests and test batteries may prove useful in identifying impairments in executive control functions.

- Given the potential limitations of psychometric data, it is particularly important that the assessment of frontal functions be supplemented by medical information and history, observational data, and the incorporation of information about past and current functioning in natural contexts.
- The incorporation of observational and questionnaire data targeting the day-to-day demonstration of executive control can be extremely valuable.

Regardless of the intervention approach adopted, the first stage in developing a rehabilitation plan is to characterize the nature of the disorder. A critical evaluation of the neuropsychological assessment of executive function is beyond the scope of this chapter, but some issues are particularly relevant to rehabilitation and are mentioned here. First and foremost, it is important to be aware of some of the inherent problems in assessing the executive functions. Lezak pointed out that psychometric testing protocols, by their nature, typically provide structure, cues for the initiation and maintenance of on-task behaviour, minimization of distractions, and identification of explicit goals, obviating the need for many of the executive control capacities that are required for everyday functioning (Lezak, 1982, 1993). In addition, the measurement of the cognitive processes carried out by the frontal region is hampered by the complex and interactive nature of these processes, and by the extensive interconnections between the frontal lobes and other regions of the brain (Stuss et al., 1995). Many of the component cognitive functions that have been ascribed to the executive control system, such as inhibitory control or working memory, are not easily operationalized and their measurement almost always involves some dependence on other cognitive abilities such as visual recognition or reading. Clinical tests that show deficits in patients with frontal lobe lesions typically require multiple component processes and lack performance measures that are specific to individual cognitive processes. Though any two frontal tests may each be sensitive to frontal lesions, they may load heavily on different nonfrontal processes. In addition, different frontally sensitive tests may require the function of anatomically and functionally separate systems within the frontal lobes. Finally, not only are correlations between different frontal measures low, but the variability of performance on a single frontal measure is often high. Indeed, Stuss (1991b) has suggested that variability of performance is a characteristic of frontally impaired individuals.

With these caveats in mind, there is a large number of psychometric tests which appear to have some sensitivity to frontal/executive functions in some individuals. Psychometric measures which have been shown to have some sensitivity to frontal involvement often include the need for problem solving, use of feedback, mental flexibility and/or set shifting (e.g. Wisconsin Card Sorting Test, Tower of Hanoi, Trail Making B, Six Elements Test), working memory (e.g. Consonant Trigrams Test, self-ordered pointing measures, delayed response alternation measures), inhibition of prepotent responding (e.g. Stroop Test, Go–NoGo measures); and flexible, generative output (e.g. verbal and nonverbal fluency tests). Though prospective memory has been less commonly assessed, portions of the Rivermead Everyday Memory Test (Wilson, Cockburn and Halligan, 1985) and the Prospective Memory Screening (Sohlberg and Mateer, 1989a) can be used to gain insight into the capacity to remember to initiate previously intended actions. Given the problems with sensitivity and specificity of frontal measures noted in the introduction to this section, it is important to rely on multiple rather than single measures, and to recognize both that individuals with damage to nonfrontal areas of the brain may do poorly on the measures, and that some individuals with known or suspected frontal injury may do well.

Recently, numerous test batteries incorporating multiple measures for assessment of executive functioning have been introduced. The Behavioural Assessment of Dysexecutive Syndrome (BADS; Wilson et al., 1996) includes six subtests designed to address everyday problems in organization, planning and problem solving. A standardized version of the Six Elements Test has been incorporated that had been shown to be quite sensitive to the problems with organization and disinhibition (Shallice and Burgess, 1991b).

The Executive Interview (Royall, Mahurin and Gray, 1992) was designed for use as a clinical bedside screener for frontal involvement. It tests for frontal release signs, motor or cognitive perseveration, verbal intrusions, disinhibition, loss of spontaneity, imitation behaviour, environmental dependency and utilization behaviour.

It is important to recognize that while impaired performance on a particular measure may reliably indicate frontal involvement, it may tell you little about how that impairment is manifest in day-to-day activity. Numerous useful observational and questionnaire approaches to the evaluation of executive function, as it is manifest in day-to-day function, have been developed and one or more should be incorporated into the assessment. Most of these approaches provide an opportunity for ratings/judgements by both the patients themselves and by family members or rehabilitation staff who know the individuals well and/or who have had an opportunity to observe them in a variety of settings. The BADS (Wilson et al., 1996) contains a 20-item Dysexecutive Questionnaire (the DEX) to be completed by the patient and a family member. The Profile of the Executive Control System (Sohlberg, 1992) provides for staff and family ratings of behaviour on seven scales (Goal Selection, Planning/Sequencing, Initation, Execution, Time Sense, Awareness of Deficits and Self-Monitoring). The Brock Adaptive Functioning Questionnaire (Dywan and Segalowitz, 1996) provides for self and other report on 12 scales. Research with this instrument has identified two factors: one reflecting capacity for planning and initiation, believed to be related to dorsolateral prefrontal systems, and one more dependent on social monitoring and control of arousal, thought to be more orbitofrontally mediated. The use of these measures can increase an understanding and appreciation of how the individual is functioning on a day-to-day basis in terms of executive control.

Finally, there are several measures that have been designed to look specifically at the level of awareness demonstrated by brain-injured individuals. Such information can be important in relation to assessing individuals' motivation for change and their commitment to involvement in rehabilitation. These include the Change Assessment Questionnaire by Lam et al. (1988), and the Self-Awareness of Deficits Interview by Fleming, Strong and Ashton (1996).

The evaluation of executive functions is challenging. An increased understanding of the various frontally based functions will probably lead to more theoretically driven measures. At the present time, the assessment is most likely to provide a meaningful picture of the individual if it incorporates a range of appropriate psychometric measures, behavioural observations, collateral information from family and/or caregivers, and medical history.

Management and remediation of executive disorders: theoretical considerations

- The process of rehabilitation involves the implementation of environmental manipulations, the training of compensatory activities, and/or the application of activities designed to restore or improve underlying abilities.
- Some approaches focus on factors external to the patient, whereas others focus on changing the abilities, compensatory activities and/or perceptions of the patients themselves.
- The selection of specific intervention strategies should be based on the individual's level of environmental dependency, the constellation of preserved and impaired executive functions, and their level of self-awareness.
- Rehabilitation can be conceptualized as a set of activities which assist the individual in moving from a more dependent, externally monitored/supported state, to a more independent, internally supported and self-regulated state.

The goal of rehabilitation should be to improve the adaptive functioning of individuals in the setting in which they will be living and working. Following an evaluation of the cognitive and behavioural profile, and the probable real-world impact of the deficits, it is necessary to establish specific goals given current and anticipated future circumstances. An approach to intervention is then selected, the intervention plan or programme is delivered, and data are kept on performance or behaviour as appropriate. Generalization strategies should be developed and implemented from the begin-

ning of treatment. Finally, there should be an evaluation of the efficacy of the intervention and determination made about the impact of functioning in natural contexts (Sohlberg and Mateer, 1989b). Typically, the process of rehabilitation involves the implementation of environmental manipulations, the training of compensatory activities which allow the individual to function more effectively despite the impairments, and the application of activities designed to restore or improve underlying abilities. Some of these approaches focus on factors external to the patient, as in the case of environmental alterations, whereas others focus on changing the patient's abilities, activities and/or perceptions.

Environmental manipulations

One set of approaches to rehabilitation focuses on manipulating or altering the environment. Such 'external manipulations' alter factors external to the patients with minimal or no expectation of underlying change in their capacities. Included in this category are such manipulations as altering demands on the patient. This might be accomplished by simplifying tasks, eliminating the need to do certain tasks or allowing longer time frames to complete activities. Other manipulations consistent with this approach would include the provision of more salient cues for behaviour in the form of oral or written cue systems or checklists to follow. Yet another manipulation in this vein is the altering of environmental parameters such as the reduction of noise, clutter or other potential distractions. There is an inherent assumption that such external manipulations would need to remain in place if the change in functioning or behaviour is to continue, although it is possible that behaviours might become more routine and thereby gain habit strength. Externally mediated compensations are put into place by someone other than the patient. They are typically rather inflexible and require a high level of dependency on another person.

The use of behavioural interventions might also be considered to be an external manipulation, at least at the outset. Behavioural interventions typically have as their goal an increase or decrease in the frequency of certain behaviours or a change in their quality through the use of response contingencies (positive or negative reinforcement). In some instances, implementation of such programmes may result in a change in behaviour that stabilizes, so that the contingency can be withdrawn. In other cases, however, it is necessary to maintain the behavioural programming indefinitely, or to move into another phase of training to effect behaviour change in a different context.

Compensatory approaches

In contrast to approaches which focus on environmental manipulations or the modification of factors external to the patient, there are approaches which have as a goal a primary change in the behaviour or actions of the patients themselves, such that they are performing a task in another way. A compensation might include a new behaviour or substitute skill (such as using a memory notebook), and/or an increase in time and/or effort employed (such as in studying). Approaches which attempt to increase self-awareness, or which teach self-regulatory or metacognitive strategies, could also be included here. Individuals may also adapt to their new situation by changing self-expectations, selecting alternative activities, or relaxing the criteria for success. Whether patients are taught to use the compensation or develop it on their own, they are active participants in its application and continued use.

Direct interventions

Direct interventions involve the use of procedures which have as a goal improving or restoring some underlying ability or cognitive capacity (Meier, Benton and Diller, 1987). They would include a myriad of approaches for improving underlying cognitive skills, such as attention, prospective memory or problem solving. Sohlberg and Mateer (1989b) applied what they termed a 'process oriented approach' to the rehabilitation of some cognitive impairments. The basic tenets of this approach included a solid understanding of the specific cognitive area involved and a detailed analysis of the nature of impairments in that area. This was followed by hierarchical training exercises designed to provide structured opportunities to practise and thereby strengthen particular

cognitive skills. Repetition was believed to be critical to the re-automatization of such abilities.

Given the complex constellations of behavioural and cognitive difficulties demonstrated by frontally impaired patients, it is important to match the profile of the patient with the intervention approach (Sohlberg, Mateer and Stuss, 1993b; Stuss, Mateer and Sohlberg, 1994; Mateer, 1997). In general, patients who demonstrate little behavioural initiative or flexibility, who are environmentally dependent with apparently minimal response to internal cues, and/or who are minimally aware of their deficits, tend to respond better and more consistently to external manipulations. For these patients, environmental manipulations, behavioural strategies and external cueing systems are often effective in increasing function. Patients who demonstrate greater behavioural initiative and flexibility, who initiate and direct their own behaviour to some degree, and who are somewhat aware of the changes in their abilities resulting from their injury, are more likely to benefit from specific cognitive training, training in the use of compensatory devices such as memory books, and training in the use of self-instructional and metacognitive strategies. These last-mentioned strategies have been described and used extensively with learning disabled children who have difficulty with self-regulation of organized strategic behaviours.

In many cases it is useful to start out with predominantly external approaches and then to move to more internally focused approaches as gains are realized and/or behavioural flexibility, initiative and insight improve. It may be useful to conceptualize rehabilitation on a continuum. During coma, for example, the management of the individual is almost entirely in the hands of medical staff. In the early stages of recovery, when individuals are agitated, confused and/or minimally aware of their circumstances, hospital staff and caregivers must assume substantial responsibility for the safety and behaviour of the brain-injured patient. Over time, the brain-injured person, with support and assistance, gradually can and should be expected to assume an increasing share of the responsibility for his or her own behaviour and function. Interventions shift their focus from techniques which require little involvement on the part of the patient to techniques which

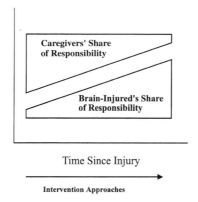

Time Since Injury

Intervention Approaches

Primarily 'External'   Primarily 'Internal'

Environmental modifications   Cognitive–behavioural interventions

Behavioural strategies   Metacognitive/self-regulatory strategies

Cues, prompts and checklists   Train use of compensation strategies

Teaching task-specific routines   Practice in task management

Pharmacological interventions   Awareness training and psychotherapy

Fig. 20.1 Diagram illustrating a theoretical model of rehabilitation. The relative amount of responsibility for the injured person which falls to rehabilitation staff and caretakers gradually decreases over time, while the relative amount of responsibility the injured person can assume increases over time. Different intervention strategies are most effective at different stages of recovery. The illustration is hypothetical, and the beginning and end points on the continuum will vary from individual to individual.

require active participation in the treatment and increasing demands on self-regulation. Figure 20.1 illustrates these shifts in the share of responsibility of behaviour over the course of recovery and indicates some of the strategies which are likely to be most useful along the continuum. Of course, each individual will recover at a different rate and to a different extent, so that the 'balance' of responsibility and integration of strategies must be carefully monitored. The model reflects a primary purpose of rehabilitation, which is to assist the individual in moving from a dependent, or externally supported, state to an independent, or internally supported, state. Executive functions are critical for this transition.

Finally, it has become increasingly evident that many individuals need assistance in dealing with the emotional and behavioural consequences of acquired cognitive impairment. It is often difficult to adjust to changes in one's 'thinking ability', and fear, frustration and feelings of loss are common. The importance of providing assistance in dealing with the emotional responses to these changes in functioning on the part of both the affected individuals and their families cannot be overestimated. Education of the family and significant others in how to respond to a person with cognitive impairments is also very important. An appreciation of the organic and nonvolitional nature of the behaviour is often helpful in alleviating the fears and misconceptions of family members and caregivers.

Specific approaches to the rehabilitation of impairments in executive control

- Considerable evidence exists for the efficacy of interventions that address various components of executive control.
- Impairments in initiation and sequencing of action can be targeted through a variety of cueing techniques, training of task-specific routines, and a variety of self-regulatory and self-monitoring strategies.
- Impaired inhibitory control has been shown to improve with the implementation of a variety of behavioural, cognitive–behavioural and self-regulatory procedures and strategies.
- Substantial evidence exists for improvements in attention skills with targeted practice in this area. The strongest support is for improved sustained attention and working memory, with less strong but promising support in the areas of selective attention, shifting of attention and divided attention. Task-specific gains, functional gains and changes in electrophysiological correlates of attention have been demonstrated following specific training on appropriate attentional functions.
- There is some evidence that prospective memory functions can be improved with targeted training.
- There is some evidence to support improvements in problem-solving skills, task analysis and planning

with training and practice, but limited generalization of such interventions to functional tasks.

- Limitations in awareness are often acknowledged to compromise rehabilitation efforts. Although some approaches to improving awareness have been described, further work in the conceptualization, the measurement, and the modification of awareness is needed.

In the following sections, rehabilitation in several cognitive and behavioural domains commonly disrupted following frontal injury will be discussed. Some rehabilitation specialists have focused on the larger picture, attempting to improve such overarching executive functions as planning, problem solving and organizing, whereas others have focused efforts on the so-called subservient or support processes which presumably underlie and support the more global capacities. Included here are approaches that address and attempt to improve initiation, working memory, prospective memory and awareness. This latter approach is consistent with recent views elaborating the fractionization of frontal processes into separable components (Shallice and Burgess, 1991a; Stuss et al., 1995; Baddeley, 1996; West, 1996). Such separability of functions argues for specificity in rehabilitation. Finally, the frequency of multiple, interrelated problems of an affective, behavioural and cognitive nature among individuals with executive function compromise requires the use of multicomponential, integrative interventions.

Techniques to improve the initiation and sequencing of action

Behaviours can be categorized into those actions that stem from internal motivations, and those that are made in response to external stimulation (Frith, 1987). Many investigators have emphasized the need to distinguish between poverty of action associated with difficulty starting an intended behaviour (initiation), and poverty of action associated with a lack of desire to engage in behaviour (volition) (Liddle, 1993). Thus, there may be a dissociation between stated intent or the verbal ability to define the action intended, and the person's ability to carry out the behaviour based on that knowledge (Stuss and Benson, 1986; Tranel et al., 1994).

Individuals with problems with initiation and/or volition often respond quite well to external cues or prompts to begin activity. For example, if patients are failing to initiate steps in grooming, they might be provided with prompts in the form of verbal reminders and alarm systems, which can function to prompt behaviour. In many cases it is profitable initially to focus on teaching task-specific routines. The assumption here is that the patient will not be capable of a wide variety of different action plans in different settings because of a failure to see the need to initiate activity, stimulus boundedness, perseveration, related cognitive disorders of attention or memory, or extremely limited insight and awareness.

Frontally impaired individuals may also show marked impairment in the sequencing of behaviour. Schwartz and her colleagues (1993; Schwartz, 1995) have developed a system for coding errors of action which can be very helpful in identifying errors of omission, commission and order on everyday functional activities. In terms of intervention, training of particular behavioural sequences for standard highly repetitive functional activities, such as grooming and dressing, has been shown to be possible (Craine, 1982). Extensive use is made of cues and checklists to guide behaviour. Another example of a specific routine that might be taught is the preparation of a simple breakfast. The patient might be taught a simple sequence for preparing juice, toast and cereal, which could be done in much the same way each day. A limited number of food items is utilized and the emphasis is on the avoidance of potential dangers such as the use of the stove or waste disposers. Geyer (1989) prepared a handbook for teaching such task-specific routines for just this purpose. Behavioural techniques involving the shaping of behaviour and reinforcement are commonly a complementary adjunct to such functional skills training approaches (Wood, 1987; Giles and Clarke-Wilson, 1988).

Another interesting approach was described by Gervin (1991), who systematically paired external cues in the form of song lyrics with an accompanying tempo and melody used for pacing. In the first phase of treatment, the therapist gathered baseline data during dressing. The information gathered was used to develop a series of one-stage and two-stage commands which were combined with an original melody. During the intervention phase, the therapist sang the commands and played a guitar while the client completed the task. The pace of the song was matched to the person's abilities and the intervention continued until the time to complete the task stabilized. At this point, the song was recorded for continued use by the client.

Another approach to working on initiation and volition involves the use of metacognitive or self-regulatory techniques. These techniques are based on the observation that it is possible to regulate one's own behaviour through self-talk (Meichenbaum, 1977; Graham and Harris, 1989; Harris, 1990; Borkowski and Muthukrishna, 1992). A small case study report by Stuss, Delgado and Guzman (1987) was one of the first to describe the use of this type of approach in an individual with acquired neurological impairment. Stuss et al. used a verbal self-regulation strategy in an individual with motor impersistence who could not maintain a simple motor movement over time. The patient demonstrated the ability to maintain movement during a period of active self-reminding. However, he continued to need to be cued to initiate and to maintain the self-regulation strategy.

Cicerone and Wood (1987) reported the successful treatment of a patient, four years after head injury, who exhibited impaired planning ability and poor self-control, using self-instructional procedures before and during the execution of a training task. They used a modified version of the Tower of London as a training task. Training in the self-instructional technique involved three distinct phases involving overt verbalization of the steps needed to accomplish the task, overt self-guidance, and covert internalized self-monitoring. To promote generalization following the programme, the patient was presented with a structured interpersonal problem and asked to solve it by applying principles learned in the self-instructional training. The results supported the clinical efficacy of verbal mediation training. The authors noted, however, that generalization of training occurred only after direct, extended training using real-life situations. Additional work in the use of self-instructional strategies has been carried out by Cicerone and Giacino (1992).

Burke and his colleagues (1991) described work with three people with traumatic brain injury who demonstrated problems with initiation in the workplace. In the first phase of treatment, the patient's job was broken down into a series of daily tasks which could be completed in the same order each day. During a baseline phase, a job coach provided prompts (verbal initiation cues) as to what needed to be done next. After five days of baseline, the intervention was implemented. The intervention consisted of an 'initiation checklist' (external cue) on which the day's tasks had been written in the order they needed to be completed. The job coach provided just one demonstration of how to perform the task, checked it off the initiation list, and looked at what needed to be done next. The introduction of the list reduced the amount of prompting that was required and increased the number of tasks that were completed each day. In each case, the checklists were withdrawn without deterioration in performance at a later time, suggesting that the tasks had become a matter of routine.

Some individuals with frontal system impairment may demonstrate adequate knowledge of what is going on in the environment, but show little apparent interest or involvement. Sohlberg, Sprunk and Metzelaar (1988) described an intervention with an individual who had sustained severe frontal lobe impairment and who demonstrated marked initiation problems. As a consequence, he appeared apathetic and socially unresponsive and isolated, despite a demonstrated understanding of what was going on around him. The goal of the intervention was to increase the patient's self-awareness of the behaviours involved in two types of social responding. The patient was shown to respond differentially when he was given cues for the two separate targets of self-analysis. During a group activity, the patient was provided with a cue at which time he was to ask himself whether or not he had recently initiated conversation. His verbal interactions in group during the time he received these cues increased significantly over a baseline period. An increase in verbal initiations over baseline was maintained during a posttreatment phase when cues were no longer provided. Experimental control of behaviour was demonstrated by means of comparison to another measured behaviour, response acknowledgements; these responses did not increase during the baseline or initial intervention stage, but only when response acknowledgements were specifically trained and then cued by a similar prompted self-evaluation system.

To summarize, techniques for increasing initiation and drive typically begin with a focus on providing external cues and prompts. As gains are achieved, the focus shifts to the use of more internally generated strategies and self-monitoring approaches.

Techniques for dealing with problems of disinhibition

Loss of executive skills can impair patients' ability to monitor their own performance and/or to utilize feedback to exert control over their own behaviour. Blake, Bogod and Newbigging (1995) used a discrimination training technique to provide cues for appropriate and inappropriate behaviour on a rehabilitation unit. The subject, who had sustained severe frontotemporal injury, was constantly interrupting conversations and others' work in order to speak with staff. Verbal cues and reminders about when it was appropriate to talk were not effective and only served to increase the behaviour. As an intervention, a programme was initiated in which the patient was only reinforced, by being engaged in conversation, when he approached staff members who were wearing a large green square; approaches to staff wearing a red square were ignored. The patient learned and began initiating contacts only with the appropriately tagged staff. The cues for this discrimination training initially needed to be highly salient, but were successfully reduced in size and obviousness over the training period. This intervention led to increased inhibitory control on the part of the patient, who was then less disruptive on the unit and better able to participate in the treatment programme.

Alderman and his colleagues (Alderman and Burgess, 1990; Burgess and Alderman, 1990; Alderman and Ward, 1991) have demonstrated effective use of several behaviour-modification techniques in assisting individuals to increase inhibitory control. In a response–cost paradigm, for example, the patient is given a number of tokens which are subsequently exchanged for tangible rewards. However, in the interim, whenever a targeted negative behaviour is observed, the individual is prompted to give staff one token and state the reason for its loss. The advantages of this procedure are that it facilitates directing patients' attention to aspects of their behaviour which they are not monitoring. It has been hypothesized that this technique facilitates the extraction of salient feedback from the environment, while placing a minimal load on memory. It also appears to facilitate procedural learning and increase awareness. Alderman and his colleagues (Alderman, Fry and Youngson, 1995) described greater effectiveness of a response–cost programme, as opposed to a time-out programme, in reducing inappropriate verbalizations in a brain-injured woman. Although inhibition of disruptive speech output was obtained in the institutional training environment through the response–cost technique, results did not automatically transfer to a second environment. A new programme of self-monitoring training was successfully implemented to teach inhibitory control in the new environment. This training involved teaching the woman to recognize inappropriate verbalizations and then to reduce them. The importance of keeping accurate behavioural data and carefully monitoring behavioural consequences was emphasized. These results suggested that even severe disorders of behaviour could come under specific control in patients with frontal compromise through the use of a variety of traditional behavioural management techniques. A key was drawing the individual's attention to the behaviour and to a set of consequences.

Other investigators have also emphasized the importance of drawing attention to behaviour, whether it be for the purposes of increasing or inhibiting behaviours. Fasotti, Bremer and Eling (1992) investigated the influence of text encoding on arithmetic word problem solving after frontal lobe damage. They suggested that, secondary to impulsiveness, patients with left frontal involvement tended to begin performing arithmetic operations on only the first fragment of information that catches their attention. They hypothesized that frontally impaired subjects would perform better in a cued condition designed to facilitate a more complete encoding of the text. They found that subjects with left frontal involvement benefited from cueing, whereas those with left posterior involvement did not. (Subjects with right frontal involvement were at the level of control subjects.) Despite the improvement seen with cueing in the experimental session, there was no transfer of learning to a follow-up session.

In summary, techniques for increasing inhibitory control have in common the implementation of cues and consequences which serve to slow down or halt the behaviour as well as drawing the individual's attention to the behaviour and to its consequences. As was the case for improving initiation, the clinician attempts to move from using a more external cue or manipulation to one involving the patient's self-regulated control and monitoring.

Techniques for improving attention and working memory

Many patients with frontal lobe impairments demonstrate problems with attention and concentration. They often demonstrate problems with sustained attention to task, and are likely to have difficulty with distractibility and with the smooth and effective allocation of attentional resources on more complex tasks (Van Zomeren and Brouwer, 1987, 1994). They are also likely to have difficulty shifting and dividing attention (Stuss et al., 1985; Stuss et al., 1989; Stablum et al., 1994).

Many brain-injured individuals, including those with significant frontal lobe impairment, have been shown to benefit substantially from exercise and training of attentional skills (Kewman et al., 1985; Ben-Yishay, Piasetsky and Rattok, 1987; Ethier, Baribeau and Braun, 189a; Gray and Robertson, 1989; Niemann, Ruff and Baser, 1990; Gray et al., 1992; Sturm et al., 1997). Sohlberg and Mateer (1987, 1989b) developed and evaluated the efficacy of a package of attention training materials (Attention Process Training) which was based on a hierarchical model with five levels of attention: focused, sustained, selective, alternating, and divided attention. A large set of both auditory and visual tasks designed to exercise and challenge different aspects of attention was used in treatment sessions over periods of six to eight weeks in length. The efficacy of this training in improving attentional capacities has been supported in a series of single-case designs and in group pretreatment and posttreatment comparisons (Sohlberg and

Mateer, 1987; Mateer, Sohlberg and Youngman, 1990). It was also demonstrated that improved attentional function was associated with improved anterograde memory function in individuals who received attention but not memory training (Mateer and Sohlberg, 1988; Mateer, 1992). In a recent larger scale study of 23 patients who received training with the Attention Process Training materials, gains were seen in multiple outcome measures on the Paced Auditory Serial Addition Test (Park, Proulx and Towers, 1999). These researchers have hypothesized that attention training improves working memory capacity. In another recent well controlled cross-over design study in 14 subjects, training with Attention Process Training materials improved performance on measures of executive function while a supportive placebo condition improved aspects of psychosocial function (Sohlberg et al., 1998). Finally, on a neurophysiological index using evoked potential data, subjects with traumatic brain injury showed a delayed P300 response prior to training and reduced latency following training of attentional skills (Baribeau, Ethier and Braun, 1989; Ethier, Baribeau and Braun, 1989a; Ethier, Braun and Baribeau, 1989b).

Recently, Sturm and his colleagues (1997) addressed the issue of specificity in attention training in a group of patients with lateralized focal vascular lesions. The domains of alertness, vigilance, selective attention and divided attention were evaluated, and subjects received consecutive training in the two most impaired of the four attentional domains. There were significant training effects for both alertness and vigilance; in addition, subjects demonstrated shorter response times on selection attention tasks, and reduced error rates on divided selective attention tasks. Interestingly, the study not only revealed a high degree of specific training effects, but also a substantial number of deteriorations in performance after inadequate or nonspecific training. The authors suggested a negative effect of training when the treatment focused on complex aspects of attention (e.g. selectivity training) when basic aspects of attention (e.g. alertness and/or vigilance) had not been trained. These results supported the hypothesis of a hierarchical organization of attentional functions and the need to incorporate this information into treatment paradigms.

There is growing agreement that certain aspects of attention, particularly sustained attention and working memory, can be improved with targeted training. However, questions remain about the nature and the underlying source of the change. Whereas some of the electrophysiological data cited above suggest underlying neurophysiological changes, others have argued that attention training can serve as a forum for gaining insight regarding attentional failures. Indeed, recent developments in attention training programmes have emphasized not only practice on attention tasks, but also activities which require patients to monitor and evaluate attentional failure and successes. These programmes also focus on assisting individuals to become more knowledgeable and active in managing situations so as to enhance their capacity to attend (Attention Process Training II; Sohlberg et al., 1993a). This reflects a shift to techniques which increase self-awareness and enhance a sense of self-control and mastery over cognitive weaknesses. The reader is referred to Mateer and Mapou (1996), Mateer and Raskin (1999), and Robertson (Chapter 19) for more extensive reviews of recent literature regarding the assessment and management of attentional impairments following traumatic brain injury.

Techniques for improving prospective memory

In everyday terms, memory or the act of remembering involves two different aspects: remembering what one has done and remembering what one has to do (Neisser, 1982). Individuals with frontal lobe impairment frequently fail to act on future intended actions. They may have formed an intent to do something, but at the time that the action is required they may fail to remember to act. Prospective memory, the term used to refer to this ability to 'remember to remember', requires the person to carry out a particular action at a specified time in the future based on a self-initiated and internally generated plan of action. Prospective memory can involve such practical and useful activities as remembering to take medications, remembering to make a phone call, or remembering to bring home items when shopping. This capacity may differ sharply from performance on more traditional measures of anterograde, semantic or epi-

sodic memory, which are traditionally tested by providing a cue or prompt for recall (Winograd, 1988; Dobbs and Reeves, 1996). Performance on specific prospective memory tasks has been shown to be more closely correlated with functional independence in the community than has performance on more traditional measures of cued recall (Wilson, 1991, 1992).

A number of prospective memory training studies have been conducted in brain-injured adults. The goal of prospective memory training is to increase the amount of time after an instruction that the patient can remember to carry out an action. Training typically starts with no intervening task between the instruction and the carrying out of the action; over the period of training, distracting information and/or intervening tasks are gradually added during this time interval. Sohlberg et al. (1992a) reported results from two case studies of individuals who had sustained severe closed head injuries. A 29-year-old female underwent 58 prospective memory training sessions; her performance increased from 0 per cent accuracy on a one-minute prospective memory task at the start of training to between 40 and 80 per cent accuracy on eight-minute prospective memory tasks. A 39-year-old man's ability to carry out a prospective memory task progressed from four minutes to eight minutes over the course of 32 training sessions. For both cases, the training generalized to prospective memory performance in everyday life, as family members reported improvements on tasks such as relaying telephone messages and remembering to utilize memory books. To verify that the improvements in prospective memory were due to the training efforts, Sohlberg et al. (1992b) utilized an A-B-A-B within-subject design. Gains were seen on a variety of naturalistic tasks after the treatment phases. Though still severely impaired, this patient was capable of a higher level of independence after the training. With improved prospective memory, the capacity to utilize other memory and organizational systems and to move from room to room or task to task while maintaining an intention is enhanced. Prospective memory can also be partially compensated for by systematic training in the use of memory books or daily planners/organizers (Sohlberg and Mateer, 1989b, 1989c), and/or by use of cueing devices such as watch alarms or paging systems.

In a further study using the same form of prospective memory training, Stone and Raskin (1996) used electro-physiological measures (EEG) as a measure of efficacy. Quantified EEGs were recorded in a resting state prior to initiation of the training and after the completion of the training. Two subjects showed abnormal distribution of alpha activity predominating in frontal regions prior to training. Both showed a return to a more normative posterior distribution after training, as well as improvement on treatment tasks and on generalization measures of prospective memory functioning in everyday life. Raskin (1996) also measured the classic P3, using an auditory odd-ball paradigm, before and after prospective memory training. The classic P3 is maximal at parietal sites in normal subjects, and is thought to reflect the maintenance of working memory (Polich and Kok, 1995). Two subjects with traumatic brain injury showed delayed P3 prior to training and reduced latency following training. These results suggest that prospective memory training may serve to promote recovery rather than merely teaching a compensatory skill and may, in some cases, be an important part of the treatment plan for an individual with executive function impairments.

Techniques for improving problem-solving abilities

These approaches focus on complex and integrated cognitions, skills and behaviours, such as organizing, planning, sequencing and problem solving. Von Cramon and Matthes-von Cramon (1991) described positive results in a series of patients with frontal lobe dysfunction using a training procedure which focused on assisting patients to reduce the complexity of a multi-stage problem by breaking it down into a series of manageable steps. Problem-solving training incorporated four modules. The first involved the generation of goal-directed ideas, a kind of 'brainstorming' designed to produce a variety of alternatives to a given problem. The second module involved training in systematic and careful comparison of information provided about a problem to be solved. The third consisted of tasks requiring simultaneous analysis of information from multiple sources (such as the patient comparing catalogues from several tourist offices in order to find the most favourable trip to England for a family of four). The

fourth module focused on improving the patient's abilities to draw inferences. The authors utilized short detective stories and the patients uncovered discrepancies and detected 'clues' about how crimes could have been committed. The authors reported significant psychometric as well as functional gains in a group receiving this training as opposed to a group receiving more generic memory training.

Crepeau et al. (1995) described a therapy activity designed to improve strategic time sharing on a multiple-step task in three patients with executive function compromise. The remediation technique was based on the model of executive impairment described by Shallice and Burgess (1991b) in their description of frontally impaired patients on the Six Element Task. The rationale of the approach was to reduce demands on the Supervisory Attentional System by making routine certain specific behaviours (e.g. the recording of starting and ending times on a task, or the shifting from one activity to another after a self-directed delay). Although the authors were cautious about their findings due to the small number of subjects, they did find an increased number of subtasks carried out (suggesting greater flexibility), and a decrease in time allocated to one subtask (suggesting improved strategy application). In addition, one subject demonstrated improved ability to monitor time passage and one demonstrated a decrease in rule breaking.

Although many rehabilitation programmes incorporate exercises designed to work on everyday problem-solving skills (e.g. finding/following a bus route, finding information from a telephone directory, planning an event or activity), there is little evidence reported to date that these sorts of activities generalize to other contexts or settings, or how they might best be structured and delivered. Depending on whether functional problems on such tasks are related to memory problems, distractibility, impulsivity, poor prospective memory or other factors, the most effective approaches to dealing with the problems may be quite different.

Techniques for facilitating self-awareness

Insight, self-awareness and self-regulatory capacity are felt to reflect the highest level of frontal lobe activity (Prigatano, 1991; Stuss, 1991a). In the field of rehabilitation, awareness usually refers to the ability of patients to possess knowledge about their deficits and to understand the implications of these deficits. As many people with frontal lobe damage demonstrate limited awareness of and insight into their difficulties, they often have limited motivation to comply with, or apparent investment in, therapy (Fleming et al., 1996). Motivation has been found to be related to successful outcome in rehabilitation (Herbert and Powell, 1989), as has involvement of the brain-injured person in setting goals for the rehabilitation programme (Bergquist and Jacket, 1993). Thus, treatment in this area presents a tremendous challenge for the rehabilitation professional.

The documentation and measurement of deficits in awareness remain problematic. Several researchers have compared patients' ratings of their difficulties with the ratings of rehabilitation staff (Fordyce and Roueche, 1986; Prigatano and Altman, 1990; Godfrey et al., 1993), and found that underestimation of abilities by patients with traumatic brain injury is fairly common. Patients seem to be in agreement with relatives when rating their abilities to perform certain routine self-care activities but not when rating cognitive abilities such as memory (Oddy et al., 1985), or their behaviours in more complex social situations (e.g. noting when they have said something to upset someone, controlling their temper, handling arguments) (Prigatano, Altman and O'Brien, 1990).

Making judgements about the self must involve combining objective information concerning external reality with subjective information about inner experience. Kihlstrom and Tobias (1991) suggest that brain-injured individuals may lack the ability to benefit from personal experience in order to construct their own ideas about their abilities. Certainly, many theories about the mechanisms of awareness imply an organic cause of the inability to be aware of or to monitor one's behaviour. However, this lack of awareness has also been seen as an adaptation in some patients who may be unable to cope with their disability. Crosson and colleagues (1989) define psychological denial as a subconscious process that spares the patient the psychological pain of accepting the serious consequences of a brain injury and its unwanted effects on everyday life. It is likely that defensive denial plays a role in some 'unawareness' phenomena exhibited by some patients with brain damage. In many cases, emotional and moti-

vational factors may interact with organically produced unawareness to produce a very complicated symptom picture.

Awareness training can take a variety of forms. Usually, a direct approach is taken such that patients are given didactic information about the nature of their injury, the way in which it affects their behaviour, and the reasons why a particular behaviour is or is not appropriate or acceptable. Such information may help patients to perceive the reasons for disparate ratings of behaviour carried out by themselves and their significant others and to see some of the ways that the deficit is impacting their life and those around them. Although sometimes helpful and often necessary, such didactic training is usually not sufficient to bring about the desirable change in behaviour (Crosson et al., 1989).

One approach to increasing self-awareness is to inform patients that they exhibit a particular behaviour, be it desirable or undesirable (e.g. escalating to a loud voice, limited eye contact). Patients are then told to mark a piece of paper every time they exhibit the behaviour during a designated time period. This recording can be done during a spontaneous conversation, in a one-on-one session, or during a group session. The clinician simultaneously keeps track of the behaviour; videotapes may be made as an additional source of information. The patients' awareness may be increased by comparing their observations with those of the clinician or observed on a tape. Quantitative feedback and encouraging patients to draw a graph of their own scores may help them to see improvement (Klonoff et al., 1989). The more familiar and quantifiable the task, the more likely it is that awareness of the deficit and its implications will be achieved (Langer and Padrone, 1992). Heightening of awareness is often a first step in implementing cognitive–behavioural interventions focusing on such self-regulatory abilities as anger management and self-management of anxiety and stress. Once individuals are aware of the internal and external cues that trigger or signal emotional states, they can begin to use self-regulatory strategies for self-management.

In supported risk taking or planned failure, patients attempt to do something they believe is within their capabilities; patients are then provided with a supportive environment in which to experience and process the failure. Godfrey and colleagues (1993) provide evidence that the onset of emotional dysfunction often coincides with increased awareness of deficits and their implications. Langer and Padrone (1992) suggest that when unawareness is neuropsychologically based, the therapist should work on building structures to support knowledge. As awareness increases and/or when emotional denial is prominent, therapeutic intervention should strengthen the patient's ego functions and coping skills. Confronting the denial head-on may result only in withdrawal and frustration. Given a strong therapeutic alliance, the person who has demonstrated prominent levels of unawareness may begin to question the therapist and to begin to integrate honest feedback. Supportive counselling in both individual and group therapy can play an important role in assisting patients to develop realistic self-appraisals and rebuild self-esteem. Exercises designed to achieve a more balanced perspective, and to begin to use language that reflects more realistic statements about the self, can be usefully incorporated into treatment with individuals who present with rigid or black-and-white thinking. Ponsford, Sloan and Snow (1995) state that the ultimate goal of therapy is the attainment of some degree of acceptance, and an ability to like the 'new' person who has survived the injury. With respect to executive functioning, the capacity for self-awareness and reflectiveness is thought to represent the highest level of ability. Increasing self-awareness can have a significant impact in that it may open the door for the implementation of many self-regulatory strategies and techniques. Given the importance of awareness to the process of rehabilitation, it is imperative that researchers develop more comprehensive conceptualizations of self-awareness and a wider range of approaches to the assessment of this construct. Only then will a wider range of, and more effective, interventions for individuals with limitations in self-awareness be developed.

Conclusions

Individuals with executive function compromise present with a myriad of challenges to effective functioning in social, cognitive and behavioural domains. Although the study of executive function has often focused on higher level organizational and planning difficulties, these problems are often secondary to underlying disorders of component systems involving initiation, inhibition, working memory, prospective memory and awareness. The rehabilitation literature has begun to document the effectiveness of a variety of approaches designed to address impairments in each of these areas. Both complex, overarching abilities and basic elements/components of executive control can be targeted for intervention. In general, intervention for individuals with these disorders begins with techniques to manipulate the saliency of external cues and the implementation of behavioural strategies, and moves to a focus on techniques which are designed to establish and maintain internally focused self-regulatory control. The process of rehabilitation can be seen as a strategic and structured shift of responsibility from the therapist/caretaker to the individual. Intervention techniques are selected to assist the individual in moving from a relatively dependent, externally supported state to a more independent, internally directed state. This continuum is particularly relevant to, and evident in, the rehabilitation of executive functions.

References

Alderman, N. and Burgess, P.W. 1990. Integrating cognition and behaviour: a pragmatic approach to brain injury rehabilitation. In *Cognitive Rehabilitation in Perspective*, ed. R.L. Wood and I. Fussey, pp. 204–28. Basingstoke: Taylor Francis.

Alderman, N., Fry, R.K. and Youngson, H.A. 1995. Improvement of self-monitoring skills, reduction of behaviour disturbance and the dysexecutive syndrome: comparison of response cost and a new programme of self-monitoring training. *Neuropsychol Rehabil* 5(3), 193–221.

Alderman, N. and Ward, A. 1991. Behavioural treatment of the dysexecutive syndrome: reduction of repetitive speech using response cost and cognitive overlearning. *Neuropsychol Rehabil* 1, 65–80.

Baddeley, A.D. 1996. Exploring the central executive. *Q J Exp Psychol A* 49, 5–28.

Baribeau, J., Ethier, M. and Braun, C. 1989. A neurophysiological assessment of attention before and after cognitive remediation in patients with severe closed head injury. *J Neurol Rehabil* 3, 71–92.

Ben-Yishay, Y., Piasetsky, E.B. and Rattok, J. 1987. A systematic method for ameliorating disorders in basic attention. In *Neuropsychological Rehabilitation*, ed. M.J. Meyer, A.L.

Benton, and L. Diller, pp. 165–81. Edinburgh: Churchill Livingstone.

Bergquist, T.F. and Jacket, M.P. 1993. Awareness and goal setting with the traumatically brain injured. *Brain Inj* **7**, 275–82.

Blake, G., Bogod, N.M. and Newbigging, T. 1995. Establishing stimulus control over the attention seeking behaviors of a memory impaired, brain injured adult. Presented at meeting of the International Applied Behavioral Analysis Conference, Washington, DC.

Borkowski, J. and Muthukrishna, N. 1992. Moving cognition into the classroom: 'working models' and effective strategy teaching. In *Promoting Academic Competency and Literacy in School*, ed. M. Pressley, K.R. Harris, and J. Guthrie, pp. 477–501. San Diego: Academic Press.

Burgess, P.W. and Alderman, N. 1990. Rehabilitation of dyscontrol syndromes following frontal lobe damage: a cognitive neuropsychological approach. In *Cognitive Rehabilitation in Perspective*, ed. R. Li. Wood and I. Fussey, pp. 183–203. London: Taylor & Francis.

Burke, W.H., Zenicus, A.H., Wesolowski, M.D. and Doubleday, F. 1991. Improving executive function disorders in brain-injured clients. *Brain Inj* **5**, 25–8.

Cicerone, K.D. and Giacino, J.T. 1992. Remediation of executive function deficits after traumatic brain injury. *Neuropsychol Rehabil* **2**, 12–22.

Cicerone, K.D. and Wood, J.C. 1987. Planning disorder after closed head injury: a case study. *Arch Phys Med Rehabil* **68**, 111–15.

Cockburn, J. 1996. Failure of prospective memory after acquired brain damage: preliminary investigation and suggestions for future research. *J Clin Exp Neuropsychol* **18**, 304–9.

Craine, S.F. 1982. The retraining of frontal lobe dysfunction. In *Cognitive Rehabilitation: Conceptualization and Intervention*, ed. L.E. Trexler, New York: Plenum Press.

Crepeau, F., DeCourcy, R., Scherzer, P. and Charette, G. 1995. Toward a remediation approach to improve strategic time-sharing. Poster presented at the Baycrest Conference on Frontal Lobe Functions. Toronto.

Crosson, B., Crosser, B., Barco, P.P., Velozo, C.A. et al. 1989. Awareness and compensation in post-acute head injury rehabilitation. *J Head Trauma Rehabil* **4**, 46–54.

Dempster, F.N. 1991. Inhibitory processes: a neglected dimension of intelligence. *Intelligence* **15**, 157–73.

Dempster, F.N. 1993. Resistance to interference: developmental changes in a basic processing mechanism. In *Emerging Themes in Cognitive Development*, ed. M.L. Howe and R. Pasnak, pp. 3–27. New York: Springer Verlag.

Diamond, A. 1988. Abilities and neural mechanisms underlying AB performance. *Child Dev* **59**, 523–7.

Dobbs, A.R. and Reeves, M.B. 1996. Prospective memory: more than memory. In *Prospective Memory: Theory and Applications*, ed. M. Brandimonte, G.O. Einstein and M.A. McDaniel, pp. 199–222. Mahwah: Lawrence Erlbaum Associates.

Duffy, J.D. and Campbell, J.J. 1994. The regional prefrontal syndromes: a theoretical and clinical overview. *J Neuropsychiatry* **6**, 379–87.

Duncan, J. 1995. Attention, intelligence, and the frontal lobes. In *The Cognitive Neurosciences*, ed. M.S. Gazzaniga, pp. 721–33. Cambridge, MA: MIT Press.

Dywan, J. and Segalowitz, J. 1996. Self- and family ratings of adaptive behavior after traumatic brain injury: psychometric scores and frontally generated ERPs. *J Head Trauma Rehabil* **11**, 79–95.

Ethier, M., Baribeau, J.M.C. and Braun, C.M.J. 1989a. Computer-dispensed cognitive–perceptual training of closed head injury patients after spontaneous recovery. Study 2: non-speeded tasks. *Can J Rehabil* **3**, 7–16.

Ethier, M., Braun, C.M.J. and Baribeau, J.M.C. 1989b. Computer-dispensed cognitive–perceptual training of closed head injury patients after spontaneous recovery. Study 1: speeded tasks. *Can J Rehabil* **2**, 223–33.

Fasotti, L., Bremer, J.J.C.B. and Eling, P.A.T.M. 1992. Influence of improved text encoding on arithmetical work problem-solving after frontal lobe damage. *Neuropsychol Rehabil* **2**, 3–20.

Fleming, J.M., Strong, J. and Ashton, R. 1996. Self-awareness of deficits in adults with traumatic brain injury: how best to measure? *Brain Inj* **10**, 1–15.

Fordyce, D.J. and Roueche, J.R. 1986. Changes in perspective of disability among patients, staff, and relatives during rehabilitation of brain injury. *Rehabil Psychol* **31**, 217–29.

Frith, C.D. 1987. The positive and negative symptoms of schizophrenia reflect impairments in the perception and initiation of action. *Psychol Med* **17**, 631–48.

Frith, C.D., Friston, K., Liddle, P.F. and Frackowiak, R.S.J. 1991. Willed action and the prefrontal cortex in man: a study with PET. *Proc R Soc Lond B* **244**, 241–6.

Fuster, J.M. 1989. *The Prefrontal Cortex: Anatomy, Physiology, and Neuropsychology of the Frontal Lobe*, 2nd edn. New York: Raven Press.

Gervin, A.P. 1991. Music therapy compensatory technique using song lyrics during dressing to promote independence in the patient with brain injury. *Music Ther Persp* **9**, 87–90.

Geyer, S. 1989. *Training Executive Function Skills*. Puyallup, WA: Good Samaritan Hospital.

Giles, G.G. and Clarke-Wilson, J. 1988. The use of behavioral techniques in functional skills training after severe brain injury. *Am J Occup Ther* **42**, 658–65.

Godfrey, H.P.D., Patridge, F.M., Knight, R.G. and Bishara, S. 1993. Course of insight disorder and emotional dysfunction following closed head injury: a controlled cross-sectional follow-up study. *J Clin Exp Neuropsychol* **15**, 503–15.

Goldman-Rakic, P.S. 1987. Circuitry of primate prefrontal cortex and regulation of behavior by representational memory. *Hdbk Physiol – Nerv Sys* **5**, 373–417.

Graham, S. and Harris, K.R. 1989. A components analysis of cognitive strategy instruction: effects on learning disabled students' compositions and self-efficacy. *J Educ Psychol* **81**, 353–61.

Gray, J.M. and Robertson, I. 1989. Remediation of attentional difficulties following brain injury: three experimental single case designs. *Brain Inj* **3**, 163–70.

Gray, J.M., Robertson, I., Pentland, B. and Anderson, S. 1992. Microcomputer-based attentional retraining after brain damage: a randomised group controlled trial. *Neuropsychol Rehabil* **2**, 97–115.

Harris, K.R. 1990. Developing self-regulated learners: the role of private speech and self-instructions. *Educ Psychol* **25**, 35–50.

Herbert, C.M. and Powell, G.E. 1989. Insight and progress in rehabilitation. *Clin Rehabil* **3**, 125–30.

Ishii, N., Nishihara, Y. and Imamura, T. 1986. Why do frontal lobe symptoms predominate in vascular dementia with lacunes? *Neurology* **36**, 340–5.

Jouandet, M. and Gazzaniga, M.S. 1979. The frontal lobes. In *Handbook of Behavioral Neurology*. Vol. 2 *Neuropsychology*, ed. M.S. Gazzaniga, pp. 25–59. New York: Plenum Press.

Kewman, D.G., Seigerman, C., Kinter, H., Chu, S., Henson, D. and Reeder, C. 1985. Stimulation and training of psychomotor skills: teaching the brain-injured to drive. *Rehabil Psychol* **30**, 11–27.

Kihlstrom, J.F. and Tobias, B.A. 1991. Anosognosia, consciousness, and the self. In *Awareness of Deficits After Brain Injury*, ed. G.P. Prigatano and D.L. Schacter, pp. 198–222. New York: Oxford University Press.

Klonoff, P.S., O'Brien, K.P., Prigatano, G.P., Chiapello, D.A. and Cunningham, M. 1989. Cognitive retraining after traumatic brain injury and its role in facilitating awareness. *J Head Trauma Rehabil* **4**, 37–45.

Knight, R.T. and Grabowecky, M. 1995. Escape from linear time: prefrontal cortex and conscious experience. In *The Cognitive Neurosciences*, ed. M.S. Gazzaniga, pp. 1357–71. Cambridge, MA: MIT Press.

Lam, C.S., McMahon, B.T., Priddy, D.A. and Gehred-Schultz, A. 1988. Deficit awareness and treatment performance among traumatic head injury adults. *Brain Inj* **2**, 235–42.

Langer, K.G. and Padrone, F.J. 1992. Psychotherapeutic treatment of awareness in acute rehabilitation of traumatic brain injury. *Neuropsychol Rehabil* **2**, 59–70.

Lezak, M. 1982. The problem of assessing executive functions. *Int J Psychol* **17**, 281–97.

Lezak, M. 1993. Newer contributions to the neuropsychological assessment of executive functions. *J Head Trauma Rehabil* **8**(1), 24–31.

Liddle, P.F. 1993. The psychomotor disorders: disorders of the supervisory mental processes. *Behav Neurol* **6**, 5–14.

Luria, A.R. 1966. *Higher Cortical Functions in Man.* London: Tavistock.

Mateer, C.A. 1992. Systems of care for post-concussive syndrome. In *Rehabilitation of Post-Concussive Disorders*, ed. L.J. Horn and N.D. Zasler, pp. 143–60. Philadelphia: Henley & Belfus.

Mateer, C.A. 1997. Rehabilitation of individuals with frontal lobe impairment. In *Neuropsychological Rehabilitation: Fundamentals, Innovations and Directions*, ed. J. Leon-Carrion, pp. 285–300. Delray Beach, FL: GR/St Lucie Press.

Mateer, C.A. and Mapou, R. 1996. Assessment and management of attentional disorders following closed head injury. *J Head Trauma Rehabil* **11**, 1–16.

Mateer, C.A. and Raskin, S. 1999. Cognitive rehabilitation. In *Rehabilitation of the Adult and Child with Traumatic Brain Injury*, 3rd edn., ed. M. Rosenthal, E.R. Griffith, J.S. Kreutzer and B. Pentland. Philadelphia: F.A. Davis Company. (In press.)

Mateer, C.A. and Sohlberg, M.M. 1988. A paradigm shift in memory rehabilitation. In *Neuropsychological Studies of Nonfocal Brain Injury: Dementia and Closed Head Injury*, ed. H. Whitaker, pp. 202–25. New York: Springer-Verlag.

Mateer, C.A., Sohlberg, M.M. and Youngman, P. 1990. The management of acquired attentional and memory disorders following mild closed head injury. In *Cognitive Rehabilitation in Perspective*, ed. R. Wood, pp. 68–95. London: Taylor and Francis.

Meichenbaum, D. 1977. *Cognitive Behavior Modification: an Integrative Approach.* New York: Plenum Press.

Meier, M., Benton, A. and Diller, L. 1987. *Neurophysiological Rehabilitation.* New York: Guilford Press.

Neisser, H. 1982. *Memory Observed: Remembering in Natural Contexts.* San Francisco: W.H. Freeman.

Niemann, H., Ruff, R.M. and Baser, C.A. 1990. Computer assisted attention training in head injured individuals: a controlled efficacy study of an outpatient program. *J Clin Consult Psychol* **58**, 811–17.

Oddy, M., Coughlan, T., Tyerman, A. and Jenkins, D. 1985. Social adjustment after closed head injury: a further follow-up seven years after injury. *J Neurol Neurosurg Psychiatry* **48**, 564–8.

Park, N.W., Proulx, G.B. and Towers, W. in press. Evaluation of the Attention Process Training Program. *Neuropsych Rehab* (in press).

Polich, J. and Kok, A. 1995. Cognitive and biological determinants of P300: an integrative review. *Biol Psychol* **41**, 103–46.

Ponsford, J., Sloan, S. and Snow, P. 1995. *Traumatic Brain Injury: Rehabilitation for Everyday Adaptive Living*. East Sussex: Lawrence Erlbaum.

Prigatano, G.P. 1991. Disturbances of self-awareness of deficit after traumatic brain injury. In *Awareness of Deficit after Brain Injury: Clinical and Theoretical Perspectives*, ed. G.P. Prigatano and D.L. Schacter, pp. 111–26. New York: Oxford University Press.

Prigatano, G.P. and Altman, I.M. 1990. Impaired awareness of behavioral limitations after traumatic brain injury. *Arch Phys Med* **71**, 1058–62.

Prigatano, G.P., Altman, I.M. and O'Brien, K.P. 1990. Behavioral limitations traumatic brain injured patients tend to underestimate. *Clin Neuropsychol* **4**, 163–76.

Raskin, S. 1996. P300 as a measure of brain reorganization following cognitive rehabilitation. Poster presented at the Cognitive Neuroscience Society Meetings. San Francisco, CA.

Robertson, I.H. 1999. Theory-driven neuropsychological rehabilitation: the role of attention and competition in recovery of function after brain damage. In *Attention and Performance XVII*, ed. D. Gopher and A. Koriat, Cambridge, MA: MIT Press.

Royall, D.R., Mahurin, R.K. and Gray, K.F. 1992. Bedside assessment of executive dyscontrol: the Executive Interview (EXIT). *J Am Geriatr Soc* **40**, 1221–6.

Schwartz, M.F. 1995. Re-examining the role of executive functions in routine action production. *Ann NY Acad Sci* **769**, 321–35.

Schwartz, M.F., Mayer, N.H., FitzpatrickDeSalma, E.J. and Montgomery, M.W. 1993. *J Head Trauma Rehabil* **8**, 59–72.

Shallice, T. and Burgess, P.W. 1991a. Higher-order cognitive impairments and frontal-lobe lesions in man. In *Frontal Lobe Function and Injury*, ed. H. Levin, H.M. Eisenberg, and A.L. Benton, pp. 125–38. Oxford: Oxford University Press.

Shallice, T. and Burgess, P.W. 1991b. Deficits in strategy application following frontal lobe damage in man. *Brain* **114**, 727–41.

Sohlberg, M.M. 1992. *Manual for the Profile of Executive Control System*. Puyallup, WA: Association for Neuropsychological Research and Development.

Sohlberg, M.M., Johnson, L., Paule, L., Raskin, S.A. and Mateer, C.A. 1993a. *Attention Process Training-II: a Program to Address Attentional Deficits for Persons with Mild Cognitive Dysfunction*. Puyallup, WA: Association for Neuropsychological Research and Development.

Sohlberg, M.M. and Mateer, C.A. 1987. Effectiveness of an attention training program. *J Clin Exp Neuropsychol* **19**, 117–30.

Sohlberg, M.M. and Mateer, C.A. 1989a. *Prospective Memory Screening*. Puyallup, WA: Association for Neuropsychological Research and Development.

Sohlberg, M.M. and Mateer, C.A. 1989b. *Introduction to Cognitive Rehabilitation: Theory and Practice*. New York: Guilford Press.

Sohlberg, M.M. and Mateer, C.A. 1989c. Training use of compensatory memory books: a three stage behavioral approach. *J Clin Exp Neuropsychol* **11**, 871–91.

Sohlberg, M.M., Mateer, C.A. and Stuss, D.T. 1993b. Contemporary approaches to the management of executive control dysfunction. *J Head Trauma Rehabil* **8**(1), 45–58.

Sohlberg, M.M., McLoughlin, K.A., Pavese, A., Heidrich, A. and Posner, M.I. 1998. *Evaluation of Attention Process Training in Persons with Acquired Brain Injury*. Technical Report No. 98–08, pp. 1–69. Oregon: University of Oregon, Institute of Cognitive and Decision Services.

Sohlberg, M.M., Sprunk, H. and Metzelaar, K. 1988. Efficacy of an external cueing system in an individual with severe frontal lobe damage. *Cogn Rehabil* **6**, 36–40.

Sohlberg, M.M., White, O., Evans, E. and Mateer, C.A. 1992a. Background and initial case studies into the effects of prospective memory training. *Brain Inj* **5**, 129–38.

Sohlberg, M.M., White, O., Evans, E. and Mateer, C.A. 1992b. An investigation of the effects of prospective memory training. *Brain Inj* **5**, 139–54.

Stablum, F., Leonardi, G., Mazzoldi, M., Unilta, C. and Morra, S. 1994. Attention and control deficits following closed head injury. *Cortex* **30**, 603–18.

Stone, S. and Raskin, S. 1996. Training prospective memory in an individual with anoxic brain damage. Poster presented at the International Neuropsychology Society Meetings, Chicago, IL.

Sturm, W., Willmes, K., Orgass, B. and Hartje, W. 1997. Do specific attention deficits need specific training? *Neurophysiol Rehab* **7**, 81–103.

Stuss, D.T. 1991a. Self, awareness and the frontal lobes: a neuropsychological perspective. In *The Self: an Interdisciplinary Approach*, ed. J. Strauss and G.R. Goethals, pp. 255–78. New York: Springer-Verlag.

Stuss, D.T. 1991b. Interference effects on memory functions in postleukotomy patients: an attentional perspective. In *Frontal Lobe Function and Dysfunction*, ed. H.S. Levin, H.M. Eisenberg and A.L. Benton, pp. 157–72. New York: Oxford University Press.

Stuss, D.T. and Benson, D.F. 1986. *The Frontal Lobes*. New York: Raven Press.

Stuss, D.T. and Benson, D.F. 1987. The frontal lobes and control of cognition and memory. In *The Frontal Lobes Revisited*, ed. E. Perecman, pp. 141–54. New York: IRBN Press.

Stuss, D.T., Delgado, M. and Guzman, D.A. 1987. Verbal regulation in the control of motor impersistence. *J Neurol Rehabil* **1**, 19–24.

Stuss, D.T., Ely, P., Hugenholtz, H. et al. 1985. Subtle neuropsychological deficits in patients with good recovery after closed head injury. *Neurosurgery* **17**, 41–7.

Stuss, D.T., Mateer, C.A. and Sohlberg, M.M. 1994. Innovative approaches to frontal lobe deficits. In *Brain Injury Rehabilitation: Clinical Considerations*, ed. A. Finlayson and S. Garner, pp. 212–37. Baltimore, MD.: Williams & Wilkins.

Stuss, D.T., Shallice, T., Alexander, M.P. and Picton, T.W. 1995. A multidisciplinary approach to anterior attentional functions. *Ann NY Acad Sci* **769**, 191–212.

Stuss, D.T., Stethem, L.L., Hugenholtz, H., Picton, T., Pivik, J. and Richard, M.T. 1989. Reaction time after head injury: fatigue, divided and focused attention, and consistency of performance. *J Neurol Neurosurg Psychiatry* **52**, 742–8.

Tranel, D., Anderson, S.W. and Benton, A. 1994. Development of the concept of 'executive function' and its relationship to the frontal lobes. In *Handbook of Neuropsychology*, Vol. 9, ed. F. Boller and J. Grafman, pp. 125–48. Amsterdam: Elsevier.

Van Zomeren, A.H. and Brouwer, W.H. 1987. Head injury and concepts of attention. In *Neurobehavioral Recovery from Head Injury*, ed. H.J. Levin, J. Grafman and H.M. Eisenberg, pp. 398–415. New York: Oxford University Press.

Van Zomeren, A.H. and Brouwer, W.H. 1994. *Clinical Neuropsychology of Attention*. New York: Oxford University Press.

Von Cramon, D.Y., Matthes-von Cramon, G. and Mai, N. 1991. Problem solving deficits in brain injured patients: a therapeutic approach. *Neuropsychol Rehabil* **1**, 45–64.

West, R.L. 1996. An application of prefrontal cortex function theory to cognitive aging. *Psychol Bull* **120**, 272–92.

Wilson, B. 1991. Long-term prognosis of patients with severe memory disorders. *Neuropsychol Rehabil* **1**, 117–34.

Wilson, B. 1992. Recovery and compensatory strategies in head injured memory impaired people several years after insult. *J Neurology Neurosurg Psychiatry* **55**, 177–80.

Wilson, B.A., Alderman, N., Burgess, P.W., Emslie, H.C. and Evans, J.J. 1996. *The Behavioural Assessment of the Dysexecutive Syndrome*. Bury St Edmunds, Suffolk: Thames Valley Test Company.

Wilson, B.A., Cockburn, J. and Halligan, P. 1985. *The Rivermead Everyday Memory Test*. Bury St Edmunds, Suffolk: Thames Valley Test Company.

Winograd, E. 1988. Some observations on prospective remembering. In *Practical Aspects of Memory: Current Research and Issues*, Vol. 1, *Memory in Everyday Life*, ed. M.M. Gruneberg, P.E. Morris and R.N. Sykes, pp. 348–53. Chichester: John Wiley & Sons.

Wood, R.L.I. 1987. *Brain Injury Rehabilitation: a Neurobehavioural Approach*. London: Croom Helm.

21

Memory rehabilitation in brain-injured people

Barbara A. Wilson

Introduction

Unlike the study of memory itself, or the interest shown in memory performance and the effects of loss of memory, there has been, until quite recently, little scientific enquiry into the remediation or amelioration of memory problems after brain injury. Neither has there been much effort, prior to the mid 1980s, to relate theory to the practical experiences of memory-impaired people, or vice versa.

With less than two decades of real interest from a section of the scientific community, memory rehabilitation has nevertheless made significant strides towards providing solutions to many of the everyday problems faced by memory-impaired people. Publications such as *Clinical Management of Memory Problems* (Wilson and Moffat, 1984, 1992), *Memory Rehabilitation for Closed Head Injured Patients* (Berg, 1993), and 'A practical framework for understanding compensatory behaviour in people with organic memory impairment' (Wilson and Watson, 1996) have attempted to provide practical guidelines for managing memory problems. These texts have been supported by a theoretical framework that is itself little more than the shaky beginnings of a scaffolding. Faced by very large numbers of memory-impaired people requiring assistance in their daily lives, memory rehabilitation workers have, out of necessity, continued to invent and develop new programmes that have been tested and, of these, some have been confirmed as effective in remediating or ameliorating some of the burdens confronted daily by brain-injured people. With this developing body of work to guide them, workers in memory rehabilitation can look forward to further improvements in this field resulting from the combined efforts of practitioners and academic theorists who are also keen to see their work bearing fruit in the world beyond book shelves.

It is the intention in this chapter to describe the various guidelines that have been established during the past two decades of memory rehabilitation, and to highlight any practical success that has been achieved. Reference is made to the role of theory in those cases in which it has been shown that its influence has led to improvement in the management of memory problems. It is hoped that some of the guidelines and descriptions of memory impairment in practice provided will encourage readers to apply a theoretical critique that in itself might encourage further debate of a positive kind.

There have been three major approaches to memory rehabilitation in recent years, and these can be summarized as involving: (1) environmental adaptations, (2) new learning, and (3) new technology. The contribution of each of these is described in the following pages, followed by a description of a group of other strategies that in themselves do not form a major approach but are nevertheless important additions to the store of methods that can be implemented by the rehabilitation therapist. The chapter concludes with a section dealing with memory therapy as the author sees it in practice.

Environmental adaptations

- People whose memory systems have ceased to function adequately can be helped to meet the demands of daily living by restructuring their environment.

- Behaviour modification suggests that it is possible to change a situation which, if left unaltered, would continue to stimulate undesirable or unhelpful behaviour.
- Although environmental control is open to abuse if its restrictions merely obliterate the need for intellectual functioning, it may, when used properly, offer the only solution to some severely intellectually impaired people.

Kolb (1995) notes that animals (and probably humans) brought up in unstimulating environments do less well at cognitive tasks than those brought up in stimulating environments. This unsurprising observation can be applied to the environment in which memory-impaired people find themselves, and this chapter describes the modification or restructuring of environments to enable people to cope with the sophisticated demands of daily living without trying to rely upon memory systems that have ceased to function adequately to meet those demands.

Some designers have recognized that the correct use of any object should be so obvious that users will find it almost impossible to make an error. Turning on cookers and showers or opening doors and boxes are examples that Norman (1988) discusses in his stimulating book which puts forward the idea that knowledge should be in the world and not in the head. By this, he means that good ergonomic design would avoid problems with cookers, showers, doors and so forth. Norman's ideas can be extended to help people with organic memory impairment. For example, clients can be provided with kettles, cookers and electric lights which turn themselves off after a certain interval, thereby avoiding dangers for those who are very forgetful. Many memory-impaired people forget where domestic objects are kept in the home and frequently cannot remember which room is which in their own house. Labelling cupboards and doors is a very effective way of making the environment more easily remembered by these people. Even directions within the house can be hard to follow for some memory-impaired people, so signposts appropriately positioned, or even arrows directing people from, for instance, the dining room to the garden can be of help.

Positioning objects so they cannot be missed is also worth trying. For example, clipping a notebook to a waist-belt or using a neck cord for spectacles will prevent people from leaving them in some place soon forgotten. It may be possible to reduce or eliminate repetitive behaviour by identifying and eliminating environmental situations or verbal questions that trigger repetitions.

The environmental adaptation model argues for the avoidance of problems that arise because of memory impairment. Gross and Schutz (1986) called this the environmental control model, the origins of which can be found within the discipline of behaviour modification. Murphy and Oliver (1987) remind us that restructuring the environment is a useful procedure for decreasing undesirable behaviour in people with developmental learning disabilities. They say that the operant view of behaviour is that it is determined by both consequences and antecedents. If it becomes clear that undesirable behaviour occurs in one situation, it may be possible to modify that situation in order to prevent the behaviour reoccurring. Although this can be a very rapid and effective way of eradicating or reducing such behaviours, it is not always possible to achieve. There is also an ethical argument against a methodology that might involve undue restriction to a point at which, let us say, the environment is made so restrictive that no demands are made upon memory at all, and the memory-impaired person is never required to exercise his or her powers of memory however much they may be weakened. Like many psychiatric and psychological methods of management, environmental control is open to abuse. Nevertheless, there is little doubt that for many severely intellectually impaired people, environmental control is their best chance of obtaining some degree of independence. For example, one woman with anoxic brain damage lives in a health authority home where her day is structured to the extent that staff tell her when to get up, when to get washed, and when to go to the day room, etc. She lives quite happily in these circumstances, with the staff acting as an environmental substitute for her damaged memory. Kapur (1995) also addresses the issue of environmental memory aids. One of the most exciting developments in environmental control is the designing of 'smart' houses in which technology is used to disable the disabling environment, and these are considered in more detail in the next section.

New learning

- Memory-impaired people need to learn new information, and studies show that it is possible to use well-documented strategies that enhance, for example, the learning of names.
- Certain strategies from the field of study techniques and learning disability have been used successfully in neuropsychological rehabilitation.
- Errorless learning has proved to be an effective way to teach new skills to people with learning difficulties.
- It is suggested that one reason for failures and anomalies in implicit learning studies when applied to memory-impaired people is that implicit learning is poor at eliminating errors.
- A number of recent studies are quoted to show that amnesic subjects learn better when they are prevented from making mistakes during the learning process.
- Further studies are required to assess whether errorless learning is more effective when combined with expanding rehearsal, and whether the errorless learning advantage is maintained over time.

Although external aids and environmental adaptations can be of great assistance to the memory-impaired person, it is unlikely that they will offer sufficient support throughout all the demands of daily living. Memory-impaired people need to learn new information on certain occasions. For example, although people's names can be written down in a notebook, reference to the notebook would not help in a normal social setting when people need to be greeted by name. Referring to a notebook in such a situation would seriously affect natural communication and also be embarrassing. While it is true that learning names is particularly difficult for people with organic memory impairment, there are a number of studies showing that it is possible to teach names to amnesic people using strategies that enhance learning. Wilson (1987) evaluated the strategy of visual imagery to teach names and demonstrated that it is virtually always superior to rote repetition. Thoene and Glisky (1995) also found visual imagery superior to other methods for teaching people's names to amnesic subjects. More recently, Clare et al. (1999) were able to teach a 74-year-old man in the early stages of Alzheimer's disease the names of his colleagues at a social club. They used a combination of strategies, including finding a distinctive feature of the face together with backward chaining and expanding rehearsal. For example, one of the subject's colleagues was named Sylvia and this name was learned using a combination of all three methods described above. The distinctive feature selected was her silvery hair, which the subject was asked to associate with the name Sylvia. At the same time, backward chaining was employed so that the subject was given written versions of his colleague's name with progressively more letters omitted, as in the following example: SYLVIA, SYLVI_, SYLV_, and so on. The subject completed the missing letters and eventually learned the name without any cues. These two strategies were combined with expanding rehearsal, otherwise known as spaced retrieval, in which the information to be remembered is first presented, then tested immediately, tested again after a very brief delay, tested again after a slightly longer delay and so on. This is a form of distributed practice described in the introduction and is a fairly powerful learning strategy in memory rehabilitation (Lorge, 1930, as cited in Johnson and Solso, 1971; Baddeley and Longman, 1978). The method of expanding rehearsal owes much to the work of Landauer and Bjork (1978). Clare et al.'s patient learned the names of his colleagues using photographs in his memory therapy sessions, and demonstrated generalization by greeting his colleagues by name at a social club. The results can be seen in Fig. 21.1.

Certain strategies from the field of study techniques (e.g. Robinson, 1970), and learning disability (e.g. Yule and Carr, 1987) have been used in neuropsychological rehabilitation (Wilson, 1991), and work along these lines continues to be applied in the search for improved methods of learning. One series of potentially important studies in recent years has involved errorless learning. This is a method for teaching new skills to people with learning difficulties (Sidman and Stoddard, 1967; Jones and Eayrs, 1992), but until quite recently its principles had not been applied to any great extent to neurologically impaired adults. As the name implies,

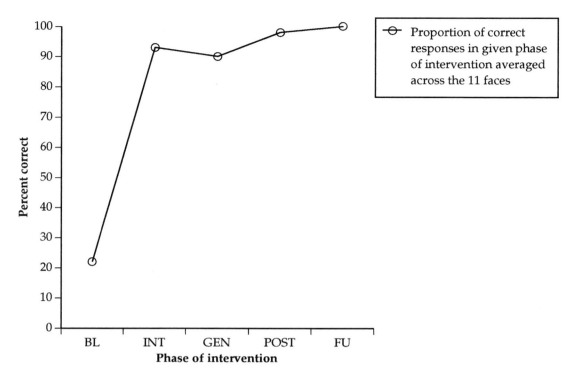

Key for phase of intervention:
    BL   baseline
    INT   intervention
    GEN   generalization
    POST   post-training baseline
    FU   follow-up (one, three and six months)

Fig. 21.1 Learning names through errorless learning principles.

errorless learning involves learning without errors or mistakes. Most of us can learn or benefit from our errors because we can remember and thus avoid them in our future efforts to learn. However, people without episodic memory cannot remember their mistakes so fail to correct them. Furthermore, the very fact of engaging in a behaviour may strengthen or reinforce it even though that behaviour is errorful. Consequently, for someone with a severe memory impairment, it makes sense to ensure that any behaviour that is going to be reinforced is correct rather than incorrect.

Work on errorless learning in memory-impaired adults has been influenced by studies of implicit learn-

ing from the field of cognitive neuropsychology as well as by the earlier studies from the field of learning disability. There have been numerous studies showing that amnesic subjects can learn some things normally or nearly normally, even though they may have no conscious recollection of learning anything at all (Brooks and Baddeley, 1976; Graf and Schacter, 1985; Glisky and Schacter, 1987). Glisky and Schacter tried to use the implicit learning abilities of amnesic subjects to teach them computer technology, and although some success was achieved this was at considerable expense of time and effort. These attempts, and others that try to build on the relatively intact skills of memory-impaired people, have, on the whole, been disappointing. One reason for failures and anomalies could be that implicit learning is poor at eliminating errors. Error elimination is a function of explicit not implicit memory and consequently when subjects are forced to rely upon implicit memory (as amnesic subjects are), the subsequent trial-and-error learning becomes a slow and laborious procedure.

In 1994, Baddeley and Wilson published the first study demonstrating that amnesic subjects learn better when they are prevented from making mistakes during the learning process. This was a theoretical study in which a stem completion task was used to teach lists of words to severely memory-impaired patients. All of the 16 amnesic patients in the study showed better learning when they were prevented from making mistakes, that is, prevented from guessing, than when they were forced to guess, that is, forced to make errors. The conclusions to this study were (1) errorless learning appears to be superior to trial-and-error learning; (2) the effect is greater for amnesic subjects than it is for controls; and (3) amnesic subjects show less forgetting with errorless learning. Since then, several single-case studies have been conducted with memory-impaired patients, comparing errorful and errorless learning for teaching practical, everyday information (Wilson et al., 1994). In the majority of cases, errorless learning proved to be superior to trial-and-error learning. Squires, Hunkin and Parkin (1996), and Wilson and Evans (1996) report further studies. The latter paper also discusses some of the potential problems connected with errorless learning.

Results from recent work (Evans et al., in press) involving ten errorless learning experiments suggest that tasks and situations that depend upon implicit memory (such as stem completion or retrieving a name from a first letter cue) are more likely to benefit from errorless learning methods than tasks requiring explicit recall of new situations. Nevertheless, Wilson et al. (1994) demonstrated new explicit learning in a memory-impaired, head-injured patient. Clare et al. (1999), mentioned above, also demonstrated explicit learning in a man with Alzheimer's disease. The Evans et al. (submitted) studies found that the more severely

amnesic patients benefited to a greater extent from errorless learning methods than did those who were less severely impaired, although this may only apply when the interval between learning and recall is relatively short, i.e. within an hour or so, which was the length of the individual experimental session. How long the errorless learning advantage is maintained has not yet been tested. One of the implications from this finding is that errorless learning should be combined with expanding rehearsal to enhance its effectiveness. This prediction is currently being tested with patients attending a memory clinic.

New technology

- 'Smart' houses, (involving the use of new technology) that are being designed to increase the independence and activity of confused elderly people may be adapted to suit the needs of other groups with cognitive impairments.
- NeuroPage, a simple, portable paging system which reminds memory-impaired people to take certain actions throughout the day, is proving to be effective.
- Interactive Task Guidance Systems are used to provide a set of cues to guide subjects through the sequential steps of an everyday task.
- All new developments in technology will need to be evaluated critically to see if they stand up to the test of transfer and generalization.

As in many other areas, the growth in new technology is benefiting memory rehabilitation in several ways. 'Smart' houses employ computers and video cameras to monitor and control the living environments of people with dementia. The aim is to use and perhaps modify new technology in order to increase independence and activity and thus the quality of life of confused elderly people. If success is achieved with the elderly population, then it is possible that 'smart' houses will be adapted to suit the needs of other groups with cognitive impairments.

Two 'smart' houses have been started in Norway (Slaven, 1996, personal communication) which target problems such as falls, disorientation, inadequate meals, poor hygiene, emergencies, and limited home management. Examples of 'smart' house technology, often adapted from appliances that are readily available to the general householder, include the following.

Use of the telephone.

1. Photographs of ten people important in the client's network are pasted on to the telephone buttons. Each button is programmed to dial the number of the person in the photograph.
2. A video-phone link is provided between the patient's home and the care centre or main helper.
3. A big red 'Help' button is provided to call the day centre or a relative.

Entrances and exits.

1. A floodlight is installed by the front door that lights up when someone approaches.
2. A movement detector can be connected to a verbal message that indicates someone is approaching.
3. An infrared key is provided for opening doors.
4. Environmental control systems may be installed to open and close doors from a distance.

Temperature control.

1. A fitted control system for showers and baths can ensure that water is neither too hot nor too cold.
2. A central control can be used to regulate the temperature of rooms.

Alarm systems.

1. Alarms can be fitted to sound when the cooker or other electric appliances are left on and unused for a certain length of time.
2. An alarm system can sound when the person leaves the house in order to prevent wandering.
3. In case of fire or any other emergency, an alarm rings in an alarm or care centre. A voice message is relayed to the client telling him or her to leave the house because of the emergency.

With the rapid development of technology, it is possible that 'smart' houses will become more important in the future and their design requirements could open up fruitful dialogue between psychologists, engineers, architects and computer programmers.

A simple and portable paging system, designed in California by an engineer father of a head-injured son working together with a neuropsychologist, is proving to be an effective tool in memory rehabilitation. Known as NeuroPage, it uses a computer linked by a modem and telephone to a paging company. The scheduling of reminders or cues for each individual is entered into the computer, from which point no further human interaction is necessary (Hersh and Treadgold, 1994). On the appropriate date and time, NeuroPage automatically transmits the reminder information to the paging company, which transmits the message to the individual's pager.

A major advantage of NeuroPage is that the system avoids many of the difficulties faced by memory-impaired people when they attempt to use a compensatory aid or strategy. Obviously, using aids or strategies involves exercising memory, so the very people who need them most have the greatest difficulty in managing their complexities. Memory-impaired people may forget to make use of their aids, or find that programming them is too difficult; they may use them unsystematically, or might even be embarrassed by having to refer to them in public. In contrast, NeuroPage is controlled by one large button which is easy to press even for those with motor difficulties. It is highly portable and has an audible or vibratory alarm, depending on the user's preference. It has an accompanying explanatory message and, like other pagers, is viewed as a prestigious possession rather than an embarrassment.

NeuroPage was evaluated in a recent study with 15 brain-injured people whose memory difficulties followed head injury, stroke or tumour (Wilson et al., 1997). Using an ABA design whereby the first A phase was the pretreatment period, and the second A phase was the posttreatment baseline period, it was demonstrated that all 15 subjects benefited significantly from using NeuroPage. The average number of problems tackled for the group as a whole was 3.86, with a range of one to seven, and a mode of four. Typical reminders included: 'Take your medication', 'Today is . . .', 'Make sure you have your spectacles', and 'Check your diary'. Results from the study can be seen in Fig. 21.2

The mean percentage success for completing tasks in the first baseline period, for the group as a whole, was 37.05; in the treatment phase this rose to 85.46. Using an Odds Ratio Test (Everitt, 1995), which takes into account different underlying success rates for each target and calculates an average improvement factor, it was found

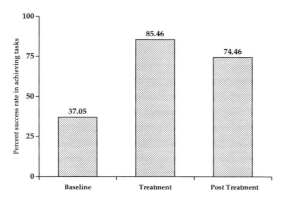

Fig. 21.2 Results of 15 memory-impaired people using NeuroPage.

that each subject showed a significant improvement. However, there were wide individual differences, with some subjects changing from 0 per cent success to over 90 per cent success in the treatment period, and others having more modest changes such as 6.67 per cent in the baseline stage to 22.93 per cent in the treatment stage.

Wide variations were also noted between subjects in the posttreatment baseline phase. The mean success of the group as a whole was 74.46 per cent, which is better than in the first baseline phase. The Odds Ratio Test indicated that 11 of the 15 subjects were significantly better than in the baseline phase and four were not. The implications here are that some subjects 'learn' to do what is expected during treatment, that is, they learn to take their medication, feed the dog, pack their school bag etc., whereas other people remain dependent on reminders to help them complete the tasks. At present, the team is in the process of setting up a paging service for people with everyday memory problems arising from organic amnesia and/or planning, attentional or organizational difficulties. NeuroPage should also prove beneficial to normal elderly people as well as to some children with memory problems and possibly to patients with schizophrenia.

Another developing area for new technology is in the use of computers as Interactive Task Guidance Systems (Kirsch et al., 1987) to provide a set of cues to guide patients through sequential steps of an everyday task such as cooking or cleaning. The computer acts as a compensatory device providing step-by-step instructions. Little knowledge of computer operations is needed by the subject. One example is provided by Bergman and Kemmerer (1991), who describe how a 54-year-old woman with a number of cognitive problems learned to use a computerized task guidance system. The patient had a left-sided neglect, so only the right side of the screen was employed. She also had poor visual acuity, so the colours of the screen were adjusted to make it more discriminable. An audible tone was included to enhance arousal and attentiveness. The patient learned to use the computerized system in three one-hour training sessions and employed it for: (1) writing lists of things to do or buy; (2) writing instructions or requests to her companion helper; (3) making notes about telephone calls and letters; and (4) money management, such as printing out cheques to pay her electricity bill. Bergman and Kemmerer reported that the patient's self-sufficiency increased and her emotional distress decreased as a result of the system.

Glisky (1995) discusses issues involved in the use of computers for memory rehabilitation. She argues that computers are likely to play an increasingly important role as new technologies are developed, and the interface between computer and user is improved. She reminds us of the problems of transfer and generalization and emphasizes the need for critical evaluation of new applications.

Other strategies for managing memory problems

- Despite little evidence that restoration of function occurs once the period of natural recovery is over, there is some slight evidence that partial recovery can occur over time for some subjects.
- It may also be possible to slow down the rate of decline in patients with progressive conditions.
- No strong evidence is provided to suggest that anatomical reorganization of the brain takes place as far as memory functioning is concerned.
- Functional adaptations or compensatory approaches, using external aids, are probably the most effective and popular approaches in memory rehabilitation.
- The use of external memory aids will be most efficient

when taught rigorously, recognizing factors such as age, severity of memory impairment, and additional cognitive deficits.

- Mnemonics are systems for teaching memory-impaired people new information and enabling people to organize, store and retrieve information more efficiently.
- Most brain-injured people will not use mnemonics spontaneously.
- Several suggestions are offered to ensure greater effectiveness in the teaching of mnemonics.

As suggested earlier, there is little evidence that restoration of function occurs once the period of natural recovery is over. However, in a long-term follow-up study of 50 memory-impaired people with nonprogressive brain injury (Wilson, 1991), some partial recovery appeared to occur in almost a third of patients reassessed five to ten years postinjury. Arkin (1991, 1992) also suggests that it might be possible to slow down the rate of decline in patients with progressive conditions. She made tape recordings of important personal information for Alzheimer patients and used this information in a quiz. After repeatedly listening to the tapes and being quizzed, patients learned some of the information. Although Arkin's evidence is very tentative, her ideas would be well worth evaluating in a larger study.

Another approach to memory rehabilitation is to encourage anatomical reorganization. Although detailed discussion is beyond the scope of this chapter, it is perhaps worth noting in passing that despite Kolb's (1995) very persuasive arguments that the brain is far more plastic than was once believed, there is still no strong evidence that anatomical reorganization of the brain takes place as far as memory functioning is concerned.

It is sometimes worth considering an alternative means to a final goal in much the same way that Luria did with his principle of functional adaptation (Luria, 1963), or Zangwill with his principle of compensation (Zangwill, 1947). In memory rehabilitation, such compensation is often achieved through the use of external memory aids such as notebooks, lists, diaries, tape recorders etc. Most people use external memory aids and they are, perhaps, the most useful strategy for

people with organic memory impairment. Some patients resist using such aids because they feel that it is cheating, or that any natural recovery will be slowed down by reliance upon them. These feelings should be discouraged as it is normal to use compensatory aids and there is neither evidence nor reason to believe their use will have a slowing down effect upon recovery. A bigger problem is the difficulty memory-impaired people have in remembering to use their aids efficiently or even at all. This issue is addressed above in the discussion of new technology. Wilson (1991) found that memory-impaired people were far more likely to be using compensatory aids five to ten years postrehabilitation than they were during or at the end of rehabilitation. This was despite the fact that much of their rehabilitation emphasized the use of such aids. Furthermore, those patients using six or more aids or strategies were significantly more likely to be independent than those using five or fewer. The numbers of people using each kind of compensation can be found in Wilson (1995). The most popular aid was writing notes, and the least popular was tying a knot in a handkerchief (analogous to the American custom of tying a string round a finger).

Despite general agreement that a compensatory approach is probably the most effective one to adopt, there is uncertainty about why some people use external aids efficiently and others do not. Simply providing aids and expecting them to be used appropriately is likely to lead to failure for many memory-impaired people, and patience and ingenuity are required when teaching their use. Kime, Lamb and Wilson (1996), and Sohlberg and Mateer (1989) describe ways of teaching the use of aids. More recently, Wilson and Watson (1996) described a theoretical framework influenced by the work of Bäckman and Dixon (1992). This framework proposed four stages in the development of compensatory behaviour: (1) origins, (2) forms, (3) mechanisms, and (4) consequences. Wilson and Watson (1996) discussed how these steps might apply to brain-injured people with memory problems who might be trying to compensate for their difficulties. They went further, however, by using data from a long-term follow-up study and showed that age, severity of memory impairment and additional cognitive deficits are important variables in predicting independence and the use of compensations several years postrehabilitation.

Rehearsal strategies such as expanding rehearsal (described above), and other procedures from the field of study techniques have all been successfully employed to teach new information to memory-impaired people. For further discussion of these strategies, see Wilson (1987).

Mnemonics are systems that enable people to organize, store and retrieve information more efficiently. Some people use the term mnemonics to refer to anything that helps people remember, including external aids. In memory rehabilitation, however, the term is used for methods involving the mental manipulation of material. For example, in order to remember how many days there are in each month, most people use a system of mnemonics. In the UK and much of the USA, people recite a rhyme: 'Thirty days hath September . . .'. In other parts of the world, people use their knuckles to refer to 'long' months and the dips between the knuckles to refer to the 'short' months. Mnemonics are often employed to learn the names of cranial nerves, notes of music, colours of the rainbow, and other ordered material. (See Wilson (1987) and Moffat (1989) for further discussion of mnemonics in memory rehabilitation, and West (1995) for the use of these strategies in people with age-related memory impairment.)

The following suggestions are offered to those wishing to employ mnemonics with memory-impaired people.

1. Mnemonics are useful for teaching new information. However, most brain-injured people will not use them spontaneously.
2. Dual coding, i.e. using two methods rather than one, will probably result in more efficient learning than the use of one method alone.
3. Information or the component skills of a new task should be taught one step at a time.
4. If visual imagery is employed, i.e. transforming a name or word to be learned into a picture (such as remembering Barbara as a barber), it is better for the memory-impaired person to see a drawing of the picture on paper or card rather than to rely on a mental image.

5. Information to be learned should be realistic and relevant to the everyday needs of patients or clients. Thus, it is better to teach people things they really need to know rather than material from a workbook.
6. Individual styles, needs and preferences should be recognized. Not everyone will benefit from the same strategy.
7. Generalization issues need to be addressed. If a patient learns to use a notebook in the psychology department, this does not necessarily mean the book will be used outside the department unless this is specifically taught.

It is wrong to think that memory-impaired people are taught how to use mnemonics and then go on to employ them in novel situations, because brain-injured people find it extremely difficult to use mnemonics spontaneously. In fact, the real value of mnemonics is that they are useful for *teaching* memory-impaired people new information, and they almost invariably lead to faster learning than rote rehearsal.

Games and exercises can also help people use their residual skills more effectively, although this is probably less likely to be because they improve memory and more likely to be because they enable people to realize they can do better if they use a strategy. The games and exercises also provide opportunities to try out these strategies in enjoyable situations.

Memory therapy in practice

- Personality, awareness, motivation, anxiety, depression, lifestyle, and additional cognitive problems must be taken into account in memory rehabilitation.
- Families require straightforward information, explanations and reassurance.
- Cognitive–behavioural therapy, group and individual psychotherapy are all recommended for alleviating depression, anxiety and social isolation.
- Brain-injured people may have multiple cognitive problems which must be assessed accurately by employing detailed neuropsychological assessments.

Although some recovery of memory functioning can be expected during the early stages following head injury and other nonprogressive brain damage, memory-impaired people and their families should not be led to believe that significant improvement will occur once the period of natural recovery is over. However, this does not mean that nothing can be done to help. As indicated above, people can be taught to avoid problems, compensate for their difficulties, and learn more efficiently. Their distress can be reduced and their awareness and understanding can be increased. 'Memory rehabilitation does not occur in a vacuum' (Prigatano, 1995). Personality factors, awareness, motivation, levels of anxiety, depression, lifestyle, and additional cognitive problems may all affect the way memory problems are experienced and subsequently dealt with in everyday life. Kopelman and Crawford (1996) found depression in over 40 per cent of 200 consecutive referrals to a memory clinic. Evans and Wilson (1992) found anxiety to be common in attenders at a weekly memory group meeting. Prigatano (1995) found that the methods of treatment employed in rehabilitation were influenced by social factors, and that the personality of patients influenced their approach to rehabilitation activities. Prigatano suggested that patients with low motivation and low awareness after brain injury were the most difficult to treat.

Listening to what families have to say and providing straightforward information or explanations are therapeutic in themselves. Family members commonly ask why it is that their memory-impaired relative can remember what happened 20 years earlier but cannot remember what happened an hour before, or variations on that theme. They should be given simple explanations such as the fact that old memories are stored differently in the brain. For some relatives, this will not be enough and they will demand a fairly detailed anatomical or biochemical explanation; when such demands occur, the therapist should be sufficiently knowledgeable and confident to be able to provide an explanation.

Anxiety in family members can be reduced by offering reassurance that their relative is experiencing a typical pattern of difficulties found in most memory-impaired people. Written information is also appreciated by families. There is a number of useful pamphlets and books available, such as *Memory Problems after Head Injury* (Wilson, 1989), written for the National Head Injuries Association, *Managing Your Memory. A Self-help Manual for Improving Everyday Memory Skills* (Kapur, 1991), and *Coping with Memory Problems: a Practical Guide for People with Memory Impairments, their Relatives, Friends and Carers* (Clare and Wilson, 1997). A useful reference on the topic of self-help and support groups for memory-impaired people and their carers is by Wearing (1992), who graphically illustrates the failure of resources for memory-impaired people. For example, Wearing (1992, p. 281) writes:

A woman in Worthing had been looking after her amnesic husband for many years after his head injury. She herself was chronically sick and needed a break for her own treatment, so a place was found for him in respite care. Ten days later he and two respite staff were back on the doorstep. 'We're very sorry,' explained the staff, 'we cannot cope with your husband any longer because he is aggressive.' So this sick lady was left to cope alone with him.

Relaxation therapy can be useful in reducing anxiety, and its benefits may last even though treatment sessions have been forgotten. Relaxation audiocassette tapes can be bought or made for patients so that they do not need to rely upon memory in order to carry out exercises. One word of caution here, though. When tense-and-release exercises (Bernstein and Borkovec, 1973) are employed for relaxation, therapists need to be aware that some brain-injured people, particularly those with motor difficulties, may have problems. Tensing muscles can cause a spasm or increase spasticity. It is best, therefore, to discuss the advisability of such exercises with a physiotherapist treating the particular patient or, alternatively, to look for another form of relaxation such as that recommended by Ost (1987) or those described by Clark (1989).

Memory functioning can be impaired by depression in those without brain injury (Watts, 1995), probably because of diminished resources available as a result of emotional preoccupations. For similar reasons, depression may well exacerbate difficulties in people with organic memory impairment. It is possible that cognitive–behavioural therapy approaches such as those employed by Beck (1976) would be appropriate for brain-injured patients, although there do not appear to be any studies reporting this. Psychotherapy, on the other hand, is a well-established intervention with brain-injured people. Prigatano et al. (1986) firmly believe in group and individual psychotherapy with brain-injured patients, and use principles from the school of Jung. Jackson and Gouvier (1992) provide descriptions and guidelines for group psychotherapy with brain-injured adults and their families.

Social isolation among brain-injured people is common (Talbott, 1989; Wearing, 1992). Wearing suggests some of the reasons for this isolation are connected with the fact that a memory-impaired person's social network falls away when visits and conversations are forgotten, when that person is unable to go out alone for fear of getting lost, or may not be able to control inappropriate behaviour.

An immediate solution to such isolation is to form memory groups. Wilson and Moffat (1992b) describe various groups for patients. Moffat (1989) reports on a relatives' memory group for people with dementia, and Wearing (1992) provides suggestions for setting up self-help groups. Psychotherapy groups can achieve the same ends (Jackson and Gouvier, 1992). Evans and Wilson (1992) discuss the value of memory groups and also comment on the reduction in anxiety that can follow attendance. The author has been involved in running many groups over the past years and has come to the conclusion that the main value of such groups is that they encourage a reduction in the emotional sequelae that follow memory impairment. Reminiscence and Reality Orientation groups may achieve similar ends.

Brain-injured people may well have multiple cognitive problems that will need to be tackled in rehabilitation. People with a pure amnesic syndrome are relatively rare, and most patients present with attentional deficits, word-finding problems or executive difficulties of planning and organization. Memory problems may, in fact, be secondary to other cognitive deficits or they may both be present but separate from each other. Detailed neuropsychological assessment will probably be necessary to obtain an accurate picture of a person's cognitive strengths and weaknesses before a coherent and sensible memory therapy programme can be designed. More detailed information on the neuropsychological assessment of memory can be found in Mayes (1995), Howieson and Lezak (1995), and Wilson (1996). Information from detailed neuropsychological assessment needs to be supplemented with a behavioural assessment defining the real-life, everyday problems to be targeted for treatment. Numerous publications address the issue of cognitive rehabilitation, including memory. A recent summary can be found in Wilson (1995). Many articles in the journal *Neuropsychological Rehabilitation* are also concerned with the management and remediation of cognitive deficits.

Conclusions

Although restoration of memory functioning is unlikely to occur, there is a considerable amount that can be done to enable memory-impaired people and their relatives to come to terms with their difficulties and surmount a number of them by using various strategies and aids.

Environmental modifications can be of considerable help to people whose memory functioning is impaired, and new technology has an increasingly important role to play in the future management of memory problems. As discussed, some technological aids such as pagers and computers are already proving to be beneficial. When a variety of technological aids are set to work cooperatively in the same building, we have what has become known as a 'smart' house, and it is possible that such dwellings will be developed in increasing numbers and greater sophistication for the benefit of elderly and cognitively impaired people in the future.

Nonelectronic external memory aids such as diaries, notebooks, tape records etc. are widely used but are often problematic for memory-impaired people simply because reliance upon them demands exercising memory. However, the successful use of these aids is possible through carefully structured teaching, particularly with people who are younger, have less severe memory problems, or have fewer additional cognitive impairments. Others may need more intensive therapy or rehabilitation to ensure efficient usage.

Internal strategies such as mnemonics and rehearsal techniques can be employed to teach new information, and although they almost always lead to faster learning than rote repetition, it must be recognized that most memory-impaired people will be unable to use mnemonics spontaneously. Instead, relatives, carers and therapists will have to employ mnemonics to encourage learning among memory-impaired people.

Errorless learning is usually more effective than trial-and-error learning for memory-impaired people. This is because, in order to benefit from our mistakes, we need to be able to remember them, and this is something which most memory-impaired people will not be able to do. In the absence of episodic memory, making an error may strengthen or reinforce the erroneous response.

In addition to poor memory, many brain-injured people will have other cognitive problems which will need to be addressed. The emotional sequelae of memory impairment such as anxiety, depression and loneliness will also have to be reduced by providing written information, counselling, anxiety-management techniques and treatment in memory or psychotherapy groups.

Although we cannot restore lost memory functioning, we can help people to bypass problems and compensate for their difficulties. We can help them learn more efficiently and we can reduce the effects of their problems in their daily lives. We must also educate society so that there is a greater understanding of what it means to have severe organic memory impairment.

References

Arkin, S.M. 1991. Memory training in early Alzheimer's disease: an optimistic look at the field. *Am J Alzheimer's Care Related Disord Res* **July/August**, 17–25.

Arkin, S.M. 1992. Audio-assisted memory training with early Alzheimer's patients: two single subject experiments. *Clin Gerontol* **12**, 77–96.

Bäckman, L. and Dixon, R.A. 1992. Psychological compensation: a theoretical framework. *Psychol Bull* **112**, 259–83.

Baddeley, A.D. and Longman, D.J.A. 1978. The influence of length and frequency on training sessions on the rate of learning to type. *Ergonomics* **21**, 627–35.

Baddeley, A.D. and Wilson, B.A. 1994. When implicit learning fails: amnesia and the problem of error elimination. *Neuropsychologia* **32**, 53–68.

Beck, A.T. 1976. *Cognitive Therapy and Emotional Disorders*. New York: International Universities Press.

Berg, I. 1993. *Memory Rehabilitation for Closed Head Injury Patients*. The Hague: CIP-Data Koninklijke Bibliotheek.

Bergman, M.M. and Kemmerer, A.G. 1991. Computer-enhanced self sufficiency: Part 2. Uses and subjective benefits of a text writer for an individual with traumatic brain injury. *Neuropsychology* **5**, 25–8.

Bernstein, D.A. and Borkovec, T.D. 1973. *Progressive Relaxation Training*. Champaign, IL: Illinois Research Press.

Brooks, D.N. and Baddeley, A. 1976. What can amnesic patients learn? *Neuropsychologia* **14**, 111–22.

Clare, L. and Wilson, B.A. 1997. *Coping with Memory Problems: a Practical Guide for People with Memory Impairments, their Relatives, Friends and Carers*. Bury St Edmunds, Suffolk: Thames Valley Test Company.

Clare, L., Wilson, B.A., Breen, E.K. and Hodges, J.R. (1999). Learning face–name associations in early Alzheimer's disease. *Neurocase* **5**, 37–46.

Clark, D.M. 1989. Anxiety states: panic and generalized anxiety. In *Cognitive Behaviour Therapy for Psychiatric Problems*, ed. K. Hawton, P.M. Salkovskis, J. Kirk and D.M. Clark, pp. 52–97. Oxford: Oxford Medical Publications.

Evans, J.J. and Wilson, B.A. 1992. A memory group for individuals with brain injury. *Clin Rehabil* **6**, 75–81.

Evans, J.J., Wilson, B.A., Schuri, U. et al. (in press). A comparison of 'errorless' and 'trial and error' learning methods for teaching individuals with acquired memory deficits. *Neuropsychol Rehabil*.

Everitt, B. 1995. *Cambridge Dictionary of Statistics in the Medical Sciences*. Cambridge: Cambridge University Press.

Glisky, E.L. 1995. Computers in memory rehabilitation. In *Handbook of Memory Disorders*, ed. A.D. Baddeley, B.A. Wilson and F.N. Watts, pp. 557–75. Chichester: John Wiley & Sons.

Glisky, E.L. and Schacter, D.L. 1987. Acquisition of domain-specific knowledge in organic amnesia: training for computer-related work. *Neuropsychologia* **25**, 893–906.

Graf, P. and Schacter, D.L. 1985. Implicit and explicit memory for new associations in normal and amnesic subjects. *J Exp Psychol Learn Mem Cogn* **11**, 501–18.

Gross, Y. and Schutz, L.E. 1986. Intervention models in neuropsychology. In *Clinical Neuropsychology of Intervention*, ed. B.P. Buzzell and Y. Gross, pp. 179–205. Boston: Martinus Nijhoff.

Hersh, N. and Treadgold, L. 1994. NeuroPage: the rehabilitation of memory dysfunction by prosthetic memory and cueing. *NeuroRehabilitation* 4, 187–97.

Howieson, D.B. and Lezak, M.D. 1995. Separating memory from other cognitive problems. In *Handbook of Memory Disorders*, ed. A.D. Baddeley, B.A. Wilson and F.N. Watts, pp. 411–26. Chichester: John Wiley & Sons.

Jackson, W.T. and Gouvier, W.D. 1992. Group psychotherapy with brain-damaged adults and their families. In *Handbook of Head Trauma: Acute Care to Recovery*, ed. C.J. Long and L.K. Ross, pp. 309–27. New York: Plenum Press.

Jones, R.S.P. and Eayrs, C.B. 1992. The use of errorless learning procedures in teaching people with a learning disability. *Ment Handicap Res* 5, 304–12.

Kapur, N. 1991. Managing your Memory. A Self-help Memory Manual for Improving Everyday Memory Skills. Available from the author at the Wessex Neurological Centre, Southampton General Hospital, Southampton.

Kapur, N. 1995. Memory aids in the rehabilitation of memory disordered patients. In *Handbook of Memory Disorders*, ed. A.D. Baddeley, B.A. Wilson and F.N. Watts, pp. 533–56. Chichester: John Wiley & Sons.

Kime, S.K., Lamb, D.G. and Wilson, B.A. 1996. Use of a comprehensive program of external cueing to enhance procedural memory in a patient with dense amnesia. *Brain Inj* 10, 17–25.

Kirsch, N.L., Levine, S.P., Fallon-Krueger, M. and Jaros, L.A. 1987. The microcomputer as an 'orthotic' device for patients with cognitive deficits. *J Head Trauma Rehabil* 2, 77–86.

Kolb, B. 1995. *Brain Plasticity and Behaviour*. Hillsdale, NJ: Lawrence Erlbaum.

Kopelman, M. and Crawford, S. 1996. Not all memory clinics are dementia clinics. *Neuropsychol Rehabil* 6, 187–202.

Landauer, T.K. and Bjork, R.A. 1978. Optimum rehearsal patterns and name learning. In *Practical Aspects of Memory*, ed. M.M. Gruneberg, P.E. Morris and R.N. Sykes, pp. 625–32. London: Academic Press.

Lorge, I. 1930. Influence of regularly interpolated time intervals upon subsequent learning. Cited in Johnson, H.H. and Solso, R.L. 1971. *An Introduction to Experimental Design in Psychology: a Case Approach*, pp. 7–8. New York: Harper & Row.

Luria, A.R. 1963. *Recovery of Function after Brain Injury*. New York: Macmillan.

Mayes, A.R. 1995. The assessment of memory disorders. In *Handbook of Memory Disorders*, ed. A.D. Baddeley, B.A. Wilson and F.N. Watts, pp. 367–91. Chichester: John Wiley & Sons.

Moffat, N. 1989. Home based cognitive rehabilitation with the elderly. In *Everyday Cognition in Adulthood and Late Life*, ed. L.W. Poon, D.C. Rubin and B.A. Wilson, pp. 659–80. Cambridge: Cambridge University Press.

Murphy, G. and Oliver, C. 1987. Decreasing undesirable behaviours. In *Behaviour Modification for People with Mental Handicaps*, ed. W. Yule and J. Carr, pp. 102–42. London: Croom Helm.

Norman, D.A. 1988. *The Psychology of Everyday Things*. New York: Basic Books.

Ost, L.G. 1987. Applied relaxation: description of a coping technique and review of controlled studies. *Behav Res Therapy* 25, 397–410.

Prigatano, G.P. 1995. Personality and social aspects of memory rehabilitation. In *Handbook of Memory Disorders*, ed. A.D. Baddeley, B.A. Wilson and F.N. Watts, pp. 603–14. Chichester: John Wiley & Sons.

Prigatano, G.P., Fordyce, D.J., Zeiner, H.K., Roueche, J.R., Pepping, M. and Wood, B.C., eds. 1986. *Neuropsychological Rehabilitation after Brain Injury*. Baltimore: Johns Hopkins University Press.

Robinson, F.P. 1970. *Effective Study*. New York: Harper and Row.

Sidman, M. and Stoddard, L.T. 1967. The effectiveness of fading in programming simultaneous form discrimination for retarded children. *J Exp Analysis Behav* 10, 3–15.

Sohlberg, M.M. and Mateer, C. 1989. Training use of compensatory memory books: a three-stage behavioural approach. *J Clin Exp Neuropsychol* 11, 871–91.

Squires, E.J., Hunkin, N.M. and Parkin, A.J. 1996. Memory notebook training in a case of severe amnesia: generalising from paired associate learning to real life. *Neuropsychol Rehabil* 6, 55–65.

Talbott, R. 1989. The brain injured person and the family. In *Models of Brain Injury Rehabilitation*, ed. R.L. Wood and P. Eames, pp. 3–16. London: Chapman and Hall.

Thoene, A.I.T. and Glisky, E.L. 1995. Learning of name–face associations in memory impaired patients: a comparison of different training procedures. *J Int Neuropsychol Soc* 1, 29–38.

Watts, F.N. 1995. Depression and anxiety. In *Handbook of Memory Disorders*, ed. A.D. Baddeley, B.A. Wilson and F.N. Watts, pp. 293–317. Chichester: John Wiley & Sons.

Wearing, D. 1992. Self help groups. In *Clinical Management of Memory Problems*, 2nd edn, ed. B.A. Wilson and N. Moffat, pp. 271–301. London: Chapman and Hall.

West, R.L. 1995. Compensatory strategies for age-associated memory impairment. In *Handbook of Memory Disorders*, ed. A.D. Baddeley, B.A. Wilson and F.N. Watts, pp. 481–500. Chichester: John Wiley & Sons.

Wilson, B.A. 1987. *Rehabilitation of Memory*. New York: Guilford Press.

Wilson, B.A. 1989. *Memory Problems after Head Injury*. Nottingham: National Head Injuries Association.

Wilson, B.A. 1991. Long term prognosis of patients with severe memory disorders. *Neuropsychol Rehabil* 1, 117–34.

Wilson, B.A. 1995. Memory rehabilitation: compensating for memory problems. In *Compensating for Psychological Deficits and Declines: Managing Losses and Promoting Gains*, ed. R.A. Dixon and L. Bäckman, pp. 171–90. Hillsdale, NJ: Lawrence Erlbaum.

Wilson, B.A. 1996. Assessment of memory. In *Assessment in Neuropsychology*, ed. L. Harding and J.R. Beech, pp. 135–51. London: Routledge.

Wilson, B.A., Baddeley, A.D., Evans, J.J. and Shiel, A. 1994. Errorless learning in the rehabilitation of memory impaired people. *Neuropsychol Rehabil* 4, 307–26.

Wilson, B.A. and Evans, J.J. 1996. Error free learning in the rehabilitation of individuals with memory impairments. *J Head Trauma Rehabil* 11, 54–64.

Wilson, B.A., Evans, J.J., Emslie, H. and Malinek, V. 1997. Evaluation of NeuroPage: a new memory aid. *J Neurol Neurosurg Psychiatry* 63, 113–15.

Wilson, B.A. and Moffat, N. eds. 1984. *Clinical Management of Memory Problems*. London: Croom Helm.

Wilson, B.A. and Moffat, N., eds. 1992a. *Clinical Management of Memory Problems*, 2nd edn. London: Chapman and Hall.

Wilson, B.A. and Moffat, N. 1992b. The development of group memory therapy. In *Clinical Management of Memory Problems*, 2nd edn, ed. B.A. Wilson and N. Moffat, pp. 243–73. London: Chapman and Hall.

Wilson, B.A. and Watson, P.C. 1996. A practical framework for understanding compensatory behaviour in people with organic memory impairment. *Memory* 4, 465–86.

Yule, W. and Carr, J. eds. 1987. *Behaviour Modification for People with Mental Handicaps*. London: Croom Helm.

Zangwill, O.L. 1947. Psychological aspects of rehabilitation in cases of brain injury. *Br J Psychol* 37, 60–9.

22

Memory rehabilitation in the elderly

Elizabeth L. Glisky and Martha L. Glisky

Introduction

- The ageing population is heterogeneous.
- Compensatory mechanisms and other variables that contribute to cognitive competence in ageing should be incorporated into rehabilitation programmes.

Memory problems are among the most common complaints of people as they get older, and although much has been learned in recent years about the nature of age-related memory decline, little is yet known about how to prevent, reduce or compensate for the problems. Among the ageing population, there is considerable heterogeneity in cognitive function (Weintraub, Powell and Whitla, 1994). Some individuals are vigorous and cognitively competent at age 80, whereas others are struggling to maintain function at age 60. Moreover, some abilities seem to hold up well or even increase with age, while others diminish. The reasons for this variability are as yet unknown, but some researchers (Dixon and Bäckman, 1993) have speculated that at least part of the interindividual variability may be attributable to different internal compensatory mechanisms that are differentially available to different individuals. Additionally, differences may arise as a result of any number of biological, psychological, environmental or lifestyle variables. To the extent that these variables and compensatory mechanisms can be determined, it may be possible to incorporate them into rehabilitation programmes to enhance the functioning of less cognitively capable elderly individuals.

This chapter explores ways in which older adults might be trained to use some of these compensatory strategies and to take advantage of other important variables that might improve their memory functioning. The bulk of the chapter is organized around three broad goals or approaches to rehabilitation: (1) external compensation for lost function, (2) optimization of residual function, and (3) substitution of intact function. Within each of these general approaches to rehabilitation, remedial techniques are outlined that are consistent with the approach, the theoretical rationale and empirical findings that support each technique, the strengths and weaknesses of each methodology, and the individual difference variables that might moderate the effectiveness of each intervention. Finally, the chapter looks to the future and suggests directions for continued research. Before beginning the discussion of memory rehabilitation in the elderly, the nature of the memory changes that are most often associated with normal ageing is summarized briefly.

Memory changes in normal ageing

- Age-related neurobiological changes in medial temporal and prefrontal cortices may account for memory changes.

Although considerable variability is observed in the memory performance of older adults, there appears to be little doubt that, *on average*, episodic memory – memory for relatively recent events or episodes – begins to show some declines when people are in the 40s and 50s and drops precipitously beyond the age of 70 (Albert, Duffy and Naeser, 1987; Salthouse, 1991). These deficiencies are probably related to atrophy or shrinkage in medial temporal and/or prefrontal regions of the brain (Coffey et al., 1992; Raz et al., 1997) and to reductions in blood flow and glucose metabolism, which are most marked in the same areas (Martin et al., 1991). Although memory processes have been linked to both medial temporal and prefrontal cortices, the exact mapping between neuroanatomical structures and specific mnemonic functions has only begun to be examined (Shallice et al., 1994; Tulving et al., 1994; Schacter et al., 1996a). With respect to the elderly, the first reports from functional neuroimaging studies indicate that, when performing memory tasks, older adults show reduced activation relative to young adults, both in the hippocampal regions (Grady et al., 1995) and in prefrontal cortex (Schacter et al., 1996b).

It has also become evident that not all kinds of memory tasks are affected equally by ageing (for reviews, see Craik and Jennings, 1992; Kausler, 1994; Craik et al., 1995; Howard, 1996). In general, age decrements tend to be largest in tasks that require free recall of unrelated pieces of information, such as lists of unrelated words or paired associates, and least in tasks that require only recognition of previously experienced events. Older adults also seem to experience more difficulty remembering contextual or source information than focal or core information, and are particularly disadvantaged relative to young adults when material is novel and not well organized conceptually. Although they show little loss of memory when information merely has to be passively held in short-term memory (e.g. forward digit span), they commonly experience problems when that material has to be manipulated or reorganized in some way (e.g. backward digit span) – what is referred to as working memory. General knowledge of the world, vocabulary and well-learned skills are well retained with age, and older adults are as able as young adults to learn new skills or procedures, although they are much slower to acquire new factual information. They generally show little, if any, declines in implicit memory or priming tasks, such as word-fragment completion or tachistoscopic identification of recently presented materials.

These patterns of impaired and preserved functions as well as the findings of substantial individual differences in age-related memory decline have suggested a number of different approaches to memory rehabilitation in the elderly. Three of these approaches provide the organizational framework for the discussion of rehabilitation techniques that follows.

External compensation for lost function

Although the concept of 'compensation' has had a variety of meanings and applications in the psychological literature (Dixon and Bäckman, 1995), the term is used here, as it has frequently been used in neuropsychological rehabilitation, to refer to external or environmental changes that help to bypass or alleviate memory problems. This approach requires no assumptions concerning whether declining neural or cognitive mechanisms can be altered or reorganized. There is no attempt to restore or otherwise remediate any internal mnemonic processes. Instead, the approach focuses on ways to achieve functional or behavioural outcomes that place minimal cognitive demands on the user. For these reasons, most of these compensations can be used by all older adults, no matter what their level of cognitive function.

External aids

External memory aids can take a variety of forms and serve a variety of purposes (for reviews, see Harris, 1978, 1992; Kapur, 1995). Diaries, notebooks and lists can be used to record and store information so that it is easily retrievable when needed. Calendars, appointment books, alarm watches and timers can provide prompts and reminders for future actions. Many older adults appear to make good use of these kinds of external aids. In several real-world studies of prospective memory – memory for future intentions – it has been reported that older individuals frequently outperform young people, partly because they rely to a greater extent on reliable external reminders (Moscovitch, 1982) rather than on fallible internal strategies.

A device that would appear to have potential as an external aid for older adults is the microcomputer (Glisky, 1995). Given its capability to store large quantities of information and to retrieve such information on command, the computer would seem to be an ideal device for people with declining memories. This potential, however, has gone largely untapped. Surveys have indicated that few adults over the age of 65 know how to use computers or have easy access to them. The few studies that have examined computer learning in elderly individuals reported that older people required much more assistance and took significantly longer than young people to learn computer tasks such as word processing (e.g. Elias et al., 1987). As the present generation of computer-literate middle-aged people ages, however, such problems will probably become less critical and the computer may well come to have an important compensatory function for older adults.

Demonstrations of the important use of external aids in everyday life have been provided by studies of medication compliance (for review, see Park and Kidder, 1996). Park et al. (1992) found that providing older adults with a seven-day medication organizer and an organizational chart describing how medications were to be taken significantly improved medication adherence in a group of old–old adults (more than 70 years of age). Such aids to medication use may both reduce the memory load associated with multiple medication regimens and also provide feedback concerning whether medication has been taken. This latter problem – one of source monitoring – is known to present particular difficulties for older adults.

Environmental support

Another type of external compensation for declining memory abilities in the elderly is what Craik (1986; Craik et al., 1995) has referred to as environmental support. Craik has argued that memory involves an interaction between internal mnemonic processes and external environmental influences. As people age, they become increasingly less able to initiate encoding and retrieval operations on their own, perhaps because of declining cognitive resources, and are therefore increasingly more reliant on environmental support. To the extent that the environment provides effective encoding and retrieval cues, age decrements in performance are likely to be small. When the environmental context is relatively uninformative, however, age differences would be expected to be more substantial. A number of empirical findings are consistent with this view. For example, the findings of greater age deficits in free recall than in cued recall or recognition (Craik and McDowd, 1987) may be attributable to the relative lack of cue information available to guide retrieval processes in free recall. Reports of reduced age effects when semantic encoding instructions are provided (West and Boatwright, 1983) suggest that older adults do not spontaneously engage in the kind of elaborate encoding activities that produce durable memories, but can benefit from them when they are provided. Further evidence comes from findings that age differences are reduced or eliminated when the memory task itself seems to drive meaningful processing such as when subjects are required to manipulate objects in some way (Bäckman, 1985) or study complex pictures (Park, Puglisi and Smith, 1986). Although results across studies have not been entirely consistent, it nevertheless appears that if cues are presented at *both* encoding and retrieval (Craik, Byrd and Swanson, 1987), age differences are minimal.

In a related vein, the poorer recall of contextual or source information observed among older adults (McIntyre and Craik, 1987; Craik et al., 1990) may result from a failure to initiate the appropriate encoding and retrieval operations necessary to integrate events with their context. Although cues, in some cases, may be adequate to guide the retrieval of target information, the retrieval of source information is usually less direct and may require more demanding search and decision processes. Finally, in prospective memory tasks, the elderly have been found to be unimpaired when cues are available as reminders to perform certain actions, but show deficits when they are required to initiate retrieval activities in the absence of specific cues (Einstein and McDaniel, 1996).

The environmental support view suggests that in planning rehabilitation strategies for older adults, it may be particularly important to ensure that good cues are available at both encoding and retrieval and that the encoding context is reinstated at retrieval as closely as possible. The provision of such cues may elicit relatively automatic responses that do not tax the limited resource system. For example, conceptual cues may induce appropriate semantic elaborations of to-be-learned materials at encoding, and automatically activate matching trace information at retrieval, thereby reducing the need for effortful search processes. In effect, the provision of cues may provide an external source of direction and control to individuals whose internal source of control has been weakened with age.

Optimization of residual function

An alternative or complementary approach to rehabilitation focuses on optimizing the residual function of older adults rather than on providing external support. Some older individuals feel that relying on external aids may weaken their already compromised memory capacities; and although there is no evidence that this is the case, training of more active, mnemonic processes may be an approach that has greater face validity and is therefore more acceptable to older people. Implicit in this approach is the notion that neural and cognitive processes that were previously part of an individual's biological and behavioural repertoire are no longer being used as efficiently as they once were. This has been referred to as a production deficit: older people fail to engage in appropriate mnemonic activities although they are capable of doing so. There may be a variety of reasons why this occurs: (a) internal mnemonic strategies may be resource demanding and therefore avoided; (b) skills may have declined because of lack of practice, or (c) older adults may have fewer processing resources to allocate to memory tasks.

The methods that fall within this approach assume that previously used mnemonic processes can be retrained or increased in efficiency. Most of the techniques involve extensive practice of encoding strategies; however, there has been at least one recent attempt to retrain retrieval processes. Other methods have tried to achieve more general mnemonic benefits through practice or exercise. Because this approach relies on residual function, these techniques are likely to be most effective for relatively high-functioning older adults.

Training mnemonic strategies

Probably the most commonly used method for rehabilitating memory dysfunction is the teaching of

mnemonic strategies (for reviews, see Wilson, 1987; Harris, 1992; West, 1995). Many of these are techniques that have proved effective with young adults and that everyone may use to a greater or lesser extent in everyday life. Most focus on creating encodings that are meaningful and elaborate and on providing potential cues that will be readily available at the time of retrieval. Although one might suppose that verbal strategies would be effective for older adults, given that most older people retain good verbal skills throughout their lives, little research has explored their use amongst the elderly. The discussion here, therefore, focuses on the most common mnemonic technique used for memory training in older adults – visual imagery.

In general, this technique requires the formation of distinctive, interactive visual images of material to be remembered, which are then linked to some easily retrievable cue – well-learned places as in the method of loci, a set of keywords as in the peg-word method, or features of a face when trying to learn name–face associations. These methods have been found to be effective for remembering names, lists and locations, but little in the way of long-term maintenance or generalization of the strategies has been demonstrated (Poon, 1985; West and Tomer, 1989; West, 1995). Further, visual imagery is not a technique that can be used by all older adults. Some older people have considerable difficulty forming visual images (Winograd and Simon, 1980) and others find many of the techniques too difficult to learn (Yesavage et al, 1990). Even those who are able to learn the methods tend not to use them spontaneously, probably because they are too resource demanding.

To get around some of these problems, investigators have tried a number of modifications: providing visual imagery training prior to the teaching of the mnemonic strategies (Yesavage, 1983), demonstrating the use of the techniques on multiple tasks using video instruction (West and Crook, 1992), giving extensive practice (Hill, Sheikh and Yesavage, 1988), and including attentional and relaxation pretraining (Yesavage and Rose, 1983; Yesavage, 1984). Although these manipulations have enabled somewhat greater success, real long-term benefits have still been difficult to demonstrate. For example, Anschutz et al. (1985) found that about half of their subjects spontaneously used the method of loci two months after training, but only one individual was still using it three years later (Anschutz et al., 1987). West and Crook (1992) found that, following interactive imagery training, general instructions to use strategies promoted maintenance within the laboratory a week later, but transfer to other tasks was minimal. Scogin and Bienias (1988) reported no maintenance of initial improvements in memory performance at a three-year follow-up. However, Sheikh, Hill and Yesavage (1986) reported maintenance of gains after a six-month interval when pretraining had been provided.

The most impressive finding of long-term benefits was reported by Neely and Bäckman (1993a, 1993b). These investigators used a multifactorial memory-training programme, which combined training in the use of interactive imagery and the method of loci with attentional and relaxation training. They reported significant memory improvements on the trained tasks, which were maintained up to 3.5 years later, although the training effects were relatively task specific (Neely and Bäckman, 1995). However, the subjects that received mnemonic instruction without attention and relaxation training also showed equivalent long-term benefits, so it does not appear that multimodal training is essential.

In summary, it appears that many older adults can benefit from mnemonic training to improve their memory performance on specific tasks, but there is little evidence of generalization to untrained tasks (Verhaeghen, Marcoen and Goosens, 1992). In addition, the techniques may only be appropriate for the highest functioning older adults. More research is needed to isolate the key factors in the successful use of imagery mnemonics and to find ways to improve transfer.

Training recollective processes

Jacoby (1991) has recently suggested a distinction between two components of remembering – one that reflects automatic influences and the other that relies on consciously controlled processes – both of which may be operating in any memory situation. Jacoby and his colleagues have demonstrated, in a series of experiments (Jennings and Jacoby, 1993; Jacoby, Jennings and Hay, 1996), that older adults are impaired in the con-

trolled, recollective component of memory but have no deficits in the more automatic, familiarity-based component. These investigators have therefore suggested that rehabilitation efforts might be most beneficial if focused on the retraining of recollection.

In a preliminary study, Jacoby et al. (1996) used a shaping procedure to train older people to override the automatic influences of familiarity. The task for subjects was to reject repeated occurrences of distractor items in a recognition test. At the start of training, subjects were unable to recognize a repetition when more than a single item intervened between the first and second presentations. After seven days of training, however, during which correct responses were reinforced and the interval between repetitions gradually increased, older adults were able to perform accurately across an interval of 28 intervening items. Although these initial findings suggest that some control processes can be trained, the results are clearly preliminary. Whether the findings represent actual changes in a recollective component of memory or whether they may signal attentional improvement, for example, could not be ascertained from the reported findings, and questions of long-term maintenance or generalization have yet to be addressed. Nevertheless, initial findings with this procedure are encouraging and warrant further investigation.

Practice, experience, time and effort, schooling

There is also a number of more general ways to try to optimize residual memory function in older adults. For example, it has been suggested that older adults are disadvantaged on many laboratory tests of memory because they are unpractised at memorizing or they are undermotivated to perform on tasks that have little apparent ecological validity (Denney, 1982). However, most reports suggest that older adult volunteers are, if anything, more motivated to succeed than young college students (Craik et al., 1995), and although they perform better on memory tasks in which materials are familiar or relevant rather than novel, young adults do so also. Similarly, practice usually improves performance in older adults, but it does not eliminate age differences (Salthouse, 1991). Older adults can also improve their memory substantially if they are given extra study time (Wahlin, Bäckman and Winblad, 1995) or they are effortfully involved in the learning process, either by generating the target stimuli (Rabinowitz, 1989) or by engaging in the manipulation of objects (Bäckman, 1985), although only in the latter case are age differences reported to be eliminated.

At the same time, there appear to be minimal age differences in memory for information relevant to an area of expertise. Evidence that experience buffers the effects of ageing was obtained in a study by Shimamura et al. (1995). These investigators found no age differences among university professors in prose recall, although age deficits were observed in memory for unrelated paired associates. They suggested that the lack of age differences in the recall of meaningful text may be attributable to the fact that professors are continually acquiring and retrieving conceptual knowledge. Thus, in some sense they are experts at integrating new, meaningful information into existing knowledge structures. The learning of arbitrary associations, however, does not draw on this well-practised skill.

These findings suggest that older adults may be able to use their residual memory function more effectively by maintaining memory-relevant activities into the later years. An optimal way to do this may be through continued schooling. Parks, Mitchell and Perlmutter (1986) suggested that being a student provides opportunities to use and practise memory skills; therefore, individuals currently in school should have an advantage on laboratory tests of memory. However, evidence supporting the beneficial effects of current schooling for older adults is mixed (Zivian and Darjes, 1983; Parks et al. 1986). Nevertheless, a number of studies have shown that education is positively correlated with maintenance of memory function in old age (Zelinski, Gilewski and Schaie, 1993; Albert et al., 1995; Hill et al., 1995).

Practice may achieve its effects by allowing some task components to be carried out automatically, thus enabling processing resources to be devoted to other, more demanding aspects of a task; automatic processes may also be less susceptible to the effects of interference. At a neurobiological level, practice may help to maintain neural circuitry (Woodruff-Pak and Hanson, 1995). Alternatively, practice may facilitate the development of new, more efficient strategies (see below). As was demonstrated with mnemonic strategies, however, practice and experience may provide specific rather than general memory advantages – that is, benefits may accrue only to the tasks practised (e.g. prose memory but not paired associate memory in college professors). Findings of specificity are consistent with the notion that once processes become automatic, they may be tightly bound to a particular context and not available to be used flexibly in multiple tasks (Singley and Anderson, 1989).

Activity, physical fitness, exercise

One of the oldest theories of cognitive ageing (Foster and Taylor, 1920) is the theory of disuse, which accounts for age-related cognitive decline and individual differences among older adults in terms of differential activity levels (Salthouse, 1991). The basic tenet of this view is that as people get older, activities are reduced, there are fewer demands on cognitive processes, and cognitive function begins to deteriorate.

In support of this hypothesis, a number of studies have found that various measures of social, domestic and leisure activity levels are positively correlated with memory functioning in older adults (Winocur, Moscovitch and Freedman, 1987; Cockburn and Smith, 1991; Halpern, 1994). Other studies have reported a relation between physical fitness and various aspects of memory. For example, Clarkson-Smith and Hartley (1989) and Abourezk (1989) found that older subjects who exercised had better working memories than nonexercisers. There is also evidence to suggest that cognitive tasks that are particularly difficult or that require effortful processing may be more sensitive to the effects of fitness than those that require automatic processing (Craik, Byrd and Swanson, 1987; Chodzko-Zajko, 1991; Chodzko-Zajko et al., 1992).

Berger and Hecht (1989) have noted that elderly people who exercise also have higher levels of education, are more health conscious, and come from higher socioeconomic backgrounds than nonexercising elderly, and these other variables may account for some of the variability in cognitive performance. Clarkson-

Smith and Hartley (1990), however, using a structural equation model, demonstrated that after taking into account the indirect effects of age, education, health and well-being, there still remained an independent contribution of exercise to working memory. Similarly, the MacArthur Studies of Ageing (Albert et al., 1995) found that strenuous activity and peak pulmonary expiratory flow rate (i.e. lung capacity) together with education were direct predictors of cognitive change (including measures of verbal and nonverbal memory) over a two-year period.

However, only a few studies have used exercise specifically as an intervention. Dustman and colleagues (1984) randomly assigned previously sedentary older adults to an aerobic exercise group (exercise three times/week), an exercise control group (stretching three times/week) or a nonexercise control group. Subjects in the aerobic group showed clear cardiovascular improvements accompanied by significant increases in performance on neuropsychological tests, including tests of short-term memory. The control groups showed no such improvements. Hill, Storandt and Malley (1993) also found that older adults who participated in a 9–12-month exercise programme scored significantly higher on a verbal memory task relative to a nonexercising control group. However, differences in performance were attributable to declines in the control group rather than to increases in the exercise group, suggesting that the exercise training may have served to prevent the normal age-related memory decline. In a recent study, Glisky (1998) found evidence for both effects. After participating in a four-month aerobic exercise regimen, older adults showed increases on measures of verbal fluency, whereas a nonexercising control group showed declines on both verbal memory and verbal fluency tasks.

The mechanisms involved in the improvement of cognition from exercise are not well understood. One possibility is that the effects are mediated through an increase in processing speed; this suggestion is consistent with findings of improvement on speeded tasks. Animal studies suggest that improved aerobic fitness and increased physical activity can result in an increase in neurotransmitter levels, an increase in speed of information transmission, and changes in brain structure

and vasculature (MacRae et al., 1987). Alternatively, improved cardiovascular strength and increased oxygen transport may lead to more efficient cerebrovascular functioning (Hawkins, Kramer and Capaldi, 1992; Shay and Roth, 1992).

Although studies relating activity and fitness levels to cognitive functioning are suggestive, they are largely correlational and have produced inconsistent findings (Perri and Templer, 1985; for null results, Blumenthal et al., 1989; Emory and Gatz, 1990). Additional studies are needed to evaluate further the conditions under which exercise regimens are likely to be most beneficial and to explore the underlying mechanisms mediating the relation between cognition and activity.

Time of day

Recent studies (May, Hasher and Stoltzfus, 1993) have shown that older and younger adults experience peak circadian arousal levels at different times of day: most older people are at their peak early in the day (i.e. they are morning-type people) whereas most young adults experience their peak in the late afternoon (i.e. they are evening-type people). Moreover, recent studies have demonstrated that the effectiveness of certain cognitive processes is correlated with circadian arousal levels. For example, in a difficult test of recognition memory, May et al. (1993) found that older adults (as well as young adults) performed significantly more accurately when tested in their peak arousal period, and that there were no age-related deficits when testing occurred in the morning (that is, at the optimal time of day for the elderly and the nonoptimal time for the young). Hasher, Zacks and May (1999) have since shown that time of day may be particularly important for cognitive tasks that require inhibitory control or the suppression of dominant responses, and may have little if any effect on tasks that require the relatively automatic retrieval of well-learned information. Because inhibitory processes are assumed to be necessary for the efficient operation of working memory (Hasher and Zacks, 1988), any cognitive activities that require working memory are likely to show deficits when attempted at off-peak times.

These findings have a straightforward message for

rehabilitation: learning and memory tasks are likely to be performed most accurately and efficiently if carried out during an individual's optimal time of day, which for most older adults is in the morning. Further, if tasks are well practised or well supported contextually (e.g. recognition memory), time of day should have little impact.

Pharmacological interventions

Normal ageing is accompanied by a loss of neurons and synapses in the brain, and by a reduction in neuronal metabolism and information transmission, all of which may affect learning and memory performance. To compensate for these losses and to enhance residual function, a number of pharmacological interventions have been attempted. Although beneficial effects of various chemical agents, particularly those that enhance cholinergic activity, have been demonstrated in animals, clinical trials with humans have produced inconsistent results (Woodruff-Pak and Hanson, 1995). Other drugs, such as amphetamines, have produced some positive outcomes, possibly as a result of increased arousal levels, which may enable better use of residual memory capacities (Lombardi and Weingartner, 1995).

The administration of glucose has also been found to enhance performance on episodic memory tasks in the elderly (Manning, Hall and Gold, 1990; Gold, 1992). Although the exact mechanism of this effect is uncertain, findings suggest that poor regulation of glucose and impaired uptake of glucose from blood to brain are associated with memory deficits. Further, it appears that the beneficial effects of glucose may be selective to memory tasks that depend on the hippocampus rather than on prefrontal cortex (Winocur, 1995).

Substitution of intact function

This approach to rehabilitation (Rothi and Horner, 1983) assumes that memory processes normally used by young adults may no longer be available to older adults or may be sufficiently compromised as to be nonfunctional. To overcome these deficits, other intact processes, not normally used in the performance of episodic memory tasks, may have to be recruited (Bäckman and Dixon, 1992). This reorganization of function at the cognitive/behavioural level is assumed to be supported by a reorganization of function at the neural level (Luria, 1963; Woodruff-Pak and Hanson, 1995). Although such neural reorganization remains somewhat speculative, recent findings using neuro-imaging techniques have suggested that the brain may be able to compensate for reduced function in one area by using an alternative area, either a homologous region in the other hemisphere (Petersen, 1996) or another structure not normally involved in the behaviour (e.g. Grady et al., 1994).

Implicit memory

In the memory domain, numerous studies have demonstrated that implicit memory performance holds up well with age, despite the reliable findings of decline in explicit memory (for review, see Howard, 1996). These results are consistent with findings from recent neuro-imaging studies that have implicated extrastriate occipital cortex in implicit memory tasks (Buckner et al., 1995; Schacter et al., 1996a) – a region of the brain that is minimally affected by age – and hippocampal and prefrontal areas in explicit memory – areas that show substantial age-related declines. These findings have led a number of researchers to suggest that a reasonable strategy for rehabilitation might be to try to recruit intact implicit memory processes and structures to compensate for the explicit functions that have been compromised by age (Howard, 1996). This approach is in some ways the complement to the Jacoby approach outlined above. Whereas Jacoby and colleagues have attempted to retrain damaged control processes, these methods attempt to tap into automatic processes. This tactic has been used with some success among brain-injured patients (for review, see Glisky, 1997), but as yet, little is known about its potential for use with the elderly. Brief descriptions of three of these methods are outlined below.

Spaced retrieval

The spaced retrieval technique (Landauer and Bjork, 1978) is a relatively simple rehearsal method in which to-be-learned information is rehearsed repeatedly at gradually increasing delays. The technique has not, to the authors' knowledge, been tested with normally ageing elderly individuals, but Camp and colleagues (Camp, 1989; Camp and McKitrick, 1992) have demonstrated its effectiveness with Alzheimer's disease patients, who were able to learn people's names and the locations of objects and to retain them over a period of several weeks. The procedure has also been used successfully with amnesic and other neurological populations (Schacter, Rich and Stampp, 1985; Moffat, 1992). Camp and McKitrick (1992) speculated that learning by this method, which appears to be relatively effortless, may rely on automatic or implicit memory processes.

Errorless learning

Baddeley and Wilson (1994; Baddeley, 1992) suggested that implicit memory is particularly susceptible to proactive interference. Therefore, it is important for memory-impaired individuals, who rely on implicit memory processes to learn new information, to avoid errors early in the learning process. If errors are generated during initial learning, they may be difficult to eliminate without access to explicit memory. Wilson and colleagues (1994; Baddeley and Wilson, 1994) have demonstrated that memory-impaired patients can learn people's names and other pieces of factual information much more readily if they use an errorless learning technique. To the authors' knowledge, the benefits of errorless learning have not been demonstrated with the elderly. There is evidence to suggest, however, that older adults are prone to interference, and so any technique that reduces interference may provide benefits.

Vanishing cues

The method of vanishing cues (Glisky, Schacter and Tulving, 1986) was designed specifically to take advantage of the preserved priming or implicit memory processes demonstrated by amnesic patients. The technique involves the use of partial information as a cue or prompt, which is gradually withdrawn across learning trials. It has been used primarily to teach memory-impaired patients complex domain-specific knowledge relevant to a variety of everyday tasks (for

review, see Glisky, Schacter and Butters, 1994).

In an attempt to explore whether the method would be effective for older adults, a study was designed to teach older people rare words and their definitions, and compared the method of vanishing cues to a standard method of anticipation. In a conceptually similar study with amnesic patients (Glisky et al., 1986), a significant advantage for the vanishing cues procedure had been found. However, no such advantage was found among the normal elderly subjects, who took twice as many trials as the young people to learn the vocabulary items, although there was no difference between the two training methods. Although it is not clear why older subjects did not benefit from the method of vanishing cues, one possibility concerns the number of errors. Older adults tended to guess in the presence of letter cues, thus making many more errors in the vanishing cues condition. Further, the number of errors correlated with perseverative errors on the Wisconsin Card Sorting Test ($r = 0.64$), suggesting that the method may have been particularly problematic for older adults with reduced frontal control. If, as Baddeley and Wilson have suggested, the method of vanishing cues derives its benefits by constraining responding and reducing errors, its lack of effectiveness in this study may be attributable to its failure to meet these criteria. Because the stimuli were novel as opposed to familiar words, the constraints on potential responses were relatively few in this study.

To try to reduce errors in the vanishing cues condition, a subsequent study switched to a computer-related vocabulary. In this case, the target stimuli were familiar words paired with novel definitions. This manipulation successfully reduced the guessing/error rate in the faded-cueing condition, but still no advantage was found for the vanishing cues method. It was speculated that the method of vanishing cues allows people to use implicit memory processes to learn new information but that it may be useful only for individuals with severe impairments in explicit memory, such as amnesic or dementia patients. For people with only mild or moderate deficits, such as the normal elderly, relying on implicit memory processes, which are largely automatic and prone to error and interference, may be less reliable than using residual explicit memory processes, particularly for individuals with declining frontal lobe function.

In general, then, although the idea to substitute preserved implicit memory function for impaired explicit memory function is appealing, there is as yet little indication that it can be accomplished successfully in normal elderly individuals.

Expertise

Bäckman has suggested that one way to compensate for deficits in basic cognitive abilities is to use 'substitutable skills' (Bäckman and Dixon, 1992, p. 262). Evidence for the use of new skills in the performance of old tasks comes from studies of expertise. Experts tend to maintain performance in their specific domain of expertise across the lifespan. For example, Salthouse (1984) found that typists were able to maintain typing speed into their 70s, despite the fact that the component skills required for typing, such as finger-tapping speed and choice reaction time, had declined. Salthouse determined that expert typists were able to maintain overall performance levels by looking further ahead at material to be typed. They were thus substituting an intact process, not normally used by skilled typists, to compensate for age-related declines in other processes. Similarly, Charness (1989) reported that older chess experts were as accurate as young experts in selecting the next best move in a chess game despite their less efficient working memory capacities. Charness suggested that the older experts developed more efficient chunking and search strategies, which limited working memory demands and enabled them to maintain performance.

The studies of expertise have some important implications for rehabilitation in older adults. First, they demonstrate that there may be several ways to perform any particular task and that deficits in some processes may be offset by the substitution of alternative processes that are less affected by age. Second, they suggest that extensive practice may mitigate age-related declines by allowing for more efficient processing of some task components. Third, they imply that knowledge, which increases with age, may be able to compensate for age-related deficits in encoding, retrieval or other speeded processes. Finally, they suggest, in a practical sense, that older people with extensive experience in a particular field (e.g. a job) may be able to maintain performance in that domain despite declining function in other domains (Park, 1994).

Conclusions

Although research concerning the rehabilitation of memory function in normally ageing older adults is relatively sparse, some suggestive patterns of findings are noteworthy. First, unlike amnesic patients, older adults have considerable residual memory function that they may be able to use more efficiently given appropriate training. Such training may take the form of the teaching and practice of specific encoding and retrieval strategies or it may involve the engagement of more general activities or exercise regimens. Although most evidence suggests that practice effects are highly specific and do not generalize to unrelated tasks, the preliminary findings of beneficial effects of aerobic exercise suggest that general benefits may be possible, although they may be moderated by a host of individual difference variables. Second, memory performance can be improved through the use of external aids or environmental supports. Such assistance may enable older people to bypass altogether the need to engage in effortful memory processes or may allow some memory processes to be initiated and carried out automatically. Third, older adults may be able to learn new cognitive skills that can be substituted for other age-dependent mnemonic skills that have declined. Although the use of implicit memory enhances learning in neurological patients, including those with Alzheimer's disease, it has yet to prove differentially effective for the normal elderly. Fourth, to compensate for reduced memory function, older people may have to exert more time and effort, take optimal advantage of their prior knowledge and expertise, keep active and involved, and plan their most cognitively demanding activities at their optimal time of day.

Most of the research on memory rehabilitation in the elderly is based on principles and findings derived from cognitive psychology and theories of ageing. Yet, despite this solid empirical and theoretical grounding, the rehabilitation techniques have produced relatively modest outcomes. This limited success may be attributable to the heterogeneity of the ageing population. Cognitive psychologists, to a large degree, have ignored individual difference variables, choosing to treat them as error variance. This variability, however, may be critical in the design of interventions. If different functions age differently across individuals, then it may be necessary to tailor remedial programmes to the individual.

Recent findings using neuroimaging techniques have demonstrated that both the hippocampal formation and the prefrontal cortex are involved in memory, but in different capacities (Tulving et al., 1994; Nyberg et al., 1996; Schacter et al., 1996a). Both of these brain regions are also particularly susceptible to the effects of ageing (Coffey et al., 1992; Raz et al., 1997), although substantial individual differences may exist. In an ongoing longitudinal study of normal elderly adults in the authors' laboratory, it was found that medial temporal lobe and frontal lobe functions show different ageing patterns both within and across individuals (Glisky, Polster and Routhieaux, 1995), and that these patterns differentially predict performance on various memory tasks. Other investigators have noted a relation between the existence and extent of white matter lesions in healthy elderly individuals and disruptions in frontal lobe function (Boone et al., 1992). The interindividual variability in cognitive performance that occurs with age may thus be partly attributable to variability in brain ageing. Increased intraindividual variability in memory performance across time has also been noted among older adults (Hertzog, Dixon and Hultsch, 1992). Although reasons for this variation are not well understood, it may represent changes in internal states such as health or mood, environmental influences such as life events, and other psychosocial variables such as anxiety and stress (Winocur, Moscovitch and Freedman, 1987). These factors may have direct effects on memory performance or they may interact with neurological changes. Alternatively, declining brain function may itself contribute to lack of stability in performance over time.

This increased variability that occurs with age makes it unlikely that any single remedial technique will work for everyone. Instead, it seems important to consider what neurobiological, cognitive and psychosocial factors might be contributing to an individual's performance and to design interventions with these variables in mind. Rehabilitation methodologies that are constructed to address specific cognitive problems and to take account of individual differences should produce more consistent and successful outcomes in the future.

References

Abourezk, T. 1989. The effects of regular aerobic exercise on short-term memory efficiency in the older adult. In *Aging and Motor Behavior*, ed. A.C. Ostrow, pp. 105–13. Indiana: A.C. Benchmark Press.

Albert, M., Duffy, F.H. and Naeser, M. 1987. Nonlinear changes in cognition with age and their neuropsychologic correlates. *Can J Psychol* 41, 141–57.

Albert, M.S., Jones, K.S. Savage, C.R. and Berkman, L. 1995. Predictors of cognitive change in older persons: MacArthur studies of successful aging. *Psychol Aging* 10, 578–89.

Anschutz, L., Camp, C.J., Markley, R.P. and Kramer, J.J. 1985. Maintenance and generalization of mnemonics for grocery shopping by older adults. *Exp Aging Res* 11, 157–60.

Anschutz, L., Camp, C.J., Markley, R.P. and Kramer, J.J. 1987. Remembering mnemonics: a three-year follow-up on the effects of mnemonics training in elderly adults. *Exp Aging Res* 13, 141–4.

Bäckman, L. 1985. Further evidence for the lack of adult age differences on free recall of subject-performed tasks: the importance of motor action. *Hum Learn J Pract Res Appl* 4, 79–87.

Bäckman, L. and Dixon, R.A. 1992. Psychological compensation: a theoretical framework. *Psychol Bull* 112, 259–83.

Baddeley, A.D. 1992. Implicit memory and errorless learning: a link between cognitive theory and neuropsychological rehabilitation. In *Neuropsychology of Memory*, ed. L.R. Squire and N. Butters, pp. 309–21. New York: Guilford Press.

Baddeley, A.D. and Wilson, B.A. 1994. When implicit learning fails: amnesia and the problem of error elimination. *Neuropsychologia* 32, 53–68.

Berger, R.G. and Hecht, L.M. 1989. Exercise, ageing, and psychological well-being: the mind–body question. In *Aging and Motor Behavior*, ed. A.C. Ostrow, pp. 117–57. Indiana: A.C. Benchmark Press.

Blumenthal, J.A., Emory, C.F., Madden, D.J. et al. 1989. Cardiovascular and behavioral effects of aerobic exercise training in healthy older men and women. *J Gerontol* 44, M147–57.

Boone, K.B., Miller, B.L., Lesser, I.M. et al. 1992. Neuropsychological correlates of white-matter lesions in healthy elderly subjects. *Arch Neurol* **49**, 549–54.

Buckner, R.L., Petersen, S.E., Ojemann,J.G., Miezin, F.M., Squire, L.R. and Raichle, M.E. 1995. Functional anatomical studies of explicit and implicit memory retrieval tasks. *J Neurosci* **15**, 12–29.

Camp, C.J. 1989. Facilitation of new learning in Alzheimer's disease. In *Memory, Aging, and Dementia*, ed. G.C. Gilmore, P.J. Whitehouse and M.L. Wykle, pp. 212–25. New York: Springer Verlag.

Camp, C.J. and McKitrick, L.A. 1992. Memory interventions in Alzheimer's-type dementia populations: methodological and theoretical issues. In *Everyday Memory and Aging: Current Research and Methodology*, ed. R.L. West and J.D. Sinnott, pp. 155–72. New York: Springer Verlag.

Charness, N. 1989. Age and expertise: responding to Talland's challenge. In *Everyday Cognition in Adulthood and Late Life*, ed. L.W. Poon, D.C. Rubin and B.A. Wilson, pp. 437–56. Cambridge: Cambridge University Press.

Chodzko-Zajko, W.J. 1991. Physical fitness, cognitive performance, and aging. *Med Sci Sports Exerc* **23**, 868–72.

Chodzko-Zajko, W.J., Schuler, P., Solomon,J., Heinl, B. and Ellis, N.R. 1992. The influence of physical fitness on automatic and effortful memory changes in aging. *Int J Aging Hum Dev* **35**, 265–85.

Clarkson-Smith, L. and Hartley, A.A. 1989. Relationship between exercise and cognitive abilities in older adults. *Psychol Aging* **4**, 183–9.

Clarkson-Smith, L. and Hartley, A.A. 1990. Structural equation models of relationships between exercise and cognitive abilities. *Psychol Aging* **5**, 437–46.

Cockburn, J. and Smith, P.T. 1991. The relative influence of intelligence and age on everyday memory. *J Gerontol* **46**, P31–6.

Coffey, C.E., Wilkinson, W.E., Parashos, I.A. et al. 1992. Quantitative cerebral anatomy of the ageing human brain: a cross-sectional study using magnetic resonance imaging. *Neuropsychology* **42**, 527–36.

Craik, F.I.M. 1986. A functional account of age differences in memory. In *Human Memory and Cognitive Capabilities, Mechanisms and Performances*, ed. F. Klix and H. Hagendorf, pp. 409–22. Amsterdam: Elsevier.

Craik, F.I.M., Anderson, N.D., Kerr, S.A. and Li, K.Z.H. 1995. Memory changes in normal ageing. In *Handbook of Memory Disorders*, ed. A.D. Baddeley, B.A. Wilson and F.N. Watts, pp. 211–41. Chichester: John Wiley & Sons.

Craik, F.I.M., Byrd, M. and Swanson, J.M. 1987. Patterns of memory loss in three elderly samples. *Psychol Aging* **2**, 79–86.

Craik, F.I.M. and Jennings, J.M. 1992. Human memory. In *The Handbook of Aging and Cognition*, ed. F.I.M. Craik and T.A. Salthouse, pp. 51–110. Hillsdale, NJ: Lawrence Erlbaum.

Craik, F.I.M. and McDowd, J.M. 1987. Age differences in recall and recognition. *J Exp Psychol Learn Mem Cogn* **13**, 474–9.

Craik, F.I.M., Morris, L.W., Morris, R.G. and Loewen, E.R. 1990. Relations between source amnesia and frontal lobe functioning in older adults. *Psychol Aging* **5**, 148–51.

Denney, N.W. 1982. Aging and cognitive changes. In *Handbook of Developmental Psychology*, ed. B.B. Wolman and G. Stricker, pp. 807–27. Englewood Cliffs, NJ: Prentice Hall.

Dixon, R.A. and Bäckman, L. 1993. The concept of compensation in cognitive aging: the case of prose processing in adulthood. *Int J Aging Hum Dev* **36**, 199–217.

Dixon, R.A. and Bäckman, L., eds. 1995. *Compensating for Psychological Deficits and Declines*. Mahwah, NJ: Lawrence Erlbaum.

Dustman, R.E., Ruhling, R.O., Russell, E.M. et al. 1984. Aerobic exercise training and improved neuropsychological function of older individuals. *Neurobiol Aging* **5**, 35–42.

Einstein, G.O. and McDaniel, M.A. 1996. Retrieval processes in prospective memory: theoretical approaches and some new empirical findings. In *Prospective Memory*, ed. M. Brandimonte, G.O. Einstein and M.A. McDaniel, pp. 115–41. Mahwah, NJ: Lawrence Erlbaum.

Elias, P.K., Elias, M.F., Robbins, M.A. and Gage, P. 1987. Acquisition of word-processing skills by younger, middle-age, and older adults. *Psychol Aging* **2**, 340–8.

Emory, C.F. and Gatz, M. 1990. Psychological and cognitive effects of an exercise program for community-residing older adults. *The Gerontologist* **30**, 184–8.

Foster, J.C. and Taylor, G.A. 1920. The applicability of mental tests to persons over 50. *J Appl Psychol* **4**, 39–58.

Glisky, E.L. 1995. Computers in memory rehabilitation. In *Handbook of Memory Disorders*, ed. A.D. Baddeley, B.A. Wilson and F.N. Watts, pp. 557–75. Chichester: John Wiley & Sons.

Glisky, E.L. 1997. Rehabilitation of memory dysfunction. In *Behavioral Neurology and Neuropsychology*, ed. T.E. Feinberg and M.J. Farah, pp. 491–5. New York: McGraw-Hill.

Glisky, E.L., Polster, M.R. and Routhieaux, B.C. 1995. Double association between item and source memory. *Neuropsychology* **9**, 229–35.

Glisky, E.L., Schacter, D.L. and Butters, M.A. 1994. Domain-specific learning and remediation of memory disorders. In *Cognitive Neuropsychology and Cognitive Rehabilitation*, ed. M.J. Riddoch and G.W. Humphreys, pp. 527–48. Hove, UK: Lawrence Erlbaum.

Glisky, E.L., Schacter, D.L. and Tulving, E. 1986. Learning and retention of computer related vocabulary in memory-impaired patients: method of vanishing cues. *J Clin Exp Neuropsychol* **8**, 292–312.

Glisky, M.L. 1998. The effects of aerobic exercise and cognitive training on cognitive and psychosocial functioning in older adults. *J Int Neuropsychol Soc* (Abstract) **4**(1), 50.

Gold, P.E. 1992. Modulation of memory processing: enhancement of memory in rodents and humans. In *Neuropsychology of Memory*, ed. L.R. Squire and N. Butters, pp. 402–14. New York: Guilford Press.

Grady, C.L., Maisog, J.M., Horwitz, B. et al. 1994. Age-related changes in cortical blood flow activation during visual processing of faces and location. *J Neurosci* **14**, 1450–62.

Grady, C.L., McIntosh, A.R., Horwitz, B. et al. 1995. Age-related reductions in human recognition memory due to impaired encoding. *Science* **269**, 218–21.

Halpern, D.F. 1994. Exercise and everyday remembering: are they related in older adults? Paper read at 35th Annual Meeting of The Psychonomic Society, at St Louis, MO.

Harris, J.E. 1978. External memory aids. In *Practical Aspects of Memory*, ed. M.M. Gruneberg, P.E. Morris and R.N. Sykes, pp. 172–9. London: Academic Press.

Harris, J.E. 1992. Ways to help memory. In *Clinical Management of Memory Problems*, ed. B.A. Wilson and N. Moffat, pp. 59–85. London: Chapman & Hall.

Hasher, L. and Zacks, R.T. 1988. Working memory, comprehension, and aging: a review and a new view. In *The Psychology of Learning and Motivation*, ed. G.H. Bower, pp. 193–225. New York: Academic Press.

Hasher, L., Zacks, R.T. and May, C.P. 1999. Inhibitory control, circadian arousal, and age. In *Attention and Performance XVII: Cognitive Regulation of Performance: Interaction of Theory and Application*, ed. D. Gopher and A. Koriat, pp. 653–75. Cambridge, MA: MIT Press.

Hawkins, H.L., Kramer, A.F. and Capaldi, D. 1992. Aging, exercise, and attention. *Psychol Aging* **7**, 643–53.

Hertzog, C., Dixon, R.A. and Hultsch, D.F. 1992. Intraindividual change in text recall of the elderly. *Brain Lang* **42**, 248–69.

Hill, R.D., Sheikh, J.I. and Yesavage, J. 1988. Pretraining enhances mnemonic training in elderly adults. *Exp Aging Res* **14**, 207–11.

Hill, R.D., Storandt, M. and Malley, M. 1993. The impact of long-term exercise training on psychological function in older adults. *J Gerontol Psychol Sci* **48**, P12–17.

Hill, R.D., Wahlin, A., Winblad, B. and Bäckman, L. 1995. The role of demographic and life style variables in utilizing cognitive support for episodic remembering among very old adults. *J Gerontol Psychol Sci* **50B**, P219–27.

Howard, D.V. 1996. The aging of implicit and explicit memory. In *Perspectives on Cognitive Change in Adulthood and Aging*, ed. F. Blanchard-Fields and T.M. Hess, pp. 221–54. New York: McGraw-Hill.

Jacoby, L.L. 1991. A process dissociation framework: separating automatic from intentional uses of memory. *J Mem Lang* **30**, 513–41.

Jacoby, L.L., Jennings, J.M. and Hay, J.F. 1996. Dissociating automatic and consciously controlled processes: implications for diagnosis and rehabilitation of memory deficits. In *Basic and Applied Memory Research: Theory in Context*, ed. D.J. Herrmann, C. McEvoy, C. Hertzog, P. Hertel and M.K. Johnson, pp. 161–93. Mahwah, NJ: Lawrence Erlbaum.

Jennings, J.M. and Jacoby, L.L. 1993. Automatic versus intentional uses of memory: aging, attention, and control. *Psychol Aging* **8**, 283–93.

Kapur, N. 1995. Memory aids in the rehabilitation of memory disordered patients. In *Handbook of Memory Disorders*, ed. A.D. Baddeley, B.A. Wilson and F.N. Watts, pp. 534–56. Chichester: John Wiley & Sons.

Kausler, D.H. 1994. *Learning and Memory in Normal Aging*. New York: Academic Press.

Landauer, T.K. and Bjork, R.A. 1978. Optimum rehearsal patterns and name learning. In *Practical Aspects of Memory*, ed. M.M. Gruneberg, P.E. Morris and R.N. Sykes, pp. 625–32. London: Academic Press.

Lombardi, W.J. and Weingartner, H. 1995. Pharmacological treatment of impaired memory function. In *Handbook of Memory Disorders*, ed. A.D. Baddeley, B.A. Wilson and F.N. Watts, pp. 577–601. Chichester: John Wiley & Sons.

Luria, A.R. 1963. *Restoration of Function after Brain Injury*. New York: Macmillan.

MacRae, P.G., Spirduso, W.W., Walters, T.J., Farrar, R.P. and Wilcox, R.E. 1987. Endurance training effects on striatal D2 dopamine receptor binding and striatal dopamine metabolism in presenescent older rats. *Psychopharmacology* **92**, 236–40.

Manning, C.A., Hall, J.L. and Gold, P.E. 1990. Glucose effects on memory and other neuropsychological tests in elderly humans. *Psychol Sci* **1**, 307–11.

Martin, A.J., Friston, K.J., Colebatch, J.G. and Frackowiak, R.S.J. 1991. Decreases in regional cerebral blood flow with normal ageing. *J Cereb Blood Flow Metab* **11**, 684–9.

May, C.P., Hasher, L. and Stoltzfus, E.R. 1993. Optimal time of day and the magnitude of age differences in memory. *Psychol Sci* **4**, 326–30.

McIntyre, J.S. and Craik, F.I.M. 1987. Age differences in memory for item and source information. *Can J Psychol* **41**, 175–92.

Moffat, N. 1992. Strategies of memory therapy. In *Clinical Management of Memory Problems*, ed. B.A. Wilson and N. Moffat, pp. 86–119. London: Chapman & Hall.

Moscovitch, M. 1982. A neuropsychological approach to perception and memory in normal and pathological aging. In *Aging and Cognitive Processes*, ed. F.I.M. Craik and S. Trehub, pp. 55–79. New York: Plenum Press.

Neely, A.S. and Bäckman, L. 1993a. Long-term maintenance of gains from memory training in older adults: two 3½-year follow-up studies. *J Gerontol Psychol Sci* **48**, P233–7.

Neely, A.S. and Bäckman, L. 1993b. Maintenance of gains following multifactorial and unifactorial memory training in late adulthood. *Educ Gerontol* **19**, 105–17.

Neely, A.S. and Bäckman, L. 1995. Effects of multifactorial memory training in old age: generalizability across tasks and individuals. *J Gerontol Psychol Sci* **50B**, P134–40.

Nyberg, L., McIntosh, A.R., Houle, S., Nillson, L.-G. and Tulving, E. 1996. Activation of medial temporal structures during episodic memory retrieval. *Nature* **380**, 715–17.

Park, D.C. 1994. Aging, cognition, and work. *Hum Perform* **7**, 181–205.

Park, D.C. and Kidder, D.P. 1996. Prospective memory and medication adherence. In *Prospective Memory: Theory and Applications*, ed. M. Brandimonte, G.O. Einstein and M.A. McDaniel, pp. 369–90. Mahwah, NJ: Lawrence Erlbaum.

Park, D.C., Morrell, R.W., Frieske, D. and Kincaid, D. 1992. Medication adherence behaviors in older adults: effects of external cognitive supports. *Psychol Aging* **7**, 252–6.

Park, D.D., Puglisi, J.T. and Smith, A.D. 1986. Memory for pictures: does an age-related decline exist? *Psychol Aging* **1**, 11–17.

Parks, C.W. Jr., Mitchell, D.B. and Perlmutter, M. 1986. Cognitive and social functioning across adulthood: age or student status differences? *Psychol Aging* **1**, 248–54.

Perri, S. and Templer, D.I. 1985. The effects of an aerobic exercise program on psychological variables in older adults. *Int J Aging Hum Dev* **20**, 167–71.

Petersen, S.E. 1996. Using words to probe cognitive function: imaging and lesion–behavior studies. Paper read at 6th Annual Rotman Research Institute Conference on Functional Neuroimaging, at Toronto, Canada.

Poon, L.W. 1985. Differences in human memory with aging: nature, causes and clinical implications. In *Handbook of the Psychology of Aging*, ed. J.E. Birren and K.W. Schaie, pp. 427–62. New York: Van Nostrand Reinhold.

Rabinowitz, J.C. 1989. Judgments of origin and generation effects: comparisons between young and elderly adults. *Psychol Aging* **4**, 259–68.

Raz, N., Gunning, F.M., Head, D. et al. 1997. Selective aging of the human cerebral cortex observed *in vivo*: differential vulnerability of the prefrontal gray matter. *Cereb Cortex* **7**, 268–82.

Rothi, L.J. and Horner, J. 1983. Restitution and substitution: two theories of recovery with application to neurobehavioral treatment. *J Clin Neuropsychol* **5**, 73–81.

Salthouse, T.A. 1984. Effects of age and skill in typing. *J Exp Psychol Gen* **113**, 345–71.

Salthouse, T.A. 1991. *Theoretical Perspectives on Cognitive Aging*. Hillsdale, NJ: Lawrence Erlbaum.

Schacter, D.L., Alpert, N.M., Savage, C.R., Rauch, S.L. and Albert, M.S. 1996a. Conscious recollection and the human hippocampal formation: evidence from positron emission tomography. *Proc Natl Acad Sci* **93**, 321–5.

Schacter, D.L., Rich, S.A. and Stampp, M.S. 1985. Remediation of memory disorders: experimental evaluation of the spaced-retrieval technique. *J Clin Exp Neuropsychol* **7**, 79–96.

Schacter, D.L., Savage, C.R., Alpert, N.M., Rauch, S.L. and Albert, M.S. 1996b. The role of hippocampus and frontal cortex in age-related memory changes: a PET study. *NeuroReport* **7**, 1165–9.

Scogin, F. and Bienias, J.L. 1988. A three-year follow-up of older adult participants in a memory-skills training program. *Psychol Aging* **3**, 334–7.

Shallice, T., Fletcher, P., Frith, C.D., Grasby, P., Frackowiak, R.S.J. and Dolan, R.J. 1994. Brain regions associated with acquisition and retrieval of verbal episodic memory. *Nature* **368**, 633–5.

Shay, K.A. and Roth, D.L. 1992. Association between aerobic fitness and visuospatial performance in healthy older adults. *Psychol Aging* **7**, 15–24.

Sheikh, J.I., Hill, R.D. and Yesavage, J.A. 1986. Long-term efficacy of cognitive training for age-associated memory impairment: a six-month follow-up study. *Dev Neuropsychol* **2**, 413–21.

Shimamura, A.P., Berry, J.M., Mangels, J.A., Rusting, C.L. and Jurica, P.J. 1995. Memory and cognitive abilities in university professors: evidence for successful aging. *Psychol Sci* **6**, 271–7.

Singley, M.K. and Anderson, J.R. 1989. *The Transfer of Cognitive Skill*. Cambridge, MA: Harvard University Press.

Tulving, E., Kapur, S., Craik, F.I.M., Moscovitch, M. and Houle, S. 1994. Hemispheric encoding/retrieval asymmetry in episodic memory: positron emission tomography findings. *Proc Natl Acad Sci* **91**, 2016–20.

Verhaeghen, P., Marcoen, A. and Goosens, L. 1992. Improving memory performance in the aged through mnemonic training: a meta-analytic study. *Psychol Aging* **7**, 242–51.

Wahlin, A., Bäckman, L. and Winblad, B. 1995. Free recall and recognition of slowly and rapidly presented words in very old age: a community-based study. *Exp Aging Res* **21**, 251–71.

Weintraub, S., Powell, D.H. and Whitla, D.K. 1994. Successful cognitive ageing: individual differences among physicians on a computerized test of mental state. *J Ger Psychiatry* **27**, 15–34.

West, R.L. 1995. Compensatory strategies for age-associated memory impairment. In *Handbook of Memory Disorders*, ed. A.D. Baddeley, B.A. Wilson and F.N. Watts, pp. 481–500. Chichester: John Wiley & Sons.

West, R.L. and Boatwright, L.K. 1983. Age differences in cued recall and recognition under varying encoding and retrieval conditions. *Exp Aging Res* **9**, 185–9.

West, R.L. and Crook, T.H. 1992. Video training of imagery for mature adults. *Appl Cogn Psychol* **6**, 307–20.

West, R.L. and Tomer, A. 1989. Everyday memory problems of healthy older adults: characteristics of a successful intervention. In *Memory, Aging and Dementia: Theory, Assessment and Treatment*, ed. G.C. Gilmore, P.J. Whitehouse and M.L. Wykle, pp. 74–98. New York: Springer Verlag.

Wilson, B. 1987. *Rehabilitation of Memory*. New York: Guilford Press.

Wilson, B.A., Baddeley, A.D., Evans, J. and Shiel, A. 1994. Errorless learning in the rehabilitation of memory impaired people. *Neuropsychol Rehabil* **4**, 307–26.

Winocur, G. 1995. Glucose-enhanced performance by aged rats on a test of conditional discrimination learning. *Psychobiology* **23**, 270–6.

Winocur, G., Moscovitch, M. and Freedman, J. 1987. An investigation of cognitive function in relation to psychosocial variables in institutionalized old people. *Can J Psychol* **41**, 257–69.

Winograd, E. and Simon, E.W. 1980. Visual memory and imagery in the aged. In *New Directions in Memory and Aging: Proceedings of the George A. Talland Memorial Conference*, ed. L.W. Poon, J.L. Fozard, L.S. Cermak, D. Arenberg and L.W. Thompson, pp. 485–506. Hillsdale, NJ: Lawrence Erlbaum.

Woodruff-Pak, D.S. and Hanson, C. 1995. Plasticity and compensation in brain memory systems in aging. In *Compensating for Psychological Deficits and Declines*, ed. R.A. Dixon and L. Bäckman, pp. 191–217. Mahwah, NJ: Lawrence Erlbaum.

Yesavage, J.A. 1983. Imagery pretraining and memory training in the elderly. *Gerontology* **29**, 271–5.

Yesavage, J.A. 1984. Relaxation and memory training in 39 elderly patients. *Am J Psychiatry* **141**, 778–81.

Yesavage, J.A. and Rose, T.L. 1983. Concentration and mnemonic training in elderly with memory complaints: a study of combined therapy and order effects. *Psychiatry Res* **9**, 157–67.

Yesavage, J.A., Sheikh, J.I., Friedman, L. and Tanke, E. 1990. Learning mnemonics: roles of aging and subtle cognitive impairment. *Psychol Aging* **5**, 133–7.

Zelinski, E.M., Gilewski, M.J. and Schaie, K.W. 1993. Individual differences in cross-section and 3-year longitudinal memory performance across the adult life span. *Psychol Aging* **8**, 176–86.

Zivian, M.T. and Darjes, R.W. 1983. Free recall by in-school and out-of-school adults: performance and memory. *Dev Psychol* **19**, 513–20.

Epilogue. The future of cognitive rehabilitation

Ian H. Robertson, Donald T. Stuss and Gordon Winocur

The research reviewed in this book shows that cognitive rehabilitation can work, and this is in line with the results of research on the rehabilitation of motor deficits. For cognitive rehabilitation to develop further, however, we must develop a better understanding of how it works. Any phenomenon can be addressed at multiple levels of analysis. The remark of one Nobel Prize winner when addressing a meeting of biochemists – 'everything is physics – all else is Social Work' – is clearly as wrong as it is hubristic. Without an adequate model of how rehabilitation works, the refinement and improvement of rehabilitation methods on scientific principles will be impossible.

Billions of dollars each year are spent worldwide in attempting to change behaviour – and, by implication, to change the brain – through a whole range of therapies offered to people who have suffered some type of damage or disease in the brain. Yet hardly any of this enormous enterprise is based on well-developed theory at any level of analysis. It has been shown in this book that it is impossible to pursue cognitive rehabilitation without very close links to the biological characteristics of the brain, and it is critical that a theoretical framework be developed for the behavioural level of analysis. For cognitive rehabilitation is about nothing if it is not about learning, and the determinants of learning, though accessible to some extent at the molecular and cellular levels, are most fruitfully addressed at the behavioural level if one is to yield principles with which to guide the clinical practice of the hundreds of thousands, if not millions, of people worldwide offering therapy to brain-damaged people. Biological levels of analyses are limited in the extent to which they can be heuristically useful in generating hypotheses about interventions at the behavioural level of analysis.

A behavioural level of analysis is required to generate hypotheses about the nature of the behavioural strategies needed to accelerate the recovery of function, though, of course, such a theoretical model must be able to intersect with neurophysiological levels of analysis also. The great Russian neuropsychologist Luria (1963; Luria et al., 1975) was one of the few to formulate such a theoretical model. He proposed that 'functional reorganization' underpins behavioural recovery, with surviving neural circuits reorganizing to achieve the given behaviour in a different way. Dixon and Bäckman have reviewed this type of compensatory reorganization in Chapter 4 of this volume. The question is: can cognitive rehabilitation also aspire to restitute cognitive function?

In Chapter 1, Kolb and Gibb show clearly how experience changes the brain. Partially lesioned neural networks may, under certain circumstances, reconnect, providing that appropriate stimulation and input are provided to these networks. The problems posed by this new field of cognitive rehabilitation include the questions of how one decides when a compensatory versus a restitutive approach to cognitive rehabilitation is advisable and, when a restitutive approach is chosen, how one decides what is the optimal stimulation needed to foster the repair of lesioned circuits? Robertson and Murre (under review) have proposed a theoretical framework within which such questions may be answered, but they have not addressed some issues which pose an even greater theoretical challenge, namely, how these lesioned circuits and impaired cognitive functions interact with the whole person in his or her perceived social environment.

One advance which has been made, and which has been amply demonstrated in this book, is the fact that precision in the planning of the behavioural input to the brain will influence the likelihood of reconnection – or at least of the saving of existing connections – following damage. A good example of guided recovery comes from the work of Nudo et al. (1990), who showed that, following lesion to the motor cortex of the squirrel monkey, hand movement representations adjacent to the area of infarct that were spared from direct injury underwent further loss of cortical territory. Nudo et al. argued that such losses in the representational area of the hand over and above those caused by the direct lesion are the result of a diminished use of the affected hand. Nudo and his colleagues also demonstrated that intensive behavioural training of skilled hand use resulted in a prevention of the loss of the hand territory adjacent to the infarct. In some instances, the hand representations expanded into regions formerly occupied by representations of the elbow and shoulder. Furthermore, this functional reorganization of the undamaged motor cortex was accompanied by behavioural recovery of skilled hand function. The conclusion was that rehabilitative training can shape subsequent reorganizaton in the adjacent intact cortex.

In Chapter 13, Uswatte and Taub show parallel results of how the recovery of limb function can occur as a result of discouraging the use of the intact arm, and encouraging the use of the hemiparetic limb. Robertson and Murre (under review) have argued that whereas such precise input can aid brain repair and behavioural recovery, some types of behavioural intervention may hinder such recovery, particularly when circuits which inhibit the damaged parts of the brain are activated by the therapy. As has been shown in the psychotherapy literature, if a therapy is potent enough to produce positive results it almost certainly can, under certain circumstances, lead to negative consequences also. Finding the correct behavioural input to the malfunctioning brain circuit may also be difficult, even if one can be certain that there is no inadvertent inhibition of that circuit through the stimulation of competitor networks. This is where cognitive neuroscience can make a great contribution to cognitive rehabilitation by showing the functional architecture of interacting cognitive systems. Knowledge, for instance of the close connections between a right hemisphere alertness system on the one hand, and a posterior spatial orientation system on the other (Robertson et al., 1998), has led directly to the effective rehabilitation of spatial problems by manipulating their separate but functionally connected alertness circuits (Robertson et al., 1995).

It is likely also that the attentional circuits of the brain will be shown to have a privileged role in the plastic reorganization of the brain. Merzenich and his colleagues, for example, have shown that sensory stimulation results in synaptic remodelling only if the animal pays attention to the stimulation. When such stimulation occurs passively, plastic reorganization usually does not occur (Recanzone, Schreiner and Merzenich, 1992). This may explain why lesions to the frontal lobe predict very poor recovery from a range of different disorders, though it may also be the case that the effects of frontal lesions on self-awareness, motivation and emotion are highly relevant to this poor prognosis (Stuss, 1991; Stuss and Gow, 1992; Stuss et al. 1995).

Plastic reorganization of the brain is also strongly affected by the availability of neuromodulators such as norepinephrine and acetylcholine, as the work of Feeney and others has shown (Feeney, 1997). Integrating such findings to all these other variables will pose a formidable theoretical challenge, which must nevertheless be met for the promise of cognitive rehabilitation to be fulfilled.

Chapters 4, 10, 11 and 12 show how various manipulations such as transplantation and pharmacological intervention can foster repair in damaged circuits. It seems ultimately desirable that cognitive rehabilitation be tied in with such interventions – indeed, it may sometimes be the case that neither class of approach can be effective except in conjunction with the other. To give an example of this, Mayer et al. (1992) showed that rats given striatal neural transplants only benefited from the transplants when they were given the opportunity for perceptuomotor learning: in the absence of such behavioural 'driving' of the neural tissue, the necessary connectivity did not develop sufficiently to produce behavioural improvements. What seemed most exciting about this future direction was the specificity of the type and timing of pharmacological interventions, and dovetailing this with the type and timing of cognitive rehabilitation. For example, the 'executive' deficits may be most effectively addressed behaviourally when the patient has recovered to a degree at which these deficits are isolated, but the pharmacological interventions may be relevant earlier, and at the time of functional rehabilitation. Combining research into the recovery and deterioration of function may be the best way truly to understand the relationship between the physical brain, the chemical brain, and the cognitive and functional expression of both.

It is a clinical truism to say that the person's attitude to his or her disability influences the outcome of rehabilitation. Motivation, emotion and social support all intersect with this 'attitude', to change the person, and to change that person's brain. Prigatano in Chapter 15 highlights the importance of these psychological variables pertaining to motivation, emotion and self-concept. The motivation of the rehabilitation specialist and the rehabilitation team may also be critical, as Mills and Alexander suggest in Chapter 10. The practical effect of this is evident in the brain injury programme of Christensen and Caetano, in which the teamwork approach allows the development of a therapeutic milieu with an integrated treatment approach. In other words, the environment can become the motivation for the patient, by being provided externally or by using the milieu to develop and guide internal motivation. A very similar concept is embedded in Proulx's stress on the new family context in rehabilitation in Chapter 16.

Establishing the context for improvement of motivation and emotion is important, but the key factor remains the patient. Chapters 14 and 15, by Feinstein and Prigatano, emphasize different aspects of individual motivation. Feinstein notes that damage in specific regions of the brain can directly affect motivation, resulting in apathy, which may be a major impediment to rehabilitation, especially to generalization. The areas suggested as causing apathy are related to the frontal systems. As noted above, this may mean that in a very structured environmental context, the patient may perform well. However, if the patient is left alone or is

required to generalize the learning, apathy may impede the implementation of action. Prigatano notes that psychotherapy may help, though this may be effective in only some patients. What may be required is a comprehensive approach, including psychopharmacological interventions. The job of the rehabilitation team is to discover the many factors impeding recovery, and to develop and implement the appropriate prodedures.

The need to consider motivational and emotional factors in developing effective strategies for cognitive rehabilitation is de facto recognition of the multifactorial basis of cognitive impairment in individuals with brain dysfunction. Head trauma patients, for example, confront catastrophic changes in their lives that severely limit their experiences, accomplishments and aspirations. Failure to adapt effectively to these changes impacts profoundly on the patient's ability to function and, conceivably, could affect cognitive processes. In some respects, research on the elderly has led the way in identifying extraneous factors that interact with reduced brain function to exacerbate cognitive difficulties. Apart from health-related and lifestyle-related factors, there is growing evidence that personal and social variables may also affect cognitive performance. In an illustrative example, Marilyn Albert and her colleagues (1995) investigated predictors of cognitive change in older people and found that activity levels and personal feelings of self-efficacy were among the key predictors. This literature is reviewed in Chapter 6 by Dawson, Winocur, and Moscovitch, who also refer to evidence from a longitudinal study that other psychosocial factors (e.g. optimism, locus of control) contribute significantly to cognitive ageing. It is reasonable to expect that the factors that influence cognitive decline in the elderly operate similarly in many brain-injured patients.

Dawson, Winocur and Moscovitch sketch a model for cognitive rehabilitation that reflects the comprehensive approach advocated. The proposal is for an intervention programme that incorporates training in cognitive, psychosocial and lifestyle domains. The cognitive component is the critical element to such a programme and recently developed, sophisticated protocols are extremely promising (see Wilson, Chapter 21; Glisky and Glisky, Chapter 22; and also Jacoby, Jennings and

Hay, 1996). Supplementary interventions in the psycho-social and lifestyle areas (see Chapter 6) may be what is necessary to raise the ceiling of cognitive enhancement in head-injured patients, as well as in other populations (e.g. normal elderly) who experience cognitive losses.

Conclusions

The contributors have not only reviewed the literature, they have also expressed the challenges for the future. Is there a theoretical basis for cognitive neurorehabilitation? While it is important to appreciate these complex influences on brain plasticity and behavioural change, the attempt to build a theoretical framework for cognitive rehabilitation would probably be doomed to failure if one tried to incorporate all these many levels of analysis at the first stage. Research in these different realms will have to proceed in parallel, albeit while ensuring considerable cross-referencing, for advances to be made. Wertz, in Chapter 17, for example, has clearly shown the chasm that exists between theoretical models of cognitive function on the one hand and techniques for behaviour change on the other. Nevertheless, there can be little doubt that both endeavours should strive to interact in a mutually beneficial way.

The book contains issues about the adequacy of the methodologies used, and how the deficiencies to move forward might be overcome. One reverberating theme is the necessity of a multidisciplinary approach, which would incorporate an understanding of the pathophysiology underlying cognitive disorders; the combination of directed pharmacological treatment with, where appropriate, different clinical approaches, including psychotherapy, to address problems such as motivation; and the importance of valid and reliable outcome measures of cognitive, behavioural and functional domains. To achieve this requires a dramatic change from traditional approaches to the science and practice of cognitive neurorehabilitation. Basic scientists from the biological (including genetic) level to the psychological theorists must work hand in hand with clinician–scientists and practitioners who apply this fundamental knowledge to the practical domain. The flip side of this theme is the emphasis on the integration, not just of approaches, but also of the recipient of cognitive rehabilitation – an approach to the whole person.

One matter has been left to the last: the financing of rehabilitation. In times of financial restraint, cost may be the main factor which determines whether or not rehabilitation is made available, in spite of the human suffering and loss of function entailed. It behoves the rehabilitation scientist and practitioner to demonstrate that a properly scientifically grounded and practically feasible cognitive rehabilitation can both reduce long-term financial costs and improve the quality of life of the tens of millions of people worldwide suffering from impaired brain function.

References

Albert, M., Jones, K., Savage, C. et al. 1995. Predictors of cognitive change in older persons: MacArthur studies of cognitive ageing. *Psychol Aging* **10**, 578–89.

Feeney, D.M. 1997. From laboratory to clinic: noradrenergic enhancement of physical therapy for stroke or trauma patients. *Adv Neurol* **73**, 383–94.

Jacoby, L.L., Jennings, J.M. and Hay, J.F. 1996. Dissociating automatic and consciously controlled processes: implications for diagnosis and rehabilitation of memory deficits. In *Basic and Applied Memory Research: Theory in Context*, ed. D. Herrmann, C. McEvoy and C. Hertzog, pp. 161–93. Mahwah, NJ: Lawrence Erlbaum.

Luria, A.R. 1963. *Restoration of Function after Brain Injury*. Oxford: Pergamon Press.

Luria, A.R., Naydin, V.L., Tsvetkova, L.S. and Vinarskaya, E.N. 1975. Restoration of higher cortical functions following local brain damage. In *Handbook of Clinical Neurology*, ed. P.J. VInken and G.W. Bruyn, pp. 368–433. New York: Elsevier.

Mayer, E., Brown, V.J., Dunnett, S.B. and Robbins, T.W. 1992. Striatal graft-associated recovery of a lesion-induced performance deficit in the rat requires learning to use the transplant. *Eur J Neurosci* **4**, 119–26.

Nudo, R.J., Wise, B.M., Si Fuentes, F. and Milliken, G.W. 1990. Neural substrates for the effects of rehabilitative training on motor recovery after ischemic infarct. *Science* **272**, 1754–91.

Recanzone, G.H., Schreiner, C.E. and Merzenich, M.M. 1992. Changes in the distributed temporal response properties of s1 cortical-neurons reflect improvements in performance on a temporally based tactile discrimination task. *J Neurophysiol* **67**, 1071–91.

Robertson, I.H., Mattingley, J.B., Rorden, C. and Driver, J. 1998.

Phasic alerting of right-hemisphere neglect patients overcomes their spatial deficit in visual awareness. *Nature* **395**, 169–72.

Robertson, I.H. and Murre, J.M.J., in press. Rehabilitation of brain damage: brain plasticity and principles of guided recovery. *Psychol Bull.*

Robertson, I.H., Tegnér, R., Tham, K., Lo, A. and Nimmo-Smith, I. 1995. Sustained attention training for unilateral neglect: theoretical and rehabilitation implications. *J Clin Exp Neuropsychol* **17**, 416–30.

Stuss, D.T. 1991. Self-awareness and the frontal lobes: a neuropsychological perspective. In *The Self: Interdisciplinary Approaches*, ed. J. Strauss and G.R. Goethals, pp. 255–78. New York: Springer Verlag.

Stuss, D. and Gow, C.A. 1992. Frontal dysfunction after traumatic brain injury. *Neuropsychiatry Neuropsychol Behav Neurol* **5**, 272–82.

Stuss, D.T., Shallice, T., Alexander, M.P. and Picton, T.W. 1995. A multidisciplinary approach to anterior attentional functions. *Ann NY Acad Sci* **769**, 191–212.

Index

abulia 236, 237

accelerometers 223–4, 226

accommodation 61, 63
  in memory impairment 66

acetylcholine (ACh) 363
  ACh-producing cells, intracerebral grafts 39, 40
  in brain trauma 120
  in medial temporal lobe function 127
  as pharmacological target 27–8, 163–5
  in prefrontal cortex function 126
  see also cholinergic system; basal forebrain

acetylcholinesterase inhibitors 27, 163–5

acrobat rats 20

The Action Research Arm Test 205

activities of daily living
  efficacy of rehabilitation 292
  evoking aggression 255
  scales 205–6, 225–6

Activity Monitors 223–4

Actual Amount of Use Test 222–3, 226

adenosine 84

adenovirus, nerve growth factor gene delivery 39

β-adrenergic receptor blockers 146

Adult Memory and Information Processing Battery
    204

affect
  cognitive function in old age and 97–8, 103
  constraint-induced movement therapy and 225
  pseudobulbar 235
  see also mood

affective disorders 231–5
  see also depression; mania

age
  aphasia recovery and 268
  neuroplasticity and 16–17, 18, 23
  recovery from diffuse axonal injury and 287, 288

age-related cognitive decline 94–6, 102–4
  Canadian Aging Research Network (CARNET) study
      98–100
  cognitive neurorehabilitation 100–2, 103–4
  compensation for 60, 65
  individual differences 29, 347, 357
  psychosocial well-being and 7, 96–8
aged animals 28–9
  brain structural changes 14
  fetal tissue grafts 30–4
  gene transfer studies 36, 37, 38
aggression
  activities of daily living evoking 255
  in Alzheimer's disease 162
  case study 148–9
  in traumatic brain injury 136, 140, 144–5
ageing
  basal forebrain cholinergic system 26–8
  brain changes 95
  memory changes 347–8
  sex differences 76–7
  see also elderly
agitation
  in Alzheimer's disease 156–8
  in traumatic brain injury 140
agnosia, auditory 50–1
AK295 122
akathisia, neuroleptic-induced 157, 162
akinetic mutism 236, 237
alanine aminotransferase (ALT), serum 164
albumin solutions 79
alertness training 307–8, 324
alliance, therapeutic 246–7, 248–9
α-2-adrenergic agonists 124–6, 145, 146
Alzheimer's disease (AD) 153–67
  α-2 agonists 126
  animal models, see animal models of Alzheimer's disease
  basal forebrain cholinergic system 27–8
  behavioural problems 156–62, 255
  cholinergic-enhancing agents 127, 163–5
  clinical characteristics 153–4
  compensatory brain activation 67–8
  depression 159–61, 232
  diagnosis 154–5
  memory rehabilitation 340, 355
  mood disorders 232
  neuropathological changes 155
  oestrogen therapy 88
  ondansetron 127
  pharmacological therapy 27–8, 112, 155–67

amantadine 145
α-amino-3-hydroxy-5-methyl-4-isoxazole propionate (AMPA)
      receptors 115
  modulation, in brain trauma 118
2-amino-5-phosphovaleric acid (APV) 117
21-aminosteroids, in head injury 121
amitriptyline 144–5, 235
amnesia
  anterograde 283
  posttraumatic, see posttraumatic amnesia
  see also memory, deficits
amphetamine
  in memory deficits 354
  in traumatic brain injury 120, 145, 147
amputation 53
amygdala, neurotransmitter modulation 126–7
β-amyloid protein 165
animal models of Alzheimer's disease 28–30
  behavioural assessment 40–1
  fetal tissue grafts 26, 30–4, 39–40
    cell savings and fibre regeneration 30–1, 32
    functional recovery 31–4
  gene transfer 34–9, 40
  intraventricular nerve growth factor 34
  neurotransmitter-secreting cell grafts 39, 40
  trophic factor-secreting cell grafts 35–9, 40
    cell savings 35–6
    functional recovery 37–8
    neural progenitor cells in 38–9
    regeneration of pathways 37
anosognosia 244
  see also awareness, of deficits
anoxic–hypotensive brain injury 175
anterior cingulate cortex 230–1, 315
  attention system 303
  lesions 231, 315
anticholinergic agents 120
anticonvulsants 143–4, 145, 150
antidepressants 234
  in Alzheimer's disease 160
  in traumatic brain injury 144–5, 148
  see also selective serotonin reuptake inhibitors
antidiuretic hormone 78
antipsychotic agents, see neuroleptics
anxiety 235
  in Alzheimer's disease 161
  assessment 207–8
  in memory problems 342
apathy 231, 235–7, 364
  assessment and treatment 236–7

depression and 236
  medical illness and 236
  primary and secondary 236
  see also motivation, impaired
aphasia 265–76
  determinants of recovery 265–71, 276
    age at onset 268
    experience over time 268–9
    lesion size 269
    reactive brain changes 269–71
    time since onset 266–8
  functional neuroimaging 49–50
  mood assessment in 208, 233
  neurobehavioural theory of/for therapy 274–6
  role of theory in therapy 263, 271–6
    theories 'for' therapy 271–2
    theories 'of' therapy 271, 272–4
  sex differences 76
  spontaneous recovery 266, 267, 276
apoptosis, in brain trauma 113
apraxia, sex differences 76
arginine vasopressin (antidiuretic hormone) 78
arithmetic, text encoding technique 323–4
Arm Motor Ability Test 218, 221–2
arousal
  circadian variations 353
  performance and 242–3
Ashworth Scale, modified 203
Assessment of Motor and Process Skills 207
assessments, for rehabilitation 178, 185
  case study 179–81
  for day programme 192–4
assimilation 53, 61
attention 302–11
  assessment 209, 307
  deficits 263, 302–3, 314
    in elderly 95
    spatial, *see* neglect, unilateral
  divided 307–8, 324
  role in neuroplasticity 363
  selective 302, 307–8, 310, 324
  sustained 302, 308, 315
    assessment 308
    training 308–9, 310, 325
  training 303–11, 324–5
    efficacy 292, 310–11
    nonspecific 303–7
    specific nonlateralized 307–9
    in unilateral neglect 309–10
attention deficit hyperactivity disorder 125

auditory system
  functional neuroimaging 50–1
  stimulation, in aphasia 273
autistic children 65
automatic processing 64, 255–6
  in memory problems 352
awareness 174
  assessment of 317–18, 327
  in compensation 61, 63–4
  of deficits 63–4
    in frontal dysfunction 314
  learning without 255–6
  training 104, 326–8
  see also self-awareness
axons, development 13–14

B-HT920 124
baby hamster kidney (BHK) cells, nerve growth factor-
    producing 36, 37, 38
backward chaining technique 335
balance performance monitor 203
Barthel Index 205
basal forebrain cholinergic system, *see* cholinergic system,
    basal forebrain
basal ganglia stroke 51, 232
Beck Depression Inventory 207
Behavioural Assessment of Dysexecutive Syndrome (BADS)
    209, 317
behavioural compensation 66, 69
behavioural disorders
  activities of daily living evoking 255
  in Alzheimer's disease 156–62, 255
  family interventions 255
  in traumatic brain injury, *see* traumatic brain injury,
    behavioural disorders
  see also destructive behaviour
Behavioural Inattention Test 209
behavioural observation 140
behavioural therapy
  in elderly 103–4
  in executive disorders 318–19, 321, 323
  family interventions 255
  in memory problems 334
  promoting structural brain changes 17, 19–20
  in traumatic brain injury 150
benzodiazepines
  in agitated dementia patients 148, 158
  in Alzheimer's disease 161
  in anxiety 161
  in delirium 141

benzodiazepines (*cont.*)
  in sleep disturbances 161
bethanecol 162, 163
biological model, recovery in traumatic brain injury 289–90
bipolar affective disorder 158, 234–5
blindness, cortical 244
brain
  compensatory activation 67–8, 69
  development 13
  sex differences in function 75–7
  sexual dimorphism 74–5
brain-derived neurotrophic factor (BDNF)-producing cells, intracerebral grafts 36
brain reorganization 5, 363
  in aphasia 269–771
  compensatory 67–8, 362
  constraint-induced movement therapy and 219–20
  in cortical regions near damaged area 47
  cortical representational maps 53
  exogenous treatments stimulating 9, 19–21, 23, 289–90
  neuroimaging 6, 48–53
  recruiting new networks/using alternate networks 47
  remaining circuits 9, 16–17
  sex hormones and 77–8
  underlying functional recovery 16–17, 23
  within existing network 47
brain structure
  age-related changes 95
  changes in injured brain 5, 16–17
  changes underlying recovery 11–12, 23
  compensatory changes 67
  developmental changes 13–14
  experience-dependent changes 14–16
  fetal tissue grafts and 30–1
  human, evidence for changes 15–16
  manipulation of changes 17–21
  measuring changes 12
  sex differences 15, 74–5
  sex hormone-dependent changes 74–5
breast cancer 88
Brock Adaptive Functioning Questionnaire 317
bupropion 160
buspirone   .
  in agitated dementia patients 148, 157, 158
  in Alzheimer's disease 161
  in traumatic brain injury 145, 146–7
BW1003C87 119

calcium-channel blockers 119, 166
calcium ions (Ca²⁺), in brain trauma 115–16

calpain inhibitors 122
Canada, rehabilitation services 182
Canadian Aging Research Network (CARNET) study 98–100, 103
canary, singing centres 74
carbamazepine 143–4, 145
  in agitation 157, 158
3-(2-carboxypiperizin-4yl)-propyl-1-phosphonic acid (CPP) 117
caregivers
  in Alzheimer's disease 166
  compensation by 65
  see also family
case manager 184
catastrophic reactions 156
catecholamines
  in brain trauma 120
  see also norepinephrine; dopamine
Catherine Bergego Scale 209
Center for Epidemiologic Studies Depression Scale 207
Center for Rehabilitation of Brain Injury, Copenhagen 173, 188, 189–98
cerebral oedema
  ischaemic 81–2
  mechanisms of progesterone actions 86–7
  posttraumatic 78–81, 82–4
CG-3703 120
CGS19755 117, 119
Change Assessment Questionnaire 317–18
chess players, expert 356
chloral hydrate 161
choline 162, 163
choline acetyltransferase (ChAT)
  in Alzheimer's disease 27
  ChAT-producing cells, intracerebral grafts 39
cholinergic mechanisms
  medial temporal lobe function 127
  prefrontal cortex function 126
cholinergic system, basal forebrain 26–8
  in aged animals 28–9
  in ageing/Alzheimer's disease 27–8
  experimentally lesioned animals 29–30
    fetal tissue grafts 30–4
    gene transfer studies 34–9
  as pharmacological target 27–8
cholinergic treatments
  in Alzheimer's disease 163–5
  in brain trauma 120
cholinesterase inhibitors 27, 163–5
circadian rhythms, *see* diurnal rhythms

clonidine 124, 125
   in traumatic brain injury 145, 146
clozapine 124, 143, 234–5
   in agitation 157, 158
cognitive–behavioural therapy 342–3
Cognitive Failures Questionnaire 208
cognitive function
   age-related decline, see age-related cognitive decline
   assessment 203, 204, 208–9
   complex problems 179
   posttraumatic 283–4
   sex differences 75–6
cognitive neuropsychological theory 271–2
cognitive tests
   constraint-induced movement therapy and 225
   in elderly 99
   in rodent brain injury models 114–15
cognitive training
   in day rehabilitation programme 195, 197
   in elderly 104
collagen, nerve growth factor-producing cells embedded in
      37, 38
coma 283
   duration 283, 284, 285–6, 287
   emergence from 141, 283
   pattern of recovery 284, 285
   rehabilitation strategies 290, 296, 297
communication skills, for families 257
Communicative Activities of Daily Living 209
community-based rehabilitation 183
community-dwelling old people
   cognitive function 96, 98–9, 100
compensation (in neuroscience) 60
compensation (in psychology) 6–7, 59–70, 362–3
   areas of research 60–1
   awareness and 61, 63–4
   behavioural, for organic cognitive impairment 66, 69
   brain activation 67–8, 69
   in cognitive neurorehabilitation 65–9
   consequences of 61, 64–5
   in executive disorders 319
   failure to develop 63
   history of use 59–60
   interactions between brain/behavioural 68–9
   mechanisms 61, 63
   in memory rehabilitation 66, 340–1, 348–50, 356
   model of process 62
   origin 61–3
   principal features of process 61–5
   working definition 61

Compensation Questionnaire 64
complex cognitive problems, patients with 179
computed tomography (CT), in Alzheimer's disease 154
   see also neuroimaging
computers
   in attention training 303–7
   in memory rehabilitation 337–9, 348–9
   skills learning, in elderly 102, 348–9
concussion 284
conditioned responses, monkeys with deafferented limbs 216
confusional state, posttraumatic 283, 284
   rehabilitation strategies 290, 296–7
constraint-induced movement therapy 215–26, 363
   initial motor ability of patients 219
   measurement of efficacy/compliance 220–5
      cognitive and affective measures 225
      laboratory range of motion measures 220–2
      real-world measures 222–4
      real-world versus motor ability measures 225
   neurophysiological mechanisms 219–20
   research with humans 217–19
   research with monkeys 216–17
context in assessment 257
continuum of care 182–3
control
   locus of 97, 99
   for patients and families 257
contusion injury, cerebral 282–3
   behavioural disorders after 138
   effect of progesterone on outcome 78–81
   mechanisms of progesterone actions 86–7
   natural history/outcome 288
   pharmacological interventions 128
   progesterone therapy in males 80–4
corpus luteum 89
cortical shock 216
cost effectiveness, rehabilitation programmes 189, 190
costs
   cognitive neurorehabilitation 183, 185–6
   constraints, in traumatic brain injury 280
   reduction strategies 186
   traumatic brain injury 279
   see also financing
counselling
   for caregivers 166
   in elderly 103–4
   see also cognitive–behavioural therapy; psychotherapy
'Craig bed' 141
crying, pathological 235
cued-procedural learning approach 181

cues
    in elderly 102, 349–50
    in executive disorders 318, 321–4
    in memory deficits 325, 338–9
    vanishing 355–6
customers, cognitive neurorehabilitation programmes 183
6-cyano-7-nitroquinoxaline-2,3-dine (CNQX) 118
cytotoxic T-cells, effects of progesterone 86

databases, clinical and administrative 185
day programme for cognitive rehabilitation 173, 188–99
    activities 194, 195–8
    evaluation procedures 192–4
    holistic neuropsychological approach 188–90
    promoting motivation 242
    selection procedures 191–2
    theoretical premises 190–1
    treatment approach 194–8
deafferentation, limb 216
defect, see deficit
deferoxamine 121
deficit 59, 61
    awareness of 63–4
        see also anosognosia
    compensation originating in 61–3
Delighted–Terrible Faces Scale 208
delirium
    management 141–2
    medications causing 137, 138, 141
    in traumatic brain injury 140–2
delusions
    in Alzheimer's disease 158–9
    in traumatic brain injury 142–3, 145
dementia
    assessment of mood 208
    behavioural problems 156–62, 255
    depression presenting as 148, 233–4
    differential diagnosis 155
    family education 253
    prevalence 153
    in traumatic brain injury 147–8
    see also Alzheimer's disease; elderly
dendrites
    development 13–14
    experience-dependent changes 14, 15–16
    functional recovery and 16–17, 23
    in injured brains 16, 17, 18
    measuring changes 12
    sex hormone-dependent changes 74–5
    treatments stimulating growth 17–21

denial 244–5, 249, 327
L-deprenyl, see selegiline
depression 231–4
    in Alzheimer's disease 159–61, 232
    apathy and 236
    assessment 207–8, 232–4
    in caregivers 166
    cognitive function in elderly and 97–8
    constraint-induced movement therapy and 225
    diagnosis 234
    differential diagnosis 155, 233–4
    frequency 231–2
    in frontal system pathology 231–2
    history (clinical) 232–3
    in memory problems 342
    in traumatic brain injury 144, 148, 232
    treatment of 234
desferrioxamine (deferoxamine) 121
desipramine 160
destructive behaviour 140–50
    case study 148–9
    nonpharmacological management 149–50
    pharmacological management 140–9
    see also behavioural disorders
development, neuronal changes during 13–14
dexamethasone
    ischaemic brain oedema and 81
    suppression test 234
dextroamphetamine, see amphetamine
dextromethorphan 117
dextrorphan 117
diagnosis, rehabilitation 176–7, 178
diagonal band of Broca 26, 27
diaries, daily home treatment 222
diaschisis 216
dichotic listening 269–70
diffuse axonal injury 281–2
    behavioural disorders after 139
    natural history 283–4
    pharmacological strategies 127–8
    predicting outcome 284–7
    severity, recovery and 284, 285
    stages of recovery 283–4
    versus focal contusion 288
diffuse brain injury 281–2
    behavioural disorders after 138–9
    natural history/outcome 283–7
disability
    definition 201, 254
    family education 254–5

measures 204–9, 210–11
   role of rehabilitation 202
Disability Rating Scale 210
disconnection syndromes 145–6
discrimination training technique 323
disinhibition 273, 314, 315
   techniques for managing 323–4
distractibility 315
diurnal rhythms
   in Alzheimer's disease 161
   behavioural disorders 139
   memory rehabilitation and 353–4
divalproex, see valproate
dizocilopine 117
donepezil 162, 163, 164–5
dopamine
   in motivation disorders 231
   in prefrontal cortex function 123–4
   receptors 123–4
dopamine agonists 123, 124
   in apathy 237
   in traumatic brain injury 145, 147, 297
dorsal root ganglia, effects of progesterone 85
dorsolateral prefrontal cortex 230–1
dorsolateral prefrontal syndrome 231, 315
dressing skills, assessment 206
drugs, see medications; pharmacological therapy
dynamometry 203
dyslexia, neglect 310
dystonia, neuroleptic-induced 157

eating behaviour, disturbances in 161–2
eclampsia 118
Edinburgh Functional Communication Profile 209
education
   cognitive decline in old age and 96
   dendritic structure and 15
   family 179, 253–5, 342
   in memory rehabilitation 351–2
EEG, see electroencephalography
elderly
   aphasia recovery 268
   cognitive neurorehabilitation 100–2, 103–4
   functional neuroimaging 51–3, 348, 357
   memory deficits 95, 264, 347–8
   memory rehabilitation 264, 347–57
      external compensation 348–50
      optimizing residual function 350–4
      substitution of intact function 354–6
   pharmacological therapy 155–6

psychosocial factors in cognitive function 7, 94–104, 364
   see also aged animals; ageing
electroconvulsive therapy (ECT) 160–1, 234
electroencephalography (EEG)
   in Alzheimer's disease 154, 159
   in aphasia 269
   portable devices 226
   prospective memory training and 326
Emerson, R.W. 59, 60
emopamil 119
encephalitis 175
enriched environments 334
   dendritic structural changes 14–15
   glial cell changes 12
   responses to brain injury and 19–20, 21
entorhinal cortex lesions 75
environment, physical
   aphasia recovery and 268
   cognitive decline in old age and 96, 98–9, 100
   context specificity in assessment/treatment 257
   in dementia 156, 257
   enrichment, see enriched environments
   in executive disorders 318
   in memory rehabilitation 333–5, 343, 349–50, 354
   promoting learning 256
   in traumatic brain injury 139, 141, 150
Environmental Status Scale 210
epilepsy
   catamenial 84
   posttraumatic 138
      drug therapy 145
      progesterone and 84–5
errorless learning 256, 335–7, 344
   in elderly 102, 355
estrogen, see oestrogen
Everyday Memory Questionnaire 208
excitatory amino acids (EAA)
   effects of progesterone 86–7
   metabotropic receptors 116
      modulation in traumatic brain injury 118–19
   modulation, in traumatic brain injury 117–19
   neurotoxicity 115–16
   in posttraumatic cognitive dysfunction 116–17
   receptors
      antagonists, neuroprotective effects 117–18
      in traumatic brain injury 115–17
   release inhibitors, in traumatic brain injury 119
executive control functions 314
   assessment 316–18
   attentional system interactions 303

executive control functions (*cont.*)
  conceptualization 315–16
executive disorders 263–4, 314–28
  in elderly 95
  in frontal dysfunction 314–15
  rehabilitation 293, 303, 318–28
    compensatory approaches 319
    direct interventions 319–20
    environmental manipulations 318–19
    specific approaches 320–8
    theoretical aspects 318–20
Executive Interview 317
exercise
  cognitive decline in old age and 97
  in cognitive rehabilitation 100–1, 103
  in memory rehabilitation 352–3, 356
  see also physical activity
Expanded Disability Status Scale 204
experience
  aphasia recovery and 268–9
  brain structural changes 14–15
    in humans 15–16
    in injured brains 19–20
  in memory rehabilitation 351–2
  traumatic brain injury recovery and 289–90
  trophic factor production and 21
expertise, in elderly 356
explosive disorder, intermittent 145
Extended Activities of Daily Living Scale 205–6
extrapyramidal side-effects 157

face perception, in elderly 51–2
family 174, 252–8, 364
  central role in rehabilitation 252–5
  education 179, 253–5, 342
  in memory rehabilitation 255–6, 342
  preventive interventions 255–7
feedback, in day rehabilitation programme 194, 195, 196
females
  in research studies 73–4
  see also sex differences
fetal tissue, intracerebral grafts 26, 30–4, 39–40
fibroblast growth factor, basic (bFGF) 21, 122
fibroblasts
  mouse 3T3, nerve growth factor-secreting 35–6
  primary
    acetylcholine-producing 39
    nerve growth factor-secreting 35, 36, 37–8
  rat 208F, nerve growth factor-secreting 35

fimbria–fornix cholinergic pathway 26, 27
  -lesioned animals 29
    fetal tissue grafts 30–1, 32
    gene transfer studies 35–9
financing 365
  acute care 182
  postacute rehabilitation 182, 183, 184, 253
  rehabilitation programme design and 179
  see also costs
finger opposition task 48–9, 53
finger-tapping speed 247–8, 249
fingers, cortical neurons representing 15, 16
fluoxetine 144, 160
fluphenazine 157, 158
focal brain injury 282–3
  brain contusion, *see* contusion injury, cerebral
  natural history/outcome 288
'forced use' techniques
  in motor problems 293
  see also constraint-induced movement therapy
Franz, S.I. 240–1
free radicals
  effects of progesterone 86–7
  inhibitors, in brain trauma 120–1
Frenchay Activities Index 205–6
Frenchay Arm Test 205
frontal cortex
  executive control functions 315–16
  lesions
    behavioural recovery 11, 17
    brain structural changes 16, 17, 18, 22
    compensatory brain activation 68
    promoting recovery 19–20
    sex hormone effects 77–8, 79–84, 86–7
  see also prefrontal cortex
frontal eye fields 230
frontal lobes
  age-related changes 95
  executive control functions 314, 315–16
  lesions/dysfunction 314–15, 363
    age-dependent effects 17
    aphasia recovery and 270
    assessment 316–17
    in elderly 95–6
    impaired self-awareness 244, 248, 314
    mood disorders 232
    motivational disorders 236, 248
    rehabilitation 318–28
    in traumatic brain injury 145–6

subcortical circuits 54, 230–1
    behavioural effects of lesions 231
    mechanisms of behavioural change 231
Fugl–Meyer Poststroke Motor Recovery Test 220–1
functional abilities, assessment 205–7, 226–7
Functional Ambulation Category 204
Functional Assessment Measure 206
Functional Communication Profile 209
Functional Independence Measure 205, 206, 207
Functional Limitations Profile 207
functional neuroimaging, *see* positron emission tomography;
        single photon emission computed tomography
functionally based treatment 264, 293
    in aphasia 273
    in traumatic brain injury 293

GABA receptors, effects of progesterone 86
gender differences, *see* sex differences
gene transfer 6, 26, 33–9
    in animal models of Alzheimer's disease 34–9, 40
    ex vivo 34–9
    in vivo 34, 39
General Health Questionnaire (GHQ) 208
gestures, in aphasia therapy 273, 275
Glasgow Coma Scale, predicting outcome 284, 285,
        286
glial cells
    effects of progesterone 85–6
    measurement of changes 12
glial fibrillary acidic protein 85–6
glucocorticoids, in head injury 79, 83–4, 121
glucose and memory performance 354
glutamate 86, 115
goal setting 198
Goldstein, K. 188–9
Golgi-type stains 12
grip strength 203, 247
groups
    in day rehabilitation programme 194, 196–8
    in memory rehabilitation 343
growth factors, *see* trophic factors
guanfacine 124, 125–6
GYKI 52466 118

habituation task 38
haemorrhages, intracerebral 282, 283
hallucinations 159
hallucinosis, secondary 142–3
haloperidol

in agitated dementia patients 157, 158
    in traumatic brain injury 141, 144
handicap
    definition 201–2, 254
    family education 254–5
    measures 210–11
    role of rehabilitation 202
happiness, in elderly 99–100
Hauser Ambulation Index 204
head injury
    management guidelines 78–9
    outcome measures 207
    secondary brain injury 113–14
    see also traumatic brain injury
heat shock proteins 117–18
Hebb, D.O. 17, 242–3
herniation, brain 282–3
high-altitude sickness 87
hippocampus
    age-related changes 95, 357
    cholinergic innervation 26–7
    neuronal losses, in brain trauma 116–17
    neuronal regeneration 21, 30–1, 37
    neurotransmitter modulation 126–7
    sex differences 74–5
holistic approach
    cognitive neurorehabilitation 173, 188–99, 365
    definition 190
home
    adaptations 257, 334, 337–8
    aphasia recovery at 268
Hospital Anxiety and Depression Scale 207
hospitals
    acute
        efficacy of rehabilitation 294
        postacute care services 184
        transfer from 182, 291
        in traumatic brain injury 291
    chronic 182
houses, 'smart' 337–8, 343
5-HT, *see* serotonin
5-HT$_{1A}$ agonists 145
5-HT$_3$ receptor antagonists 126, 127
HU-211 (7-hydroxy-tetrahydrocannabinol 1,1-dimethylheptyl)
        117
Huntington's disease 34, 232
hydergine 162, 165
hyoscine (scopolamine) 120, 126
hypothermia, in brain trauma 121–2, 127

hypoxic–ischaemic brain injury
    behavioural disorders after 138–9
    diffuse 282
    focal 282

IgG-saporin (immunotoxin)-lesioned animals 29–30,
        36
imipramine 160
immune cells, effects of progesterone 85–6
immunotoxin (IgG-saporin)-lesioned animals 29–30, 36
impairment
    definition of 201, 254
    family education 254–5
    measures 203–4, 211
    role of rehabilitation 202
impulsivity 314, 315
individual differences, age-related changes 29, 347, 357
individual therapies, day rehabilitation programme 194,
        195–6, 198
indole-2-carboxylic acid (I2CA) 118
indomethacin 162, 166
infants
    brain reorganization after injury 9, 19–20
    neuroplasticity 16–17
    tactile stimulation 14–15, 19–20
inflammatory reactions, effects of progesterone 86
inflexible behaviour 314, 315
inhibition 315
initiation 314, 315
    techniques to improve 321–3
insight 195, 326–7
insomnia, in Alzheimer's disease 161
institutional care, long-term 291
institutionalized elderly
    cognitive function 96, 98–9, 100
    rehabilitation programme 104
insurance money 183
intensive care unit, rehabilitation in 294
Interactive Task Guidance Systems 339
interference control 315–16
internal capsule lesions 48–9, 53
International Classification of Impairments, Disabilities and
        Handicap 201
intersystemic reorganization 273, 274–5
intrasystemic reorganization 273, 274–5
iron, in brain trauma 120, 121
irritability, in traumatic brain injury 140
8-isoprostaglandin $F_{2\alpha}$ (8-isoPGF$_{2\alpha}$) 86–7

kainate (KA) receptors 115
    modulation, in brain trauma 118
Katz Adjustment Scale 139
Katz Index 205
Kennard principle 16–17, 47
ketamine 117–18
Kluver–Bucy syndrome 162
Korsakoff's syndrome 125
Kurtzke Multiple Sclerosis Rating Scale 203–4, 207
kynurenate (KYNA) 118, 119

L1-producing cells, intracerebral grafts 40
lamotrigine derivatives 119
language
    assessment scales 209
    cerebral localization
        functional neuroimaging 49–50
        sex differences 76, 77
    disorders
        compensation in 60
        unawareness 244
        see also aphasia
Lashley, K. 241
laughing, pathological 235
lazeroids, in head injury 121
leadership
    definition of 184
    rehabilitation programmes 178, 183–4
learned nonuse
    measures in hemiparesis 220–5
    mechanism of overcoming 216–17, 218
    model of development 217
    in stroke patients 217
    techniques for overcoming 217–19
learning
    deficits
        assessment in animal models 40–1, 114–15
        cholinergic hypothesis 27
        fetal tissue grafts and 31–3
    errorless, see errorless learning
    in memory problems 335–7, 351–2, 354
    model, recovery in traumatic brain injury 289–90
    without awareness 255–6
left hemisphere
    lesions
        right hemisphere recruitment 48–51, 269–70
        sex differences in effects 76
    sex differences in function 77

leisure participation, assessment 206
levodopa 235
Lieberman's Index 203
limb
    activation treatments, in neglect 310
    deafferentation 216
    hemiparesis, *see* upper-extremity hemiparesis
linguistic model, aphasia therapy 273
lipid peroxidation 86–7, 120–1
lithium 235
    in Alzheimer's disease 157, 158, 160
    in traumatic brain injury 143, 146
London Handicap Scale 210
long-term potentiation 116
lorazepam 141, 157, 161
losses, social and personal developmental 60
Luria, A.R. 189, 190–1, 195, 362
    aphasia therapy approach and 273, 274–5
    on role of motivation 241
Luria Neuropsychological Investigation 190
lymphocytes, effects of progesterone 86

magnesium ions (Mg^{2+})
    in brain trauma 116
    NMDA receptor modulation therapy 118
magnetic resonance imaging (MRI) 2
    in Alzheimer's disease 154
    constraint-induced movement therapy and 219
    functional, sex differences 76
management
    definition 184
    rehabilitation programmes 183–6
mania, secondary 143–4, 234–5
mannitol 78–9
mastectomy, timing in females 88
medial frontal–anterior cingulate syndrome 231, 315
medial temporal lobe
    age-related changes 95, 347–8
    assessment of function in animals 123
    cognitive function 122–3
    neurotransmitter modulation 126–7
medications
    causing anxiety 235
    causing cognitive problems 137, 138, 141
    causing depression 233
    compliance 349
    see also pharmacological therapy
medroxyprogesterone 162

Melodic Intonation Therapy 273, 274–5
memory
    assessment
        in animal models 40–1, 114, 115
        clinical measures 204, 208
    deficits 264
        in Alzheimer's disease 154
        behavioural compensation 66, 340–1, 348–50, 356
        cholinergic hypothesis 27
        compensatory brain activation 67–8
        in elderly 95, 264, 347–8
        fetal tissue grafts and 31–3
        neuroimaging in elderly 52–3, 348, 357
        other cognitive problems 343, 344
    episodic, in elderly 52, 347–8
    explicit, in elderly 95
    groups 343
    implicit 255–6
        in elderly 95–6
        in errorless learning 336–7, 355
        in memory rehabilitation 354–6
    prospective 316, 317
        techniques for improving 325–6
    rehabilitation 292, 333–44
        in elderly 264, 347–57
        environmental adaptations 333–5, 343
        family interventions 255–6, 342
        new learning 335–7, 344
        new technology 337–9, 343
        other strategies 339–41, 343–4
        in practice 341–3
    remote, preservation 256
    source, in elderly 95
    working 315
        in elderly 95, 348
        rehabilitation 324–5
memory aids, external 325–6, 340–1, 343
    case study 180–2
    in elderly 104, 348–9, 356
    paging system 338–9
Memory Failures Questionnaire 208
menstrual cycle
    breast cancer surgery and 88
    cognitive performance changes 75–6
mental retardation, dendritic morphology in 17
mental state examination 233
meta-analysis 203, 211
metacognitive techniques 322

method of loci technique 101
α-methyl-4-carboxyphenylglycine (MCPG) 118–19
N-methyl-D-aspartate receptors, see NMDA receptors
methylphenidate
    prefrontal cortex function and 123
    in traumatic brain injury 145, 147, 297
methylprednisolone, in head injury 79, 83–4, 121
metrifonate 165
microglia, effects of progesterone 86
middle cerebral artery
    occlusion 81–4
    stroke 17, 48, 54
milieu, treatment, see therapeutic milieu
mineral deficiencies 97
minimally conscious stage 283, 284
    rehabilitation strategies 296–7
minor-hemisphere mediation model, aphasia therapy
        273
MK801 (dizocilopine) 117
mnemonics 341, 343–4
    in elderly 101–2, 104, 350–1
    visual imagery, see visual imagery mnemonics
modality model, aphasia therapy 273
monoamine oxidase inhibitors (MAOIs) 160
mood 174, 230–7
    assessment measures 207–8
    disorders 231–5
    frontal subcortical lesions and 231
    see also affect; depression
mood-stabilizing drugs 234–5
'morning meetings' 196–8
Morris water maze 11, 38
    in rodent models of brain injury 114–15
    sex differences 75
    sex hormone influences 82
motivation 174, 230–7, 327, 364
    behavioural measures 248, 249
    definition 242
    effect on recovery 240, 241–2, 246, 248–9
    excessive 242, 248
    in frontal subcortical lesions 231
    impaired 235–7, 240–9
        clinical examples 245–6
        historical perspective 240–2
        role of psychotherapy 246–7
        see also apathy
    mechanisms 247–8
    process of promoting 242
    theoretical and research observations 242–4

Motor Activity Log 218, 222, 226
Motor Assessment Scale 203
Motor Club Assessment 203
motor cortex
    lesions 10–11, 16
        functional neuroimaging 48, 53
        reorganization of representations 53, 363
    reorganization after therapy 220
motor deficits
    constraint-induced movement therapy 215–26
    in diffuse axonal injury 284
    efficacy of rehabilitation 293
    functional neuroimaging 48–9, 53, 55
motor function assessment 215
    disability measures 204–5
    impairment measures 203–4
motor vehicle accidents 281–2
Motricity Index 203, 221
mountain sickness 87
multidimensional approach 174, 365
    in elderly 102, 103
multiple sclerosis
    mood disorders 232
    outcome measures 203–4, 207
Multiple Sclerosis Quality of Life 54 Instrument 210
muscarinic receptor agonists 163
muscarinic receptors 27–8, 126
muscle
    strength assessment 203
    tone assessment 203
mutism, akinetic 236, 237

nadolol 146
nalmefene 120
naloxone 119–20
names, learning techniques 335
nefazodone 160
neglect, unilateral 303, 308, 309–10
    assessment measures 208–9
    efficacy of rehabilitation 310
    functional neuroimaging 51
    limb activation treatments 310
    sustained attention training 308–9
    visual scanning training 51, 309
Neglect Alert Device 310
nerve growth factor (NGF) 6
    adenovirus vector (Ad-NGF), intracerebral injection 39
    in Alzheimer's disease 162, 165
    in brain trauma 122

grafted fetal cells producing 31
intraventricular infusion 31, 34, 37
NGF-secreting cells, intracerebral grafts 35–9, 40
stimulating dendritic changes 21, 22
neuritic plaques 155
Neurobehavioral Functioning Inventory 209
Neurobehavioral Rating Scale 209
neurobehavioural theory, in aphasia therapy 274–6
neurofibrillary tangles 155
neuroimaging 6, 47–55
in Alzheimer's disease 154, 159
in aphasia 49–50
compensatory brain activation 67–8
constraint-induced movement therapy and 219
in depression 232
implications for rehabilitation 54–5
memory function in elderly 52–3, 348, 357
in neglect 51
recruitment of new networks 48–53
reorganization within existing network 48–53
sensorimotor representations 53
sex differences 76–7
neuroleptics (antipsychotics)
adverse effects 157–8
in agitated dementia patients 148, 157–8
in delirium 141
in psychosis 142–3, 159
in secondary mania 143, 234–5
neurological disorders, compensation in 60
neurological examination, in traumatic brain injury 140
neurological model of rehabilitation 136, 176–7
case study 179–82
versus traditional approaches 177–8
neurons
developmental changes 13–14
experience-dependent changes 14–15
functional recovery and 16–17, 23
loss
in Alzheimer's disease 155
in secondary brain injury 113–14
measurement of changes 12
peripheral, effect of progesterone on repair 85
protective effects of progesterone 82, 83
regeneration 10, 21–3
after fetal tissue grafts 30–1
after gene transfer 37
sex differences in density 74
see also dendrites
NeuroPage 338–9

neuroplasticity 5, 9–23, 363
age-specific variations 16–17, 18, 23
in injured brain 16–17
measuring structural changes 12
methods of manipulation 17–23
neuroimaging 47–55
in normal brain 12–16
physical activity promoting 100–1
see also brain reorganization
neuroprotection
in acute traumatic brain injury 111, 113–22, 127
in Alzheimer's disease 165
by progesterone 82, 83
neuropsychiatric examination, in traumatic brain injury 140
Neuropsychiatric Inventory 208
neuropsychological rehabilitation 188–90
neuropsychological theory, cognitive 271–2
neurotransmitters
in disorders of mood and motivation 231
fetal tissue grafts producing 26
grafts of cells engineered to produce 39, 40
medial temporal lobe modulation 126–7
prefrontal cortex modulation 123–6
neurotrophic factors, see trophic factors
nicotinic receptors 27, 28
nimodipine 119, 162, 166
NMDA receptors
associated glycine site modulation 118
associated ionophore blockers 117–18
associated polyamine site modulation 118
in brain trauma 115, 116
competitive antagonists 117
modulation by magnesium 118
nonuse, learned, see learned nonuse
nootropic agents 165
norepinephrine (noradrenaline) 363
modulation, in brain trauma 120
in prefrontal cortex function 124–6
North-western University Disability Scales 207
Northwick Park Index 205
nortriptyline 160
Nottingham Dressing Assessment 206
Nottingham Sensory Assessment 204
nucleus basalis magnocellularis (NBM) 26–7
in Alzheimer's disease 27
lesioned animals 29
fetal tissue grafts 31, 32
gene transfer studies 35–6, 37, 38, 39
nutrition, in elderly 97, 104

object identification 54, 75
observation, behavioural 140
obsessive–compulsive disorder 54–5, 231
occipital lesions 244
occupation
    disability assessment 209
    neuronal structure and 16
oestrogen
    dendrite/synapse structure and 75
    outcome of brain injury and 77–8, 79, 80–1
    seizure-inducing effects 84
    therapy, in Alzheimer's disease 88
oestrus cycle
    brain structural changes 75
    effects of brain injury and 77–8, 79–80
olanzapine 142, 157, 158
olfactory bulb, neuronal regeneration 21
oligodendrocytes
    effects of progesterone 85–6
    progesterone production 85
ondansetron 127
opiate peptides, in brain trauma 119–20
optimism, in elderly 99–100
orbitofrontal circuit 230–1
    lesions 75, 231
orbitofrontal syndrome 231, 315
outcome 201
    determinants 254–5
    follow-up systems 185
    measurement 2, 173–4, 201–11
        future developments 210–11
        in real world 225–6
        selection of measures 202–10
        upper-extremity function 215, 220–6
    projected 177
    see also recovery
outpatient rehabilitation 183, 291
    efficacy 294–6
    see also day programme for cognitive rehabilitation
overlearning 256
Overt Aggression Scale 139
oxazepam 148, 161

P factor 247
P300 response
    in attention training 324
    in memory training 326
Paced Auditory Serial Addition Test (PASAT) 304–5, 324
paging systems 338–9

parietal lobe
    attentional system 308
    function, sex differences 76
    lesions 19, 244
parkinsonism, neuroleptic-induced 157
Parkinson's disease
    depressive disorders 232, 234
    motor assessment 203, 207
paroxetine 160
passive attitude 241
    see also apathy; motivation, impaired
pemoline 147
personality 240
    memory rehabilitation and 342
personality disorders
    interictal 145
    in traumatic brain injury 145–7
PET, see positron emission tomography
pharmacological therapy 111–12, 363–4
    in Alzheimer's disease 27–8, 112, 155–67
    guidelines for elderly 155–6
    in memory rehabilitation in elderly 354
    promoting structural brain changes 17–19, 20–1
    in traumatic brain injury 113–28, 140–9, 297, 298
phencyclidine 117
phosphatidylcholine 162, 163
cis-4-(phosphomethyl)-2-piperidine carboxylic acid (CGS19755) 117, 119
physical activity
    cognitive decline in old age and 97, 99
    in cognitive rehabilitation 100–1, 103, 104
    in day rehabilitation programme 196, 197
    in memory rehabilitation 352–3
    see also exercise
physical disability, assessment 204–5
physostigmine 159, 162, 163
pindolol 146
piracetam 162, 165
planned failure 327–8
plasticity, neural, see neuroplasticity
polyethylene glycol–superoxide dismutase (PEG–SOD) 121
polymer encapsulation, immortalized cells 35
positron emission tomography (PET) 6
    in Alzheimer's disease 154
    in aphasia 270
    applications in rehabilitation 54–5
    brain reorganization after injury 48–53
    compensatory brain activation 67–8

in depression 232
in neglect 51
sex differences 76–7
postacute care
efficacy 294–6
financing 182, 183, 184
services 182–3
in traumatic brain injury 291
postconfusional/evolving independence stage
rehabilitation strategies 297–8
traumatic brain injury 283–4
posttraumatic amnesia (PTA) 283
duration
indicating severity of injury 283
predicting outcome 284, 285–6, 287
efficacy of rehabilitation 290, 297
potassium ions (K⁺), in excitotoxicity 115, 116
practicality, outcome measures 202
praxis, sex differences 76
prazosin 124, 125
prefrontal cortex
age-related changes 347–8, 357
assessment of function in animals 123
cognitive function 122–3
dorsolateral, see dorsolateral prefrontal cortex
executive control functions 314, 315–16
memory functions 52
neurotransmitter modulation 123–6
pregnancy-related hypertension 118
premenstrual syndrome 89
primary therapist 191, 194, 195, 198
primates, non-human
aged 28–9
constraint-induced movement therapy 216–17
problem-solving skills
in elderly 95
rating scale 209
training 293, 326
Problems in Everyday Living Questionnaire 208–9
process 201
process-specific rehabilitation 264, 292–3
in aphasia 273
in executive disorders 319
Profile of the Executive Control System 317
Profile of Functional Impairment in Communication 209
progenitor cells, neural
brain-derived neurotrophic factor-producing 36
nerve growth factor-producing 38–9
neurotransmitter-producing 40

progesterone 7, 89
anxiolytic properties 84
breast cancer surgery and 88
dendrite/synapse structure and 75
excitatory amino acid/free radical metabolism and 86–7
glia/immune cells and 85–6
high-altitude sickness and 87
neuroprotective effects 82, 83
outcome of brain injury and 77–84, 87
compared to oestrogen 80–1
in male and female rats 81–4
posttraumatic epilepsy and 84–5
therapy, in traumatic brain injury 80–4, 88–9
progestins 89
prognosis, rehabilitation 177
programmes, cognitive rehabilitation 175–86
case study 179–82
clinical model and 176–8
continuum of care 182–3
development 183–4, 185
in elderly 100–2, 103–4
family interventions 255–7
holistic neuropsychological approach 173, 188–99, 365
leadership 178, 183–4
management 173, 183–6
neurological model 176–7
selection criteria 191–2
team 178–9
traditional approaches 177–8
see also day programme for cognitive rehabilitation
project groups 196, 197
propranolol (Inderal) 146, 158
Prospective Memory Screening 317
protease inhibitors 122
pseudobulbar affect 235
pseudodementia 148, 233–4
pseudopregnancy 77–8, 79–80
psychiatric disorders, in traumatic brain injury 141–2
psychological well-being, in elderly 97–8, 99–100
psychomotor disturbances, in Alzheimer's disease 162
psychosis
in Alzheimer's disease 158–9
in traumatic brain injury 142–3
psychosocial factors
cognitive function in elderly 7, 94–104, 364
neurorehabilitation programme targeting 100–2, 103–4
psychosocial tests, in elderly 99
psychostimulants 145, 147, 237

psychotherapy 343
   in day rehabilitation programme 194, 195, 196, 197
   in depression 234
   in impaired motivation/awareness 237, 246–7
   in traumatic brain injury 150
pursuit rotor task 203, 297
pyramidal neurons 12, 13

quality of life 103, 202, 210

Rancho Los Amigos levels of cognitive functioning 283, 284
randomized controlled trials 203, 211
rats, neural development 13
reading deficits 60, 307
recollection, training 351
recovery
   definition 10
   determinants in aphasia 265–71, 276
   mechanisms 5, 47–8
   multiple factors 2
   natural occurrence 10–11, 23
   neuroplasticity and 5, 9–23
   sex differences 7
   time course 189
   in traumatic brain injury, *see* traumatic brain injury, natural
      history/outcome
   see also outcome
regeneration, neuronal, *see* neurons, regeneration
Rehabilitation Accreditation Commission 185
rehearsal strategies 335, 341, 343–4, 354–5
relaxation therapy 342
reliability, outcome measures 202, 210–11
remediation 61, 63
   in memory impairment 66
reorganization, cerebral, *see* brain reorganization
residential treatment services 291
response–cost programme 323
restlessness, motor 162
restraints
   in behavioural disorders 141, 156
   limb, in deafferentation 216–17
right hemisphere
   attention system 302, 303, 308
   recruitment in left-sided lesions 48–51, 269–70
   sex differences in function 77
riluzole 119
risperidone 142, 157, 158, 234
Rivermead Activities of Daily Living Scale 205
Rivermead Behavioral Memory Test 209

Rivermead Everyday Memory Test 317
Rivermead Head Injury Follow-up Questionnaire 207
Rivermead Mobility Index 204
Rivermead Motor Assessment 203
running wheels 20

schizophrenia 125, 307
Schwann cells
   intracerebral grafts 40
   progesterone production 85
sciatic nerve lesions 85
scopolamine 120, 126
secondary brain injury
   in brain trauma 113–14, 282
   pharmacological intervention 115–22, 127
seizures
   after traumatic brain injury 138
   effects of progesterone 84–5
selective serotonin reuptake inhibitors (SSRIs) 234
   in Alzheimer's disease 160
   in apathy 237
   in traumatic brain injury 144
   see also paroxetine; fluoxetine; sertraline
selegiline (L-deprenyl) 160, 163, 165
Self Assessment Parkinson's Disease Disability Scale 207
self-awareness 244–5, 247, 316
   impaired 241, 244–5, 249
      clinical examples 245–6
      in frontal dysfunction 244, 248, 314
      mechanisms 247–8
      versus denial of disability 244, 249, 327
   techniques for promoting 104, 326–8
   see also awareness
Self-Awareness of Deficits Interview 318
self-efficacy beliefs 97
Self-Rating Depression Scale 207
self-regulation 63–4, 322
sensitivity, outcome measures 202
sensorimotor representations, reorganization 53
sensory deficits
   assessment 204
   compensation in 60
septum, medial 26, 27
sequencing of action, techniques to improve 321–3
serotonin
   antagonists 126
   in disorders of mood and motivation 231
   in prefrontal cortex function 126
sertraline 160

services, rehabilitation 182–3
    accessibility 183
    in traumatic brain injury 183, 291
sex differences 7, 73–89
    brain functions 75–7
    brain structure 15, 74–5
    lack of research on 73–4
sex hormones 7, 73–89
    brain structure and 74–5
    outcome of brain injury and 77–84
    see also oestrogen; progesterone; testosterone
sexual dimorphism, brain 74–5
sexual problems, in Alzheimer's disease 162, 166
shaping techniques, limb deafferentation 216
Short Form 36 205, 210
Sickness Impact Profile 207
singing centres, canaries 74
single-case experimental designs 202–3, 211
single photon emission computed tomography (SPECT) 154,
        270
619C89 119
Six Elements Test 317
skills training 293
        see also functionally based treatment
sleep disturbances, in Alzheimer's disease 161
'smart' houses 337–8, 343
social competence/community re-entry stage 284, 297–8
social functioning, assessment 209
social isolation 343
sodium ions (Na+), in brain trauma 115, 116
somatosensory cortex
    neuronal structure 15, 16
    reorganization of representations 53, 219–20
sound categorization task 50
spaced retrieval technique 335, 354–5
spatial learning task, delayed 77–8
spatial location matching task 51–2
spatial orientation system 302, 308, 309
        see also neglect, unilateral
speech disorders, compensation in 60
speech therapy 274
    efficacy in aphasia 266, 268–9
spinal shock 216
stem cells, neural 13, 21
stepdown care placements 182–3
stimulation-facilitation model, aphasia therapy 273
stress, prefrontal cortex function and 123
striatal lesions 48–9, 231
striate cortex, topographical reorganization 53

stroke 175
    compensatory brain activation 68
    constraint-induced movement therapy 215–26
    family support 253
    functional neuroimaging 48–51, 54
    middle cerebral artery 17, 48, 54
    mood disorders 232
    outcome measures 203, 205, 206
    time course of recovery 47
    see also aphasia
Stroke Aphasic Depression Questionnaire 208
Stroop training 306
structure 201
stuttering 49, 55
substitution
    in aphasia therapy 273, 275
    with latent process 61, 63
    in memory rehabilitation 66, 354–6
    at neuroanatomical level 67
    with novel skill 61, 63
suicide 233
superoxide dismutase, polyethylene glycol-conjugated
        (PEG–SOD) 121
supplementary motor area 48, 230, 315
supported risk taking 327–8
supramarginal gyrus, neuronal structure 15, 16
synapses
    development 13, 14
    experience-dependent changes 14–16
    measuring changes at 12
    sex hormone-dependent changes 74–5

tacrine 127, 162, 163–4
tactile stimulation, infants 14–15, 19–20
tardive dyskinesia 157–8
team
    authority 184
    interdisciplinary 178, 188–99
    leaders 178
    rehabilitation 174, 178–9, 364
        case study 179–82
        Center for Rehabilitation of Brain Injury 191, 192–4, 198
        primary therapist 191, 194, 195, 198
    training 179
technological aids, in memory rehabilitation 337–9, 343
temazepam 161
temporal lobe
    lesions 244
    medial, see medial temporal lobe

Test of Everyday Attention 209
testosterone 74, 75
thalamus 54
therapeutic alliance 246–7, 248–9
therapeutic milieu
    Center for Rehabilitation of Brain Injury 191, 198
    in traumatic brain injury 141, 150
thioridazine 157, 158, 161
thiothixene 157, 158
thyrotrophin-releasing hormone 120
time-out 150
time planner 181–2
timing
    aphasia onset, recovery and 266–8
    brain injury, sex differences in effects 77–8
    recovery 189
    of rehabilitation 189
topographical cortical maps, reorganization 53
training
    family 253–4
    rehabilitation team 179
transcranial magnetic stimulation (TMS) 219–20
transplantation, intracerebral 5–6, 10, 26–41, 363–4
    fetal tissue grafts 26, 30–4, 39–40
    genetically engineered cells 26, 33, 34–9
        cell savings and fibre regeneration 34–7
        functional recovery 37–8
        neural progenitor cells 38–9
        neurotransmitter replacement 39, 40
traumatic brain injury 263, 279–99, 364
    acute, diagnosis of severity 127–8
    behavioural disorders 136–50
        assessment 136–40
        case study 148–9
        categories 139
        clinical examination 140
        environmental factors 139
        nonpharmacological strategies 149–50
        patient evaluation 139
        pharmacological management 140–9
        premorbid function and 139
    biological versus learning models of recovery
        289–90
    constraint-induced movement therapy 217–18
    costs 279
    depression 144, 148, 232
    diagnosis and prognosis 280, 281–8, 299
    economic constraints 280
    efficacy of rehabilitation 279–80, 291–6, 299
        in acute hospital/intensive care unit 294

acute inpatient rehabilitation 294
    along treatment continuum 293–6
    functional strategies 293
    postacute rehabilitation 294–6
    process-specific strategies 292–3
family support 253
impaired self-awareness 244, 247–8
incidence 175
motivational problems 240, 243–4, 247–8
natural history/outcome 189, 283–8
pathophysiology 115–22, 281–2
pharmacological approaches 113–28, 297, 298
    behavioural disorders 140–9
    established cognitive deficits 111, 122–7
    immediate 111, 113–22, 127
progesterone effects on outcome 78–81
progesterone therapy 80–4, 88–9
recommendations for rehabilitation 280, 296–8
rehabilitation case study 179–82
rehabilitation interventions 290–1
rehabilitation services 183, 291
rodent models, cognitive tests 114–15
secondary brain injury 113–14, 282
secondary complications 137–9
sex differences in recovery 73
treatment settings 290–1
see also contusion injury, cerebral; diffuse axonal injury;
        head injury
trazodone
    in Alzheimer's disease 157, 158, 160, 161
    in traumatic brain injury 145
tricyclic antidepressants (TCAs) 160, 234
L-triiodothyronine 160
trophic factors
    in brain trauma 122
    cells producing , intracerebral grafts 35–9, 40
    fetal tissue grafts producing 26, 31
    intraventricular infusions 30–1, 34
    promoting dendritic changes 19, 20–1, 22
    stimulating neural regeneration 21–3
    see also nerve growth factor
trunk, cortical neurons representing 15, 16
typists, expert 356

U-74006F 121
UK-14,304 124
unconsciousness 283
    wakeful 283, 284
    see also coma
Unified Parkinson's Disease Rating Scale 207

United States (USA), rehabilitation services 182–3
upper-extremity hemiparesis
    constraint-induced movement therapy 215–26
    outcome measures 215, 220–6

validity
    outcome measures 202, 210–11
    real-life, therapeutic interventions 242, 257
valproate (divalproex) 144, 145, 157, 158
vanishing cues method 355–6
vegetative state 283, 284
    rehabilitation strategies 290, 296, 297
velnacrine 163
venlafaxine 160
ventricular dilatation, sex hormones and 78
Vienna Test System 305
vigilance training 307–8, 324
visual function, assessment 204
visual imagery mnemonics 335, 341
    in elderly 101, 104, 350–1

visual scanning task 51, 309
vitamin deficiencies 97
volition 315, 321

Wakefield Depression Inventory 207
walk test, timed 10 m 204
wandering in Alzheimer's disease patients 162
water maze, see Morris water maze
Webster Rating Scale 203
Wechsler Memory Scale – Revised 204
Whishaw reaching task 10–11, 19
Win 44,441-3 120
Wolf Motor Function Test 218, 221
word pair lists 52
word-stem completion task 49–50, 68, 96, 337
working memory, see memory, working
World Health Organization (WHO), handicap scales 210

YM-14673 120
yohimbine 124–5